V&R Academic

Wiener Forum für Theologie und Religionswissenschaft / Vienna Forum for Theology and the Study of Religions

Band 16

Herausgegeben im Auftrag
der Evangelisch-Theologischen Fakultät der Universität Wien,
der Katholisch-Theologischen Fakultät der Universität Wien
und dem Institut für Islamisch-Theologische Studien der Universität Wien
von Ednan Aslan, Karl Baier und Christian Danz

Die Bände dieser Reihe sind peer-reviewed.

Karl Baier / Philipp A. Maas /
Karin Preisendanz (eds.)

Yoga in Transformation

Historical and Contemporary Perspectives

With 55 figures

V&R unipress

Vienna University Press

universität
wien

MIX
Papier aus verantwortungsvollen Quellen
FSC www.fsc.org FSC® C083411

Bibliografische Information der Deutschen Nationalbibliothek

Die Deutsche Nationalbibliothek verzeichnet diese Publikation in der Deutschen Nationalbibliografie; detaillierte bibliografische Daten sind im Internet über http://dnb.d-nb.de abrufbar.

ISSN 2197-0718
ISBN 978-3-8471-0862-7

Weitere Ausgaben und Online-Angebote sind erhältlich unter: www.v-r.de

Veröffentlichungen der Vienna University Press erscheinen im Verlag V&R unipress GmbH.

Published with the support of the Rectorate of the University of Vienna, the Association Monégasque pour la Recherche Académique sur le Yoga (AMRAY) and the European Research Council (ERC).

Printed in Germany.
Titelbild: Four-armed Patañjali holding a sword. Ramamani Iyengar Memorial Yoga Institute, Pune.
© Dominik Ketz, www.dominikketz.de
Druck und Bindung: CPI books GmbH, Birkstraße 10, D-25917 Leck

Gedruckt auf alterungsbeständigem Papier.

Contents

Karl Baier / Philipp A. Maas / Karin Preisendanz
Introduction 7

Part A. Yoga in South Asia and Tibet

Dominik Wujastyk
Chapter 1: Some Problematic Yoga Sūtra-s and Their Buddhist Background 21

Philipp A. Maas
Chapter 2: "*Sthirasukham Āsanam*": Posture and Performance in Classical Yoga and Beyond 49

Jason Birch
Chapter 3: The Proliferation of *Āsana*-s in Late-Medieval Yoga Texts . . 101

James Mallinson
Chapter 4: Yoga and Sex: What is the Purpose of *Vajrolīmudrā?* 181

Marion Rastelli
Chapter 5: Yoga in the Daily Routine of the Pāñcarātrins 223

Catharina Kiehnle
Chapter 6: The Transformation of Yoga in Medieval Maharashtra 259

Philipp A. Maas / Noémie Verdon
Chapter 7: On al-Bīrūnī's *Kitāb Pātanǧal* and the *Pātañjalayogaśāstra* . . 283

Ian A. Baker
Chapter 8: Tibetan Yoga: Somatic Practice in Vajrayāna Buddhism and Dzogchen 335

Part B. Globalised Yoga

Karl Baier
Chapter 9: Yoga within Viennese Occultism: Carl Kellner and Co. 387

Joseph S. Alter
Chapter 10: Yoga, Nature Cure and "Perfect" Health: The Purity of the Fluid Body in an Impure World 439

Maya Burger
Chapter 11: Sāṃkhya in Transcultural Interpretation: Shri Anirvan (Śrī Anirvāṇa) and Lizelle Reymond 463

Anand Amaladass
Chapter 12: Christian Responses to Yoga in the Second Half of the Twentieth Century 485

Beatrix Hauser
Chapter 13: Following the Transcultural Circulation of Bodily Practices: Modern Yoga and the Corporeality of Mantras 505

Anne Koch
Chapter 14: Living4giving: Politics of Affect and Emotional Regimes in Global Yoga 529

Suzanne Newcombe
Chapter 15: Spaces of Yoga: Towards a Non-Essentialist Understanding of Yoga 549

Gudrun Bühnemann
Chapter 16: *Nāga, Siddha* and Sage: Visions of Patañjali as an Authority on Yoga 575

Contributors 623

Karl Baier / Philipp A. Maas / Karin Preisendanz

Introduction

1. Context, Scope and Structure of the Present Volume

Ever since the emergence of yoga-related practices and teachings in South Asia around 500 BCE, yoga has shown a protean flexibility and creativity, constantly reproducing itself in dependence on changing social, cultural and religious contexts. Thus, the history of yoga is a complex and multifaceted one, and still remains far from having been exhaustively investigated. Furthermore, the roughly two decades of academic research on yoga since the late 1990's have brought new insights, methodological approaches and questions concerning the history of premodern yoga, the interpretation of yoga-related literature, and the early impact of the phenomenon on other Asian cultures. What is more, the investigation of modern transnational yoga has established itself as a multidisciplinary field of study in its own right. Studies on the history and contemporary state of modern yoga have caused ongoing public and academic debates about the relation between so-called traditional and modern yoga and about issues like authenticity, authority and ownership. Moreover, the motives and experiences of contemporary practitioners and their global networks are being investigated with methods of the social sciences and cultural anthropology.[1]

In view of these vibrant developments, the editors of the present volume convened an international conference on "Yoga in Transformation: Historical and Contemporary Perspectives on a Global Phenomenon" at the University of Vienna, which took place on 19–21 September 2013.[2] For the sake of coherence and optimisation of synergies, its focus was on the exploration of the phenomenon of yoga from the point of view of South Asian studies, the study of religions,

1 The pertinent literature is far too comprehensive to be reviewed here. However, in combination the reference sections of the individual chapters of the present volume will provide a good overview of the recent special and general literature on the above-mentioned aspects of yoga research.

2 See http://yogaintransformation.wissweb.at (accessed 3 November 2017).

sociology, cultural studies, theology and history of religions. The investigation of yoga from the perspectives of psychology and medicine, interesting and relevant as they may be, thus remained outside the scope of the conference. The editors were fortunate to attract many of the key players in current yoga research of the described types as well as acknowledged specialists in the afore-mentioned areas of yoga-related research to the conference, either as speakers or as participants in the panel discussions. The vast majority of them also kindly agreed to elaborate and expand their papers and turn them into chapters of a book on the conference topic. The present volume is the fruit of their combined labours. In line with the conference agenda, it explores yoga from a broad perspective, but definitely does not aspire to be encyclopedic. Thus, the volume examines different strands and specific issues of South Asian and Tibetan yoga in the premodern period as well as developments within its practices and theories. It also investigates forms of modern yoga in their complex historical contexts and addresses recent developments and the current transformation of transnational modern yoga. Moreover, it considers aspects of the encounter of the Islamic and Christian traditions with the theory and practice of yoga in the past and present. In general, in keeping with the current trend in yoga-related studies emphasis has been put on the practice of yoga and its immediate theoretical underpinnings. Thus, even though several papers inevitably also touch upon philosophical aspects of yoga and consider, next to the social and religious contexts, also the philosophical context of the development and transformation of yoga practice, the philosophy, or rather: philosophies of yoga properly speaking do not play a prominent role in the present volume.

The volume consists of altogether sixteen chapters that make up its two parts of approximately equal size and with different historical and geographical foci. Part A, "Yoga in South Asia and Tibet", is mainly devoted to the study of premodern yoga on the basis of primary sources in several South Asian languages, in Arabic and in Tibetan, whereas Part B, entitled "Globalised Yoga", deals with aspects of modern and post-modern forms of yoga that are investigated primarily on the basis of sources in European languages and with empirical methods. The following survey is meant to provide an overview of the content of the individual chapters and at the same time to show their coherence and interrelatedness.

2. Synopsis of Part A: "Yoga in South Asia and Tibet"

The initial contribution, "Some Problematic Yoga Sūtra-s and Their Buddhist Background" by **Dominik Wujastyk** emphasises the importance and need of an informed historical and philological approach in order to arrive at a full understanding of the *Pātañjalayogaśāstra*, Patañjali's masterpiece on yoga which was composed from a Brahmanical perspective. Drawing special attention to the three technical Sanskrit terms *asaṃpramoṣa*, *anantasamāpatti* and *dharmamegha* that occur in the *sūtra* text of *Pātañjalayogaśāstra* 1.11, 2.46–47 and 4.49, respectively, Wujastyk demonstrates that these *sūtra*-s were frequently misunderstood throughout the reception history of the *Pātañjalayogaśāstra* due to a lack of awareness on the part of its interpreters about the original meaning of the above terms which were actually coined and used in the Buddhist tradition of South Asia. By drawing upon parallels to the employment of the three technical terms in Buddhist literature, Wujastyk highlights the deep intellectual influence of Buddhism on Patañjali. In this way, he defines familiarity with South Asian Buddhist thought, religious concepts and meditation practices as a necessary condition for an appropriate understanding of the *Pātañjalayogaśāstra* before its intellectual backdrop and in its original intellectual milieu in late fourth- or early fifth-century South Asia.

The chapter by **Philipp A. Maas**, "'*Sthirasukham Āsanam*': Posture and Performance in Classical Yoga and Beyond", is also largely devoted to the *Pātañjalayogaśāstra* and the history of its reception. More specifically, Maas investigates Patañjali's treatment of yogic postures (*āsana*), starting with a contextualisation of the role of *āsana*-s within the yogic path to liberation. He then analyses the passage *Pātañjalayogaśāstra* 2.46–48 and demonstrates that the two *sūtra*-s 2.46 and 2.47 should be understood as a single sentence. This is followed by a discussion of the list of posture names in the *Pātañjalayogaśāstra* as well as of the possible nature of the postures themselves from a philological perspective. Maas' critical edition of the text of *Pātañjalayogaśāstra* 2.46 provides the basis for a detailed comparison of various descriptions of posture performance in medieval commentaries on the *Pātañjalayogaśāstra* and in the authoritative Jaina yoga treatise by Hemacandra. This comparison reveals that designations of *āsana*-s and the descriptions of their performance may differ from source to source. However, all analysed sources agree in presenting *āsana* as a complex of psycho-physiological practices meant to enable the yogi to undertake long sessions of exercises, such as breath control, and of various kinds of meditation, rather than mere performances of bodily configurations as means in themselves.

"The Proliferation of *Āsana*-s in Late-Medieval Yoga Texts" by **Jason Birch** continues the investigation of yogic posture practice, which he carries on to the historical setting of late medieval South Asia. Birch bases his exposition on newly discovered Sanskrit manuscripts that list and describe a considerably larger number of yogic postures than earlier sources. Their descriptions are here for the first time analysed and compared with descriptions of *āsana*-s in earlier and roughly contemporary Haṭha and Rāja Yoga texts. In the final analysis, Birch's presentation and interpretation of the newly discovered manuscript evidence shatters the belief in a recent historical narrative concerning the origin of many modern yogic postures. According to this narrative, a radical historical rupture of *āsana* practice occurred in colonial India when all of a sudden a large number of previously undocumented complex and physically demanding postures became fashionable, exactly at the time when European body building and gymnastic exercises appeared on the stage of physical culture in South Asia. Birch's research reveals that many of the physical yoga practices allegedly introduced during the colonial period were actually not innovations, but had predecessors in the tradition that have so far remained unnoticed simply because they are not to be found in the widely known published Haṭha Yoga texts.

The aim of the chapter "Yoga and Sex: What is the Purpose of *Vajrolīmudrā?*" by **James Mallinson** is also to overcome a wide-spread preconception concerning the history of Haṭha Yoga, namely, the view that the origins of haṭhayogic practice have to be sought in Śaiva tantric sex rituals. The evidential basis for this narrative is usually considered to be the *vajrolīmudrā,* the practice of drawing up liquids through the urethra. The *vajrolīmudrā* figures prominently in Haṭha Yoga, and it seems to have an obvious connection with sex. However, by taking into consideration textual, ethnographic, experiential and anatomical data in order to determine the history, method and purpose of *vajrolīmudrā,* Mallinson arrives at the conclusion that this practice was most probably developed in a celibate ascetic milieu. Its purpose in Haṭha Yoga is the absorption of semen in the body of a practitioner who wants to enjoy intercourse, even after ejaculation. Thus, *vajrolīmudrā* emerges from Mallinson's research as a means for yogis to have sex and yet remain continent, rather than a component of tantric sex rituals.

In "Yoga in the Daily Routine of the Pāñcarātrins" **Marion Rastelli** leads her readers to the religious ambience of tantric Vaiṣṇavism or, more specifically, to that of the Pāñcarātra tradition of South India. Rastelli describes in great detail the performance, role and meaning of yoga as the fifth and final constituent of the "five times" or "five time periods", i.e., the five daily ritual duties performed by a Pāñcarātra devotee. In doing so, she surveys a wide spectrum of pertinent sources comprising the Pāñcarātra Saṃhitās, Veṅkaṭanātha's *Pāñcarātrarakṣā* and Purāṇic literature. In her final analysis, Rastelli demonstrates convincingly that yoga is an essential part of life for all followers of the Pāñcarātra tradition. Yoga may figure as a set of ritual techniques or as an autonomous practice that is largely disconnected from ritual contexts. It may be performed in many different forms daily before sleep, between two phases of sleep, or after sleep. The benefit that Pāñcarātrins derive from yoga consists in mental training, an awareness of the nature of God, and insights concerning God's relationship to man, particularly to his devotees. The time period before falling asleep and an interval of wakefulness between two phases of sleep suggest themselves as ideal times for yoga practice, because then the insights provided by yoga can be intensified during the following phase of sleep. The specific contents of these yogic insights, however, depend on the theology propounded by the devotee's particular tradition or sub-tradition.

"The Transformation of Yoga in Medieval Maharashtra" by **Catharina Kiehnle** is focussed on yoga in the context of another Vaiṣṇava tradition, different from the one discussed by Rastelli. Kiehnle deals with the role of yoga in the so-called "nominal Vaiṣṇavism" of the Vārkarī religious movement, which developed in Maharashtra during the thirteenth and fourteenth centuries. Her study is based on the Marathi-language *Jñāndev Gāthā*, a collection of songs attributed to the poet–saint Jñāndev. In these songs, multiple and partly conflicting attitudes towards yoga and other forms of religious practice are reflected. Kiehnle suggests that the Bhakti Yoga ("yoga of devotion") of the Vārkarīs was developed for lay practitioners as an alternative to forms of yoga that were practised mainly in ascetic circles. In the *Haripāṭh* and related literature of the Vārkarīs an outright rejection of yoga can even be observed. This dismissive attitude may be explained as a result of the missionary endeavour of early Vārkarīs who wanted to convince as many potential followers as possible of the advantages of their less demanding way towards liberation.

In the chapter "On al-Bīrūnī's *Kitāb Pātanğal* and the *Pātañjalayogaśāstra*" by **Philipp A. Maas** and **Noémie Verdon** the thematic focus shifts from the description and analysis of yoga in individual religious and philosophical traditions of premodern South Asia to the cultural transfer of yoga from South Asia to the Arab intellectual world in the Middle Ages. After providing an introduction to the life and work of al-Bīrūnī, the famous Perso-Muslim polymath who lived at the turn of the first millennium CE and spent some years in north-western South Asia, Maas and Verdon survey previous scholarly attempts to identify the Sanskrit source of his *Kitāb Pātanğal*, an Arab rendering of a yoga work in the tradition of Patañjali. The two authors arrive at the novel hypothesis that al-Bīrūnī may have used the *Pātañjalayogaśāstra* (i. e., the *Yogasūtra* together with the so-called *Yogabhāṣya*) as the main source of the *Kitāb Pātanğal*. This finding provides the basis for a new assessment of this work as the result of different literary transformations, some of which necessarily had to be highly creative in order to transfer the philosophical and religious content of a Sanskrit yoga work of the late fourth or early fifth century into the intellectual culture of medieval Islam. Taking into consideration these creative aspects of the *Kitāb Pātanğal*, Maas and Verdon demonstrate that the aspiration of the Perso-Muslim author was not merely to provide a translation faithful to the wording of its source text, but to make the spiritual dimension of yoga accessible to his Muslim readership.

Also **Ian A. Baker**'s "Tibetan Yoga: Somatic Practice in Vajrayāna Buddhism and Dzogchen" deals with a cultural transfer of yoga, namely, the transfer of haṭhayogic practices from South Asia to Tibet. Baker highlights the early occurrences of the word *haṭhayoga* and of haṭhayogic techniques in South Asian

Buddhist tantric literature in works such as the *Guhyasamājatantra* and the *Amṛtasiddhi.* He then describes five practices, namely the "axis of awareness", "yoga of breath and movement", the "heart essence of Tibetan yoga", "yoga of spontaneous presence", and "yoga of active perception", all of which occur in Buddhist tantric sources like the *Kālacakratantra,* the commentarial literature on them and further tantric treatises composed by Tibetan scholars. Baker then contextualises these yoga techniques in the history of Tibetan Buddhism. He concludes his detailed account of Tibetan somatic practices by suggesting that the "yoga of active perception" may be the quintessence of Tibetan yogic practice with a large potential to alter embodied experiences and to create "forms of awareness that transcend perennially limiting perspectives and preoccupations".

3. Synopsis of Part B: "Globalised Yoga"

In the initial chapter of the second part of the volume, "Yoga within Viennese Occultism: Carl Kellner and Co.", **Karl Baier** investigates the role of yoga within the occultist movement that flourished in Vienna during the last decades of the Habsburg Empire. The focus of this chapter is on the industrialist and occultist Carl Kellner. Kellner and other members of his milieu displayed a positive attitude towards Haṭha Yoga, although many influential theosophical publications of the time warned against body-centered yoga practices. Baier shows that the interpretation of yoga within the occultist movement was prompted by the teaching of certain physical exercises in the Rosicrucian tradition represented by Johann B. Krebs and Alois Mailänder. Furthermore, Baier substantiates a hypothesis concerning yoga practice and ritual sex within the so-called Inner Occult Circle of the Sovereign Sanctuary, a high-degree masonic order in which Kellner operated as financial sponsor and spiritual teacher. This small group plays an important role within the historiography of modern occultism, as time and again it is considered to be the hotbed of the later Ordo Templi Orientis. The coda of the chapter examines Herbert Silberer's views on yoga. Silberer was the most talented representative of second-generation Viennese occultism and his work foreshadows later developments such as Carl Gustav Jung's interpretation of alchemy and the Eranos circle.

Joseph S. Alter's "Yoga, Nature Cure and 'Perfect' Health: The Purity of the Fluid Body in an Impure World" discusses the correlation between purification and embodied perfection to highlight how postures (*āsana*), breathing techniques and exercises (*prāṇāyāma*) came to be understood within the framework of nature cure in modern India. Alter argues that the combination of nature cure and yoga provided a practical solution to the problem of contingency in health care. Nature cure shaped the practice of yoga and, in turn, yoga provided a justification not only of different body-centred purifying practices, but also for the purification of mind by means of meditation practices. Without doubt, this synthesis of yoga and nature cure had an enormous impact on the global practice of yoga, but it also initiated a historical development within modern India that continues until the present day. Alter builds a bridge between Swami Sivananda – an Indian medical doctor who in the first half of the twentieth century integrated elements of yoga and nature cure, renounced the world and established the Divine Life Society – and more recent political innovations in India, namely, the establishment of the Central Council for Research on Yoga and Naturopathy (CCRYN) and its incorporation under the Ministry of Ayurveda, Yoga and Naturopathy, Unani, Siddha and Homoeopathy (AYUSH).

A bridge of a different kind is addressed in the chapter "Sāṃkhya in Transcultural Interpretation: Shri Anirvan (Śrī Anirvāṇa) and Lizelle Reymond" by **Maya Burger**. Burger analyses the writings of the Bengali author Shri Anirvan (1896–1978) and the Swiss author of books on Indian spirituality Lizelle Reymond (1899–1994), who was Shri Anirvan's disciple and translator. Burger demonstrates in a paradigmatic way the tight connections between India and Europe in the modern interpretation of yoga. In this context, she draws special attention to the concepts of Sāṃkhya philosophy that Shri Anirvan employed in order to explain his experience of yoga. Steeped in the local tradition of the Bauls of Bengal, Shri Anirvan also enjoyed a classical training in Sanskrit. He was interested in modern science and (e.g., as translator of the works of Aurobindo into Bengali) familiar with Indian thinkers who reflected the confluence of cultures. Reymond was one of the intellectuals who introduced French-speaking Europe to the spiritualities of India, founding a book series that later became the important series "Les spiritualités vivantes". Burger investigates the reinterpretation of yoga that took place in the collaboration of Shri Anirvan and Reymond by analysing key terms like *prakṛti* and *puruṣa* as well as the concept of the "void" that was inspired by the Greek–Armenian occultist George Ivanovich Gurdjieff. She concludes that Shri Anirvan and Reymond presented a psychological and mystical interpretation of Sāṃkhya that made this ancient Indian philosophical tradition suitable for the modern world.

In "Christian Responses to Yoga in the Second Half of the Twentieth Century" **Anand Amaladass** addresses a further bridge provided by yoga, not between regional or national cultures, or between tradition and modernity within the same culture, but between two different religious traditions, namely, the Hindu and Christian traditions. However, his chapter shows that the Christian reception of yoga during the last century was not only rather ambiguous but by and large negative. The explanation that Amaladass offers for this state of affairs draws upon the Orientalistic typology of "the West" and "the East". Influential intellectuals like Carl Gustav Jung and Hermann Hesse, who were interested in

India and Indian studies, were nonetheless averse to Europeans having recourse to Asian methods of prayer and meditation in general and to yoga in particular. Additionally, many Christians may have had an especially reserved attitude towards yoga due to their theological presuppositions. The Christian "missionary" thrust aims at giving a unique message to the whole world, but Christian traditions were frequently not ready to receive inspiration from outside. Moreover, the distinction Christian theologians made between their "revealed" religion and all other "natural" religions put them in an asymmetrical position – religiously and culturally. The negative response to yoga is a consequence of these attitudes. Nevertheless, there were exceptional individuals who wrote appreciatively on yoga from a Christian perspective, both in India and abroad. They took to its practice seriously and profited personally from it. In line with their experiences, some Christian authorities interpreted yoga as a helpful discipline that may be resorted to by Christians for their spiritual development and can be adapted within a Christian theological framework.

Concerning the broad, truly transnational dissemination of yoga and its theoretical aspects, **Beatrix Hauser**'s "Following the Transcultural Circulation of Bodily Practices: Modern Yoga and the Corporeality of Mantras" is particularly critical of two models: that of a linear and primarily bilateral transfer from India and that of a global distribution in the form of global distribution networks. She proposes to replace these conceptualisations by introducing recent theories of global flows into Modern Yoga Studies. In her theorisation of global flows, Hauser argues that a consideration of the sentient human body as a source of recontextualisation and meaning production in its own right is of essential importance. The ethnographical part of her study investigates the chanting of mantras in contemporary yoga classes in Germany. Teachers explain the usage of mantras not only with reference to tradition but also with reference to sound as a type of energy that prompts attentiveness towards various sensorial spaces within the body. The latter point corresponds to older therapeutic concepts that were developed in Germany at the crossroads of voice training, breath therapy and autosuggestive techniques. The idea of chanting mantras for mental and physical benefit has seemingly superseded earlier concepts of vocal therapy. Hauser takes this as a confirmation of the view that yoga practitioners assess any of their somatic sensations in relation to previous experiences and sociocultural categories that shape the experiential repertoire.

The chapter "Living4giving: Politics of Affect and Emotional Regimes in Global Yoga" by **Anne Koch** explores socio-political aspects of modern yoga. She discusses a prominent social manifestation of contemporary yoga, namely the Yoga Aid World Challenge (YAWC). This public yoga event gathers thousands of people across nearly thirty countries worldwide every year. On a certain day, yoga teacher teams compete for donations by offering yoga classes in public spaces around the globe. Koch examines the political economy of this new form of organised global yoga and explains how neoliberal elements like competition permeate it. The success of YAWC depends on several factors: an emotional regime in the sense of a recognisable subcultural pattern, virtual and marketing communication, a corporate identity aesthetics, and the imagination of a global yoga space created by joint body practices. According to Koch, this new configuration of yoga is based on a transformation of social belonging and the offer of a specific purpose in life. By means of a certain "politics of affect" altruistic behaviour is generated as something distinct from late-modern spirituality that at the same time presents itself as a kind of self-empowerment concordant with it.

Similar to Beatrix Hauser's chapter, **Suzanne Newcombe**'s "Spaces of Yoga: Towards a Non-Essentialist Understanding of Yoga" interlinks questions of methodology and conceptualisation with a more empirical objective. Drawing on Jim Knott's spatial analysis of religion, she examines the physical and social spaces of contemporary yoga. At the same time Newcombe argues for an approach to yoga that introduces instrumental and situational terms instead of essentialist definitions. On this note she presents the different locations and spaces connected with the practice of yoga: the stage used for yoga performances, public schools, typical contemporary yoga studios in cosmopolitan, multicultural areas, and, last but not least the yoga mat as a sacred ritual space where physical and psychological re-orientation take place. In this way she enquires not so much into what yoga is but into where yoga is practised and into the different meanings that emerge when yoga is practised in these different spaces. Her close look at the spaces yoga occupies in contemporary society reveals a great variety. Furthermore, Newcombe concludes that yoga is neither a necessarily religious or spiritual practice, nor a purely secular activity. It can be private, but sometimes it also assumes social and political dimensions.

In the final chapter of the present volume, "*Nāga, Siddha* and Sage: Visions of Patañjali as an Authority on Yoga", **Gudrun Bühnemann** also turns to spaces where yoga is practised nowadays. She points out that statues and other visual representations of Patañjali have become an important component of the visual culture of contemporary yoga. These representations also provide a link between South Asian and globalised yoga. Bühnemann argues that two factors created the modern interest in visual representations of the legendary author of the *Yogasūtra*: (1) the canonical status that the *Yogasūtra* has gained in many modern schools of yoga and (2) the recitation of stanzas in praise of Patañjali at the beginning of yoga sessions in globalised yoga studios. Searching for links between tradition and modernity, she traces the development of Patañjali's iconography, starting with the earliest representations in the tradition of the Naṭarāja Temple at Cidambaram in Tamilnadu, South India. Against this backdrop, Bühnemann then examines the more recent iconography of Patañjali in the tradition of the twentieth-century yoga master Tirumalai Krishnamacharya. Furthermore, she treats representations of Patañjali as an accomplished being (*siddha*) absorbed in meditation, which she considers a distinct phenomenon that may also have originated in Tamilnadu. Bühnemann concludes her chapter with a look at recent representations of Patañjali that experiment with new forms and modes of expression.

4. Acknowledgements

At this place, we would like to thank the following institutions and organisations for their generous support of the conference "Yoga in Transformation: Historical and Contemporary Perspectives on a Global Phenomenon" mentioned in section 1 above which was the starting point of the present book project: the Katholisch-Theologische Fakultät, Universität Wien, the Philologisch-Kulturwissenschaftliche Fakultät, Universität Wien, the Kulturabteilung der Stadt Wien (MA 7), the Embassy of India to Austria and Montenegro and Permanent Mission of India to the International Organisations in Vienna, the Institut für Südasien-, Tibet- und Buddhismuskunde, Universität Wien, the Sammlung De Nobili – Arbeitsgemeinschaft für Indologie und Religionsforschung / The De Nobili Research Library – Association for Indology and the Study of Religion, Vienna, the Berufsverband der Yogalehrenden in Deutschland and the Österreichische Gesellschaft für Religionswissenschaft / Austrian Association for the Study of Religions, Vienna. We are also indebted to the Shanti Yoga Store, Vienna, Yoga Austria – BYO (Berufsverband der Yogalehrenden in Österreich), the Institut für Religionswissenschaft, Universität Wien, and the magazine "Ursache und Wirkung", Vienna, for their kind support and assistance. The extraordinary commitment of Alexandra Böckle, Ewa Lewandowska and Judith Starecek of the Institut für Südasien-, Tibet- und Buddhismuskunde, Universität Wien proved invaluable in the practical planning and organisation of the conference.

We would also like to express our special gratitude to Alexandra Scheuba (née Böckle), our editorial assistant, for taking care of the bulk of communication with our speakers and authors, for the professional preparation of the manuscript of the present volume, and for painstakingly copy-editing the text and participating in its proof-reading. Without her dedicated, patient and competent assistance, the volume would not have taken its present shape. We also gratefully acknowledge the support of Camilla Nielsen who assisted us in the copy-editing especially of the chapters by non-native speakers of English. Further thanks go to the reviewers of the volume, Daniel Raveh and Geoffrey Samuel, for their kind readiness to review the voluminous manuscript at rather short notice and for their pertinent comments and suggestions, and to the editorial board of the

"Wiener Forum für Theologie und Religionswissenschaft" for accepting the present volume into their series published by the Vienna University Press, a division of V&R unipress of Vandenhoeck & Ruprecht, Göttingen.

Funding for the publication of this book both in print and in digital form as an Open Access resource was kindly provided by the Association Monégasque pour la Recherche Académique sur le Yoga (Monaco Association for Academic Research on Yoga), the European Research Council and the Rectorate of the University of Vienna.

Part A.

Yoga in South Asia and Tibet

Chapter 1

Some Problematic Yoga Sūtra-s and Their Buddhist Background

Dominik Wujastyk

Contents

1. Introduction 23
1.1. Émile Senart 24
1.2. Louis de La Vallée Poussin 26
1.3. Mircea Eliade 27

2. Three *Sūtra*-s Examined 28
2.1. Samādhipāda 11: *anubhūtaviṣayāsaṃpramoṣaḥ smṛtiḥ* 28
2.2. Sādhanapāda 46–47: *sthirasukham āsanam prayatnaśaithilyānanta-samāpattibhyām* 32
2.3. Kaivalyapāda 29: *prasaṅkhyāne 'py akusīdasya sarvathāvivekakhyāter dharmameghaḥ samādhiḥ* 35

3. Patañjali's Use of *Vibhāṣā* Materials 38

4. Conclusions 42

References 42

Dominik Wujastyk

Chapter 1: Some Problematic Yoga Sūtra-s and Their Buddhist Background*

1. Introduction

In this paper, I discuss a small selection of *sūtra*-s from the *Pātañjalayogaśāstra* that are sometimes misunderstood, or mistakenly considered to be problematic, by contemporary interpreters and even some early Sanskrit commentators. Some of these interpretative difficulties arise out of a lack of specific historical knowledge, especially of the language and content of early Buddhist literature. Several of the interpretations I shall present are not entirely new to Indological studies, but their importance has been overlooked, especially by some recent interpreters. For example, the pioneering study by Émile Senart published in 1900 argued compellingly that the *Pātañjalayogaśāstra* and the Pali *Tipiṭaka* contained passages and concepts that were either parallel or even conceptually identical. Louis de La Vallée Poussin (1937) continued Senart's work, and revealed further strong influences of Buddhism discernible in the *Pātañjalayogaśāstra*.

With this background, I shall clarify some points of interpretation and discuss selected *sūtra*-s from the point of view of their value as diagnostic tests for the quality of interpreters' understandings of early yoga texts. I shall give special attention to the historical background of the technical terms *dharmamegha, asaṃpramoṣa*, and *anantasamāpatti.* I shall argue that one cannot correctly or fully understand much of what Patañjali said in his *sūtra*-s and commentary without understanding something about Buddhism, and especially the Buddhist thought and terminology that evolved to discuss meditation and the path to liberation.

---

* I am most grateful to colleagues who commented on an earlier version of this paper, especially Eli Franco, Birgit Kellner, Chlodwig Werba and Philipp A. Maas. They raised extremely interesting points that deserve much further thought and research, but I have only been able to take up their suggestions to a limited extent in this paper. I also thank Isabelle Ratié and Ferenc Rusza for their corrections and comments.

To bring this point home in a contemporary context, I would like to suggest the following parallel. Suppose you become aware of a new religious movement that is attracting members in the city where you live. Supposing further that you are handed a leaflet by an enthusiast in the street. The leaflet praises the virtuous life, encourages protecting the environment, and speaks about realizing one's personal potential. And amongst other phrases, you see the expressions, "the ten commandments" and then later, "our saviour" and "redemption". You would, I think, draw the conclusion that this new religious movement owed at least part of its thinking to a Judeo-Christian background. These key words and phrases spring out of the text like flags, immediately indicating at least one of the sources of the leaflet's inspiration.

That is what it is like for the cultural historian of India, reading Patañjali's masterpiece on Yoga. As one reads through the work, keywords from Buddhist thought leap out of the page. Given an awareness of Buddhist history and language, these signals are unmissable.

This is not a particularly new point. As mentioned, it was made over a century ago by Senart and has been repeated by many distinguished scholars throughout more than a century since then.[1] Of course it is helpful and fascinating to see how Patañjali reprocessed and integrated Buddhist ideas and language in his classic work on Yoga. And more research specifically on this topic is much needed and will prove interesting and enjoyable. But this point by itself is not the main focus of the following argument. What I am addressing in the present study is a slightly different issue. I am focussing specifically on some of the cases where *not* knowing the Buddhist background to what Patañjali said can lead one seriously astray, where one can fail to understand what Patañjali was talking about.

1.1. Émile Senart

The pioneering study by Émile Senart published in 1900 argued compellingly that the *Pātañjalayogaśāstra* and the Pali *Tipiṭaka* contained passages and concepts that were either parallel or even conceptually identical.[2]

For example, he compared the category of the *brahmavihāra*-s – benevolence (*maitrī*), compassion (*karuṇā*), sympathetic joy (*muditā*) and detachment (*upekṣā*) – that are mentioned in *Pātañjalayogaśāstra* (PYŚ) 1.33 with their

1 E.g., Senart 1900, Woods 1914: xvii–xviii *et passim*, Kimura 1934, La Vallée Poussin 1937, Larson 1989, Cousins 1992, Yamashita 1994, Larson & Bhattacharya 2008: 42–43, Angot 2008: 91–94, Bryant 2009: 69–70.

2 Following the arguments of Maas (2006, 2013), and the colophons of most manuscripts, I refer to the *sūtra*-s and their commentary, the *Bhāṣya*, as a single work, with the title *Pātañjalayogaśāstra*.

description in Buddhist texts.[3] In both contexts, these virtues are presented as the appropriate objects for meditation (*bhāvanā*).[4]

This is an example of a case where the *sūtra*-s are reasonably clear, and the fact that the key terms receive their earliest exposition in the Buddhist *Tipiṭaka* is not critical to understanding them. We can struggle through, ignoring Buddhism, and still have a pretty good idea of what the *sūtra*-s are saying, even if the nuances and cultural background escape us.

It has to be said, however, that even in so apparently obvious a case, there is a small problem that would worry the careful Sanskrit scholar. As Louis Renou (1940: 373) pointed out, the word *muditā* ("sympathetic joy") is not well-formed Sanskrit. It is a feminine of a verbal noun in *-ta*, which is not a grammatical form normally found in classical Sanskrit. It is, however, a type of word that is well known in Buddhist Hybrid Sanskrit.[5] So this keyword used by Patañjali already creates a small problem for classical Sanskrit readers, a problem only soluble by reference to Buddhist Sanskrit.

Senart himself expressed the general idea that I am addressing, namely that there are concepts used by Patañjali that are inexplicable without the Buddhist background, when he said:

> One is surprised by the strange word *dharmamegha*, "cloud of the law", which Yoga uses to designate the ultimate *samādhi* that confirms the destruction of the *kleśa*s and of *karman* (YS. IV, 28, 29). How can one separate it from Buddhist phraseology and from this "ambrosia of the law" that the Buddha's teaching causes to fall as rain upon the world?[6]

I shall look more deeply into this word *dharmamegha* below (on p. 35ff.).

3 Patañjali does not mention the actual word *brahmavihāra.*

4 Senart 1900: 353. For a depth study of the *brahmavihāra*-s, see Maithrimurthi (1999), who argues that these categories were originally absorbed by Buddhism from much earlier Brāhmaṇa sources.

5 Edgerton (1953: 434) noted that Senart thought the word might be formed from *mudutā* ← Skt. *mṛdutā* ("softness, gentleness"). Edgerton was less convinced, because the meaning of *muditā* really does seem connected with the verbal root *mud* "delight". Maithrimurthi (1999: 131) notes the difficulty and suggests that the form is analogical with *karuṇā* and *upekṣā,* or that it once qualified an unexpressed feminine substantive.

6 Senart 1900: 353: "On s'est étonné du nom si étrange de dharmamegha, 'nuage de la Loi', dont le Yoga désigne ce samadhi ultime qui assure la destruction des *kleśas* et du *karman* (YS. IV, 28, 29). Comment le séparer de la phraséologie bouddhique et de cette 'ambroisie de la Loi' que l'enseignement du Buddha fait pleuvoir sur le monde?"

1.2. Louis de La Vallée Poussin

Over thirty years later, La Vallée Poussin continued Senart's work, and delved further into the strong influences of Buddhism discernible in the *Pātañjala-yogaśāstra.*[7]

While La Vallée Poussin showed the utmost respect for Senart's work, which had after all inspired him to take the subject further, he made one very important correction to his predecessor's ideas. This concerned the question of relative chronology. Senart had written on the assumption that a developed Yoga philosophy, what Larson usefully called, "a systematic reflection that seeks overall coherence and persuasive presentation",[8] had developed before the time of the Buddha, and that the Buddha was using the ideas of classical Yoga in his teaching. Thirty years later, La Vallée Poussin already knew that this was not so, and that the direction of influence had certainly been the other way round: Buddhism was much older than the *Pātañjalayogaśāstra,* and the influence had flowed from Buddhism to Patañjali.[9]

La Vallée Poussin studied more *sūtra*-s and specific philosophical terms than Senart had done, including,

1.25 īśvara
1.33 brahmavihāra-s
1.48–49 prajñā ṛtaṃbharā
2.5 avidyā
2.12–13, 31, 34, 4.7 karman
2.15 duḥkha
2.25, 3.50, 55, 4.26–34 kaivalya
2.27 the seven prajñā-s
2.39 janmakathaṃtā
2.42 saṃtoṣa
2.47 ānantyasamāpatti
3.13, 4.12 Sarvāstivāda ideas
3.20–21 paracittajñāna
3.26 bhuvanajñāna
3.48 manojavitva
3.46 a yogi's four saṃpad-s
3.51, 4.28–29 bhūmi-s/dharmamegha
4.1 siddhi-s
4.16ff. theory of knowledge

For example, La Vallée Poussin noted that the five means to acquiring supernatural powers that are described in PYŚ 4.1 are paralleled in the Buddhist philosophical work called the *Abhidharmakośabhāṣya* (AKBh) (7.53) composed by Vasubandhu (born c 350 CE).[10] In PYŚ 4.1, a yogi is said to be able to acquire supernatural powers by virtue of the following five causes: birth (*janma*), herbs (*oṣadhi*), invocations (*mantra*), askesis (*tapas*) and meditative integration

7 La Vallée Poussin 1937.

8 Larson 1989: 131, contrasted with "speculative intuition in an environment of received authority".

9 Maharaj (2013: 77) discusses the older views of the chronological precedence of the *Pātañjalayogaśāstra* over Buddhism. See also Jacobi 1931; Keith 1932; Renou 1940.

10 La Vallée Poussin 1937: 241–242. On the much discussed issue of Vasubandhu's date I here follow the arguments of Deleanu (2006: 1.186–194). See also Anacker 1984: ch. II, Willemen et al. 1998, Kragh 2013, etc.

(*samādhi*).[11] The powers (*ṛddhi*-s) listed in the *Abhidharmakośabhāṣya* are produced through exactly the same causes, in a different sequence: meditation (*bhāvanā*), birth (*upapatti*), invocations (*mantra*), herbs (*oṣadhi*), and by certain ascetic actions (*karma*).[12] It is beyond possibility that these two lists could be independent. There must be a connection between the Buddhist Abhidharma tradition transmitted to us by Vasubandhu and the *Pātañjalayogaśāstra* of Patañjali. La Vallée Poussin noted further parallels between these two authors, and we shall return to Vasubandhu below.[13]

1.3. Mircea Eliade

Mircea Eliade had a huge effect on the study and understanding of yoga in the latter part of the twentieth century. It is no exaggeration to say that for many scholars and students, yoga was no more and no less than what Eliade said it was. His book was extraordinarily influential, as has recently been confirmed though the reception studies of Guggenbühl (2008) and Liviu Bordaş (2011, 2012). Both studies show how important Eliade was in moulding scholarship on yoga in the second half of the twentieth century. In fact, La Vallée Poussin (1937) himself was aware of the first edition of Eliade's famous book, which came out in French, just a year before La Vallée Poussin's article.

However, Eliade's book is now obsolete in many respects. While it offered new materials in the first half of the last century, it is now superseded by more accurate and insightful scholarship on almost all aspects of the history of the yoga tradition. In particular, Eliade's chapter on the relationship between yoga and Buddhism is no longer a reliable source of information or interpretation.[14] Although Eliade describes various forms of meditation, the acquisition of magical powers, and forms of metaphysical knowledge in Buddhism, he does not draw many close parallels with the classical Yoga tradition of the *Pātañjalayogaśāstra*. And for the most part, discussion of the topics raised by Eliade has simply moved on in the research literature. The trenchant criticisms offered by

11 Āgāśe 1904: 176: *janmauṣadhimantratapaḥsamādhijāḥ siddhayaḥ* || 1 || .

12 Pradhan 1975: 428–429: *avyākṛtaṃ bhāvanājaṃ trividhaṃ tūpapattijam* | *ṛddhir mantrauṣadhābhyāṃ ca karmajā ceti pañcadhā* || 7.53 || *samāsataḥ pañcavidhām ṛddhiṃ varṇayanti* | *bhāvanāphalam upapattilābhikaṃ mantrajām auṣadhajāṃ karmajāṃ ca* | . French translation by La Vallée Poussin (1923–1926: V/121–122), translated into English by Pruden (1988–1990: IV/1176). Discussed by Pines and Gelblum (1983: 281). Citing parallel passages in the *Bhagavadgītā* (*karma* in 5.11 compared with *tapas* in 17.14–16) Pines and Gelblum (ibid.) argue convincingly that Vasubandhu's use of the word *karma* can be interpreted as referring specifically to *tapas*, thus paralleling the *Pātañjalayogaśāstra* exactly.

13 La Vallée Poussin 1937: 232, 239.

14 Eliade 1970: ch. 5.

R. Gombrich (1974) have undermined all the main arguments put forward by Eliade about the relationship between Yoga and Buddhism. Eliade's views on this topic need not detain us further. The recent historiographical survey of yoga studies by Maas (2013) is the most up-to-date guide to the current state of the field.

2. Three *Sūtra*-s Examined

In what follows, the *sūtra*-s I shall discuss include
- Samādhipāda 11: *anubhūtaviṣayāsaṃpramoṣaḥ smṛtiḥ*
- Sādhanapāda 46–47: *sthirasukham āsanam prayatnaśaithilyānantasamāpattibhyām* and
- Kaivalyapāda 29: *prasaṅkhyāne 'py akusīdasya sarvathāvivekakhyāter dharmameghaḥ samādhiḥ*

These are just a small selection of the *sūtra*-s that could be chosen to exemplify the point being made in this paper.

2.1. Samādhipāda 11: *anubhūtaviṣayāsaṃpramoṣaḥ smṛtiḥ*

This *sūtra* gives Patañjali's definition of *smṛti,* a word meaning memory or mindfulness.[15] Roughly speaking, Patañjali says that memory is having no *saṃpramoṣa* (*a+saṃpramoṣa*) of the sense objects that have been experienced. What does this awkward word *saṃpramoṣa* mean? Just using common sense, we can work out that it must mean something like "forgetting", or "losing", because after all, in addition to meaning "mindfulness" or "self-remembering", *smṛti* is also an ordinary-language word in Sanskrit, often meaning "memory" in the simplest sense, as in, "I remember what I had for breakfast."[16] Patañjali is trying to firm up the definition for philosophical purposes.[17] After all, *smṛti* is one of the five *vṛtti*-s that yoga is meant to block, so he needs to clarify what exactly it is. But

15 See Wujastyk (2012) and Maharaj (2013) for recent discussions on the interpretation of yogic *smṛti.*

16 A real example: *uktam āpadgataḥ pūrvaṃ pituḥ smarasi śāsanam* || "When you get into trouble, you remember the instruction your father said before." *Mahābhārata, Bhīṣmaparvan* (6), *adhyāya* 124, verse 20 (Krishnacharya & Vyasacharya 1906–1910: 5/188).

17 Franco (1987: 373) was the first to point out that Prabhākara may have taken and used the term *pramoṣa,* in the context of discussing *smṛti,* from the *Pātañjalayogaśāstra,* when he was developing his theory of cognitions of illusions. I am grateful to Eli Franco for observing in a personal communication that *smṛti* in philosophical discourse is never a faculty of mind, but rather a momentary mental event.

if breakfast is the sense impression that I have experienced, then memory must have at least something to do with retaining knowledge of that experience, so *asaṃpramoṣa* must mean something along those lines.

The *Pātañjalayogaśāstra* commentary on this *sūtra* does not help, since it took for granted that we know the meaning of this word, and did not explain it. Sanskrit commentators are often very good at helpfully explaining and paraphrasing awkward vocabulary. The fact that Patañjali did not do this suggests that the word *saṃpramoṣa* was sufficiently obvious to him so that it never occurred to him that it would need explaining. That is interesting.

The next commentator, Śaṅkara (8th or 9th century),[18] glossed the term as "not taking away (*anapaharaṇa*)" and "not disappearing (*atirobhāva*)".[19] Like Patañjali, Śaṅkara seemed reasonably comfortable with the word, but he introduced the sense of "not taking away" or "not removing" although he had the confidence to add the more intuitive "not disappearing".

But the next main commentator, the influential Vācaspati Miśra, who lived in about 950 CE, felt a stronger need to explain the term. In his very first sentence, Vācaspati told us what he thought the word meant.[20] For him, it was "not stealing (*asteya*)". So the *sūtra* was apparently saying, "memory is the non-stealing of the sense impressions that have been experienced." This is very odd. But Vācaspati's interpretation became standard for later commentators, and indeed for modern translators.

Two examples, separated by a century, will have to stand for the scores of translations that struggle with the idea of stealing experienced impressions. Both are books of great merit. Prasāda (1910: 24) translated: "Memory is the not stealing away along with objective mental impressions (retained) (i.e., the reproducing of not more than what has been impressed upon the mind)." Bryant (2009: 43) translated: "Memory is the retention of [images of] sense objects that have been experienced." Bryant, perhaps influenced by Śaṅkara, finessed the point, noting that *asaṃpramoṣa* meant "not slipping away, retention".

Quite inexplicably, Woods (1914: 31) translated *asaṃpramoṣa* as "not-adding-surreptitiously", a translation that bears no relation that I can think

---

18 Maas 2013: 18; Harimoto 1999: 136. The identity of this Śaṅkara is still under scholarly discussion. Several of the arguments raised in the important study by Halbfass (1991: ch. 6) are still open, although Harimoto makes the telling observation that the author of the *Vivaraṇa* used the same vocabulary and ideas as Śaṅkara the theologian, and avoided using any Advaita terminology from a later period (2014: appendix "Materials for the Authorship Problem", p. 247). If the author of the *Vivaraṇa* was not *the* Śaṅkara, then the internal evidence suggests that he was a person of the same period, and therefore earlier than Vācaspati Miśra.

19 Rama Sastri & Krishnamurthi Sastri 1952: 39.

20 Āgāśe 1904: 16.

of to anything whatsoever.[21] He translates the *sūtra* as follows: "Memory (*smṛti*) is not-adding-surreptitiously (*asampramoṣa*) to a once experienced object."

Why do all these commentators and translators get stuck on the concept of "stealing"? The answer is not difficult. One of the most advanced fields of knowledge in ancient India was grammar, specifically Sanskrit grammar. And the grammarians of about the fourth century BCE developed a list of about 2000 seed-forms of words, or elements of language, called *dhātu* in Sanskrit, "roots" in English usage, from which all other words could be derived. Shortly after this list had been created, a grammarian called Bhīmasena added a word or two to each root, just to pick out its main meaning, or to disambiguate similar roots.[22] Bhīmasena's additions do not constitute a dictionary as such, but they were often used as if they were definitions, not just indicators.[23] And in this list, the root *muṣ*, that lies at the heart of *a-saṃ-pra-**moṣ**-a*, is given the meaning √*muṣ* (9.58) = *steye* "steal".[24]

The main modern dictionaries of classical Sanskrit – Monier-Williams (1899), Apte (1957–1959), Böhtlingk & Roth (1855–1875) – all give the meaning "stealing".[25]

Now we can see where the problem came from. The early commentators followed the grammarians, and so do the modern Sanskrit lexicographers. But what did Patañjali himself mean? Was he really talking about not stealing memories?

If we turn to historical phonology, we find that there is a normal Indo-Aryan root, √*mṛṣ*, whose meaning is simply, "forget".[26] This root appears in many derivative words in Middle Indo-Aryan languages, as documented in Turner's *A Comparative Dictionary of the Indo-Aryan Languages* (see Figure 1).

The pronunciation of this family of words changed in Buddhist Pali and Buddhist Hybrid Sanskrit, generating forms such as the Pali "*pamussati*", "he forgets" and "*pamuṭṭha*", "forgotten".[27] Although we have these verb forms, there

21 Perhaps Woods was thinking about Vācaspati's "stealing", as something surreptitious? And perhaps stealing is not-adding?

22 Skeat (1968: xii) noted the same use of meanings in his own etymological dictionary, "a brief definition, merely as a mark whereby to identify the word." An etymologist is not a lexicographer.

23 Bronkhorst 1981.

24 √*mūṣ* (1.707) also = *steye*.

25 Böhtlingk and Roth also give "wegnehmen", which is a bit more helpful, and under *saṃpramoṣa* (1855–1875: VII/745) give "das Nichtvergessen", but specifically citing PYŚ 1.11. Mayrhofer (1986–2001: 383 f.) relates √*muṣ* only to "stehlen, wegnehmen, rauben".

26 Werba 1997: 366, see also Mayrhofer 1986–2001: 2/332 on √*marṣ*.

27 Rhys Davids & Stede 1921–1925: V/39, 40.

8730 ***pramr̥ṣati** ' forgets '. 2. ***pramr̥ṣyati.** 3. Pp. ***pramr̥ṣṭa -- .** [*pramŕ̥ṣē* inf.,
prámamarṣa perf., *pramarṣiṣṭhāḥ* aor., *mr̥ṣyatē* RV. -- √mr̥ṣ]
1. Pk. *pamhasaï, °mhusaï, °mhuhaï* ' forgets ' (*mh* from **pamharaï* < prasmarati), Pr. *puṣ* -- ,
Dm. *pramuṣ* -- , Gaw. *plemuṣ* -- , Kal. *prāmuṣ* -- .
2. Pa. *pamussati* ' forgets ', Paš.kuṛ. *šamaš* -- (← a dialect like uzb. with *š* -- < *pr* --).
3. Pa. *pamuṭṭha* -- ' forgotten ', Pk. *pamhaṭṭha* -- , *pamhuṭṭha* -- ; Ash. *pumiṣṭ, pərmišt,*
pumušt ' forgot ', Wg. *pramuṣṭoi, pramušt* -- , Kt. *pəmiṣṭyo, prə́muštyo.*
***pramr̥ṣṭa -- , *pramr̥ṣyati** ' forgets ' see prec.

Figure 1: Turner 1966–1985: #8730.

appears to be no Pali or Prakrit noun form **pamosa.*[28] Nevertheless, other verbal and participial derivatives from this root with the prefix *pra-* do appear in Vedic Sanskrit, Pali and Prakrit, as Turner showed.[29]

What is not in doubt is that the word *asaṃpramoṣa* was used in Buddhist Hybrid Sanskrit, meaning "not forgetting".[30] The word is in fact quite common in Buddhist Sanskrit texts, including especially those from the same period as the *Pātañjalayogaśāstra.*[31] The word *asaṃpramoṣaṇa* often occurs in sentences with *smr̥ti* "memory". One text uses Patañjali's exact compound expression, *smr̥tyasaṃpramoṣaṇa.*[32] Even more striking is Asaṅga's *Abhidharmasamuccaya,* also from the same period, that uses the word *asaṃpramoṣa* in a definition of recollection (*smr̥ti*) that almost exactly parallels Patañjali's *sūtra.*[33]

We can take one clear message from all this: Patañjali's *asaṃpramoṣa* has an older and much more diverse history than the later Sanskrit commentators seem to have credited. In Buddhist circles, and amongst speakers for whom the Prakrit languages were less remote, the meaning of the word *asaṃpramoṣa* "not forgetting" was clear. Patañjali knew what it meant and felt no need to explain the

---

28 A point kindly drawn to my attention in a personal communication from my colleague Chlodwig H. Werba.

29 Across many IA languages, Turner's dictionary has a number of interesting entries related to the roots *muṣ* and *mr̥ṣ* "wipe away, forget". These suggest the possibility that words sounding like *muṣ* or *mr̥ṣ* had a primary meaning connected with "forgetting" both in very early language like that of the *R̥gveda,* and in related Iranian languages such as Pahlavi. It would be interesting to apply the methods of historical phonology to the hypothesis that an old Sanskrit formation *mr̥ṣa* "wipe away, forget" evolved into a Prakrit *moṣa,* which was then taken back into Buddhist Hybrid Sanskrit unchanged. Once in Sanskrit usage, the word's connection with *mr̥ṣ* "wipe, forget" was forgotten, and the grammarians started to try to connect it with the quite different root *muṣ* "steal".

30 Edgerton 1953: 83.

31 E.g., *Aṣṭādaśasāhasrikāprajñāpāramitāsūtra* (Conze 1974), *Bodhisattvabhūmi* (Dutt 1966: 76, 88, 142, 221, 279), and many others.

32 *Suvarṇaprabhāsottamasūtra* (Bagchi 1967: 55).

33 Pradhan 1950: 6: *smr̥tiḥ katamā | saṃsmr̥te [v. l. saṃstute] vastuni cetasaḥ asaṃpramoṣo 'vikṣepakarmikā ||*. Trans. Rahula 2001: 9: "What is mindfulness (*smr̥ti*)? It is non-forgetting by the mind (*cetas*) with regard to the object experienced. Its function is non-distraction." Cf. the same expression in *Pañcaskandhaprakaraṇam* 35.

term. But as centuries passed, its use in this sense was gradually forgotten even by the Sanskrit commentators.

Using what we have learned from the Buddhist sense of the word, Patañjali's *sūtra* means "memory is not forgetting the elements of awareness that have been experienced." There is no stealing involved. But one only arrives at this by understanding the Buddhist use of language.

2.2. Sādhanapāda 46–47: *sthirasukham āsanam prayatnaśaithilyānanta-samāpattibhyām*

As Philipp A. Maas has explained elsewhere in this volume, this *sūtra* can be translated as "A steady and comfortable posture [arises] from a slackening of effort or from merging meditatively into infinity."[34] Maas concentrated on the first part of the *sūtra,* and mentioned in passing that "merging meditatively in infinity" was connected with specifically Buddhist traditions of meditation.

The idea that this is a kind of meditation on infinity is supported by the earliest commentator on the *Pātañjalayogaśāstra,* namely Śaṅkara (8th or 9th century). In explaining this passage, he says, and I quote the translation by Philipp A. Maas and myself,

> Or, it is merged (*samāpanna*) in infinity. Infinity (*ananta*) means the All (*viśva*); infinitude (*ānantya*) is the fact of being infinite (*anantabhāva*). Being merged in that, having pervaded it, mind (*citta*), established as being the All, brings about, i. e., makes firm, the posture.[35]

There are two key points here. First, Śaṅkara was firmly describing a kind of meditation on infinity. Second, the way he expressed himself in Sanskrit makes it absolutely certain that the text of the *Pātañjalayogaśāstra* that he was looking at has the word "*ānantya*", "infinitude" and not the word "*ananta*" that means "infinite", that is printed in most modern editions of the text.

Different manuscripts of the *Pātañjalayogaśāstra* transmit two different readings of this phrase. Some say "*ananta*", while others say "*ānantya*". As Maas has said, the most conservative and original manuscripts of the *Pātañjalayoga-śāstra* have the latter reading, "*ānantya*", and Śaṅkara seems to have had access to these manuscripts.[36]

34 See the chapter by Philipp A. Maas on p. 60 of the present volume, and Maas & Wujastyk (in preparation).

35 Maas & Wujastyk (in preparation). Sanskrit text in Rama Sastri & Krishnamurthi Sastri 1952: 227.

36 See section 3.3.2 in the chapter by Maas in the present volume.

Why did the reading change from "*ānantya*" to "*ananta*"? I would like to suggest that it goes back - again - to the tenth-century commentator Vācaspati Miśra. In Indian mythology, there are stories about a snake, called "Unending" or "*ananta*" in Sanskrit. Vācaspati wanted to make this *sūtra* into a reference to some kind of meditation on the mythological snake, Ananta. In order to do this, he needed to read "*ananta*" in the *sūtra*. Vācaspati said, and again I quote the translation by Philipp A. Maas and myself,

> Alternatively [to relaxation], the mind (*citta*) produces posture when it is merged meditatively (*samāpanna*) in Ananta, the Leader of the Snakes, who supports the earth with his thousand very steady hoods.[37]

To the best of our present knowledge, Vācaspati Miśra was the first person to introduce the idea that the *Pātañjalayogaśāstra* was here talking about a mythological snake.

Several later Sanskrit commentators followed Vācaspati Miśra's interpretation, including,
- Vijñānabhikṣu (*fl.* 1550)[38]
- Bhāvagaṇeśa (*fl.* 1600)[39]
- Rāmānandasarasvatī (*fl.* 1600)[40]
- Nāgojibhaṭṭa or Nāgeśabhaṭṭa Kāḷe (*fl.* 1750)[41]

Many modern translators from the twentieth century onwards have followed Vācaspati's interpretation. Woods (1914: 192), to pick one prominent example, gave us the snake Ananta, without comment: "By relaxation of effort or by a [mental] state-of-balance with reference to Ananta-...".[42]

Prasāda (1910: 170–171), to choose another, gave the opaque translation "by thought-transformation as infinite", and Vācaspati's "Great Serpent", without comment. Prasāda's translation has been reprinted continuously up to the present time, and is widely read. Many more such translations could be cited, including some in the twenty-first century.

37 Maas & Wujastyk (in preparation). This is an image from the mythology of Ananta, the giant serpent who supports the earth. See Sörensen 1904–1925: 199b for references to the *Mahābhārata* version of the story. It also occurs in the Purāṇic literature, e.g., the *Viṣṇupurāṇa* (cited by Mani 1975: 35).

38 Nārāyaṇamiśra 1971: 263: *pṛthivīdhāriṇi sthirataraśeṣanāge samāpannaṃ.*

39 Ḍhuṇḍhirāja Śāstrī 2001: 105: *pṛthvīdhāriṇi ... śeṣanāge.*

40 Ḍhuṇḍhirāja Śāstrī 2001: 106: *nāganāyake.*

41 Ḍhuṇḍhirāja Śāstrī 2001: 105: *anante: pṛthvīdhāriṇi śeṣe.*

42 In note 1 on the word "Ananta" in the *bhāṣya*-part of PYŚ 2.47, Woods provides the following information: "Compare Bh. Gītā x.28. Ananta is Vāsuki, the Lord of Serpents. See also MBh. i.35, 5ff."

But not all later Sanskrit commentators and English translators have been comfortable with Vācaspati Miśra's snake idea. For example, the eighteenth-century south Indian commentator Sadāśivendrasarasvatī said that the meditation in question should involve a certain inwardness and commitment to mental expansion: "'I am the same as that which is infinite.' Such a meditation is steady concentration of the mind in the infinite."[43] An even more notable exception was another eighteenth-century scholar, Anantadeva. He noted that there were two different readings of the text in his manuscripts, and that these readings led to two different meanings: "'*Ananta*' means meditation on the snake, while '*ānantya*' means meditation on space (*ākāśa*)."[44]

So we see that some early interpreters were really thinking about meditative practice seriously – by which I mean mental states that engage with infinitude – and were in some cases even aware of the instability of the textual tradition they were studying. And some translators similarly preferred to stay with infinity, which seemed more appropriate in the context of meditation. But other commentators and translators have hedged their bets by retaining reference to the serpent, presumably because it was so ubiquitous in the tradition following Vācaspati Miśra and the spread of the variant reading *ananta* in the manuscripts.[45]

If we look into the earliest Buddhist sources, we find that a meditation on infinitude formed one of the very first teachings on meditation that occurred in the Buddha's life as recorded in the Pali Canon. The *Ariyaparyesanasutta* is perhaps the earliest biographical account of the Buddha's search for enlightenment and his first teaching.[46] As recorded in this work, the Buddha taught four meditations (Pali *jhāna*-s, Skt. *dhyāna*-s) followed by four further states called *āyatana*-s. All these eight meditative achievements are, in later Buddhist texts, called the eight *samāpatti*-s or "eight attainments". The fifth and sixth of these states are described in the *Ariyaparyesanasutta* as follows:

> 5. Then again the monk, with the complete transcending of perceptions of [physical] form, with the disappearance of perceptions of resistance, and not heeding perceptions of diversity, [perceiving,] 'infinite space,' enters & remains in the dimension of the infinitude of space. ...
> 6. Then again the monk, with the complete transcending of the dimension of the infinitude of space, [perceiving,] 'Infinite consciousness,' enters & remains in the di-

43 Ḍhuṇḍhirāja Śāstrī 2001: 106: *yo 'yam anantaḥ sa evāham asmīti dhyānaṃ cittasyānante samāpattiḥ*. Most of these commentators also gloss *samāpatti* as "steady concentration (*dhāraṇā*)", or "meditation (*dhyāna*)".

44 Ibid.: *ananta ānantyeti pāṭhadvaye arthadvayam | prathamapāṭhe śeṣasamāpattiḥ; dvitīye ākāśasamāpattiḥ* || 47 || .

45 Bryant (2009: 287–288), for example, keeps both explanations.

46 Wynne 2007: 2.

> mension of the infinitude of consciousness. This monk is said to have blinded Mara. Trackless, he has destroyed Mara's vision and has become invisible to the Evil One. ...[47]

These Buddhist *samāpatti*-s or "attainments" are widely discussed in the Pali Canon as part of one of the standard discourses on stages of meditation. Since two of these early Buddhist meditative attainments concern forms of infinitude, and since the words are identical to the words of the *Pātañjalayogaśāstra,* it appears that these words form part of a single discourse about meditation phenomena that has gone through a process of gradual cultural change. The *samāpatti*-s, "attainments", including *ānantyasamāpatti,* "the attainment of infinitude", form part of a world of discourse that is wider than just the *Pātañjalayogaśāstra,* and which appears in earlier Buddhist meditation treatises that pre-date the *Pātañjalayogaśāstra* by several centuries.

2.3. Kaivalyapāda 29: *prasaṅkhyāne 'py akusīdasya sarvathāvivekakhyāter dharmameghaḥ samādhiḥ*

Finally, we come to the *dharmamegha,* the cloud of *dharma.* In this *sūtra,* Patañjali was describing a particular type of *samādhi,* or integrated realisation, that is experienced by someone who has no interest or investment (*kusīda*) in contemplation (*prasaṅkhyāna*), and who has, in every respect, the realisation of discrimination.[48]

Patañjali's *sūtra* means, broadly, "he who has no investment even in contemplation, who has the realisation of discrimination in every respect, obtains *dharmamegha samādhi*".

The word *dharmamegha* is a compound of the word *dharma,* meaning "virtue, law, Buddhist doctrine", and the word *megha,* which means "cloud". This

47 Trans. Thanissaro Bhikkhu 2015. Pali text: Trenckner & Chalmers 1888–1925: 1/ sutta 26: 38. *Puna ca paraṃ bhikkhave bhikkhu sabbaso rūpa-saññānaṃ samatikkamā paṭigha-saññānaṃ attha-gamā nānattasaññānaṃ amanasi-kārā ananto ākāsoti ākāsānañcāyatanaṃ upasampajja viharati.*|| || *Ayaṃ vuccati bhikkhave bhikkhu andhamakāsi Māraṃ,*|| *apadaṃ vadhitvā Māracakkhuṃ adassanaṃ gato pāpimato.*|| || 39. *Puna ca paraṃ bhikkhave bhikkhu sabbaso ākāsānañcāyatanaṃ samatikkamma 'Anantaṃ viññāṇan' ti viññāṇañcāyatanaṃ upasampajja viharati.*|| || *Ayaṃ vuccati bhikkhave bhikkhu 'andhamakāsi Māraṃ,*|| *apadaṃ vadhitvā Māracakkhuṃ adassanaṃ gato pāpimato.*|| || Another translation: Ñānamoḷi & Bodhi 1995: 267–268.

48 Endo (2000) surveyed the history and meaning of the term *prasaṅkhyāna.* The study is valuable, although in my view Endo (pp. 78–79) failed to engage sufficiently with the *api* and alpha-privative of *a-kusīdasya* in PYŚ 4.29. Endo's interpretation that *prasaṅkhyāna* is a step towards *vivekakhyāti* does not seem to me to be what the *sūtra* says. In general, this *sūtra* and its discussion in the *Pātañjalayogaśāstra* and the *Vivaraṇa* contain many difficult and interesting points that deserve fuller treatment.

compound expression, that occurs only this one time in the *sūtra*-s, was not explained by Patañjali.[49]

The early commentator Śaṅkara explained that it is a technical term so called because the highest *dharma,* called Kaivalya, rains down.[50] As we shall see, Śaṅkara was right in his brief interpretation, although he shows no evidence of knowing the full underlying metaphor from which the expression originally arose.

If Śaṅkara's brevity does not fully satisfy, Vācaspati Miśra's explanation is little better. He had the cloud of *dharma* raining down "all kinds of knowable things (*dharma*-s)".[51]

The expression "virtue-rain (*dharmamegha*)" has continued to puzzle interpreters of Yoga since Vācaspati, including modern translators, who almost uniformly flounder with this term. When discussing this *sūtra,* Eliade had the rain of *dharma* falling on the yogi:

> a technical term that is difficult to translate, for dharma can have many meanings (order, virtue, justice, foundation, etc.) but that seems to refer to an abundance ("rain") of virtues that suddenly fill the yogin.[52]

In an article published nearly thirty years ago, Klaus Klostermaier offered an exhaustive survey of all the ways in which translators and interpreters had struggled with this term.[53] Klostermaier reminded the reader that Senart, La Vallée Poussin and others had pointed out that *dharmamegha* is explicitly mentioned in the Mahāyāna Buddhist text *Daśabhūmikasūtra,* "The Sūtra about the Ten Stages", as the last and culminating stage of spiritual awakening. It also occurs in many other Mahāyāna texts as either the name of the final or the penultimate stage of liberation. Having gathered all the necessary evidence and come tantalizingly close to solving the problem of *dharmamegha,* Klostermaier did not finally make a clear argument for the origin of the term.

The oldest occurrence of the term known in Indian literature is in a very early text, the *Milindapañha,* which may have been composed over a period of time starting in about 200 BCE. In that text, the term *dharmamegha* is introduced naturally in a beautiful metaphor describing the wise yogi:

---

49 In his remarks at PYŚ 1.2, Patañjali used the expression *dharmamegha* as a qualifier for meditation (Maas [2006: 5] *dharma-megha-dhyāna-*). In the commentary on PYŚ 3.32, he used *dharmamegha* as a synonym for *samādhi.*

50 Rama Sastri & Krishnamurthi Sastri 1952: 363: *kaivalyākhyaṃ paraṃ dharmaṃ varṣatīti dharmameghaḥ iti saṃjñā.*

51 On PYŚ 4.31 (Āgāśe 1904: 203): *ata eva sarvān dharmāñ jñeyān mehati varṣati prakāśaneneti dharmamegha ity ucyate* | Trans. Woods 1914: 343.

52 Eliade 1970: 84.

53 Klostermaier 1986.

12. 'Venerable Nāgasena, those five qualities of the rain you say he ought to take, which are they?'
'Just, O king, as the rain lays any dust that arises; just so, O king, should the strenuous yogi, earnest in effort, lay the dust and dirt of any evil dispositions that may arise within him. This is the first quality of the rain he ought to have.'
13. 'And again, O king, just as the rain allays the heat of the ground; just so, O king, should the strenuous yogi, earnest in effort, soothe the whole world of gods and men, with the feeling of his love. This, O king, is the second quality of the rain he ought to have.'
14. 'And again, O king, as the rain makes all kinds of vegetation to grow; just so, O king, should the strenuous yogi, earnest in effort, cause faith to spring up in all beings, and make that seed of faith grow up into the three Attainments, not only the lesser attainments of glorious rebirths in heaven or on earth, but also the attainment of the highest good, the bliss of Arahatship. This, O king, is the third quality of the rain he ought to have.'
15. 'And again, O king, just as the rain-cloud rising up in the hot season, affords protection to the grass, and trees, and creepers, and shrubs, and medicinal herbs, and to the monarchs of the woods that grow on the surface of the earth; just so, O king, should the strenuous yogi, earnest in effort, cultivating the habit of thoughtfulness, afford protection by his thoughtfulness to his condition of Samaṇaship, for in thoughtfulness is it that all good qualities have their root. This, O king, is the fourth quality of the rain that he ought to have.'
16. [411] 'And again, O king, as the rain when it pours down fills the rivers, and reservoirs, and artificial lakes, the caves and chasms, and ponds and holes and wells, with water; just so, O king, should the strenuous yogi, earnest in effort [yoga], pour down the rain of the Dhamma according to the texts handed down by tradition, and so fill to satisfaction the mind of those who are longing for instruction. This, O king, is the fifth quality of the rain he ought to have.'[54]

Here in the early Buddhist tradition, we find the term "cloud of *dharma*" in a beautiful and evocative literary context that makes perfect sense of the expression as a metaphor of cool, soothing abundance. This is the cool, soothing flow of virtue that rains from a wise man upon the world, dousing its flames of passion, hatred and delusion. The metaphor is an old one, central to the Buddha's opposition of his cooling, watery (*saumya*) teaching to the fiery, burning (*āgneya*) traditions of Brāhmaṇa religious practice.[55] The metaphor was still in use by the Buddhists of Patañjali's time, since it became the technical term for the tenth and highest level of a Bodhisattva's realisation. Asaṅga (*fl.* 330–405) used it in his

54 Trans. Rhys Davids 1890–1894: 356–357, with my "yogi" replacing Rhys Davids' "Bhikshu". Pali text, last paragraph (Trenckner 1880: 411): *Puna ca paraṃ mahārāja megho vassamāno nadītaḷākapokkharaṇiyo kandara-padara-sara-sobbha-udapānāni ca paripūreti udakadhārāhi, evam eva kho mahārāja yoginā yogāvacareṇa āgamapariyattiyā dhammamegham abhivassayitvā adhigamakāmānaṃ mānasaṃ paripūrayitabbaṃ.*

55 On these metaphorical oppositions, see, e.g., Gombrich 1996: ch. III; Wujastyk 2004; Jurewicz 2000, 2010.

Mahāyānasūtrālaṅkāra, and his younger half-brother Vasubandhu (*fl.* 350–430) commented on it.[56] As we shall see below, Patañjali was familiar enough with Vasubandhu's writing to cite them directly. This almost final level of attainment of Patañjali's yogi is the final level of attainment for the Buddhist meditator described in the *Daśabhūmikasūtra:*

> Thus it is said [of the enlightened Bodhisattva] that he is consecrated, has increased immeasurable merits and varieties of knowledge, and has abided in the Bodhisattva-stage called Cloud of Doctrine [*dharma-megha*]. ... Again, O son of the Conqueror, a Bodhisattva who abides in the Bodhisattva-stage (called) Cloud of Doctrine and holds the power of his own vow, raises up the cloud of great compassion and sympathy, the roar of splendor of great doctrine, ... and he tranquilizes the dust-flames of all the passions arisen from the ignorance of living beings according to their intentions by pouring down the rain of nectar of great merit. Therefore this stage is called the Cloud of Doctrine [*dharma-megha*].[57]

With this Buddhist metaphor in mind, Patañjali's use of the word in his *sūtra* as the name of the penultimate state of yoga would have made perfect sense to his contemporaries, for whom the ancient story of the wise yogi cooling the earth with the rain of his *dharma* was still a vivid image of the generosity of the realised sage.

3. Patañjali's Use of *Vibhāṣā* Materials

At the beginning of this paper (p. 26f.), I noted that La Vallée Poussin drew attention to a parallel between Vasubandhu and the *Pātañjalayogaśāstra* as long ago as his publications of 1923–1926. I also noted that the meaning and even wording of PYŚ 4.1 is directly related to Vasubandhu's text. Exciting new research is bringing to light even more parallels between Patañjali and Vasubandhu.[58]

The philosopher Vasubandhu was an Indian Buddhist monk from Gandhāra who probably lived in the period 350–430 CE. He was born in Puruṣapura, modern Peshawar, and developed initially as a thinker in the Buddhist Sarvāstivāda tradition. We have an account of his life from the scholar Paramārtha, who lived a century after Vasubandhu, as well as from much later Tibetan and Chinese authors. Under the master Saṅghabhadra, Vasubandhu studied the Vaibhāṣika

56 *Mahāyānasūtrālaṅkāra* IX.5–6, XI.46, XX–XXI.38b (ed. Lévi 1907–1911: 1.34, 66, 183, trans. Thurman et al. 2004: 74f., 83, 332). Squarcini (2015: 158f., 189) provides references to this metaphor in the *Daśabhūmikasūtra* and many other Buddhist texts of Patañjali's general period. I am grateful to Philipp A. Maas for drawing my attention to these sources. On the dating for Asaṅga and Vasubandhu see footnote 10, above.

57 Rahder 1923: 86, 89–90, trans. Honda 1968: 269–270.

58 Maas 2014.

tradition of Kashmir that had developed in the centuries before his time as a tradition of commentaries on the Abhidharma, in particular the commentaries on the *Jñānaprasthānasūtra* of Kātyāyanīputra.[59] Vasubandhu later became the abbot of Nālanda, where he was the teacher of many famous pupils, including Diṅnāga.[60]

Vasubandhu composed a treatise on the Sarvāstivāda Abhidharma that brought together his understanding of the Vibhāṣā literature. Called the *Abhidharmakośabhāṣya*, it was structured as a series of verses with Vasubandhu's own commentary (*bhāṣya*). The Sanskrit original of the work was lost for centuries, and was known only through Chinese and Tibetan translations. The work was of such importance to the history of Indian thought that in the 1930s, the great scholar Rāhula Sāṅkṛtyāyana (1893–1963) even re-translated the verses into Sanskrit, from Tibetan, and wrote his own Sanskrit commentary on them. However, during a subsequent visit to Tibet, Sāṅkṛtyāyana discovered an ancient palm leaf manuscript of 367 leaves that had not only Vasubandhu's verses, but his lost commentary.[61]

AKBh 5.25 (Pradhan 1975)	**PYŚ 3.13 (Āgāśe 1904)**
1. dharmasya-adhvasu *pra*vartamānasya	dharmasya **dharmiṇi** vartamānasya_*eva*_adhvasv
2. bhāva-anyathātvaṃ bhavati	*atītānāgatavartamāneṣu* bhāva-anyathātvaṃ bhavati
3. na dravya-anyathātvam. yathā suvarṇa-	na *tu* dravyānyathātvam. yathā suvarṇa-
4. bhājanasya bhittvā_anyathā kriyamāṇasya	bhājanasya bhittvā_anyathā-kriyamāṇasya
5. **saṃsthāna**-anyathātvaṃ bhavati na varṇa-	**bhāva**-anyathātvaṃ bhavati na **su**varṇa-
6. anyathātvam	anyathātvam *iti.*

Table 1: Patañjali's and Vasubandhu's wording compared. Reproduced from Maas 2014, with kind thanks. (Roman = identical; **bold** = important changes of sense; *italic* = unimportant variations.)

In 1967 and then in a revised edition of 1975, Pradhan finally published the original Sanskrit text of the *Abhidharmakośabhāṣya*, Vasubandhu's great work summarizing earlier traditions of the Vibhāṣā school of Buddhist philosophy.

In the past, scholars had noted the general similarity of Patañjali's text, and even some of the ways in which he seemed to be responding to Vasubandhu's

59 Dutt 1988: 383ff.

60 Dutt 1988: 390.

61 Pradhan 1975: ix.

work.[62] But impressions were based only on Tibetan and Chinese sources. However, with the discovery and publication of the original Sanskrit text of Vasubandhu's work, it has become possible to compare Patañjali's and Vasubandhu's words textually, in the original Sanskrit. The results are startling, and are just beginning to be evaluated in detail by my colleague Philipp A. Maas.[63] As we see in Table 1, there are word-for-word correspondences between Patañjali's and Vasubandhu's texts. Although the wording is very close, in fact the point being made by Patañjali is subtly different from that made by Vasubandhu, and we can be sure, because of the direction of the history of thought, and the changes in language and formulation, that it is Patañjali who is reworking Vasubandhu's view, and not vice versa.[64]

Much of Vasubandhu's *Abhidharmakośabhāṣya* narrated, in the form of miniature dialogues, a debate or conference that took place during the early second century CE, that was allegedly convened by the Śaka king Kaniṣka (*fl.* c 120 CE). The names of the chief participants in this debate are preserved: Bhadanta Vasumitra, Bhadanta Dharmatrāta, Ghoṣaka and Buddhadeva.

This becomes relevant in relation to another passage in the *Pātañjalayogaśāstra*. This is a passage that has become famous amongst historians of science because it is one of the first passages in world history that clearly mentions the combination of decimal numbers and place-value notation.

Patañjali was explaining the difference between an entity in and of itself, and the change in its significance according to its relationship to another entity. As one example, he gave the case of a woman who is a single entity in herself, yet is spoken of as a mother, a daughter or a sister, depending on her relationships to others: "And similarly, although there is singularity, a woman is called a mother, a daughter, and a sister."[65]

This passage is a reworking of the viewpoint of the Sarvāstivāda monk Bhadanta Buddhadeva, as reported by Vasubandhu.[66] See Table 2.

AKBh 5.26 (Pradhan 1975)	**PYŚ 3.13 (Āgāśe 1904)**
yathaikā strī mātā vocyate duhitā *veti*	yathā *caikatve 'pi* strī mātā cocyate duhitā *ca svasā c*eti

Table 2: Patañjali's and Vasubandhu's wording compared. (Roman = identical; *italic* = unimportant variations.)

62 Woods 1914: xvii–xviii.

63 Maas 2014.

64 Maas (ibid.) develops these points and describes the philosophical innovations that Patañjali made.

65 PYŚ commentary on 3.13 (Āgāśe 1904: 130). Other translations include Prasāda 1910: 188–193; Bryant 2009: 320–324.

66 *Abhidharmakośa* 5.26 (Pradhan 1975: 297).

Patañjali's other example was place-value notation. He said, "Just as a single stroke is a hundred in the hundreds' position, ten in the tens' position and one in the ones' position."[67] This passage has been cited as the earliest unambiguous description of written place-value notation using digits, and Patañjali's version is datable to the period 375–425.[68]

But Patañjali was in fact reworking Buddhist arguments reported by Vasubandhu about how things in the world may evolve in some respects and yet stay the same in other respects. Vasumitra said, according to Vasubandhu: "Just as a single wick (*vartikā*) thrown down into the mark of one says 'one', and in the mark of hundreds says 'hundred', and in the mark of thousands says 'a thousand'."[69]

Vasubandhu's description may refer not to writing but to placing a strip or tube on a marked board, perhaps analogous to an abacus.[70] The word *vartikā* that he used means a wick, stalk, paint-brush, or twist of cloth. It is not clear what Vasumitra was describing.[71] Bhadanta Vasumitra, to whom Vasubandhu ascribed this particular passage, may perhaps be placed in the second century CE.[72]

Once again, we see the detailed influence of Buddhist discussions on the foundations of Patañjali's yoga system.

A recurring question for historians is why Buddhism disappeared from India. Numerous social, religious and economic arguments have been put forward as explanations. In the *Pātañjalayogaśāstra,* I believe we see a conscious absorption of Buddhist meditation and philosophy doctrines into an orthodox Brāhmaṇa framework. The work re-frames the ideas as being those of an ancient yoga sage called Kapila. Text-historical scholarship shows quite clearly in many cases that Patañjali's sources were Buddhist. Yet for centuries Yoga has been a socio-religious force in India divorced from the memory of the Buddhist world that surrounded Patañjali, and that he absorbed and transformed.

67 PYŚ commentary on 3.13 (Āgāśe 1904: 130): *yathaikā rekhā śatasthāne śataṃ daśasthāne daśaikā caikasthāne.*

68 Woods 1914: 216, n. 1; Maas 2006: 65–66; Plofker 2009: 46.

69 Vasubandhu, *Abhidharmakośabhāṣya* on 5.26 (Pradhan 1975: 296): *yathaikā vartikā ekāṅke nikṣiptā ekam ity ucyate śatāṅke śataṃ sahasrāṅke sahasram iti* | (trans. Pruden 1988–1990: 3, 809).

70 See also Plofker 2009: 46.

71 One of the sources referred to by Pradhan (1975: 296), possibly the commentator Yaśomitra, gives the variant *gulikā,* meaning "little ball, pill". This variant might suggest a counting stone.

72 Anacker 1984: 12.

4. Conclusions

The *sūtra*-s of the *Pātañjalayogaśāstra* seem to speak directly across the ages to us, if sometimes mysteriously. But this is a false impression. They are deeply embedded in history and culture of their time.

Some of Patañjali's *sūtra*-s cannot be properly understood without an awareness of the Buddhist background to Indian philosophical thought at the time they were composed.

It seems that some of the earliest Sanskrit commentators, including Vācaspati Miśra, misunderstood some of Patañjali's *sūtra*-s because they had lost an awareness of Buddhist thought.

Contemporary interpreters who limit themselves to the commentarial tradition of Brāhmaṇa householders and later ascetics, but do not look at the Buddhist sources, continue to be puzzled and misled by the *Pātañjalayogaśāstra*.

References

Āgāśe, K. Ś. (Ed.). (1904). *VācaspatimiśraviracitaṭīkāsaṃvalitaVyāsabhāṣyasametāni Pātañjalayogasūtrāṇi tathā BhojadevaviracitaRājamārtaṇḍābhidhavṛttisametāni Pātañjalayogasūtrāṇi.* Ānandāśramasaṃskṛtagranthāvaliḥ 47. Puṇyākhyapattana: Ānandāśramamudraṇālaya.

Anacker, St. (Ed., Trans.). (1984). *Seven Works of Vasubandhu, the Buddhist Psychological Doctor.* Religions of Asia Series 4. Delhi: Motilal Banarsidass.

Angot, M. (2008). *Pātañjalayogasūtram* [sic]: *Le Yoga-Sūtra de Patañjali. Le Yoga-Bhāṣya de Vyāsa. Vyāsabhāṣyasametam. Avec des extraits du Yoga-Vārttika de Vijñāna-Bhikṣu. Edition, traduction et présentation.* Collection Indika 1. Paris: Les Belles Lettres.

Apte, V. Sh. (1957–1959). *Revised and Enlarged Edition of V. S. Apte's The Practical Sanskrit-English Dictionary.* Ed. by P. K. Gode … and C. G. Karve … [et al.]. 3 vols. Poona: Prasad Prakashan (repr. Kyoto: Rinsen Book Company, 1992).

Bagchi, S. (Ed.). (1967). *Suvarṇaprabhāsasūtra.* Buddhist Sanskrit Texts 8. Darbhanga: The Mithila Institute.

Böhtlingk, O. & Roth, R. (1855–1875). *Sanskrit-Wörterbuch.* St. Petersburg: Kaiserliche Akademie der Wissenschaften.

Bordaş, L. (2011). Mircea Eliade as Scholar of Yoga: A Historical Study of his Reception (1936–1954). 1st Part. In I. Vainovski-Mihai (Ed.), *New Europe College Ştefan Odobleja Program Yearbook 2010–2011* (pp. 19–73). Bucharest: New Europe College.

Bordaş, L. (2012). Mircea Eliade as Scholar of Yoga: A Historical Study of his Reception (1936–1954). 2nd Part. *Historical Yearbook. Journal of the Nicolae Iorga History Institute, 9,* 177–195.

Bronkhorst, J. (1981). Meaning Entries in Pāṇini's Dhātupāṭha. *Journal of Indian Philosophy, 9*(4), 335–357.

Bryant, E. F. (2009). *The Yoga Sūtras of Patañjali: A New Edition, Translation, and Commentary with Insights from the Traditional Commentators.* New York: North Point Press.

Conze, E. (Ed.). (1974). *The Gilgit Manuscript of the Aṣṭādaśasāhasrikāprajñāpāramitā, Chapters 70 to 82, Corresponding to the 6th, 7th and 8th Abhisamayas.* Serie Orientale Roma 46. Roma History Institute. Cited from the e-text input by Klaus Wille (Göttingen, Germany) at http://gretil.sub.uni-goettingen.de/gretil/1_sanskr/4_rellit/buddh/adsp55-u.htm. Accessed 14 October 2017.

Cousins, L. S. (1992). Vitakka/vitarka and Vicāra: Stages of samādhi in Buddhism and Yoga. *Indo-Iranian Journal, 35*(2), 137–157.

Deleanu, F. (2006). *The Chapter on the Mundane Path (Laukikamārga) in the Śrāvakabhūmi: A Trilingual Edition (Sanskrit, Tibetan, Chinese), Annotated Translation and Introductory Study.* 2 vols. Tokyo: The International Institute for Buddhist Studies.

Ḍhuṇḍhirāja Śāstrī (Ed.). (2001). *Maharṣipravarapatañjalipraṇītaṃ Yogasūtram ... Bhojarājakṛtena Rājamārtaṇḍena Bhāvāgaṇeśaviracitena Pradīpena Nāgojībhaṭṭanirmitayā Vṛttyā ... Rāmānandavihitayā Maṇiprabhayā Vidvadvarānantadaivasampāditayā Candrikayā ... Sadāśivendrasarasvatīkṛtena Yogasudhākareṇa ca Samanvitam = Yogasūtram by Maharṣi Patañjali with Six Commentaries: 1. Rājamārtaṇḍa by Bhojarāja, 2. Pradīpikā by Bhāvā-Gaṇeśa, 3. Vṛtti by Nāgoji Bhaṭṭa, 4. Maṇiprabhā by Rāmānandayati, 5. Candrikā by Anantadeva, 6. Yogasudhākara by Sadāśivendra Sarasvatī.* 3rd ed. Kashi Sanskrit Series 83. Varanasi: Caukhambha Sanskrit Sansthan.

Dutt, N. (1966). *Bodhisattvabhūmi: Being the XVth Section of Asaṅgapāda's Yogācārabhūmi.* Patna: K. P. Jayaswal Research Institute.

Dutt, N. (1988). Buddhism. In R. C. Majumdar et al. (Eds.), *The History and Culture of the Indian People* (pp. 373–392). Vol. 3. 4th ed. Bombay: Bharatiya Vidya Bhavan.

Edgerton, F. (1953). *Buddhist Hybrid Sanskrit Grammar and Dictionary.* Vol. 2. *Dictionary.* William Dwight Whitney Linguistic Series. New Haven: Yale University Press.

Eliade, M. (1936). *Yoga: Essai sur les origines de la mystique indienne.* Paris and Bucureşti: P. Geuthner etc.

Eliade, M. (1970). *Yoga: Immortality and Freedom.* Translated from the French by W. R. Trask. 2nd ed. Princeton: Princeton University Press.

Endo, K. (2000). Prasaṃkhyāna in the Yogabhāṣya. In S. Mayeda et al. (Eds.), *The Way to Liberation: Indological Studies in Japan* (pp. 75–89). Japanese Studies on South Asia 3. Delhi: Manohar Publishers & Distributors.

Franco, E. (1987). *Perception, Knowledge and Disbelief: A Study of Jayarāśi's Scepticism.* Alt- und Neu-Indische Studien 35. Stuttgart: Franz Steiner Verlag (2nd ed. Delhi: Motilal Banarsidass, 1994).

Gombrich, R. F. (1974). Eliade on Buddhism. *Religious Studies, 10*(2), 225–231.

Gombrich, R. F. (1996). *How Buddhism Began: The Conditioned Genesis of the Early Teachings.* London: Athlone Press (repr. Abingdon: Routledge, 2006).

Guggenbühl, C. (2008). *Mircea Eliade and Surendranath Dasgupta: The History of their Encounter. Dasgupta's Life, his Philosophy and his Works on Yoga. A Comparative Analysis of Eliade's Chapter on Patañjali's Yogasūtra and Dasgupta's Yoga as Philosophy and Religion.* Heidelberg: Universität Heidelberg.

Halbfass, W. (1991). Śaṅkara, the Yoga of Patañjali, and the So-Called Yogasūtrabhāṣyavivaraṇa. In W. Halbfass, *Tradition and Reflection: Explorations in Indian Thought* (pp. 205–242). Albany, NY: SUNY Press.

Harimoto, K. (1999). *A Critical Edition of the Pātañjalayogaśāstravivaraṇa: First Pāda, Samādhipāda: With an Introduction.* Unpublished Doctoral Thesis. University of Pennsylvania.

Harimoto, K. (2014). *God, Reason, and Yoga: A Critical Edition and Translation of the Commentary Ascribed to Śaṅkara on Pātañjalayogaśāstra 1.23–28.* Indian and Tibetan Studies 1. Hamburg: Department of Indian and Tibetan Studies, Universität Hamburg.

Honda, M. (1968). Annotated Translation of the Daśabhūmikasūtra. In D. Sinor (Ed.), *Studies in South, East and Central Asia Presented As a Memorial Volume to Raghu Vira* (pp. 115–176). Śata-Piṭaka Series 74. New Delhi: International Academy of Indian Culture.

Jacobi, H. (1931). Über das Alter des Yogaśāstra. *Zeitschrift für Indologie und Iranistik, 8,* 80–88.

Jurewicz, J. (2000). Playing with Fire: The pratītyasamutpāda from the Perspective of Vedic Thought. *Journal of the Pali Text Society, 26,* 77–103.

Jurewicz, J. (2010). *Fire and Cognition in the Ṛgveda.* Warszawa: Dom Wydawniczy ELIPSA.

Keith, A. B. (1932). Some Problems of Indian Philosophy. *Indian Historical Quarterly, 8*(3), 426–441.

Kimura, T. (1934). On the Influence of Patañjali upon Yogasūtra [read Buddhism? D. W.] (Particularly on Sarvāstivādin). In Celebration Committee (Ed.), *Commemoration Volume: The Twenty-fifth Anniversary of the Foundation of the Professorship of Science of Religion in Tokyo Imperial University* (pp. 304–308). Tokyo: Herald Press.

Klostermaier, K. (1986). Dharmamegha samādhi: Comments on Yogasūtra IV.29. *Philosophy East and West, 36*(3), 253–262.

Kragh, U. T. (Ed.). (2013). *The Foundation for Yoga Practitioners. The Buddhist Yogācārabhūmi Treatise and Its Adaptation in India, East Asia, and Tibet.* Harvard Oriental Series 75. Cambridge, MA: Harvard University Press.

Krishnacharya, T. R. & Vyasacharya, T. R. (Eds.). (1906–1910). *Śrīmanmahābhāratam: Saṭippaṇam. A New Edition Mainly Based on the South Indian Texts. With Footnotes and Readings.* Bombay: Nirṇayasāgara Press.

Lanman, Ch. R. (1929). *Indian Studies: In Honor of Charles Rockwell Lanman.* Cambridge, MA: Harvard University Press.

Larson, G. J. (1989). An Old Problem Revisited: The Relation Between Sāṃkhya, Yoga and Buddhism. *Studien zur Indologie und Iranistik, 15,* 129–146.

Larson, G. J. & Bhattacharya, R. Sh. (2008). *Yoga: India's Philosophy of Meditation.* Encyclopedia of Indian Philosophies 12. Delhi: Motilal Banarsidass.

La Vallée Poussin, L., de (1923–1926). *L'Abhidharmakośa de Vasubandhu: traduit et annoté.* Paris & Louvain: Paul Geuthner & J.-B. Istas.

La Vallée Poussin, L., de (1937). Le Bouddhisme et le Yoga de Patanjali. *Melanges Chinois et Bouddhiques, 5,* 232–242.

Lévi, S. (1907–1911). *Mahāyāna-Sūtrālaṃkāra: Exposé de la Doctrine du Grand Véhicule selon le système Yogācāra édité et traduit d'après un manuscrit rapporté du Népal.* Paris: Librairie Honoré Champion.

Maas, Ph. A. (2006). *Samādhipāda: Das erste Kapitel des Pātañjalayogaśāstra zum ersten Mal kritisch ediert = The First Chapter of the Pātañjalayogaśāstra for the First Time Critically Edited.* Geisteskultur Indiens. Texte und Studien 9. Studia Indologica Universitatis Halensis. Aachen: Shaker.

Maas, Ph. A. (2013). A Concise Historiography of Classical Yoga Philosophy. In E. Franco (Ed.), *Periodization and Historiography of Indian Philosophy* (pp. 53–90). Publications of the De Nobili Research Library 37. Vienna: Verein "Sammlung de Nobili, Arbeitsgemeinschaft für Indologie und Religionsforschung".

Maas, Ph. A. (2014). Sarvāstivāda Abhidharma and the Yoga of Patañjali. Presentation held at the 17th Congress of the International Association of Buddhist Studies, Vienna on 23 August 2014. https://www.academia.edu/8098284/. Accessed 10 October 2017.

Maas, Ph. A. & Wujastyk, D. (in preparation). *The Original Āsanas of Yoga.*

Maharaj, A. (2013). Yogic Mindfulness: Hariharānanda Āraṇya's Quasi-Buddhistic Interpretation of Smṛti in Patañjali's Yogasūtra I.20. *Journal of Indian Philosophy, 41*(1), 57–78.

Maithrimurthi, M. (1999). *Wohlwollen, Mitleid, Freude und Gleichmut: Eine ideengeschichtliche Untersuchung der vier apramāṇas in der buddhistischen Ethik und Spiritualität von den Anfängen bis hin zum frühen Yogācāra.* Alt- und Neu-Indische Studien 50. Stuttgart: Franz Steiner Verlag.

Mani, V. (1975). *Purāṇic Encyclopaedia: A Comprehensive Dictionary with Special Reference to the Epic and Purāṇic Literature.* Delhi: Motilal Banarsidass. First published in Malayalam language (Kottayam, 1964).

Mayrhofer, M. (1986–2001). *Etymologisches Wörterbuch des Altindoarischen.* Heidelberg: Carl Winter.

Monier-Williams, M. (1899). *A Sanskrit–English Dictionary: Etymologically and Philologically Arranged with Special Reference to Cognate Indo-European Languages by Sir Monier Monier-Williams M.A., K.C.I.E. New Edition, Greatly Enlarged and Improved with the Collaboration of Professor E. Leumann, Ph.D., Professor C. Cappeller, Ph.D. and Other Scholars.* Oxford: Clarendon Press (repr. 1970).

Ñāṇamoḷi, Bhikkhu & Bodhi, Bhikkhu (1995). *The Middle Length Discourses of the Buddha: A New Translation of the Majjhima Nikaya.* Boston: Wisdom Publications.

Nārāyaṇamiśra (1971). *Pātañjalayogadarśanam. Vācaspatimiśraviracita-Tattvavaiśāradī-Vijñānabhikṣukṛta-Yogavārtikavibhūṣita-Vyāsabhāṣyasametam. ... Śrī-Nārāyaṇamiśreṇa ṭippaṇīpariśiṣṭādibhiḥ saha sampāditam.* Vārāṇasī: Bhāratīya Vidyā Prakāśan.

Pines, Sh. & Gelblum, T. (1983). Al-Bīrūnī's Arabic Version of Patañjali's Yogasūtra: A Translation of the Third Chapter and a Comparison with Related Texts. *Bulletin of the School of Oriental and African Studies, University of London, 46*(2), 258–304.

Plofker, K. (2009). *Mathematics in India.* Princeton and Oxford: Princeton University Press.

Pradhan, P. (1950). *Abhidharma Samuccaya of Asanga. Critically Edited and Studied.* Santiniketan: Visva-Bharati.

Pradhan, P. (1975). *Abhidharmakośabhāṣyam of Vasubandhu.* Ed. by Aruna Haldar. 2nd ed. Tibetan Sanskrit Works Series 8. Patna: K. P. Jayaswal Research Institute.

Prasāda, R. (1910). *Patanjali's Yoga Sutras With the Commentary of Vyâsa and the Gloss of Vâchaspati Miśra. Translated by Râma Prasâda [...] With an Introduction from Rai*

Bahadur Śrīśa Chandra Vasu. The Sacred Books of the Hindus 4. Allahabad: Pāṇini Office (repr. New Delhi: Munshiram Manoharlal, 1998).

Pruden, L. M. (1988–1990). *Abhidharmakośabhāṣyam of Vasubandhu: Translated into French by Louis de La Vallée Poussin. English Version.* 4 vols. Berkeley: Asian Humanities Press. [Tr. of La Vallée Poussin 1923–1926.]

PYŚ. *Pātañjalayogaśāstra*
for *pāda* 1, see Maas 2006.
for *pāda*-s 2–4, see Āgāśe 1904.

Rahder, J. (1923). *Daśabhūmikasūtra et Bodhisattvabhūmi: Chapitres Vihāra et Bhūmi.* Paris & Louvain: Paul Geuthner & J.-B. Istas.

Rahula, W. (2001). *Abhidharmasamuccaya: The Compendium of the Higher Teaching (Philosophy) by Asaṅga. Originally Translated into French and Annotated by Walpola Rahula. English Version from the French by Sara Boin-Webb.* Fremont, California: Asian Humanities Press. Original French edition: Paris: École française d'Extrême-Oriente, 1971.

Rama Sastri & Krishnamurthi Sastri, S. R. (Eds.). (1952). *Pātñjala[sic]-yogasūtra-bhāṣya Vivaraṇam of Śaṅkara-Bhagavatpāda: Critically Edited with Introduction.* Madras Government Oriental Series 94. Madras: Government Oriental Manuscripts Library.

Renou, L. (1940). On the Identity of the Two Patañjalis. In N. N. Law (Ed.), *Louis de La Vallée Poussin Memorial Volume* (pp. 368–373). Calcutta: J. C. Sarkhel.

Rhys Davids, Th. W. (1890–1894). *The Questions of King Milinda.* The Sacred Books of the East 35 & 36. Oxford: Clarendon Press.

Rhys Davids, Th. W. & Stede, W. (1921–1925). *The Pali Text Society's Pali–English Dictionary.* Vol. 7. London: The Pali Text Society.

Senart, É. (1900). Bouddhisme et Yoga. *Revue de l'histoire des religions, 42,* 345–363.

Skeat, W. W. (1897–1882). *An Etymological Dictionary of the English Language.* New Edition Revised and Enlarged. Impression of 1968. Oxford: Clarendon Press.

Sörensen, S. (1904–1925). *An Index to the Names in the Mahābhārata: With Short Explanations and a Concordance to the Bombay and Calcutta Editions and P. C. Roy's Translation.* London: Williams & Norgate.

Squarcini, F. (Trans.). (2015). *Yogasūtra.* Nuova Universale Einaudi, Nuova Serie 14. Torino: Einaudi.

Thanissaro Bhikkhu (2015). Ariyapariyesana Sutta: The Noble Search (MN 26). Translated from the Pali. In J. T. Bullitt (Ed.), *Access to Insight: Readings in Theravāda Buddhism.* http://www.accesstoinsight.org/tipitaka/mn/mn.026.than.html. Accessed 20 October 2017.

Thurman, R. A. F. et al. (Ed., Trans.). (2004). *The Universal Vehicle Discourse Literature (Mahāyānasūtrālaṃkāra) by Maitreyanātha/Āryāsaṅga Together with Its Commentary (Bhāṣya) by Vasubandhu.* Treasury of the Buddhist Sciences. New York, NY: American Institute of Buddhist Studies.

Trenckner, V. (Ed.). (1880). *The Milindapañho: Being Dialogues between King Milinda and the Buddhist Sage Nāgasena. The Pali Text.* London: Williams & Norgate.

Trenckner, V. & Chalmers, R. (1888–1925). *The Majjhima-nikāya.* 4 vols. Pali Text Society Text Series 60. London: H. Frowde.

Turner, R. L. (1966–85). *A Comparative Dictionary of the Indo-Aryan Languages.* 5 vols. *Indexes* compiled by D. R. Turner (London: Oxford University Press, 1969), *Phonetic*

Analysis by R. L. and D. R. Turner (London: Oxford University Press, 1971), and *Addenda and Corrigenda* edited by J. C. Wright (London: School of Oriental and African Studies, 1985). London: Oxford University Press.

Werba, Ch. H. (1997). *Verba Indoarica: Die primären und sekundären Wurzeln der Sanskrit-Sprache.* Vol. 1. Vienna: Austrian Academy of Sciences Press.

Willemen, Ch. et al. (1998). *Sarvāstivāda Buddhist Scholasticism.* Leiden: Brill.

Woods, J. H. (Trans). (1914). *The Yoga-system of Patañjali: Or, the Ancient Hindu Doctrine of Concentration of Mind Embracing the Mnemonic Rules, Called Yoga-sūtras, of Patañjali and the Comment, Called Yoga-bhāshya, Attributed to Veda-Vyāsa and the Explanation, Called Tattvaiçāradī, of Vāchaspatimiçra.* Harvard Oriental Series 17. Cambridge, MA: Harvard University Press.

Wujastyk, D. (2004). Agni and Soma: A Universal Classification. *Studia Asiatica: International Journal for Asian Studies 4–5,* 347–370.

Wujastyk, D. (2012). The Path to Liberation through Yogic Mindfulness in Early Ayurveda. In D. G. White (Ed.), *Yoga in Practice* (pp. 31–42). Princeton: Princeton University Press.

Wynne, A. (2007). *The Origin of Buddhist Meditation.* Routledge Critical Studies in Buddhism. London: Routledge.

Yamashita, K. (1994). *Pātañjala Yoga Philosophy with Reference to Buddhism.* Calcutta: KLM Firma.

Chapter 2

“*Sthirasukham Āsanam*”: Posture and Performance in Classical Yoga and Beyond

Philipp A. Maas

Contents

1. Introduction 51

2. Posture as an Ancillary of Yoga 54

3. Patañjali's Posture Passage 55
3.1. Grammatical Analyses of the Compound *Sthirasukha* 58
3.2. The List of Postures in *Pātañjalayogaśāstra* 2.46 60
3.2.1. Patañjali's Posture Passage in Transformation 61
3.2.2. The Lotus Posture (*Padmāsana*) 62
3.2.3. The Good Fortune Posture (*Bhadrāsana*) 64
3.2.4. The Hero Posture (*Vīrāsana*) 66
3.2.5. The Lucky Mark Posture (*Svastikāsana*) 68
3.2.6. The Staff Posture (*Daṇḍāsana*) 70
3.2.7. The One with Support (*Sopāśraya*) 71
3.2.8. The Couch Posture (*Paryaṅkāsana*) 72
3.2.9. Sitting Like a Crane, Sitting Like an Elephant, and Sitting Like a Camel (*Krauñcaniṣadana, Hastiniṣadana,* and *Uṣṭraniṣadana*) 75
3.2.10. The Even Configuration (*Samasaṃsthāna*) 76
3.2.11. Steady Relaxation (*Sthiraprasrabdhi*) 77
3.2.12. As is Comfortable (*Yathāsukha*) 79
3.2.13. Additional Postures 80
3.3. The Two Means to Achieve Postures 81
3.3.1. The Slackening of Effort 81
3.3.2. Merging Meditatively into Infinity, or Meditating on the One who Supports the Earth 83
3.4. The Result of Posture Performance 85

4. Conclusions 85

Appendices 87
General Introduction to the Critically Edited Text Passages in Appendices 1, 2 and 3 87
Abbreviations Used in the Critically Edited Text Passages 87

Appendix 1: A Critical Edition of Patañjali's Passage on Postures (PYŚ 2.46–48) 88

Appendix 2: A Critical Edition of the Posture Passage of the *Pātañjalayogaśāstravivaraṇa* (*Vivaraṇa* 2.46–48) 90

Appendix 3: A Critical Edition of the Posture Passage of the *Tattvavaiśāradī* (TVai 2.46–48) 93

References 94

Philipp A. Maas

Chapter 2: "*Sthirasukham Āsanam*": Posture and Performance in Classical Yoga and Beyond*

1. Introduction

The present chapter deals with yogic postures (*āsana*-s) in Pātañjala Yoga. Starting with a brief introduction to the main sources of the chapter, i. e., to the *Pātañjalayogaśāstra* (PYŚ) and its commentaries, it initially contextualises posture practice within the yogic path to liberation. This outline provides the backdrop for a detailed analysis of PYŚ 2.46–2.48, the most pertinent source of knowledge about yogic postures and their performance in classical Yoga. This passage is here presented for the first time in a translation of the critically edited text of this passage. The translation provides the basis for an in-depth analysis. By reading the two *sūtra*-s 2.46 and 2.47 according to Patañjali's authorial intention, namely as a single sentence, the chapter shows that being steady and comfortable (*sthirasukha*) is not, as previous scholars have suggested, a general characteristic of yogic postures right from the start and by themselves, but the result either of the meditative practices of merging meditatively into infinity or of a slackening of effort in practice that lead to a steady and comfortable posture performance. Next, the chapter addresses the list of posture names in the *Pātañjalayogaśāstra* from various perspectives. At first, the textual variation of each posture name is discussed. Then, the chapter compares the various descriptions of posture performance contained in the medieval commentaries on the *Pātañjalayogaśāstra* and in the authoritative treatise on yoga (i. e., "committed activity" from a Jaina perspective) by Hemacandra, the *Yogaśāstra*. This comparison shows that the relationship between the names of yogic postures and the descriptions of their performance is a heterogeneous one. Some explanations of posture names are vague or difficult to comprehend. In other cases, slightly different postures were (or came to be) known by identical names. In still other cases, different names

* Many thanks to Jason Birch for the useful suggestions he made in order to improve on an earlier draft version of the present chapter. I am especially grateful to Karin Preisendanz for her numerous and invaluable remarks that helped to improve the present chapter even further.

were applied to the same posture. And in further cases, identical names were used for identical postures throughout the history of yoga. All descriptions agree, however, in that the postures of classical Yoga are bodily static, i.e., seated, supine or kneeling postures. The common aim of posture performance in Yoga, which cannot be reduced to the bare performance of a certain bodily configuration but has to be regarded as a complex of psycho-physiological practices, is to enable the yogi to undertake long sessions of breath control and meditations by immunizing him against unpleasant sensations like that of heat and cold, or hunger and thirst.

As is well known, the *Pātañjalayogaśāstra* is the oldest preserved systematic Sanskrit work on Yoga coming from a Brāhmaṇa milieu. It was partly composed and partly compiled at some time between the years 325 and 425 CE,[1] i.e., in the so-called classical period of South Asian cultural, intellectual, and religious history, by an author–redactor named Patañjali. The Yoga of Patañjali was, according to an account preserved in the fifth-century chronicle entitled *Mahāvaṃsa,* a rival of Buddhism at about the end of the fourth century CE.[2]

Patañjali structured his work in four chapters of different length, each consisting of two, in most cases clearly distinguishable layers of text. In the printed editions, the first layer consists of either 195 or 196 brief nominal phrases,[3] the so-called *yogasūtra*-s (YS). Patañjali probably collected the *sūtra*-s, at least in part, from older textual materials in order to arrange them in a novel way and to integrate them into his work. The *sūtra*-s serve as brief summaries or headings for the second layer of text. This layer, the so-called *bhāṣya*-part of the *Pātañjalayogaśāstra,* consists of commentaries on and explanations of the *sūtra*-text, of polemical discussions of divergent philosophical views, and of supplementary expositions and citations in support of Patañjali's view from the works of pre-classical Sāṅkhya Yoga that are today mostly lost. Some of the supplementary

1 See Maas 2006: xix.

2 The *Mahāvaṃsa,* a chronicle the earlier part of which was composed in what is now Sri Lanka probably at the end of the fifth century (according to Hinüber 1997: § 185, p. 91), narrates that the famous Buddhist commentator and author Buddhaghosa was born as a Brāhmaṇa in present-day Bihar and that he was a follower of the philosophy of Patañjali before he converted to Buddhism and emigrated to Sri Lanka (Warren & Kosambi 1950: ix–xii). However, this reference to Buddhaghosa appears in the continuation of the *Māhāvaṃsa* called *Cūḷavaṃsa,* which is of a considerably later date. Henry Warren and Damodar Kosambi argued that this biographical information must be legendary, because Buddhaghosa's works neither reveal that their author was acquainted with the geography of North India, nor that he had a Brahmanical education, nor that he was familiar with Yoga philosophy and practice. Buddhaghosa "almost certainly was a Southerner" (Hinüber 1997: § 207, p. 102). In any case, it is remarkable that the *Mahāvaṃsa* refers to Patañjali's philosophy, the reception of which is otherwise largely unknown, as being a rival to Buddhism, even though the account itself occurs in a quite late part of the *Cūḷavaṃsa* that was composed in the thirteenth century on the basis of older materials.

3 On the history of the transmission of the *Pātañjalayogaśāstra,* see Maas 2010.

expositions digress far from the topics that the respective *sūtra*-s apparently address. In comparatively late primary sources as well as in secondary literature, the second layer of text is frequently depicted as a work in its own right, namely as a commentary called the *Yogabhāṣya,* that is attributed to the mythical author Vyāsa or Veda-Vyāsa.[4]

As I have repeatedly argued elsewhere,[5] the two layers of text of the *Pātañjalayogaśāstra,* i. e., its *sūtra*- and *bhāṣya*-passages, were probably partly compiled and partly composed as a unified whole by a single author-redactor. If this is accepted, the information of the *bhāṣya* can now be used as an authoritative source to interpret the otherwise frequently enigmatic *sūtra*-s in their original context. It is this approach that I shall apply in the present chapter, the results of which are partly based on ongoing research on the early history of yoga postures that I am conducting together with my friend and colleague Dominik Wujastyk.

For our joint research, we collected references to postures connected with yoga-type practices in comparatively early Buddhist, Jaina and Brahmanical literature. The most fascinating, difficult and comprehensive account of yogic postures we have yet worked on is, without doubt, the reference to posture in the second chapter of the *Pātañjalayogaśāstra* and its three commentaries. These commentaries are (1) the *Pātañjalayogaśāstravivaraṇa* (*Vivaraṇa*) composed by a certain Śaṅkara who may or may not be identical with the author of the *Brahmasūtrabhāṣya,*[6] (2) the *Tattvavaiśāradī* (TVai), also called *Yogasūtrabhāṣyavyākhyā,* by Vācaspatimiśra I, who most probably "flourished between A. D. 950 and 1000",[7] and (3) the *Yogavārttika* (YVā) by Vijñānabhikṣu, who presumably lived in the latter half of the sixteenth century.[8] Moreover, the present chapter takes into account the description of postures in the authoritative exposition on Yoga (*Yogaśāstra*) by the Jaina monk and scholar Hemacandra (1088/1089–1172/1173 CE).[9] The following main part of the chapter first analyses the account of postures in the *Pātañjalayogaśāstra* in various contexts and from various perspectives, before it turns to these sources of information on posture performance.

4 See Maas 2013: 57–68.
5 See Maas 2006: xii–xvii and 2013: 57–68.
6 See Halbfass 1991: 207.
7 Acharya 2006: xxviii.
8 See Larson & Bhattacharya 1987: 376.
9 On the date of Hemacandra, see Vogel 1979: 335f.

2. Posture as an Ancillary of Yoga

The *Pātañjalayogaśāstra* prescribes and describes a method for achieving liberation from suffering in the cycle of rebirths that addresses exclusively male Brāhmaṇas who have renounced familial and social obligations.[10] The aspirant, frequently designated with the Sanskrit term *yogin,* devotes himself to a lifestyle that restricts a number of basic human needs. Patañjali does not mention in any detail how exactly the yogi leads his life. It is, however, possible to draw a number of conclusions from scattered references throughout his work. Among these references, the passage of the *Pātañjalayogaśāstra* starting with YS 2.29 provides particularly important information. The *sūtra* by itself consists of a series of eight terms designating the so-called ancillaries of Yoga (*yogāṅga*): "The eight ancillaries are commitments, obligations, postures, breath control, withdrawing the senses, fixation, meditation and absorption."[11]

The Sanskrit term *aṅga,* which is here translated as "ancillary", primarily means "a limb of the body",[12] or, figuratively, "a constituent part".[13] In the context of the *Pātañjalayogaśāstra* as well as in other authoritative and scholarly expositions,[14] *aṅga* designates a means to be employed for success in yoga practice.[15] The term occurs not only in yoga literature but also very prominently in early Buddhist literature. There it is part of a compound designating the eight constituents of the early Buddhist way to liberation, the "noble eightfold path". Although the series of terms characterizing the ancillaries of Yoga shares only its final component "absorption" with its Buddhist equivalent, both series serve the same purpose in their respective religious systems: they sketch the aspirant's stairway to liberation.[16]

10 Patañjali uses the Sanskrit term *brāhmaṇa* at four places in his *Pātañjalayogaśāstra* in order to refer to a yogi. See PYŚ 2.30, 2.33, 3.51 and 4.29. For more details on yogis according to the *Pātañjalayogaśāstra,* see Maas 2014: 72–77.

11 YS p. 101, l. 7f.: *yamaniyamāsanaprāṇāyāmapratyāhāradhāraṇādhyānasamādhayo 'ṣṭāv aṅgāni.*

12 See MW p. 7, column 3, s. v. *aṅga.*

13 See Apte p. 23, column 2, s. v. *aṅga.*

14 In his discussion of the meaning of *aṅga* in the *Mṛgendratantra,* Alexis Sanderson (1995: Appendix 2, p. 31), refers to Bhojarāja's commentary on YS 2.29 and a possible influence of the ritual theory of Mīmāṃsā on Bhojarāja's conception of *aṅga* in discussing the meaning of *aṅga* in the *Mṛgendratantra.*

15 In PYŚ 2.29, Patañjali glosses the term *aṅga* in *sūtra* 2.29 with the word "means" (*sādhana*) (PYŚ, p. 99, l. 3f.): "In accordance with the degree to which the means are performed, impurity is diminished" (*yathā yathā ca sādhanāny anuṣṭhīyante tathā tathā tanutvam aśuddhir āpadyate*).

16 On the Buddhist eightfold path, see Eimer 2006: 17–30. The metaphor of a stairway to liberation is used by Śaṅkara, the author of the *Pātañjalayogaśāstravivaraṇa,* in his commentary on PYŚ 2.29 (*Vivaraṇa* p. 211, l. 22f.): "The yogi who has applied himself to the commitments and obligations and is [thus] eligible [for practising yoga] through keeping commitments and

Keeping the commitments of non-violence (*ahiṃsā*), speaking the truth (*satya*), not stealing (*asteya*), chastity (*brahmacārya*), and not possessing property (*aparigraha*) is the condition for taking up the five obligations, i. e., (1) purity (*śauca*), (2) satisfaction with the personal living conditions (*saṃtoṣa*), (3) asceticism (*tapas*), (4) studying for oneself (*svādhyāya*), and (5) dedication to God (*īśvarapraṇidhāna*).[17]

According to Patañjali's explanations in PYŚ 2.30, non-violence (*ahiṃsā*) is the central conception of yogic ethics as a whole. It is the condition and the aim of all other commitments and obligations.[18]

In the further course of practice, the yogi complements the honouring of commitments and obligations step by step with the practice of further ancillaries that take him gradually to different kinds of mental training and meditation, and finally to absorption. In the ultimate stage of absorption, the yogi gains the liberating insight into the ontological difference between the Subject and Matter.

The way to liberation is a stairway on which each step brings the aspirant closer to his goal. Therefore the practice of ancillaries of yoga does not constitute a religious aim in its own right. The role and meaning of each ancillary in classical Yoga is determined by its potential to promote the yogi's spiritual progress towards liberation.

3. Patañjali's Posture Passage

With these general considerations in mind, it is now possible to turn to the passage of the *Pātañjalayogaśāstra* dealing explicitly with the practice of postures. This passage, which runs from PYŚ 2.46 to PYŚ 2.48, reads as follows:[19]

obligations attains the practice of each of the subsequent [ancillaries] after having attained a firm foothold in each of the preceding ancillaries starting with posture. For one cannot climb the following step without having climbed the first" (*yamaniyamayuktasyādhikṛtasya yogina āsanādyaṅgānāṃ pūrvapūrve sthirapadaprāptasyottarottarānuṣṭhānaṃ prāptam. na hi prathamaṃ sopānam anāruhyottaram ārodhuṃ śakyam*).

17 See YS 2.32 (p. 104, l. 12f.): *śaucasaṃtoṣatapaḥsvādhyāyeśvarapraṇidhānāni niyamāḥ*.

18 See PYŚ 2.30 (p. 102, ll. 5–10): "And the subsequent commitments and obligations, being rooted in non-violence, are taught here as being conducive to the perfection of non-violence in order to teach non-violence. They are employed only to produce a pure form of non-violence. And thus it has been authoritatively stated: 'Depending on the degree this Brāhmaṇa here wants to keep the vows, which are many, he produces non-violence in its pure form, inasmuch as he desists from the causes of violence produced out of carelessness'" (*uttare ca yamaniyamās tanmūlās tatsiddhiparatayaiva tatpratipādanāya pratipādyante. tadavadātarūpakaraṇāyaivopādīyante. tathā coktam: "sa khalv ayaṃ brāhmaṇo yathā yathā vratāni bahūni samāditsate tathā tathā pramādakṛtebhyo hiṃsānidānebhyo nivartamānas tām evāvadātarūpām ahiṃsāṃ karoti," iti*).

19 For the critically edited Sanskrit text of this passage, see Appendix 1 below.

> The commitments and obligations have already been explained [previously] together with the supernatural powers [that they generate]. Now I shall explain [the ancillaries] posture and so on. Of these, *a steady and comfortable posture* (YS 2.46) – as there are the Lotus Posture, the Good Fortune Posture, the Hero Posture, the Lucky Mark Posture, the Staff Posture, the One with Support, the Couch Posture, Sitting Like a Sarus Crane (?),[20] Sitting Like an Elephant, Sitting Like a Camel, the Even Pose, Constant Relaxation, and As is Comfortable, and so on like this – *either from the slackening of effort or from merging meditatively into infinity* (YS 2.47). "Arises" has to be supplied in this sentence. Either the posture is achieved because effort stops, so that the body does not tremble. Alternatively, the mind, merging meditatively into infinity, brings about the posture. *Because of that, one is not afflicted by the pairs of unpleasant sensations* (YS 2.48). Because one masters the postures, one is not overcome by the pairs of unpleasant sensations such as cold and heat.

The Sanskrit original of this passage contains (as YS 2.46) the famous phrase *sthirasukham āsanam* that is frequently cited in the literature of transnational postural yoga as a definition or characterisation of posture practice.[21] From the late nineteenth century up to the present date, modern translators tend, as the following more or less randomly chosen examples show, to render this phrase into English in similar ways:[22]

a) Posture (is that which is) firm and pleasant (Mitra 1883: 102)
b) Posture is steadily easy (Prasāda 1910: 169)
c) Stable-and-easy posture (Woods 1914: 191)
d) Posture is steady and comfortable (Rukmani 1983: 217)
e) Posture is to be firm and pleasant (Leggett 1990: 273)
f) A posture [as a constituent of yoga] is that which is steady and easeful (Veda Bharati 2004: 568)
g) L'assiette est qui est stable et confortable (Filliozat 2005: 229)
h) Posture should be comfortably steady (Larson 2008: 172)
i) Posture should be steady and comfortable (Bryant 2009: 283)
j) Postures (*asana*) should be firm but easy (comfortable) (Phillips 2009: 215).

The only translator who did not read the *sūtra* as a definition or characterisation of posture was James H. Woods (translation c above), who provided a virtually

20 On the problem of identifying the bird called *krauñca*, see below, p. 75.

21 A search on Google at http://google.com/ for the phrase "sthira sukham asanam" on 16 November 2017 yielded 65,300 results.

22 To the best of my knowledge, the only English translation of *sūtra*-s 2.46 and 2.47 as a syntactical unit was published in Mallinson & Singleton 2017: 97–99. This translation may be based on the explanation of the two *sūtra*-s that I first suggested in Vienna during my presentation at the conference "Yoga in Transformation: Historical and Contemporary Perspectives on a Global Phenomenon" on 19 September 2013, which James Mallinson and Mark Singleton were kind enough to attend.

unintelligible rendering that simply consists of a collocation of two English words. All other scholars understood YS 2.46 as a complete sentence that defines what a posture is (translations a, b, d, f, and g), or how a posture should be (translations e, h, i, and j). None of the above cited translators took into account that YS 2.46 actually is just the initial part of a sentence that extends - over a parenthesis in the *bhāṣya*-part of the *Pātañjalayogaśāstra* – into the following YS 2.47. This is quite surprising, because the fact that the two *sūtra*-s 2.46 and 2.47 form a single sentence is clearly expressed at the beginning of the *bhāṣya*-part of PYŚ 2.47, in which Patañjali remarks that the verbal form "'arises' (*bhavati*) has to be supplied in this sentence."[23]

Regardless of the exact meaning of the word *sthirasukham*, the two *sūtra*-s may be translated together with their supplement from the *bhāṣya* as follows: "A *sthirasukha* posture (*sūtra* 2.46) [...] from the slackening of effort or from merging meditatively into infinity (*sūtra* 2.47)." "Arises" has to be supplied in this sentence.[24]

The interpretation of the two *sūtra*-s 2.46 and 2.47 as a single sentence is in accord with the explanation presented in the following *bhāṣya*-passage of PYŚ 2.47:

> Either a posture is achieved because effort stops, whereby trembling of the body does not happen, or the mind, having merged meditatively into infinity, brings about the posture.[25]

Here Patañjali presents a commentarial paraphrase of the preceding *sūtra* 2.47 ("either from the slackening of effort or from merging meditatively into infinity", *prayatnaśaithilyānantyasamāpattibhyām*), as can be inferred from the fact that he explicitly mentions both the stopping of effort and the meditative merging into infinity as alternative causes for establishing a yogic posture. The use of the ablative case in the paraphrase of the first part of the compound indicates that Patañjali intended the ambiguous dual ending *-ābhyām* to express the ablative case with a causal meaning. Moreover, the formulations "a posture is achieved" (*āsanaṃ sidhyati*) and "brings about a posture" (*āsanaṃ nirvartayati*) may be read as auto-comments on the supplied verb form "arises" (*bhavati*) that clarify how the two mentioned practices result in a *sthirasukha* posture.

If YS 2.46 is read together with the following *sūtra* 2.47 as a single sentence, the meaning of the phrase *sthirasukham āsanam* differs from the meaning assumed in all the translations cited above. Since *sthirasukham āsanam* is not a complete

23 PYŚ 2.46, l. 6 in Appendix 1 below: *bhavati, iti vākyaśeṣaḥ*.

24 PYŚ 2.46–47, ll. 1–6 in Appendix 1 below: *sthirasukham āsanam* (YS 2.46) [...] *prayatnaśaithilyānantyasamāpattibhyām* (YS 2.47) *bhavati, iti vākyaśeṣaḥ*.

25 PYŚ 2.47, l. 6f. in Appendix 1 below: *prayatnoparamād vā sidhyaty āsanam, yena nāṅgamejayo bhavati. ānantye vā samāpannaṃ cittam āsanaṃ nirvartayati, iti*.

nominal sentence, the phrase can neither describe nor prescribe posture practice in general. The phrase is just the initial part of a sentence stating that a *sthirasukha* posture results from either of two alternative activities, i. e., from "slackening of effort" or from "merging meditatively into infinity". But what exactly is a *sthirasukha* posture?

3.1. Grammatical Analyses of the Compound *Sthirasukha*

The compound *sthirasukha* consists of the two nominal stems *sthira-* and *sukha-*. The first one is evidently an adjective with the lexical meanings, among others, "firm, not wavering or tottering, steady", and "durable, lasting, permanent, changeless".[26] The second stem, *sukha-*, may either be a noun meaning "ease, easiness, comfort, prosperity, pleasure, joy, delight in" or an adjective. In the latter case, the word means "pleasant, agreeable", or "comfortable, happy, prosperous".[27] Since all three commentators of the *Pātañjalayogaśāstra* interpret *sukha-* as an adjective, following them in this regard appears appropriate.

Vācaspati analysed the compound *sthirasukha* in his gloss of YS 2.46, where he interprets the compound to mean "steadily comfortable": "The meaning of the *sūtra* [i. e., YS 2.46] is that posture is steadily, i. e., unwaveringly, comfortable, i. e., comfort-producing."[28]

This is an interpretation of the compound as a descriptive determinative compound (*karmadhāraya*) in which the first adjective is used to qualify the second one adverbially. This interpretation corresponds to the two translations by Rāma Prasāda and Gerald Larson (translations b and h cited above). Most of the remaining translations are based on an analysis of *sthirasukha* as a *karmadhāraya* in which the meaning of the second word stem stands in apposition to the meaning of the first stem. This interpretation may have led to the translations of *sthirasukha* as "firm and pleasant" by Rajendralal Mitra, "steady and comfortable" by T. S. Rukmani, "firm and pleasant" by Trevor Leggett, "steady and easeful" by Veda Bharati, "stable et confortable" by Jean Filliozat, "steady and comfortable" by Edwin Bryant, and finally also to Steven Phillips's translation "firm but easy".

The interpretation accepted by the majority of modern translators matches the interpretation in the oldest and most informative commentary of the *Pātañjalayogaśāstra,* the afore-mentioned *Pātañjalayogaśāstravivaraṇa*. Śaṅkara

26 MW p. 1264, column 3, s. v. *sthira.*
27 MW p. 1220, column 3f., s. v. *sukha.*
28 TVai on PYŚ 2.46, l. 2f. as critically edited in Appendix 3 below: *sthiraṃ niścalaṃ yat sukhaṃ sukhāvahaṃ, tad āsanam iti sūtrārthaḥ.*

apparently took the compound *sthirasukha* to mean "steady and [yet] comfortable" when he glossed it in the following way: "One should practice that posture which produces for the person who assumes it steadiness of mind and limbs, *and* which does not result in distress."[29]

Bhojarāja, whose *Rājamārtaṇḍa* is the oldest known commentary on only the *sūtra*-part of the *Pātañjalayogaśāstra* (composed in the first half of the eleventh century CE),[30] also analysed the compound in a similar way: "So, when it (i. e., the posture) becomes steady, i. e., not trembling, *and* comfortable, i. e., not causing distress, then it counts as one of the ancillaries of yoga."[31]

Also Vijñānabhikṣu, the sixteenth-century commentator of the *Pātañjalayogaśāstra,* provided a similar interpretation of the compound *sthirasukha,* when he explained YS 2.46 as "Posture is what is steady, i. e., unwavering, *and* comfort-producing."[32]

Besides the two possible interpretations of *sthirasukha* discussed so far, there is a third one that apparently led Woods to translating YS 2.46 simply as "Stable-and-easy posture." This translation is based on Woods' analysis of the parenthesis consisting of a list of thirteen posture names that separates YS 2.46 from YS 2.47 in the *Pātañjalayogaśāstra.*[33] In the version of the *Pātañjalayogaśāstra* that was available to Woods in manuscripts and printed editions, the list contains the word *sthirasukham* in the penultimate position. The same is true for the list as it appears in the version of the *Tattvavaiśāradī* that was known to this famous translator of the *Pātañjalayogaśāstra,* which contains the word *sthirasukham* in the penultimate position. Woods understood this as a nominalised adjective and translated it accordingly with "the stable-and-easy".[34] For his interpretation of the compound *sthirasukham* in YS 2.46, Woods relied upon the commentary of Vācaspati, who, according to Woods' translation, stated that "[t]his is the one form among these [postures] which is approved by the Exalted Author of the sūtras."[35] For Woods, the compound is not an adjective specifying the word "posture" (*āsana*), but a noun in apposition to "posture".

However, as I shall argue in more detail below (see p. 77ff.), the reading *sthirasukham* in the list of postures is a secondary variant in the *Pātañjalayogaśāstra* as well as in the text of Vācaspati's commentary. This reading intruded into the two

29 *Vivaraṇa* on PYŚ 2.46, l. 2–4 as critically edited in Appendix 2 below: *yasminn āsane sthitasya manogātrāṇām upajāyate sthiratvam, duḥkhaṃ ca yena na bhavati, tad abhyasyet.*

30 On the date of Bhoja, see Pingree 1981: 336.

31 RM p. 28, l. 26f.: *tad yadā sthiraṃ niṣkampaṃ sukham anudvejanīyaṃ ca bhavati tadā yogāṅgatāṃ bhajate.*

32 YVā on PYŚ 2.46, p. 261, l. 29: *sthiraṃ niścalaṃ sukhakaraṃ ca yat tad āsanam.*

33 On this list, see below, section 3.2.

34 Woods 1914: 191.

35 Woods 1914: 192.

works in the course of their respective transmissions when it replaced the original expression "Steady" or "Permanent Relaxation" (*sthira-* or *sthitaprasrabdhi*). Therefore, *sthirasukha* of YS 2.46 cannot be the name of a specific posture or even that of the posture *par excellence.* The word is an adjective specifying "posture". However, it cannot be decided with certainty whether it is an determinative adjective compound in which the first member specifies the second one adverbially, as Vācaspati suggested, or whether the relationship of the two members of the compound is appositional, as it was understood by Śaṅkara in his *Pātañjalayogaśāstravivaraṇa,* i. e., in the oldest and most informative commentary of the *Pātañjalayogaśāstra,* and in Bhojarāja's and Vijñānabhikṣu's commentaries. Nevertheless, in view of the general superiority of the *Pātañjalayogaśāstravivaraṇa* over the *Tattvavaiśāradī,* I would tend to accept the second mentioned analysis of *sthirasukha* at least provisionally. In this case, the two *sūtra*-s 2.46 and 2.47 can be translated in the following way: "A steady and comfortable posture (YS 2.46) [arises] from a slackening of effort or from merging meditatively into infinity (YS 2.47)."

3.2. The List of Postures in *Pātañjalayogaśāstra* 2.46

In between the two *sūtra*-s 2.46 and 2.47, all known versions of the *Pātañjalayogaśāstra* transmit a list of posture names, which in a translation based on the critically edited Sanskrit text reads as follows:

– as there are
(1) the Lotus Posture (*padmāsana*),
(2) the Good Fortune Posture (*bhadrāsana*),
(3) the Hero Posture (*vīrāsana*),
(4) the Lucky Mark Posture (*svastikāsana*),
(5) the Staff Posture (*daṇḍāsana*),
(6) the One with Support (*sopāśraya*),
(7) the Couch Posture (*paryaṅkāsana*),
(8) Sitting Like a Sarus Crane (*krauñcaniṣadana*),
(9) Sitting Like an Elephant (*hastiniṣadana*),
(10) Sitting Like a Camel (*uṣṭraniṣadana*),
(11) the Even Configuration (*samasaṃsthāna*),
(12) Steady Relaxation (*sthiraprasrabdhi*), and
(13) As is Comfortable (*yathāsukha*),
and so on like this –[36]

36 PYŚ 2.46, ll. 2–5 in Appendix 1 below: – *tad yathā: padmāsanaṃ bhadrāsanaṃ vīrāsanaṃ*

This list interrupts the syntactical unit of the sentence extending over the two *sūtra*-s 2.46 and 2.47. The highly unusual and even confusing position of the list may raise doubt on whether it actually was part of Patañjali's original composition or whether it was interpolated in the course of transmission of the *Pātañjalayogaśāstra.* However, since all known textual witnesses transmit this list in this or that form, the list as such definitely belongs to the oldest reconstructable version of the *Pātañjalayogaśāstra.* The assumption that the list of posture names is derived from a scribal gloss that was copied into the common source of all presently known versions of the *Pātañjalayogaśāstra* would therefore be highly speculative. Nevertheless, the unusual position of this list in the middle of a sentence is remarkable and leads quite naturally to the question of why Patañjali expressed himself in a way that obscured the fact that *sūtra*-s 2.46 and 2.47 belong together syntactically. For the time being, I cannot provide a satisfactory answer to this question. In any case, the lack of further information on the different postures in the *Pātañjalayogaśāstra* itself may be taken as a further indication of the secondary nature of the list.

3.2.1. Patañjali's Posture Passage in Transformation

In order to discuss the reconstruction of the archetypal version of the above cited passage of the *Pātañjalayogaśāstra,* i. e., of the earliest reconstructable version of this text that most probably was the common ancestor of all other extant versions, I have to refer to the results of my previous research into the history of the transmission of the first chapter of the *Pātañjalayogaśāstra.*[37] At some time after the composition of the *Pātañjalayogaśāstra* around the fourth century and before the year 950 CE, the transmission of Patañjali's work split into two branches. In the northern part of South Asia, the *Pātañjalayogaśāstra* developed apparently along one of these branches into a version that may be called the "vulgate", because this version gained the status of a normative recension and exerted a strong contaminating influence on many other versions. It is the vulgate version that we find with some variation in virtually all printed editions of the *Pātañjalayogaśāstra.*[38] Moreover, the vulgate is also transmitted in all paper manuscripts from the northern part of India. Among the witnesses used in the present chapter, the printed edition of the *Pātañjalayogaśāstra,*[39] the manu-

---

svastikāsanaṃ daṇḍāsanaṃ sopāśrayaṃ paryaṅkāsanaṃ krauñcaniṣadanaṃ hastiniṣadanam uṣṭraniṣadanaṃ samasaṃsthānaṃ sthiraprasrabdhir yathāsukhaṃ cety evamādi –.

37 See Maas 2006: lxviii–lxxiv and 165–170, 2008: 100–105 and 2010.

38 On the transmission of the *Pātañjalayogaśāstra* in printed editions, see Maas 2006: xxxii–xxxiv.

39 Āgāśe 1904, siglum P^E in the apparatus of the critically edited text in Appendix 1 below.

scripts with the sigla B^{n1}, B^{n2}, $B^{ś}$, Jai^{n}, K^{b}, K^{n1}, K^{n2} and P^{n},[40] and the version of the *Pātañjalayogaśāstra* that Vācaspati commented upon, as far as it can be reconstructed from his commentary, are descendants of the earliest hypothetical exemplar of the vulgate version, i.e., hyparchetype α in the stemma of the *Pātañjalayogaśāstra.*[41] The remaining witnesses, i.e., the manuscripts A^{d}, M^{g2}, My^{t3}, Pc^{g} and T^{m}, and the reconstructed text commented upon in the *Pātañjalayogaśāstravivaraṇa*, are descendants of hyparchetype β, which was the starting point for the transmission along the second main branch. However, all descendants of hyparchetype β were to different degrees exposed to contamination from the vulgate. The frequent occurrence of contamination within the transmission history has consequences not only for the degree of certainty to which hyparchetype β can be reconstructed, it also makes the reconstruction of the earliest hypothetical ancestor, the archetype, at many instances difficult, i.e., uncertain.

3.2.2. The Lotus Posture (*Padmāsana*)

The manuscripts and printed edition used for the critical edition of the posture passage of the *Pātañjalayogaśāstra* transmit the name "Lotus Posture" without any substantial textual variation.

The *Pātañjalayogaśāstra* does not contain any account of how the postures that it lists are to be practised. Therefore it is necessary to turn to the commentaries and other sources in order to find information on comparatively early yogic posture practice. Probably the oldest surviving detailed account of the postures listed in the *Pātañjalayogaśāstra* is provided in the *Pātañjalayogaśāstravivaraṇa*. Śaṅkara describes the Lotus Posture in the following manner:

> In this context, the Lotus Posture is like this: drawing the left leg in towards oneself, one should then place it over the right. Likewise the right one on top of the left. And stiffening the hips, trunk and neck, with the gaze fixed on the tip of the nose,[42] like a dead or sleeping person, with the cavity of the lips (*oṣṭhasaṃpuṭa*) closed like a covered box (*samudgakavat*), not touching the top of the teeth with the teeth,[43] one's chin and chest separated by a space the measure of a fist, with the tip of the tongue placed on the interior of the front teeth, with the hands on top of one's heels, one makes either the Tortoise or Brahmāñjali gesture. The posture in which one is seated, after having once

40 For all manuscript sigla, see the sigla table in Appendix 1 below.

41 See Maas 2006: lxxiii.

42 Cf. *Bhagavadgītā* 6.13: "Holding his straight trunk, head and neck motionless, being firm, beholding the tip of his own nose and not looking around" (*samaṃ kāyaśirogrīvaṃ dhārayann acalaṃ sthiraḥ | saṃprekṣya nāsikāgraṃ svaṃ diśaś cānavalokayan || 13 ||*).

43 Cf. *Liṅgapurāṇa* 1.8.89b: "He should not touch his teeth with his teeth" (*dantair dantān na saṃspṛśet |*).

> established a configuration in this manner, having completely given up repeated effort at a particular adjustment of the limbs of the body,[44] is the Lotus Posture. And all this is the same for the other postures too. There is just a little variation.[45]

This passage describes virtually the whole body in the performance of the Lotus Posture. The legs are placed crosswise with each foot on top of the opposite thigh. The spine is erect, and the chin turned slightly towards the chest and separated from it by the space of one fist. In this way, the back of the head forms almost a straight line with the neck and the spine. The hands, which are placed on top of the heels near the navel, are folded in one of two special gestures called the Tortoise (*kacchapaka*) and Brahmāñjali gesture. It is not entirely clear to exactly which hand gesture Śaṅkara referred as the "Tortoise", because early descriptions of this gesture are rare.[46] In order to perform this gesture, the hands are obviously arranged as to resemble a tortoiseshell. Karel van Kooij cautiously suggested a connection between a Tortoise Gesture and the meditative practice of withdrawing the senses from their objects (*pratyāhāra*), for which in Upaniṣadic literature the tortoise contracting its head serves as a metaphor.[47] The second gesture to which Śaṅkara refers, the Brahmāñjali Gesture, is more commonly referred to in Sanskrit literature. In this gesture, the hands are apparently clasped.[48]

In contradistinction to the detailed account of the *Pātañjalayogaśāstravivaraṇa,* Vācaspati's comment on the name "Lotus Posture" is quite vacuous. Ac-

---

44 Here Śaṅkara refers to YS 2.47, according to which the "slackening of effort" is one of the means for a successful yogic posture practice. On the slackening of effort in yogic posture performance, see below, section 3.3.1.

45 *Vivaraṇa* on PYŚ 2.46, ll. 10–17 in Appendix 2 below: *tatra padmāsanaṃ nāma - savyaṃ pādam upasaṃhṛtya dakṣiṇopari nidadhīta, tathaiva dakṣiṇaṃ savyasyopariṣṭāt. kaṭyurogrīvaṃ ca viṣṭabhya mṛtasuptavan nāsikāgranihitadṛṣṭiḥ, samudgakavad apihitoṣṭhasaṃpuṭaḥ, dantair dantāgram aparāmṛśan, muṣṭimātrāntaraviprakṛṣṭacibukoraḥsthalaḥ rājadantāntaranihitarasanāgraḥ, hastau ca pārṣṇyor upari kacchapakaṃ brahmāñjaliṃ vā kṛtvā, sakṛdāsthāpitetthaṃsaṃsthānaḥ, punaḥpunaḥśarīrāvayavavinyāsaviśeṣaparityaktaprayatnaḥ san, yenāsīta, tat padmāsanam. etac ca sarvam anyeṣām āsanānām api tulyam. kaścid eva viśeṣaḥ.*

46 The oldest references to a hand gesture called *kacchapaka* appear, as far as I know, in Pali literature where the word "Hand Tortoise" (*hatthakacchapaka*) was used to designate a gesture of greeting. Cf. Rhys Davids & Stede 1921–1923: 728a, s. v. Hattha.

47 Kooij 1972: 14, n. 2.

48 Jan Gonda referred to the Brahmāñjali gesture as follows: "According to Manu 2, 71 the student must study while joining his hands; 'that is called *b[rahmāñjali]*.', hence translations such as 'joining the hands while repeating the Veda (= *brahma*)' or '... in token of homage of the Veda' (Monier-Williams). Kullūka however explained: 'One should study with hands closed and clasped' and Āpastamba in the Saṃskāraprakāśa p. 524: 'The left hand should be turned upwards, the right hand placed on it with the palm downwards and the fingers of both hands should firmly hold their backs'. This gesture is prescribed to a person who discharges his daily obligation, viz. recitation of the Veda (*brahmayajña*), VaiG. 1, 4; cf. 2, 13; ĀśvG. 3, 5, 11" (1980: 67 f.). The Brahmāñjali gesture is depicted in Bühnemann 1988: Appendix, plate 8.

cording to him, this posture is so widely known that the name does not require any explanation at all.[49]

It appears, however, that in the course of time, or in different geographical regions of pre-modern South Asia, various forms of the Lotus Posture came to be known. Vijñānabhikṣu described a way to perform the Lotus Posture that differs to some degree from the exposition in the *Pātañjalayogaśāstravivaraṇa*. In commenting on the word *padmāsana*, he cites the *Vasiṣṭhasaṃhitā* (VS), an early Haṭha Yoga text, which according to Jason Birch (2011: 528) dates to the twelfth or thirteenth century, in the following way:

> Oh Lord of Brahmans, one should place the soles of the feet on top of the thighs, and then hold on to one's big toes crosswise with one's hands.[50] That is the Lotus Posture which is respected by all.[51]

A third variety of the Lotus Posture occurs in the *Yogaśāstra* (YŚ) of the Jaina monk and scholar Hemacandra, who described this posture as follows:

> Now the Lotus Posture. Those who are versed in postures have declared that the Lotus Posture is the posture in which there is contact of one lower leg with the other one at its middle part. [Commentary:] The posture in which there is contact of the left or the right lower leg with the other lower leg at its middle part is the Lotus Posture.[52]

For Hemacandra, the main characteristic of the Lotus Posture is that the legs are crossed at the middle part of the lower legs. He leaves all further details open, so that the feet possibly do not rest on the opposite thighs. If this should be the case, the Jaina author knew a pose by the name Lotus Posture that differs from the one that Śaṅkara described. As I shall show below, for Hemacandra the posture that Śaṅkara called "Lotus Posture" was probably the "Hero Posture".[53]

3.2.3. The Good Fortune Posture (*Bhadrāsana*)

The transmission of the two names "Good Fortune Posture" and "Hero Posture" in Patañjali's list of postures is quite variegated. The Good Fortune Posture is missing from the list in manuscript B^{n2}, whereas the South Indian manuscripts

49 Vācaspati simply remarks that "[t]he Lotus Posture (*padmāsana*) is well known" (*padmāsanaṃ prasiddham* [TVai on PYŚ 2.46, l. 3f. in Appendix 3 below]).

50 James Mallinson (personal communication, July 2015) suggested to me that the hands probably are meant to go behind the back before they take hold of the big toes.

51 YVā on PYŚ 2.46, p. 262, ll. 3–5 (= VS 1.71, p. 21): *aṅguṣṭhau sannibadhnīyād dhastābhyāṃ vyutkrameṇa tu | ūrvor upari viprendra kṛtvā pādatale ubhe || padmāsanaṃ bhaved etat sarveṣām eva pūjitam |*.

52 YŚ 4.129, p. 1066, ll. 2–4: *jaṅghāyā madhyabhāge tu saṃśleṣo yatra jaṅghayā | padmāsanam iti proktaṃ tad āsanavicakṣaṇaiḥ || 129 || jaṅghāyā vāmāyā dakṣiṇāyā vā dvitīyayā jaṅghayā madhyabhāge saṃśleṣo yatra tat padmāsanam.*

53 See section 3.2.4 below.

Pc^{g} and T^{m}, as well as Āgāśe's 1904 edition (which is based on eight manuscripts),[54] omit the name "Hero Posture" (*vīrāsana*). Moreover, for unknown reasons manuscripts B^{n1}, $B^{ś}$, Jai^{n} and P^{n} provide the names of the two postures in an inversed sequence. In spite of these variants, it is possible to establish the sequence (1) "Good Fortune Posture" and (2) "Hero Posture" (*bhadrāsanaṃ vīrāsanaṃ*) as the reading of the archetype, because it is exactly this sequence that four witnesses with text versions derived from hyparchetype β (i.e., manuscripts A^{d}, M^{g2} and My^{t3} and the basic text commented upon in the *Pātañjalayogaśāstravivaraṇa*) share with the quite old manuscript K^{b} and with the reconstruction of the basic text commented upon in the *Tattvavaiśāradī* according to manuscript J_{TV}, whose text versions developed from hyparchetype α.

Turning now to the different explanations of the posture called "Good Fortune Posture" in the commentaries and in Hemacandra's *Yogaśāstra,* I shall first present the account of the *Pātañjalayogaśāstravivaraṇa,* which reads in the following way:

> Thus, the posture in which one is seated, having placed the right leg on top of the left, and the right hand on top of the left, is the Good Fortune Posture. Everything else is the same [as in the Lotus Posture].[55]

According to Śaṅkara's account, the Good-Fortune Posture is quite similar to the Lotus Posture. He mentions only two differences. The first one concerns the position of the feet. In the Good Fortune Posture only the right foot is placed on top of the left thigh, whereas the left foot is probably placed underneath the right thigh. Moreover, the hands of the yogi do not form the Tortoise or the Brahmāñjali Gesture but are placed above each other with the right hand on top.

This description of the Good Fortune Posture differs considerably from the one that Vācaspati provides: "The Good Fortune Posture is thus: make a hollow of the soles of the feet, close to the scrotum, and place the Hand Tortoise (*pāṇikacchapika*) above it."[56]

Vācaspati's description agrees with Hemacandra's account of the Good Fortune Posture. Hemacandra even quotes Vācaspati's commentary in support of his own view.

> Now the Good Fortune Posture: The posture, in which one should make the Hand Tortoise above the soles of the feet that make a hollow in front of the testicles, this is the

54 On the textual quality of the version of the *Pātañjalayogaśāstra* as printed in Āgāśe's edition and on the textual witnesses used in this edition, see Maas 2006: xxiii–xxv.

55 *Vivaraṇa* on PYŚ 2.46, l. 18f. in Appendix 2 below: *tathā dakṣiṇaṃ pādaṃ savyasyopari kṛtvā, hastaṃ ca dakṣiṇaṃ savyahastasyopari nidhāya, yenāste, tad bhadrāsanam. anyat samānam.*

56 TVai on PYŚ 2.46, l. 4f. in Appendix 3 below: *pādatale dve vṛṣaṇasamīpe saṃpuṭīkṛtya tasyopari pāṇikacchapikāṃ kuryād etad bhadrāsanam.*

> Good Fortune Posture. [Commentary:] This is clear. Therefore the followers of Patañjali say that the Good Fortune Posture is thus: "Make a hollow of the soles of the feet, close to the scrotum, and place the Hand Tortoise above it" (TVai on PYŚ 2.46).[57]

Vijñānabhikṣu's description, which is again a citation from the *Vasiṣṭhasaṃhitā*, slightly differs from this outline:

> A person who is extremely steady should put the ankles down underneath the testicles, at the sides of the perineum, and hold the sides of his feet firmly with his hands. That is the Good Fortune Posture. It removes all diseases and poisons.[58]

The main difference between the two descriptions of Vācaspati and Hemacandra on the one hand and that of Vijñānabhikṣu and the *Vasiṣṭhasaṃhitā* on the other concerns how the yogi positions his hands. Whereas Vācaspati describes the Good Fortune Posture as requiring a Hand Tortoise above the hollow of the feet, the *Vasiṣṭhasaṃhitā* and Vijñānabhikṣu suggest that the yogi should firmly embrace his feet. All these descriptions differ from that provided by Śaṅkara, in which the Good Fortune Posture is similar to the Lotus Posture, with the sole difference that in the later postures both feet are placed on the thighs, whereas in the former one only one foot lies on its opposite thigh. Hemacandra, for his part, mentions that some authorities call this posture the "Half Lotus Posture".[59]

3.2.4. The Hero Posture (*Vīrāsana*)

Śaṅkara described the Hero Posture quite briefly in his *Pātañjalayogaśāstra-vivaraṇa* as follows: "Thus, in the Hero Posture one of the legs is bent and the other knee is placed down on the ground. In each case, I am explaining only what is special."[60] This description is quite vague. Considering that Śaṅkara took the previously described Good Fortune Posture as his model for the description of the Hero Posture, it is, however, possible to guess. The Good Fortune Posture consists, according to Śaṅkara, in a cross-legged position with one foot upon the opposite thigh and the other foot probably placed below the other thigh. The Hero Posture differs from this pose in that one leg is bent, whereas the knee of the

57 YŚ 4.130, p. 1066, l. 5–8: *atha bhadrāsanam – saṃpuṭīkṛtya muṣkarāgre talapādau tathopari | pāṇikacchapikāṃ kuryād yatra bhadrāsanaṃ tu tat || 130 || spaṣṭam. yat pātañjalāḥ – pādatale vṛṣaṇasamīpe saṃpuṭīkṛtya tasyopari pāṇikacchapikāṃ kuryāt, etad bhadrāsanam* (TVai 2.46).

58 YVā on PYŚ 2.46, p. 232, ll. 9–11 (= VS 1.79, p. 23, with the variant readings *kṣipan* for *kṣipet* and *suniścalam* for *suniścalaḥ*): *gulphau ca vṛṣaṇasyādhaḥ sīvanyāḥ pārśvayoḥ kṣipet | pārśvapādau ca pāṇibhyāṃ dṛḍhaṃ baddhvā suniścalaḥ || bhadrāsanaṃ bhaved etat sarvavyādhiviṣāpaham |.*

59 See below, section 3.2.4.

60 *Vivaraṇa* on PYŚ 2.46, l. 20f. in Appendix 2 below: *tathākuñcitānyatarapādam avanivinyastāparajānukaṃ vīrāsanam. ucyamāna eva viśeṣaḥ sarvatra.*

other leg is placed on the ground. This may suggest that the yogi sits upon one of his legs, the knee of which touches the ground, whereas the other leg is bent towards the body.

Vācaspati apparently had a different posture in mind when he described the Hero Posture in the following way: "The Hero Posture is as follows: The person positioned [in it] places one of his legs on the ground and the other leg with a bent knee above the ground."[61]

Although this description is not very detailed, it may refer to a position in which the practitioner kneels on one of his legs that is bent so that knee and foot touch the ground, whereas the other leg is upright on the ground.

Vācaspati's account of the Hero Posture was known to Hemacandra, who, however, also described two additional varieties of the Hero Posture in the following way:

> Now the Hero Posture: The posture, suitable for heroes, in which the left foot is put above the left thigh and the right foot upon the left thigh is known to be the Hero Posture. [Commentary:] The posture, in which the left foot is put above the left thigh, and the right foot is put on the left thigh, and which is suitable for heroes, like the Jinas, not for cowards, is called the Hero Posture. The position of the right hand is the same as in the Couch Posture. Some say that this is the Lotus Posture. If only one foot is placed upon one thigh, this is the Half Lotus Posture. [...] [p. 128] He describes the Hero Posture according to a different view: Others know the Hero Posture as the position which is assumed when someone mounted on a throne remains in this position after the seat has been removed. [Commentary:] When a person mounted on a throne puts his feet on the ground, and then the throne is removed, staying in exactly this configuration is the Hero Posture. The word "others" refers to men knowledgeable about the doctrines who have explained the topics of torments of the body and austerities. The followers of Patañjali (i.e., Vācaspatimiśra), however, say that the Hero Posture is like this: one of the legs of a person who is positioned upright is placed on the ground, and the other, with a bent knee, is above.[62]

---

61 TVai on PYŚ 2.46, l. 5f. in Appendix 3: *sthitasyaikataraḥ pādo bhūnyasta ekataraś cākuñcitajānur bhūrdhvam ity etad vīrāsanam.* This is the text version of manuscript J_{TV}, emended to *-jānur* instead of *jānu* in accordance with the quotation of the passage in Hemacandra's *Yogaśāstra* (on which see below, n. 62). The text edited in Āgāśe 1904 and Nārāyaṇamiśra 1971 reads *cākuñcitajānor upari nyasta,* which would mean that the foot is placed on top of the bent knee.

62 YŚ 4.126–128, p. 1064, l. 6 – 1065, l. 10: *atha vīrāsanam – vāmo 'ṃhrir dakṣiṇorūrdhvaṃ vāmor upari dakṣiṇaḥ | kriyate yatra tad vīrocitaṃ vīrāsanaṃ smṛtam || 126 || vāmo 'ṃhrir vāmapādo dakṣiṇororūrdhvaṃ vāmasya coror upari dakṣiṇo 'ṃhrir yatra kriyate tad vīrāṇāṃ tīrthakaraprabhṛtīnām ucitam, na kātarāṇām, vīrāsanaṃ smṛtam | agrahastanyāsaḥ paryaṅkavat | idaṃ padmāsanam ity eke | ekasyaiva pādasya ūrāv āropaṇe 'rdhapadmāsanam ||* 126 || [...] *matāntareṇa vīrāsanam āha – siṃhāsanādhirūḍhasyāsanāpanayane sati | tathaivāvasthitir yā tām anye vīrāsanaṃ viduḥ ||* 128 || *siṃhāsanam adhirūḍhasya bhūmi nyastapādasya siṃhāsanāpanayane sati tathaivāvasthānaṃ vīrāsanam. anye iti said-*

The first variety of the Hero Posture that Hemacandra describes agrees with the description of the Lotus Posture in the *Pātañjalayogaśāstravivaraṇa*. Moreover, the posture that Śaṅkara described as the Good Fortune Posture was known to Hemacandra as the Half Lotus Posture. Hemacandra's second variety of the Hero Posture is the strenuous posture in which the knees of a standing person are bent to about ninety degrees as if he were sitting on a chair, but without any support for the weight of the body.

These three varieties of the Hero Posture differ again from Vijñānabhikṣu's description of the posture of the same name, for which he again quotes the *Vasiṣṭhasaṃhitā* as his authoritative source. This account is, however, far from clear: "The person positioned [thus], having placed one foot on one thigh, similarly [places the other thigh] on the other foot. That is called Hero Posture."[63] As printed in Nārāyaṇamiśra's 1971 edition of the *Yogavārttika*, this description of the Hero Posture is ungrammatical, which calls for an emendation of the text. The smallest change would be to emend the accusative *pādaṃ* in the third quarter of the verse to the locative *pāde*, and to supply the phrase "places the other thigh". Accordingly, the Hero Posture of the *Vasiṣṭhasaṃhitā* would be very similar to the posture that Śaṅkara described as the Good Fortune Posture and that Hemacandra knew as the Half Lotus Posture.

3.2.5. The Lucky Mark Posture (*Svastikāsana*)

The name "Lucky Mark Posture" (*svastikāsana*) is transmitted in the vast majority of witnesses in a contracted form as "Lucky Mark" (*svastika*), i. e., without the word "Posture" (*āsana*) as the final part of the compound.[64] Only the two witnesses Jai^{n} and M^{g2} actually read the full compound, whereas the basic text commented upon in the *Pātañjalayogaśāstravivaraṇa* apparently read the two separate words *svastikam āsanam*. Although the transmission of this posture name is thus not uniform, the reading *svastikāsanaṃ* can be established with some confidence as the archetypal reading, because according to the dictionary by Monier Monier-Williams the Sanskrit word *svastika* is invariably a masculine noun in Sanskrit literature,[65] whereas the majority of witnesses of Patañjali's list

---

dhāntikāḥ kāyakleśatapaḥprakaraṇe vyākhyātavantaḥ. pātañjalās tv āhuḥ – ūrdhvasthitasyaikataraḥ pādo bhūnyasta ekaś cākuñcitajānur ūrdhvam ity etad vīrāsanam, iti.

63 YVā on PYŚ 2.46, p. 262, l. 6f. with the emendation of *pāde* for *pādaṃ* in c: *ekapādam athaikasmin vinyasyorau ca saṃsthitaḥ | itarasmiṃs tathā pāde vīrāsanam udāhṛtam ||*. Cf. VS 1.72, p. 21: *ekaṃ pādam athaikasmin vinyasyorau ca saṃsthitam | itarasmiṃs tathaivoruṃ vīrāsanam itīritam ||* .

64 That is, in Āgāśe's 1904 edition, in manuscripts A^{d}, B^{n1}, B^{n2}, $B^{ś}$, K^{b}, K^{n1}, K^{n2}, My^{t3}, Pc^{g}, P^{n} and T^{m}, and in the version of the *Pātañjalayogaśāstra* that Vācaspati commented upon.

65 See MW p. 1283, column 1 f., s. v. *svastika*.

transmit it as the neuter noun *svastikam*. If this is true, the archetypal reading survived in a sole witness transmitting a text version derived from hyparchetype β (M^{g2}), and in another witness with a text version derived from hyparchetype α (Jai^{n}).

The sources describe the performance of the Lucky Mark Posture in very similar ways. To start with, Śaṅkara's account reads as follows:

> The posture in which one is seated with the right big toe tucked in between the left thigh and lower leg so that it cannot be seen, and with the left big toe tucked invisibly in between the right thigh and lower leg, and in such a way that the heels do not hurt the testicles, is the Posture Lucky Mark.[66]

This account agrees by and large with that of Vācaspati, who described the Lucky Mark Posture in the following way:

> The Lucky Mark is thus: one should put the bent left foot in the crook of the right thigh and lower leg, and the bent right one in the crook of the left thigh and lower leg.[67]

Hemacandra's account of the Lucky Mark Posture, which is a silent quotation of Vācaspati's explanation, reads as follows:

> Similarly the Lucky Mark Posture is the posture in which one should put the bent left foot in the crook of the right thigh and lower leg, and the bent right one in the crook of the left thigh and lower leg.[68]

Finally, Vijñānabhikṣu again quotes the *Vasiṣṭhasaṃhitā* in the following way: "Having properly placed the soles of both feet between the knees and the thighs, one is comfortably seated with the torso straight. That is considered to be the Lucky Mark."[69]

According to these four very similar accounts, the Lucky Mark Posture is a cross-legged sitting pose, in which the legs are crossed at their lower parts so that the toes can be placed into the crook of the knee. It appears that this position has been called the "Lucky Mark Posture" in yogic circles for the last 1300 years, i. e., from at least the seventh century CE up to the sixteenth century, and, as a search on the internet for depictions of the "svastikasana" reveals, up to the present day.

66 *Vivaraṇa* on PYŚ 2.46, ll. 22–24 in Appendix 2 below: *dakṣiṇaṃ pādāṅguṣṭhaṃ savyenorujaṅghena parigṛhyādṛśyaṃ kṛtvā, tathā savyaṃ pādāṅguṣṭhaṃ dakṣiṇenorujaṅghenādṛśyaṃ parigṛhya, yathā ca pārṣṇibhyāṃ vṛṣaṇayor apīḍanaṃ tathā yenāste, tat svastikam āsanam.*

67 TVai on PYŚ 2.46, ll. 6–8 in Appendix 3 below: *savyam ākuñcitaṃ caraṇaṃ dakṣiṇajaṅghorvantare kṣipet, dakṣiṇaṃ cākuñcitaṃ vāmajaṅghorvantare, tad etat svastikam.*

68 YŚ 4.133, p. 1069, l. 4f.: *tathā svastikāsanaṃ yatra savyam ākuñcitaṃ caraṇaṃ dakṣiṇajaṅghorvantare nikṣipet, dakṣiṇaṃ cākuñcitaṃ vāmajaṅghorvantare iti.*

69 YVā on PYŚ 2.46, p. 262, l. 12f. (= VS 1.68, p. 20): *jānūrvantare samyak kṛtvā pādatale ubhe | ṛjukāyaḥ sukhāsīnaḥ svastikaṃ tat pracakṣate ||.*

3.2.6. The Staff Posture (*Daṇḍāsana*)

In contradistinction to the two previously discussed posture names, the name "Staff Posture" is transmitted with just a few textual variants. The variant "Extended like a Staff" (*daṇḍāyata*) in manuscript A^d is most probably of secondary origin, as is the omission of this posture name from the list in manuscript Jai^n.[70] The different sources describe the performance of this posture largely in similar ways. To start with, Śaṅkara describes the Staff Posture as follows: "The posture in which one sits down like a stick, stretching out the feet with the ankles, big toes and knees aligned, is the Staff Posture."[71] This description is in harmony with Vācaspati's explanation:

> One should practice the Staff Posture by sitting down and stretching out the feet, lower legs and thighs in contact with the ground, with the big toes touching and the ankles touching.[72]

Also Hemacandra knew the Staff Posture in a very similar way. Moreover, in support of this, he quoted, with a slight deviation, Vācaspati's description as follows:

> Now the Staff Posture: The posture in which one should stretch out the feet with the big toes touching, and the ankles touching each other, and the thighs in contact with the ground, this is said to be the Staff Posture. [Commentary:] This is clear. On this the followers of Patañjali say that one should practice the Staff Posture by sitting down and stretching out the feet, with the big toes touching, and the ankles touching, and the lower legs in contact with the ground.[73]

Finally, also Vijñānabhikṣu quoted the explanation of the "Staff Posture" from the *Tattvavaiśāradī* almost verbatim. However, he modified the explanation of his predecessor by turning the Staff Posture from a seated posture into a supine pose:

> [The word] Staff Posture [means] lying like a staff after one has sat down and stretched out the feet with the big toes touching, the ankles touching, and with the lower legs and thighs touching the ground.[74]

---

70 The error in Jai^n was noticed by a reader or corrector and the missing word added in the margin of the manuscript.

71 *Vivaraṇa* on PYŚ 2.46, l. 25f. in Appendix 2 below: *samagulphau samāṅguṣṭhau prasārayan samajānū pādau daṇḍavad yenopaviśet, tad daṇḍāsanam.*

72 TVai on PYŚ 2.46, l. 8f. in Appendix 3 below: *upaviśya śliṣṭāṅgulīkau śliṣṭagulphau bhūmiśliṣṭajaṅghorū pādau prasārya daṇḍāsanam abhyasyet.*

73 YŚ 4.131, p. 1066, l. 10 – 1067, l. 2: *atha daṇḍāsanam – śliṣṭāṅgulī śliṣṭagulphau bhūśliṣṭorū prasārayet | yatropaviśya pādau tad daṇḍāsanam udīritam || 131 || spaṣṭam. yat pātañjalāḥ – upaviśya śliṣṭāṅgulīkau śliṣṭagulphau bhūmiśliṣṭajaṅghau ca pādau prasārya daṇḍāsanam abhyasyet* (TVai 2.46).

74 YVā on PYŚ 2.46, p. 262, l. 15f.: *daṇḍāsanam – upaviśya śliṣṭāṅgulikau śliṣṭagulphau bhūmiśliṣṭajaṅghorū pādau prasārya daṇḍavac chayanam.*

It is quite likely that Vijñānabhikṣu's description of the Staff Posture as a supine posture was innovative. If the authors of the earlier descriptions would have had in mind a completely supine posture, one would expect them to have clarified that not only the feet, lower legs and thighs should touch the ground, but also the back and the head.

Apparently Vijñānabhikṣu's view of how to practise the Staff Posture differs not only from the view of his predecessors, but also from modern types of practice, like that of Iyengar, which prescribe sitting with an upright torso and stretched legs.

3.2.7. The One with Support (*Sopāśraya*)

The next posture in Patañjali's list is called the "One with Support", because its performance involves the use of a supporting means. Śaṅkara explains this posture, whose name appears in all versions of Patañjali's list without substantial textual variants, as follows: "The One with Support is with a yoga strap or with a prop such as a crutch."[75]

Śaṅkara apparently was familiar with different devices that a yogi could use as an aid for keeping a posture. Of these, he just named the yoga strap and props like crutches.[76] Other references in yoga literature to the use of crutches (*stambha*) in meditation are not known to me, whereas the "yoga strap" (*yogapaṭṭa* or *yogapaṭṭaka*), which is a cloth ligature that is used to keep the legs of the yogi in the desired position during meditation, is mentioned not infrequently in literature and depicted also in visual representations of yogis. Apparently, the strap became the supporting device for postures *par excellence*. Thus, Vācaspati explained the posture name "The One with Support" by stating: "The One with Support is so called because of the use of the yoga strap."[77]
Hemacandra and Vijñānabhikṣu, who both knew Vācaspati's explanation of this posture, referred to the One with Support in almost identical words by quoting the comment of the famous polymath, without acknowledgement.[78]

75 *Vivaraṇa* on PYŚ 2.46, l. 27 in Appendix 2 below: *sayogapaṭṭaṃ sastambhādyāśrayaṃ vā sopāśrayam.*

76 According to James Mallinson (personal communication, June 2015), "the prop is probably a crutch of the type seen in several Mughal miniatures and still used today."

77 TVai on PYŚ 2.46, l. 9 in Appendix 3 below: *yogapaṭṭakayogāt sopāśrayam.*

78 Hemacandra (YŚ 4.133, p. 1069, l. 5f.) uses the phrase "Likewise there is a posture called 'The One with Support', which comes about because a yoga strap is used" (*tathā sopāśrayaṃ yogapaṭṭakayogād yad bhavati*), whereas Vijñānabhikṣu quotes Vācaspati when saying (YVā on PYŚ 2.46, p. 262, l. 16): "The One with Support (*sopāśraya*) is sitting by using a yoga strap" (*sopāśrayaṃ yogapaṭṭayogenopaveśanam*).

3.2.8. The Couch Posture (*Paryaṅkāsana*)

The name "Couch Posture", which very probably occurred already in the oldest reconstructable version of Patañjali's list of postures, is exclusively preserved in the basic text commented upon in the *Pātañjalayogaśāstravivaraṇa.* Manuscript My^{t3} reads *paryaṅkaniṣadanaṃ* "Sitting Like a Couch" (or, alternatively "Sitting Down or Reclining on a Couch") instead, which probably is a scribal mistake resulting from a reading error that a scribe committed when his eye jumped to the following name *hastiniṣadanaṃ* while he was actually still engaged in writing the name "Couch Posture".

The vast majority of manuscripts (i. e., A^{d}, B^{n1}, B^{n2}, B^{ś}, Jai^{n} (*ac*), K^{b}, K^{n1}, K^{n2}, M^{g2}, Pc^{g}, P^{n} and T^{m}) read the neuter nominal form *paryaṅkaṃ* instead of *paryaṅkāsanaṃ.* It is, however, highly unlikely that already Patañjali used the form *paryaṅkaṃ* when he created the *Pātañjalayogaśāstra,* because the word *paryaṅka* always has the masculine and not the neuter gender in Sanskrit. Also the words *pallaṅka* and *paliyaṃka* that correspond to Sanskrit *paryaṅka* in the Middle Indic languages Pali and Ardha Māgadhī are invariably masculine nouns.[79]

In view of the fact that the grammatically correct form *paryaṅkaḥ* occurs in the basic text commented upon in Vācaspati's commentary, it may be tempting to regard this reading (which is also found in manuscript Jai^{n} after its correction) as the oldest reconstructable version. However, it appears more probable that at Vācaspati's time the reading *paryaṅkāsanaṃ* had already been contracted in the manuscripts known to Vācaspati to *paryaṅkaṃ,* which the learned commentator then emended to *paryaṅkaḥ.*

In Buddhist literature, the Sanskrit word *paryaṅka* (as well as the Pali word *pallaṅka*) is frequently used for the cross-legged meditation posture in which both feet rest upon the opposite thighs, i. e., for a posture that is similar or even identical with the one that Śaṅkara and Hemacandra knew as the Lotus Posture. For example, when – probably in the first century CE[80] – Aśvaghoṣa described the future Buddha's struggle for awakening (*bodhi*) he said:

79 See Rhys Davids & Stede 1921–1923: 442a, s. v. *pallaṅka* and Ratnachandraji 1930: 526a, s. v. *paliyaṃka.*

80 Aśvaghoṣa also wrote a stage play entitled *Śāriputraprakaraṇa.* Heinrich Lüders (1911) studied the palaeography of a Central Asian manuscript fragment of this play more than a century ago and was able to date it to the time of either the Kuṣāṇa king Kaniṣka I or his successor Huviṣka. According to recent historical research, the reign of these two kings falls into the period between 155 and 214 CE (Golzio 2008: 89). If Lüders was correct, a manuscript tradition of at least one of Aśvaghoṣa's works must have existed by the beginning of the third century at the latest. Further recent research makes it probable that this date can be pushed back by 100 years. Jens-Uwe Hartmann (2006) has dated a manuscript fragment of the *Saundarananda* to approximately the middle of the second century CE. If one allows that some time has to pass after the composition of a poetical work before it is widely copied and

> Then he (i. e., the future Buddha) bent [his legs into] the best, unshakeable cross-legged sitting position (*paryaṅka*), which was like the solid coils of a sleeping serpent [while he vowed]: "I shall not break this posture on the earth, until I have achieved what is to be done."[81]

This passage is interesting from a historical perspective as it may contain the earliest roughly datable use of the word "posture" (*āsana*) for a bodily configuration assumed for meditation. Moreover, the comparison of the position of the seated future Buddha with "the solid coils of a sleeping serpent" indicates how Aśvaghoṣa used the word *paryaṅka* although he did not describe the posture in any detail. He apparently referred to the legs as being firmly entwined with each other, which may imply that he used the word *paryaṅka* for sitting in a cross-legged posture.

"Sitting in such a position" is also the meaning of the word *pallaṅka,* the Pali form of Sanskrit *paryaṅka.*[82] The term occurs frequently in a stock phrase describing how a Buddhist monk prepares himself for meditation as "he sits down having bent [his legs into] the *pallaṅka*".[83] The famous commentator and author Buddhaghosa,[84] who probably lived between the end of the fourth and the beginning of the fifth century CE,[85] explains this phrase in his *Visuddhimagga* ("The Way to Perfect Purity") in the following way: "'*pallaṅka*' means the posture in which (the feet) are completely attached to the thighs; 'having bent' means 'having assumed'."[86] It appears from this account that from comparatively early

---

distributed, then Aśvaghoṣa may have lived in the first half of the first century. Patrick Olivelle has noted strong thematic and textual parallels of Aśvaghoṣa's *Buddhacarita* with the *Mānavadharmaśāstra,* a work that he has dated to the second century CE (Olivelle 2005: 25). According to Olivelle, Aśvaghoṣa must have been aware of the *Mānavadharmaśāstra,* and was in some passages criticizing it. However, the ideas about *dharma* in the *Buddhacarita* and *Mānavadharmaśāstra* need not necessarily have been originally conceived by the author of the latter work. Taking into account the early Central Asian manuscript evidence that may push Aśvaghoṣa's date further back, it may be assumed that both works adopted their common ideas about *dharma* from older sources which are now lost. In this case, the dating of Aśvaghoṣa to the time around the year 50 CE may still be the best estimate, which is just slightly later than the one that Edward Johnston proposed as early as 1936 (Johnston 1936: xvii). This is also the conclusion at which Alfred Hiltebeitel (2006: 235) arrived on the basis of different arguments.

81 *Buddhacarita* 12.120, p. 144: *tataḥ sa paryaṅkam akampyam uttamaṃ babandha suptoragabhogapiṇḍitam | bhinadmi tāvad bhuvi naitad āsanaṃ na yāmi yāvat kṛtyatām iti* || 120 ||.

82 "Pallanka [...] I. sitting cross-legged, in instr. pallankena upon the hams [...]; and in phrase pallankaŋ ābhujati 'to bend (the legs) crosswise'" (Rhys Davids & Stede 1921–1923: 442a, s. v. *pallanka*).

83 The phrase *nisīdati pallaṅkaṃ ābhuñjitvā* occurs, for example, in the *Sāmaññaphalasutta,* at D ii 69, p. 71, l. 18f.

84 Cf. above, n. 2.

85 See Kieffer-Pülz 1992: 166f.

86 *Visuddhimagga* p. 223, l. 26: *[...] pallaṅkan ti samantato ūrubaddhāsanam. ābhujitvā ti bandhitvā.*

times onwards the words *pallaṅka* and *paryaṅka* were used in Buddhist works to refer to the sitting posture that is well known from Buddhist sculptures showing a seated person with the feet positioned on the opposite thighs.[87]

As mentioned above, Śaṅkara, the author of the *Pātañjalayogaśāstravivaraṇa*, knew this posture as the "Lotus Posture" (*padmāsana*) and not as the "Couch Posture" (*paryaṅkāsana*), which he described as follows: "The Couch Posture consists in lying with the arms stretched out towards the knees."[88] This description agrees with Vācaspati's explanation of the posture called "Couch": "The Couch is the lying down of someone who makes his arms stretch to their knees."[89] Also Vijñānabhikṣu explains the posture called *paryaṅka* in almost identical terms: "And The Couch is the supine posture of someone with his arms stretched down to his knees."[90]

From the three just cited commentarial glosses it appears that the tradition of Pātañjala Yoga knew the *paryaṅka* posture, at least from the seventh up to the sixteenth century, as a supine posture, in which the yogi stretches his arms out towards the knees.

Hemacandra described the Couch Posture in the following way:

> If the hands are at the region of the navel facing upwards, with the right one on the top and facing upwards, while the lower parts of the lower legs are placed on top of the feet, this is the Couch. [Commentary:] When the lower parts of the lower legs are placed on top of the feet, the two hands are near the navel, facing upwards, and the right one is on top, i. e., the right is positioned above the left. The posture in which this is so, is called "the Couch" [and] is the posture of the idols of eternal beings and of the Glorious Mahāvīra at the time of his *nirvāṇa*. Like a couch (*paryaṅka*) is positioned above its feet, so it is also the case with this posture. Therefore it is called "Couch". The followers of Patañjali (i. e., Vācaspatimiśra) say that the Couch is the lying of a person who has made his arms stretch to his knees.[91]

---

87 See, for example, the relief of a Kapardin-Buddha from circa the first century CE in Plaeschke & Plaeschke 1988: 87, fig. 50. Many thanks to Karin Preisendanz for bringing this publication to my attention.

88 *Vivaraṇa* on PYŚ 2.46, l. 28 in Appendix 2 below: *ājānuprasāritabāhuśayanaṃ paryaṅkāsanam.*

89 TVai on PYŚ 2.46, l. 9f. in Appendix 3 below: *jānuprasāritabāhoḥ śayanaṃ paryaṅkaḥ.* Note that the word *paryaṅka* is used in the masculine gender.

90 YVā on PYŚ 2.46, p. 262, l. 16: *paryaṅkaṃ ca jānuprasāritabāhoḥ śayanam.* Here the word *paryaṅka* is used as a neuter noun.

91 YŚ 4.125, p. 1064, l. 1–6: *syāj jaṅghayor adhobhāge pādopari kṛte sati | paryaṅko nābhigottānadakṣiṇottarapāṇikaḥ* || 125 || *jaṅghayor adhobhāge pādopari kṛte sati pāṇidvayaṃ nābhyāsannam uttānaṃ dakṣiṇottaraṃ yatra, dakṣiṇa uttara uparivartī yatra tat tathā, etat paryaṅko nāma śāśvatapratimānāṃ śrīmahāvīrasya ca nirvāṇakāla āsanam, yathā paryaṅkaḥ pādopari bhavati tathāyam apīti paryaṅkaḥ. jānuprasāritabāhoḥ śayanaṃ paryaṅkaḥ* (= TVai 2.46, line 26 in Appendix 2 below) *iti pātañjalāḥ.*

The Couch Posture that Hemacandra knew differs from the Buddhist *paryaṅka* in that the feet are not placed on top of the thighs but below the shanks. In the auto-commentary (*svopajñavṛtti*) on this passage, Hemacandra supplements this information by stating that in Pātañjala Yoga the *paryaṅka* is a supine posture, and he again cites Vācaspati's gloss on *paryaṅka* in support of this view.

3.2.9. Sitting Like a Crane, Sitting Like an Elephant, and Sitting Like a Camel (*Krauñcaniṣadana, Hastiniṣadana,* and *Uṣṭraniṣadana*)

The ornithological identification of birds whose names occur in Sanskrit literature is, as is well-known, a difficult task. Julia Leslie (1998) argued that the Sanskrit word *krauñca* designates the Sarus crane, whereas Ditte Bandini-König (2003) called this identification seriously into question. It is beyond the scope of the present chapter to provide a solution to this problem. In the present context it may be sufficient to note that the textual witnesses transmit this posture name, which definitely contains the name of an aquatic bird, with almost no textual variation.[92] Only the three manuscripts B^{n1}, Jai^{n} and K^{n2} transmit the name of the bird as *krońca* instead of *krauñca,* and the comparatively old palm leaf manuscript K^{b} reads *-niṣadaṃ* instead of *-niṣadanaṃ* for "sitting".

Also the word *hasti* "elephant" is uniformly transmitted in almost all witnesses. The only exception is manuscript $B^{ś}$, written in Śāradā script, that has the word *haṃsa* "goose" instead of *hasti* "elephant", probably because a scribe wrote this bird name instead of the Sanskrit word for "elephant" while still remembering the word *krauñca* that he had just written.

Finally, also the posture name "Sitting Like a Camel" is transmitted virtually without variation in all witnesses. The only exception is a manuscript in Telugu script, My^{t3}, that does not transmit this posture name at all.

The commentators do not provide much information concerning the way in which these three postures were to be practised. The *Pātañjalayogaśāstravivaraṇa* simply states that "Sitting Like a Sarus Crane, Sitting Like an Elephant and Sitting Like a Camel can be understood from their similarity to the sitting configuration of the Sarus crane, etc."[93] Also Vācaspati, whose commentary Vijñānabhikṣu used as the source of a literal quotation, advised his readers to simply look at the way in which the mentioned animals usually sit by saying that "Sitting Like a Sarus Crane and so on are to be understood from observing the configuration of seated Sarus cranes, etc."[94]

92 For the convenience of the reader, I shall stick to the translation "Sarus crane" in this chapter.
93 *Vivaraṇa* on PYŚ 2.46, l. 28f. in Appendix 2 below: *krauñcaniṣadanaṃ hastiniṣadanam uṣṭraniṣadanaṃ ca krauñcādiniṣadanasaṃsthānasādṛśyād eva draṣṭavyam.*
94 TVai on PYŚ 2.46, l. 10f. in Appendix 3 below (= YVā p. 262, l. 17f.): *krauñcaniṣadanādīni krauñcādīnāṃ niṣaṇṇānāṃ saṃsthānadarśanāt pratyetavyāni.*

The same advice is found in Hemacandra's very similar reference to animal-like yogic postures. However, the Jaina monk presented a slightly extended version of the list of animals (including the mythical bird Garuḍa) whose sitting poses a yogi may imitate, when he said that

> Sitting Like a Sarus Crane, Sitting Like a Goose, Sitting Like a Dog, Sitting Like an Elephant, Sitting Like Garuḍa and so on are to be interpreted from observing the configuration of seated Sarus cranes, etc.[95]

3.2.10. The Even Configuration (*Samasaṃsthāna*)

The posture name "Even Configuration" (*samasaṃsthāna*) is transmitted in all witnesses in a largely uniform way. One substantial variant is found in manuscript A^d, which due to a scribal mistake reads *samāsasthānaṃ* "Compound Configuration". The second substantial variant occurs in the basic text commented upon in the *Pātañjalayogaśāstravivaraṇa,* which apparently read *samasaṃsthitaṃ* "Positioned Even" instead of *samasaṃsthānaṃ*.

The descriptions of this posture vary considerably in the different sources. According to the *Pātañjalayogaśāstravivaraṇa,* "the Even Configuration (*samasaṃsthita*) consists of having the calves and thighs placed down on the ground."[96] This description is not very specific and leaves open how, according to Śaṅkara, the Even Configuration differs from the Staff Posture.

Vācaspati had a different idea of how the Even Configuration was to be performed when he wrote that "the Even Configuration is pressing against each other the two bent [legs] at the heels and forefeet."[97] Vācaspati's description is again quite elusive. It appears that pressing the heels and forefeet together implies a posture that is similar to the one that he previously described as the Good Fortune Posture. Nevertheless, Hemacandra adopted again Vācaspati's explanation when he described the Even Configuration as follows: "In the same way, the Even Configuration is the posture that consists in pressing the two bent legs against each other that touch at the heels and the tip of the feet."[98]

Finally, Vijñānabhikṣu, who may have been not entirely satisfied with Vācaspati's vague explanation, described the Even Configuration in a different way:

95 YŚ 4.133, p. 1069, l. 6f.: *tathā krauñcaniṣadanahaṃsaniṣadanaśvaniṣadanahastiniṣadanagaruḍaniṣadanādīny āsanāni krauñcādīnāṃ niṣaṇṇānāṃ saṃsthānadarśanāt pratyetavyāni.*

96 *Vivaraṇa* on PYŚ 2.46, l. 30 in Appendix 2 below: *bhūmau nyastam ūrujaṅghaṃ samasaṃsthitam.*

97 TVai on PYŚ 2.46, l. 11f. in Appendix 3 below: *pārṣṇyagrapādābhyāṃ dvayor ākuñcitayor anyonyapīḍanaṃ samasaṃsthānam.*

98 YŚ 4.133, p. 1069, l. 2f.: *tathā samasaṃsthānaṃ yat pārṣṇyagrapādābhyāṃ dvayor ākuñcitayor anyonyapīḍanam.*

"The Even Configuration means remaining without any bend in the torso, head and neck, with the two hands on top of the knees."[99]

Just like the previously discussed descriptions, this one is not very specific.

3.2.11. Steady Relaxation (*Sthiraprasrabdhi*)

The textual witnesses transmit the posture name "Steady Relaxation" with a considerable amount of variation concerning the initial (*sthira-*) as well as the final part of the compound (*-prasrabdhi*). The word-stem *sthira-* ("steady") appears as *sthita-* ("standing, permanent") in the manuscripts A^{d}, Pc^{g} and T^{m} and in the basic text commented upon in the *Pātañjalayogaśāstravivaraṇa* which all share hyparchetype β as their common ancestor. Accordingly, it is highly probable that *sthita-* was already the reading of this hyparchetype, and that the reading *sthira-* in manuscripts M^{g2} and My^{t3}, which also are descendants of hyparchetype β, results from contamination with the vulgate version of the *Pātañjalayogaśāstra.* The question of which of the two alternative readings *sthira-* and *sthita-* derived from which is difficult to answer. On the one hand, the word *sthira* is probably slightly less common than *sthita* and therefore maybe slightly more difficult. On the other hand, it is the word *sthira* that occurs in YS 2.46, which may have been on the mind of a scribe who wrote *sthira-* instead of *sthita-*. In any case, the fact that these words were confused with each other indicates that the two letters *ra* and *ta* were similar in the script of the manuscript that this scribe used as his exemplar when he introduced the variant into the transmission. Such a similarity is found, according to the tables provided by Georg Bühler, in some north Indian scripts of the late seventh and early eighth century CE.[100]

The second part of the compound is transmitted as *-sukham* in Āgāśe's 1904 edition and in manuscripts B^{n1}, B^{n2}, $B^{ś}$, Jai^{n}, K^{n1}, K^{n2}, M^{g2}, My^{t3} and P^{n}. In contrast to this, the two manuscripts A^{d} and T^{m} as well as the basic text commented upon by Śaṅkara read the word *-prasrabdhir* or a similar but meaningless derivative of this word resulting from copying errors. All three witnesses go back to hyparchetype β. Moreover, the comparatively ancient palm leaf manuscript in Old Bengali script K^{b} and the basic text commented upon in the *Tattvavaiśāradī* as reconstructed from manuscript J_{TV} (which according to the catalogue can probably be dated to the year 1143 CE), read *-prasrabdham.* This distribution of variants among witnesses belonging to both main branches of the transmission

99 YVā on PYŚ 2.46, p. 262, l. 18f.: *jānunor upari hastau kṛtvā kāyaśirogrīvasyāvakrabhāvenā-vasthānaṃ samasaṃsthānam.*

100 See Bühler 1896: plate IV, rows XVII and XX.

leads to the conclusion that *-prasrabdhir* most probably was the reading of the archetype.

The reading "Steady Relaxation" (*sthiraprasrabdhir*) is not only from a stemmatical point of view probably more original than *sthirasukhaṃ*. It is also preferable because the term "relaxation" (*prasrabdhi*) occurs almost exclusively in Buddhist Sanskrit literature.[101] It is also quite frequently found in the form *passaddhi*, the Pali equivalent to *prasrabdhi* or *praśrabdhi*, in the Buddhist literature composed in Pali.[102] Therefore, the replacement of the expression "relaxation" (*prasrabdhi*), which is quite unusual outside Buddhist contexts, with the more usual word "comfort" (*sukha*) is a much more likely scenario than that of the opposite replacement.

Śaṅkara explains the posture name "Permanent Relaxation" (*sthitaprasrabdhi*) as follows:

> When [a posture] in any form whatsoever, which may be conceived of by oneself, leads to permanent relaxation, i.e., to ease (lit. non-exertion), this is also a posture, which is called Permanent Relaxation.[103]

According to this explanation, Śaṅkara does not interpret "Permanent Relaxation" as a term referring to any well defined posture. Rather, he takes it as an umbrella term that covers a number of postures with the common characteristic of leading the practitioner to relaxation. Śaṅkara leaves it to the individual practitioner to invent or find himself bodily configurations that serve this purpose best. This indicates that according to Śaṅkara individual practitioners of yoga were qualified to find or invent new practices.

Vācaspati's explanation of the posture called *sthiraprasrabdha* is similar:

> A posture is Steadily Relaxed when a configuration leads to the accomplishment of steadiness which is comfortable, for the person who has adopted it. The venerable author of the Sūtra agrees with this.[104]

Also Vācaspati does not define the posture Steadily Relaxed by describing the configuration of the body, but by pointing to the result of the posture. It appears, however, that Śaṅkara's explanation leaves more room for the yogi's ingenuity to invent new useful postures than Vācaspati's gloss.

The final part of Vācaspati's comment, namely that the author of the Sūtra agrees with this posture, may have led to the textual change in some versions of

---

101 See BHSD p. 388a, s. v. *praśrabdhi, prasra°*.

102 See Rhys Davids & Stede 1921–1923: 447b, s. v. Passaddhi.

103 *Vivaraṇa* on PYŚ 2.46, l. 31 f. in Appendix 2 below: *sthitaprasrabdhiḥ – anyenāpi prakāreṇa svayamutprekṣyā sthitaprasrabdhir anāyāso yena bhavati tad apy āsanaṃ sthitaprasrabdhir nāma.*

104 TVai on PYŚ 2.46, l. 12–14 in Appendix 3 below: *yena saṃsthānenāvasthitasya sthairyaṃ sukhaṃ sidhyati tad āsanaṃ sthiraprasrabdham. tatra bhagavataḥ sūtrakārasya saṃmatam.*

the *Pātañjalayogaśāstra* (as well as in some versions of the *Tattvavaiśāradī*) from *sthiraprasrabdhir* (via the intermediate form *-prasrabdhaṃ*) to the reading *sthirasukham* "Steadily Comfortable", which is the reading of the vulgate. This reading, which corresponds exactly to the wording of YS 2.46 (*sthirasukham āsanam*), is apparently the result of a hypercorrection that one or more scribes who were unfamiliar with the Sanskrit words *prasrabdhi* and *prasrabdha* applied in order to restore what they thought would be the original text. Once the textual change from *-prasrabdhir* to *-sukham* had been introduced into the transmission, it appeared completely unobjectionable to all further scribes and readers of the work. Therefore Vijñānabhikṣu, who was well aware of Vācaspati's comment, referred to this posture just very briefly by stating that "And the Steady and Comfortable One is adopted from the *sūtra*."[105]

James H. Woods, the famous translator of the *Tattvavaiśāradī* and the *Pātañjalayogaśāstra,* did not question the originality of this reading. When translating YS 2.46 as "Stable-and-easy posture," he apparently thought of a scenario opposite to that assumed by Vijñānabhikṣu. For Woods, the *bhāṣya* does not quote from the *sūtra,* but the author of the *sūtra* uses the name of the posture "Stable-and-easy" for his explanation of the term *āsana.* "Stable-and-easy" would then be the name of the *āsana par excellence.*

3.2.12. As is Comfortable (*Yathāsukha*)

The final name of a posture in the list of the *Pātañjalayogaśāstra,* i.e., "As is Comfortable", occurs in almost all textual witnesses without major textual deviation. The only exception is the paper manuscript in Śāradā script from Baroda ($B^{ś}$), which omits this name, apparently incidentally, from the list.

According to the *Pātañjalayogaśāstravivaraṇa,* the name "As is Comfortable", just like the previous posture name "Permanent Relaxation", does not designate any specific posture, but serves as a generic term to cover a variety of different postures with a common characteristic. Śaṅkara explained the posture as follows: "And 'As is Comfortable'. As is Comfortable is that form which produces comfort for the seated person."[106] According to this explanation, every posture producing a comfortable feeling for the practising yogi can be named "As is Comfortable".

Vācaspati and Vijñānabhikṣu do not regard "As is Comfortable" as a separate posture name in its own right, but take the word as a commentarial gloss of the previous name.[107]

105 YVā on PYŚ 2.46, p. 262, l. 19: *sthirasukhaṃ ca sūtropāttam.*

106 *Vivaraṇa* on PYŚ 2.46, l. 33 in Appendix 2 below: *yathāsukhaṃ ca – yena rūpeṇāsīnasya sukhaṃ bhavati tad yathāsukham.*

107 Vācaspati states that "its clarification (i.e., that of the posture 'Constant Relaxation') is: 'and

3.2.13. Additional Postures

All witnesses, with the exception of the reconstructed basic text commented upon by Vācaspati, attest the occurrence of the word "et cetera" (*ādi*) at the end of the list of posture names. This indicates that the list is not a complete recording of all posture names known to the author of this passage, but that it includes only the most important designations of yogic poses. According to Śaṅkara, the word "et cetera" refers to all further postures that were taught by "the teacher" or "the teachers": "From the use of the expression 'et cetera' one can see that also any other posture is meant that has been taught by the teacher (or: the teachers)."[108]

Śaṅkara does not specify which persons he thought qualified to teach additional postures. He either may have had the authoritative representatives of the Yoga tradition in mind, i. e., the authors of normative Yoga scriptures, or just any teacher in the lineage of teachers and pupils.[109]

Vijñānabhikṣu, who must have known a large variety of postures from Haṭha and Rāja Yoga sources, took the expression "et cetera" to refer to exactly this plethora of yogic poses when he commented on the word as follows: "The word 'et cetera' refers to the Peacock Posture, et cetera. This is a summary of the fact that there are exactly as many postures as there are kinds of living beings."[110] In the final part of his explanation, Vijñānabhikṣu apparently refers to the fact that the number of postures that have their names derived from animals, of which the *Pātañjalayogaśāstra* lists three, i. e., Sitting Like a Sarus Crane, Sitting Like an Elephant and Sitting Like a Camel,[111] can easily be manifolded by taking the sitting poses of other species as a model for specific modes of positioning the body. In support of this view, Vijñānabhikṣu cites the *Vivekamārtaṇḍa*, a Haṭha Yoga work from the twelfth to thirteenth centuries,[112] which states that "[...]

[a posture] as is comfortable'" (*tasya vivaraṇam – yathāsukhaṃ ceti* [TVai on PYŚ 2.46, l. 14 in Appendix 3 below]). Vijñānabhikṣu expresses himself very similarly by saying "Its explanation is 'a [posture] as is comfortable'" (*tasya vyākhyānaṃ yathāsukham* [YVā on PYŚ 2.46, p. 262, l. 20]).

108 *Vivaraṇa* on PYŚ 2.46, l. 33 f. in Appendix 2 below: *ādiśabdād anyad api yathācāryopadiṣṭam āsanaṃ draṣṭavyam.*

109 Śaṅkara refers to Yoga authorities with the word *ācārya* for example in his commentary on PYŚ 1.1 (p. 8, l. 18).

110 YVā on PYŚ 2.46, p. 263, l. 20 f.: *ādiśabdena māyūrādyāsanāni grāhyāṇi. yāvatyo jīvajātayas tāvanty evāsanānīti saṃkṣepaḥ.*

111 See above, section 3.2.9.

112 According to the information that James Mallinson kindly provided in a personal communication (June 2015), the *Vivekamārtaṇḍa* is attributed to Gorakṣa(deva) in its earliest manuscript that is dated to 1477 CE.

there are as many postures as there are kinds of living beings. Maheśvara knows all their varieties."[113]

3.3. The Two Means to Achieve Postures

All the postures discussed so far become, according to PYŚ 2.47, steady and comfortable yogic postures, i. e., *āsana*-s in the technical meaning of the word, by means of one out of two kinds of practices, namely either from the slackening of effort or from merging meditatively into infinity. This indicates that yogic posture practice does not primarily consist of assuming a certain bodily configuration, but of a complex combination of psycho-physiological practices that enable the practitioner to take up further means on the path to spiritual liberation.

3.3.1. The Slackening of Effort

Patañjali refers only very briefly to the slackening of effort in yogic posture practice: "Either a posture is achieved because effort stops, by which the body does not tremble."[114] The key to an interpretation of how a slackening of effort may cause a steady and comfortable posture is Patañjali's reference to the trembling of the body. It may be possible that he thought of a tremor, which is, according to modern physiological conceptions, caused by muscle overstrain that may occur when a yogi forces himself into an unfamiliar and exhausting position. In the progressive course of training, the effort needed to hold a posture for a prolonged time is reduced, until finally a complete cessation of effort may lead to a steady and comfortable posture.

Śaṅkara's comments on Patañjali's explanation support this interpretation:

> Either it (i. e., a posture) is achieved because effort stops, that is, by not making any effort at a time after the posture has been taken up, or else by not making any effort. "By which the body does not tremble." "By which", that is, by the cessation of effort. For by investing effort, one makes the body shake. This means "by which the yogi's posture becomes motionless".[115]

---

113 *Vivekamārtaṇḍa* 8 as critically edited in Jason Birch's chapter in the present volume, n. 16 on p. 108: *āsanāni ca tāvanti yāvatyo jīvajātayaḥ | eteṣām akhilān bhedān vijānāti maheśvaraḥ* || 8 ||.

114 PYŚ 2.47, l. 6f. in Appendix 1 below: *prayatnoparamād vā sidhyaty āsanam, yena nāṅgamejayo bhavati.*

115 *Vivaraṇa* on PYŚ 2.47, ll. 37–39 in Appendix 2 below: *prayatnoparamād* āsanabandhottarakālaṃ prayatnākaraṇād *vā sidhyati. yena nāṅgamejayo bhavati. yena* prayatnopatameṇa, prayatnena hy aṅgaṃ kampayati, yenācalitāsano bhavatīty arthaḥ. Here as well as in some of the following notes, quotations of the basic text (i. e., of the *Pātañjalayogaśāstra*

In this passage, Śaṅkara may have referred to the muscular effort needed to assume and hold a yogic posture when he stated that "by investing effort, one makes the body shake."

Vācaspati, however, held a different view on the role of effort in posture practice. According to him, the yogi has to replace natural effort with a special yogic effort that finally leads to the perfection of postures:

> After all, a natural effort to hold up the body does not bring about the ancillary of yoga, that is, the posture which is to be taught here; if it did bring about that posture, instruction would be pointless, because it could be achieved all by itself. Therefore, this natural effort does not bring about the posture that is to be taught. And natural effort is counter-productive, because it impedes restraint in posture inasmuch as it is the cause of spontaneous postures. Therefore, a person who is practising the posture that has been taught should make an effort to slacken natural effort. The posture that has been taught cannot be achieved any other way. And so it is that slackening natural effort causes the achievement of the posture.[116]

This explanation appears, however, quite fanciful and unconvincing, simply because the passage of the *Pātañjalayogaśāstra* on which Vācaspati bases his comment does not at all presuppose the existence of two kinds of effort, i.e., a natural and a special yogic kind of effort, of which the former is counter-productive to posture practice, whereas the latter is essential.

Vijñānabhikṣu apparently also found Vācaspati's explanation not compelling. In any case, he disregarded the exposition of his predecessor completely in his own commentary. For Vijñānabhikṣu, the *Pātañjalayogaśāstra* indeed refers to the tremor of the body due to physical exercise:

> He explains the slackening of effort as the way to this [steadiness]. "By which the body does not [tremble]." If one practises a posture immediately after a lot of activity, the posture will not become steady because the body is shaking. That is what is intended.[117]

Unfortunately, Vijñānabhikṣu does not inform his readers on the precise kind of activity that he regards as harmful to a successful posture practice. Possibly he

in the present case) are set in *italics*, whereas the commentarial passages (i. e., passages from the *Vivaraṇa* in the present cases) are set in roman font.

116 TVai on PYŚ 2.47, ll. 16–21 in Appendix 3 below: *sāṃsiddhiko hi prayatnaḥ śarīradhārako na yogāṅgasyopadeṣṭavyasyāsanasya kāraṇam, tasya tatkāraṇatva upadeśavaiyarthyāt, svarasata eva siddheḥ. tasmād upadeṣṭavyasyāsanasyāyam asādhako viruddhaś ca svābhāvikaḥ prayatnaḥ, tasya yādṛcchikāsanahetutayāsananiyamopahantṛtvāt. tasmād upadiṣṭam āsanam abhyasyatā svābhāvikaprayatnaśaithilyāya prayatna āstheyaḥ. nānyathopadiṣṭam āsanaṃ sidhyati, iti svābhāvikaprayatnaśaithilyam āsanasiddhihetuḥ.*

117 YVā on PYŚ 2.47, p. 263, l. 6f., with the emendation of the unacceptable reading *prayatnaśaithilyasya dvāram* to *prayatnaśaithilyam asya dvāram*: *prayatnaśaithilyam asya dvāram āha – yena nāṅgeti.* bahuvyāpārānantaraṃ ced āsanaṃ kriyate tadāṅgakampanād āsanasthairyaṃ na bhavatīty āśayaḥ.

thinks of any kind of physical exercise like manual labour or walking longer distances.

3.3.2. Merging Meditatively into Infinity, or Meditating on the One who Supports the Earth

The second cause of a successful posture practice mentioned in YS 2.47 (as well as in the *bhāṣya*-part of PYŚ 2.47) is merging meditatively into infinity (*ānantya*), or, according to the majority of witnesses, a meditation on the mythical serpent Ananta ("the Infinite"). The reading "infinity" (*ānantya*) of the *sūtra* is transmitted only in the reconstructed basic text commented upon in the *Pātañjalayogaśāstravivaraṇa,* and in the two palm leaf manuscripts A^d and T^m. All other witnesses read the word "infinite" (*ananta*) instead. The distribution of the two variants among the textual witnesses is similar also for the *bhāṣya*-part of PYŚ 2.47. The manuscripts A^d, K^b, Pc^g and T^m, as well as the basic text commented upon in the *Pātañjalayogaśāstravivaraṇa,* read "infinity" (*ānantya*), whereas the 1904 edition of Āgāśe, manuscripts B^{n1}, B^{n2}, $B^{ś}$, Jai^n, K^{n1}, K^{n2}, M^{g2}, My^{t3} and P^n, and the basic text commented upon in the *Tattvavaiśāradī* transmit the word *ananta.*

According to Vācaspati, the word *ananta* refers to the name of a mythical serpent king who is believed to live in a certain underworld where he carries the earth on top of his thousand hoods.[118] Vācaspati explains that the mind of the yogi, on entering meditatively into Ananta, produces a posture:

> Alternatively, the mind produces a posture when it has merged meditatively into Ananta, the very steady one, the Leader of the Snakes, who supports the orb of the earth with his thousand hoods.[119]

Although Vācaspati does not specify how exactly this practice leads the yogi into a successful posture, it appears that the meditation aims at a transfer of bodily strength from the mythical serpent, the One who Supports the Earth, to the yogi. This view is in any case the basis of one of Vijñānabhikṣu's explanations of the word "infinite":

> "Infinite". Alternatively, even if one is making an effort, the mind brings about the posture when it has meditatively merged into the very steady serpent Śeṣa who supports the earth, when it has obtained his nature through mental fixation (*dhāraṇā*) on him. And the alternative is that it happens because of the grace of Ananta or because of the

118 See Sörensen 1904–1925: 199b for references to the version of the Ananta myth recorded in the *Mahābhārata.*

119 TVai on PYŚ 2.47, l. 22f. in Appendix 3 below: *anante vā nāganāyake sthiratare phaṇāsahasravidhṛtaviśvaṃbharāmaṇḍale samāpannaṃ cittam āsanaṃ nirvartayati, iti.*

power of meditating on an object belonging to a similar category, or because of the power of a special unseen force (*adṛṣṭa*).[120]

For Vijñānabhikṣu, fixing the mind on Ananta may lead to an increase of strength in the yogi's body. This, however, is not the only way in which a meditation on the serpentine supporter of the earth may lead to success in posture practice. A steady and comfortable posture may equally result from the grace that Ananta bestows upon the yogi, or from the mental fixation on a superhuman being that is as strong as Ananta. Finally, a perfect posture may result from some inexplicable force as the result of mental fixation.[121]

Although meditation on the mythological serpent Ananta apparently played an important role at least in the theory of South Asian yogic posture practice for several hundred years,[122] it is quite likely that Patañjali himself thought of the altogether different meditation of merging meditatively into infinity when he composed PYŚ 2.27.[123]

The term "merging meditatively into infinity" (*ānantyasamāpatti*) appears to be related to a series of prominent Buddhist meditation techniques called "Attainments of Formlessness" (*ārūpyasamāpatti* in Sanskrit and *āruppasamāpatti* in Pali),[124] which consist in meditations on the four so-called spheres of formlessness. According to Alexander Wynne, these meditations are of Brahmanical origin and were taught to the future Buddha by his two spiritual teachers Āḷāra Kālāma and Uddaka Rāmaputta.[125] In any case, even if these forms of spiritual training were developed a very long time before Patañjali composed and compiled the *Pātañjalayogaśāstra,* it is highly probable that at his time they were still very prominent.

The first sphere that the practitioner encounters in the Attainments of Formlessness is the "sphere of the infinity of space" (Skt. *ākāśānantyāyatana,* Pali *ākāsānañcāyatana*), which is followed by the "sphere of infinity of consciousness" (Skt. *vijñānānantyāyatana,* Pali *viññāṇānañcāyatana*). The aim of entering these stages of meditation is the cessation of sensations that in the course of the subsequent two attainments leads to contentless, i.e., uninten-

120 YVā on PYŚ 2.47, p. 263, ll. 6–10: *ananteti. atha vā prayatnaśālitve 'pi pṛthivīdhāriṇi sthiratarāśeṣanāge samāpannaṃ taddhāraṇayā tadātmatāpannaṃ cittam āsanaṃ niṣpādayatītyarthaḥ. tac cānantānugrahād vā sajātīyabhāvanāvaśād vādṛṣṭaviśeṣād vety anyad etat.*

121 On the concept of an unseen and inexplicable force (*adṛṣṭa*) see Halbfass 1991: 311–323.

122 In her chapter in the present volume (p. 577f.), Gudrun Bühnemann remarks that the nineteenth-century commentator Brahmānanda quotes a stanza recommending the veneration of Ananta as a means to success in *āsana* practice in his commentary on *Haṭhayogapradīpikā* 2.48. Even in modern *āsana*-centred yoga classes, the veneration of Ananta and Patañjali, who is frequently regarded as an incarnation of Ananta, is a common practice.

123 See also the chapter by Dominik Wujastyk in the present volume, p. 32ff.

124 See BHSD p. 104a, s. v. *ārūpya* and CPD p. 179b, s. v. *āruppa,* as well as Eimer 2006: 64.

125 See Wynne 2007, especially chapter 6.

tional, consciousness. If one considers the overlap between the Buddhist terms and the term *ānantyasamāpatti,* it is therefore very likely that Patañjali was familiar with the Buddhist formless attainments that he summarily called "merging meditatively in infinity".

Śaṅkara's commentary on PYŚ 2.47 supports this hypothesis:

> "Or from merging meditatively into infinity". Infinite means the All (*viśva*); infinity means being infinite. The steady mind (*citta*), being the All, having merged into that, i.e., having pervaded it (i.e., infinity), brings about, i.e., makes firm, the posture.[126]

According to this explanation, the mind of the yogi meditatively pervades the universe. This idea is strikingly similar to that of entering the "sphere of infinity of consciousness", even though the Buddhist notion of consciousness differs considerably from the Yoga conception of a material mind.

3.4. The Result of Posture Performance

According to YS 2.48, the primary effect of posture performance is "being not afflicted by the pairs of unpleasant sensations".[127] The term "pairs of unpleasant sensations" refers to sensations like that of heat and cold, or of extremes like hunger and thirst. The absence of these sensations enables the yogi to take up breath control and subsequently to stay in meditation for extended periods of time, possibly in a more or less unsheltered place, like, according to Śaṅkara's exposition, "in a pure place like a temple, mountain cave or sandbank of a river, that is not close to fire or water, where there are no people, and that is free from blemishes."[128]

4. Conclusions

In classical Yoga, the steady and comfortable posture is the outcome of two alternative practices. The posture may either result from a slackening of the yogi's effort, or from a meditation by which the mind merges into infinity. The aim of posture performance is to enable the yogi to stay in meditation for long

126 *Vivaraṇa* on PYŚ 2.47, ll. 39–41 in Appendix 2 below: *ānantye vā samāpannam* – anantaṃ viśvam, anantabhāva ānantyam, tasmin *samāpannam,* vyāpya viśvabhāvaṃ sthitaṃ *cittam āsanaṃ nirvartayati* draḍhayati.

127 PYŚ 2.48, l. 7f. in Appendix 1 below: *tato dvandvānabhighātaḥ* (YS 2.48) śītoṣṇādibhir dvandvair āsanajayān nābhibhūyate, iti.

128 *Vivaraṇa* on PYŚ 2.46, l. 5f. in Appendix 2 below: *śucau devanilayagiriguhānadīpulinādau jvalanasalilāsamīpe jantuvivarjite niraṅgaṇe.*

periods of time without sensations of his environment and without having to care for beverage or food. Accordingly, the technical term "posture" (*āsana*) refers in classical Yoga not only, or not even primarily, to a certain configuration of the body, but to a complex of psycho-physiological practices.

Patañjali does not provide detailed information on which postures yogis may perform. His work contains only a list of thirteen posture names that occurs at a highly unusual position in the middle of two parts of a single sentence. It is therefore very much conceivable, although not certain, that this list was interpolated in the *Pātañjalayogaśāstra* from a commentarial gloss on the word *āsana*. This gloss may have been motivated by a progressive diversification of posture practice in Yoga that had occurred between the fourth and the seventh centuries, or, in any case, before Śaṅkara composed his *Pātañjalayogaśāstravivaraṇa* and before the oldest common ancestor of all surviving manuscripts of the *Pātañjalayogaśāstra* was written.

In the course of the history of the theory of yoga practice as it is documented in the commentaries to Patañjali's work, slightly different postures were (or came to be) known by identical names. In still other cases, different names were applied to the same pose. And finally, one and the same name was used for an identical posture throughout the history of yoga. For example, the most famous yogic pose, the posture in which both feet rest on the opposite thighs is called "Lotus Posture" by Śaṅkara, whereas in Buddhist contexts this posture is called *paryaṅka,* and the Jaina scholar Hemacandra, as well as later sources, knows this pose under the name "Hero Posture". Moreover, the performance of the Good Fortune Posture that Śaṅkara describes differs considerably from the way it is described by Vācaspati, Hemacandra and Vijñānabhikṣu, who describe this posture in similar terms. Śaṅkara's description of the Good Fortune Posture agrees with Hemacandra's account of the Half Lotus posture and it is similar to Vijñānabhikṣu's description of the Hero Posture. All three commentators of the *Pātañjalayogaśāstra* agree in their explanations of the terms Lucky Mark Posture (or Lucky Mark) and Couch Posture (or Couch).

In spite of these differences, all descriptions agree in that the common characteristic of all postures whose names are listed in the *Pātañjalayogaśāstra* is their static nature, i.e., the absence of any bodily movement during their performance. Moreover, the large majority of postures, according to all four accounts, are seated poses. This differentiates the *āsana*-s of classical Yoga from many postures that became common in later yoga traditions.[129]

129 On innovations in posture practice during the late Middle Ages, see the chapter by Jason Birch in the present volume.

Appendices

General Introduction to the Critically Edited Text Passages in Appendices 1, 2 and 3

For the convenience of the reader, the text passages critically edited below include the numeration of *sūtra*-s found in other editions of the text even though the most important manuscripts do not have any numeration at all, whereas the numerations in less relevant manuscripts, mostly paper manuscripts, frequently differ from each other.

In the critically edited text, wavy underlines indicate that the reconstruction of the text is uncertain and that at least one viable alternative exists among the recorded variants. These variants are also highlighted in the critical apparatus by a wavy underline if there is more than one variant to the critically edited text.

The word forms resulting from the application of the euphonic rules of Sanskrit (*sandhi*) have been standardised in the critically edited text, regardless of which word forms occur in the manuscripts. Moreover, punctuation marks have been introduced that are based on the interpretation of the text; the actual punctuation marks, if any, in the manuscripts were not taken into consideration.

The critical apparatuses are arranged according to lemmata extracted from the critically edited text in order to record variant readings. The variants are recorded for all witnesses in the following way: First, the sigla of witnesses supporting the reading of the critically edited text are listed. Then, separated by a semicolon, the first variant reading is recorded. This is followed by a list of sigla of witnesses that read this variant, etc. Sometimes the reading of a certain witness is not available due to a longer lacuna in the text or because the reconstruction of the basic text commented upon in a commentary is impossible due to a lack of reference to this text portion. In this case, the lack of information is indicated by a dagger (†) in place of the reading of the respective witness.

The recording of variants is limited to substantial variants. This means that the apparatus does not contain minor variants that can be interpreted as simple scribal slips, unless such variants can be used to infer the existence of significant variants in an exemplar of the respective witness.

Abbreviations Used in the Critically Edited Text Passages

ac ante correctionem, i e., the reading of a manuscript before a correction was applied.
em. emendation, i. e., the reading is the result of a correction or improvement made by the editor in cases when all witnesses transmit an unacceptable text version.
om. omitted, i. e., the text of the lemma is missing in the listed witness(es).

^{2}pc The reading of a manuscript post correctionem after a correction was made by a second hand, i. e., by a different person than the original scribe of the manuscript.

Appendix 1: A Critical Edition of Patañjali's Passage on Postures (PYŚ 2.46–48)

This edition is based on the following sixteen witnesses of the *Pātañjalayoga-śāstra:*

Siglum	Witness
P^{E}	The *Pātañjalayogaśāstra* as edited in Āgāśe 1904, pp. 110, l. 1 – p. 111, l. 9 (edition no. 5 in Maas 2006: xxiii–xxv).
A^{d}	Digital images of a Xerox copy of a ms. of the *Pātañjalayogaśāstra* in Devanāgarī script on palm leaf. Lālbhaī Dalpatbhaī Saṃskṛti Vidyāmandir, Ahmedabad. Acc. no. 344.
B^{n1}	Microfilm images of the *Pātañjalayogaśāstra* in Devanāgarī script on paper. Central Library, Baroda. Acc. no. 11088, serial no. 64 (in Nambiyar 1942) (ms. no. 1 in Maas 2006: xxxix).
B^{n2}	Microfilm images of the *Pātañjalayogaśāstra* in Devanāgarī script on paper. Central Library, Baroda. Acc. no. 341, serial no. 61 (in Nambiyar 1942) (ms. no. 2 in Maas 2006: xxxixf.).
$B^{ś}$	Microfilm images of the *Pātañjalayogaśāstra* in Śāradā script on paper. Central Library, Baroda. Acc. no. 1831, serial no. 62 (in Nambiyar 1942) (ms. no. 3 in Maas 2006: xli).
Jai^{n}	Digital images of the *Pātañjalayogaśāstra* in Devanāgarī script on paper. Maharaja Sawai Man Singh II Museum, Jaipur. Ms. no. 2285 (in Bahura 1976).
K^{b}	NGMPP microfilm images of the *Pātañjalayogaśāstra* in Old Bengali script on palm leaf. National Archives, Kathmandu. Ms. no. 5–2672, reel no. B 40/2 (ms. no. 8 in Maas 2006: xlvf.).
K^{n1}	NGMPP microfilm images of the *Pātañjalayogaśāstra* in Devanāgarī script on paper. National Archives, Kathmandu. Ms. no. 61, reel no. A 61/11 (ms. no. 5 in Maas 2006: xliii.).
K^{n2}	NGMPP microfilm images of the *Pātañjalayogaśāstra* in Devanāgarī script on paper. National Archives, Kathmandu. Ms. no. 1–1337, reel no. A 62–32 (ms. no. 6 in Maas 2006: xliv).
M^{g2}	Digital images of the *Pātañjalayogaśāstra* in Grantha script on palm leaf. Government Oriental Manuscript Library, Chennai. Shelf no. R 1508, serial no. 11606 (in Kuppuswami Sastri & Subrahmanya Sastri 1938).
My^{t3}	Digital images of the *Pātañjalayogaśāstra* in Telugu script on palm leaf. Oriental Research Institute, Mysore. Shelf no. P 1560/5, serial no. 35065 (in Marulasiddhaiah 1984) (ms. no. 24 in Maas 2006: lxvi).
P^{n}	Digital images of the *Pātañjalayogaśāstra* in Devanāgarī script on paper. Jayakar Knowledge Resource Centre, Savitribai Phule Pune University (formerly Jayakar Library). Shelf no. 2742 (ms. no. 19 in Maas 2006: lix).

(Continued)

Siglum	Witness
Pc^{g}	Digital images of the *Pātañjalayogaśāstra* in Grantha script on palm leaf. École Française d'Extrême-Orient, Centre de Pondichéry, Pondicherry. Shelf no. 287 (ms. no. 15 in Maas 2006: liv).
T^{m}	Digital images of the *Pātañjalayogaśāstra* in Malayāḷam script on palm leaf. Oriental Research Institute, Thiruvananthapuram (Trivandrum). Shelf no. 622, serial no. 14371 (in Bhaskaran 1984) (ms. no. 21 in Maas 2006: lx–lxii.).
TV	The basic text of the *Tattvavaiśāradī* as reconstructed from the critical edition in Appendix 3.
YVi	The basic text commented upon in the *Pātañjalayogaśāstravivaraṇa*, reconstructed according to the critical edition in Appendix 2 below.

Beginning of text in the manuscripts and in the printed edition: A^{d} 38v1, B^{n1} 17r10, B^{n2} 22v10, B^{ś} 14r9, Jai^{n} 29v4, K^{b} 31r3, K^{n1} 12r6, K^{n2} 36v1, M^{g2} 22v5, My^{t3} 13v6, P^{E} p. 110, l. 13, P^{n} 42r4, Pc^{g} 25r2, T^{m} 61r4.

uktāḥ saha siddhibhir yamaniyamāḥ, āsanādīnīdānīṃ vakṣyāmaḥ. tatra *sthirasukham āsanam* (*sūtra* 2.46) – tad yathā: padmāsanaṃ bhadrāsanaṃ vīrāsanaṃ svastikāsanaṃ daṇḍāsanaṃ sopāśrayaṃ paryaṅkāsanaṃ krauñcaniṣadanaṃ hastiniṣadanam uṣṭraniṣadanaṃ samasaṃsthānaṃ sthiraprasrabdhir yathāsukhaṃ cety evamādi – *prayatnaśaithilyānantyasamāpattibhyām* (*sūtra* 2.47) bhavati, iti vākyaśeṣaḥ. prayatnoparamād vā sidhyaty āsanam, yena nāṅgamejayo bhavati, ānantye vā samāpannaṃ cittam āsanaṃ nirvartayati, iti. *tato dvandvānabhighātaḥ* (*sūtra* 2.48) śītoṣṇādibhir dvandvair āsanajayān nābhibhūyate, iti.

Variant readings: **2.46 āsanādīnīdānīṃ**] *em.*; āsanādīn ādānīṃ A^{d}; īdānīm āsanādīnī YVi; āsanam īdānīṃ Jai^{n} TV; āsanādīni P^{E} B^{n1} B^{n2} B^{ś} K^{b} K^{n1} K^{n2} M^{g2} My^{t3} P^{n} Pc^{g} T^{m} **tad yathā**] *not reflected in the Vivaraṇa* **bhadrāsanaṃ vīrāsanaṃ**] A^{d} K^{b} M^{g2} My^{t3} TV YVi; vīrāsanaṃ bhadrāsanaṃ B^{n1} B^{ś} Jai^{n} K^{n1} K^{n2} P^{n}; bhadrāsanaṃ P^{E} Pc^{g} T^{m}; vīrāsanaṃ B^{n2} **svastikāsanaṃ**] Jai^{n} M^{g2}; svastikam āsanam YVi; svastikaṃ P^{E} A^{d} B^{n1} B^{n2} B^{ś} K^{b} K^{n1} K^{n2} My^{t3} Pc^{g} P^{n} T^{m} TV **daṇḍāsanaṃ**] P^{E} B^{n1} B^{n2} B^{ś} Jai^{n} (^{2}*pc*) K^{b} K^{n1} K^{n2} My^{t3} M^{g2} Pc^{g} P^{n} T^{m} YVi TV; daṇḍāyataṃ A^{d}; *om.* Jai^{n} (*ac*) **paryaṅkāsanaṃ**] YVi; paryaṅkaṃ P^{E} A^{d} B^{n1} B^{n2} B^{ś} Jai^{n} (*ac*) K^{b} K^{n1} K^{n2} M^{g2} Pc^{g} P^{n} T^{m}; paryaṃkaḥ Jai^{n} (^{2}*pc*) TV; paryaṅkaniṣadanaṃ My^{t3} **krauñca-**] P^{E} A^{d} B^{n2} B^{ś} K^{b} K^{n1} M^{g2} My^{t3} P^{n} Pc^{g} T^{m} YVi TV; kroṃca B^{n1} Jai^{n} K^{n2} **-niṣadanaṃ**] P^{E} A^{d} B^{n1} B^{n2} B^{ś} Jai^{n} K^{n1} K^{n2} M^{g2} My^{t3} P^{n} Pc^{g} T^{m} YVi TV; niṣadaṃ K^{b} **hastiniṣadanam uṣṭraniṣadanaṃ**] *glossed with* -ādīni *in the TVai* **hasti-**] P^{E} A^{d} B^{n1} B^{n2} Jai^{n} K^{b} K^{n1} K^{n2} M^{g2} My^{t3} P^{n} Pc^{g} T^{m} YVi; haṃsa B^{ś}; † TV **-niṣadanaṃ**] P^{E} A^{d} B^{n1} B^{n2} B^{ś} Jai^{n} K^{n1} K^{n2} M^{g2} My^{t3} P^{n} Pc^{g} T^{m} YVi; niṣadaṃ K^{b}; † TV **uṣṭraniṣadanaṃ**] P^{E} A^{d} B^{n1} B^{n2} B^{ś} Jai^{n} K^{b} K^{n1} K^{n2} M^{g2} P^{n} Pc^{g} T^{m} YVi; *om.*

My^{t3}; † TV **samasaṃsthānaṃ**] P^E B^{n1} B^{n2} $B^{\text{ś}}$ Jai^n K^b K^{n1} K^{n2} M^{g2} My^{t3} P^n Pc^g T^m TV; samasaṃsthitam YVi; samāsasthānaṃ A^d **sthira-**] P^E B^{n1} B^{n2} $B^{\text{ś}}$ Jai^n K^b K^{n1} K^{n2} M^{g2} My^{t3} P^n TV; sthita A^d Pc^g T^m YVi **-prasrabdhir**] YVi; prasyabdhir T^m; prasravidhiḥ A^d; prasrabdhaṃ K^b TV; prajñaṃ Pc^g; sukhaṃ P^E B^{n1} B^{n2} $B^{\text{ś}}$ Jai^n K^{n1} K^{n2} M^{g2} My^{t3} P^n **yathāsukhaṃ**] P^E A^d B^{n1} B^{n2} $B^{\text{ś}}$ Jai^n K^b K^{n1} K^{n2} M^{g2} Pc^g P^n T^m YVi TV; *om.* $B^{\text{ś}}$ **cety evamādi**] A^d B^{n1} B^{n2} $B^{\text{ś}}$ K^{n2} Jai^n M^{g2} Pc^g; cety evamādiḥ K^{n1}; caivam ity ādi T^m; ceti TV; cetyādi K^b My^{t3} YVi (?); cety evamādīni P^E P^n

2.47 -śaithilyānantya-] T^m YVi; saithilyānantya A^d; śaithilyānanta P^E B^{n1} B^{n2} $B^{\text{ś}}$ Jai^n K^{n1} K^{n2} M^{g2} My^{t3} Pc^g P^n TV; † K^b **bhavati ... bhavati**] *not reflected in the TVai* **bhavati, iti**] P^E A^d B^{n1} B^{n2} $B^{\text{ś}}$ Jai^n K^b K^{n1} K^{n2} M^{g2} My^{t3} Pc^g P^n YVi; bhavati T^m; † TV **vākya-**] P^E A^d B^{n2} Jai^n K^b K^{n1} K^{n2} M^{g2} My^{t3} Pc^g P^n T^m YVi; vākye B^{n1}; *om.* $B^{\text{ś}}$; † TV **vā**] A^d M^{g2} T^m YVi; *om.* P^E B^{n1} B^{n2} $B^{\text{ś}}$ Jai^n K^b K^{n1} K^{n2} My^{t3} P^n Pc^g; † TV **āsanam**] *not reflected in the Vivaraṇa*; † TV **nāṅgamejayo**] P^E A^d B^{n1} B^{n2} $B^{\text{ś}}$ Jai^n K^b K^{n1} K^{n2} M^{g2} My^{t3} P^n YVi; aṃgajayo Pc^g; aṅgamejayo T^m; † TV **bhavati**] P^E A^d B^{n1} B^{n2} $B^{\text{ś}}$ Jai^n K^b K^{n1} K^{n2} M^{g2} P^n Pc^g T^m YVi; na bhavati My^{t3}; † TV **ānantye**] A^d K^b T^m YVi; evānantye Pc^g; anante P^E B^{n1} B^{n2} $B^{\text{ś}}$ Jai^n K^{n1} K^{n2} M^{g2} My^{t3} P^n TV **samāpannaṃ**] P^E A^d B^{n1} B^{n2} $B^{\text{ś}}$ Jai^n K^{n1} K^{n2} M^{g2} My^{t3} P^n T^m YVi TV; samāpanna K^b Pc^g **nirvartayati**] P^E B^{n1} B^{n2} $B^{\text{ś}}$ Jai^n K^b K^{n1} K^{n2} M^{g2} My^{t3} TV YVi; nivartayati A^d Pc^g P^n T^m **iti**] P^E B^{n1} B^{n2} $B^{\text{ś}}$ Jai^n K^{n1} K^{n2} M^{g2} My^{t3} P^n Pc^g T^m TV; *om.* A^d YVi; † K^b

2.48 dvandvānabhighātaḥ] P^E A^d B^{n1} B^{n2} $B^{\text{ś}}$ Jai^n K^{n1} K^{n2} M^{g2} Pc^g P^n T^m YVi TV; dvandvābhighātaḥ My^{t3}; † K^b **śītoṣṇādibhir ... nābhibhūyate**] *not reflected in the TVai* **śītoṣṇādibhir**] P^E A^d B^{n1} B^{n2} Jai^n K^{n1} K^{n2} My^{t3} M^{g2} Pc^g P^n T^m YVi; śītoṣṇādi $B^{\text{ś}}$; † TV **āsanajayān**] *not reflected in the Vivaraṇa* **nābhibhūyate**] P^E A^d B^{n1} B^{n2} $B^{\text{ś}}$ Jai^n K^b K^{n1} K^{n2} M^{g2} My^{t3} Pc^g P^n YVi TV; nabhibhūta T^m **iti**] A^d $B^{\text{ś}}$ K^b M^{g2} My^{t3} Pc^g T^m; *om.* P^E B^{n1} B^{n2} Jai^n K^{n1} K^{n2} P^n; *not reflected in the Vivaraṇa*; † TV

Appendix 2: A Critical Edition of the Posture Passage of the *Pātañjalayogaśāstravivaraṇa* (*Vivaraṇa* 2.46–48)

This edition is based on the following witnesses of the *Pātañjalayogaśāstra-vivaraṇa:*

Siglum	Witness
M^E	*Pātañjala-Yogasūtra-Bhāṣya-Vivaraṇa of Śaṅkara-Bhagavatpāda, Critically Edited with Introduction by [...] Polakam Sri Rama Sastri [...] and S. R. Krishnamurthi Sastri [...].* Madras Government Oriental Series 94. Madras: Government Oriental Manuscript Library, 1952, pp. 225, l. 10 – 227, l. 13 (for details, see Harimoto 2014: 24f.).

(Continued)

Siglum	Witness
L	Digital images of the *Pātañjalayogaśāstravivaraṇa* on palm leaf in Malayāḷam script. Punjab University Library, Lahore. Serial no. 428 (in Sahai Shastri & Ram 1941), fols. 80r9 - 81r10 (for details, see Harimoto 2014: 19f.).
T_m	Digital images of the *Pātañjalayogaśāstravivaraṇa* on palm leaf in Malayāḷam script from the Oriental Manuscript Library, Trivandrum. Serial no. 14385 (in Bhaskaran 1984), ms. no. L 662, fols. 80v5 - 81r8 (for details, see Harimoto 2014: 20–23).

2.46 *uktāḥ saha siddhibhir yamaniyamāḥ. idānīm āsanādīni vakṣyāmaḥ - tatra sthirasukham āsanam* (*sūtra* 2.46). sthiraṃ sukhaṃ cāsanam. yasminn āsane sthitasya manogātrāṇām upajāyate sthiratvam, duḥkhaṃ ca yena na bhavati tad abhyasyet. tathā śāstrāntaraprasiddhāni nāmāni padmāsanādīni pradarśyante.

tatra śucau devanilayagiriguhānadīpulinādau jvalanasalilāsamīpe jantuvivarjite niraṅgaṇe śuciḥ samyag ācamya parameśvaram akhilabhuvanaikanātham abhivandhyānyāṃś ca yogeśvarān ātmagurūṃś ca praṇipatya, cailājinakuśottaram aduḥkhakaraṃ prāṅmukha udaṅmukho vā viṣṭaram adhiṣṭhāya, anyatamad eṣām āsanaṃ nirbadhnīyāt.

tatra *padmāsanaṃ* nāma - savyaṃ pādam upasaṃhṛtya dakṣiṇopari nidadhīta, tathaiva dakṣiṇaṃ savyasyopariṣṭāt. kaṭyurogrīvaṃ ca viṣṭabhya mṛtasuptavan nāsikāgranihitadṛṣṭiḥ, samudgakavad apihitoṣṭhasaṃpuṭaḥ, dantair dantāgram aparāmṛśan, muṣṭimātrāntaraviprakṛṣṭacibukoraḥsthalaḥ rājadantāntaranihitarasanāgraḥ, hastau ca pārṣṇyor upari kacchapakaṃ brahmāñjaliṃ vā kṛtvā, sakṛdāsthāpitetthaṃsaṃsthānaḥ, punaḥpunaḥśarīrāvayavavinyāsaviśeṣaparityaktaprayatnaḥ san, yenāsīta, tat padmāsanam. etac ca sarvam anyeṣām āsanānām api tulyam. kaścid eva viśeṣaḥ.

tathā dakṣiṇaṃ pādaṃ savyasyopari kṛtvā, hastaṃ ca dakṣiṇaṃ savyahastasyopari nidhāya, yenāste, tad *bhadrāsanam*. anyat samānam.

tathākuñcitānyatarapādam avanivinyastāparajānukaṃ *vīrāsanam*. ucyamāna eva viśeṣaḥ sarvatra.

dakṣiṇaṃ pādāṅguṣṭhaṃ savyenorujaṅghena parigṛhyādṛśyaṃ kṛtvā, tathā savyaṃ pādāṅguṣṭhaṃ dakṣiṇenorujaṅghenādṛśyaṃ parigṛhya, yathā ca pārṣṇibhyāṃ vṛṣaṇayor apīḍanaṃ tathā yenāste, tat *svastikam āsanam*.

samagulphau samāṅguṣṭhau prasārayan samajānū pādau daṇḍavad yenopaviśet, tad *daṇḍāsanam.*

sayogapaṭṭaṃ sastambhādyāśrayaṃ vā *sopāśrayam.*

ājānuprasāritabāhuśayanaṃ *paryaṅkāsanam. krauñcaniṣadanaṃ hastiniṣadanam uṣṭraniṣadanaṃ* ca krauñcādiniṣadanasaṃsthānasādṛśyād eva draṣṭavyam.

bhūmau nyastam ūrujaṅghaṃ *samasaṃsthitam.*

sthitaprasrabdhiḥ – anyenāpi prakāreṇa svayamutprekṣyā sthitaprasrabdhir anāyāso yena bhavati tad apy āsanaṃ sthitaprasrabdhir nāma.

yathāsukhaṃ ca – yena rūpeṇāsīnasya sukhaṃ bhavati tad yathāsukham. *ādi*śabdād anyad api yathācāryopadiṣṭam āsanaṃ draṣṭavyam.

2.47 tadāsanajayābhyupāya idānīm upapādyate – *prayatnaśaithilyānantyasamāpattibhyām (sūtra* 2.47), *bhavatīti vākyaśeṣaḥ.* āsanaṃ dṛḍhaniṣpannaṃ bhavatīty upaskāraḥ. *prayatnoparamād* āsanabandhottarakālaṃ prayatnākaraṇād *vā sidhyati. yena nāṅgamejayo bhavati.* yena prayatnoparameṇa, prayatnena hy aṅgaṃ kampayati, yenācalitāsano bhavatīty arthaḥ. *ānantye vā samāpannam* – anantaṃ viśvam, anantabhāva ānantyam, tasmin *samāpannam.* vyāpya viśvabhāvaṃ sthitaṃ *cittam āsanaṃ nirvartayati* draḍhayati.

2.48 tato dvandvānabhighātaḥ (sūtra 2.48). tataḥ āsanasthirībhāvāt. idaṃ dṛṣṭam ānuṣāṅgikam, yac chītoṣṇādibhir dvandvair nābhibhūyate.

Variant readings: **2.46 tathā**] L T_m; tadyathā M^E **deva-**] M^E T_m; daiva L **niraṅgaṇe**] *em.*; nirāṃgake L T_m; nira(ṅga)śmake M^E **abhivandhyānyāṃś**] M^E T_m; abhivadhyānaṃś L **mṛta-**] *em.*; mṛ(ga)ta M^E; mṛga L T_m **samudgakavad-**] M^E T_m; samutgavad L **cibukoraḥ-**] M^E L; citbukoras T_m **rājadantāntara**] T_m; rājaddantāntara M^E L **ca**] L_m; *om.* M^E T_m **vinyāsaviśeṣa**] *em.*; śarīravinyāsaviśeṣa M^E; viśeṣavinyāsaviśeṣa L T_m **savyaṃ**] M^E; savyama L T_m **sayoga-**] L T_m; (na)yoga M^E **-paṭṭaṃ**] L T_m; paṭṭa M^E **sa-**] L T_m; saṃ[sthaṃ] M^E **sopāśrayam**] M^E; sāpāśrayam T_m; sāpāśram L **krauñcādi**] L T_m; kauñcādi M^E **nyastam ūrujaṅghaṃ**] *em.*; nyastorujaṅghaṃ L M^E T_m **-saṃsthitam**] L T_m; saṃsthānam M^E **utprekṣyā**] L T_m; utprekṣya M^E

Appendix 3: A Critical Edition of the Posture Passage of the *Tattvavaiśāradī* (TVai 2.46–48)

This edition is based on the following witnesses of the *Tattvavaiśāradī:*

Siglum	Witness
J_{TV}	Digital images of the *Tattvavaiśāradī* in Devanāgarī on palm leaf. Ms. no. 395/2 in the *Jinabhadrasūri tāḍapatrīya graṃth bhaṃḍār - jaisalmer durg* (in Jambuvijaya 2000), fols. 91r5 - 92r3.
P^E	Printed ed. Āgāśe 1904, p. 110, l. 26 - p. 112, l. 13.
V^E	Printed ed. Nārāyaṇamiśra 1971, p. 261, l. 14 - p. 263, l. 14.

2.46 uktāḥ saha siddhibhir yamaniyamāḥ. *āsanam idānīṃ vakṣyāmaḥ. tatra sthinam. sthiraṃ* niścalaṃ yat sukhaṃ sukhāvahaṃ tad āsanam iti sūtrārthaḥ. āsyata āste vānenety āsanam. tasya prabhedān āha - *tadyatheti. padmāsanaṃ* prasiddham. pādatale dve vṛṣaṇasamīpe saṃpuṭīkṛtya tasyopari pāṇikacchapikāṃ kuryād etad *bhadrāsanam.* sthitasyaikataraḥ pādo bhūnyasta ekataraś cākuñcitajānur bhūrdhvam ity etad *vīrāsanam.* savyam ākuñcitaṃ caraṇaṃ dakṣiṇajaṅghorvantare kṣipet, dakṣiṇaṃ cākuñcitaṃ vāmajaṅghorvantare, tad etat *svastikam.* upaviśya śliṣṭāṅgulīkau śliṣṭagulphau bhūmiśliṣṭajaṅghorū pādau prasārya *daṇḍāsanam* abhyasyet. yogapaṭṭakayogāt *sopāśrayam.* jānuprasāritabāhoḥ śayanaṃ *paryaṅkaḥ. krauñcaniṣadanā*dīni krauñcādīnāṃ niṣaṇṇānāṃ saṃsthānadarśanāt pratyetavyāni. pārṣṇyagrapādābhyāṃ dvayor ākuñcitayor anyonyapīḍanaṃ *samasaṃsthānam.* yena saṃsthānenāvasthitasya sthairyaṃ sukhaṃ sidhyati tad āsanaṃ *sthiraprasrabdham.* tatra bhagavataḥ sūtrakārasya saṃmatam. tasya vivaraṇam - *yathāsukhaṃ ceti.*

2.47 āsanasvarūpam uktvā tatsādhanam āha - *prabhyām.*

sāṃsiddhiko hi prayatnaḥ śarīradhārako na yogāṅgasyopadeṣṭavyasyāsanasya kāraṇam, tasya tatkāraṇatva upadeśavaiyarthyāt, svarasata eva siddheḥ. tasmād upadeṣṭavyasyāsanasyāyam asādhako viruddhaś ca svābhāvikaḥ prayatnaḥ, tasya yādṛcchikāsanahetutayāsananiyamopahantṛtvāt. tasmād upadiṣṭam āsanam abhyasyatā svābhāvikaprayatnaśaithilyāya prayatna āstheyo nānyathopadiṣṭam āsanaṃ sidhyati, iti svābhāvikaprayatnaśaithilyam āsanasiddhihetuḥ.

anante vā nāganāyake sthiratare phaṇāsahasravidhṛtaviśvaṃbharāmaṇḍale samāpannaṃ cittam āsanaṃ nirvartayati, iti.

24 2.48 āsanavijayasūcakam āha – *tataḥ*. nigadavyākhyātaṃ bhāṣyam. āsanam apy uktaṃ viṣṇupurāṇe – ekaṃ bhadrāsanādīnāṃ samāsthāya guṇair yutam | iti (*Viṣṇupurāṇa* 6.7.39ab).

Variant readings: **2.46 āsanam idānīṃ**] J_{TV} āsanādīni P^E V^E **vakṣyāmaḥ**] J_{TV} P^E; vakṣyāma iti V^E **tatra sthinaṃ**] J_{TV}; tatra sthirasukham āsanam P^E V^E **yad**] P^E V^E; (sra)dyat J_{TV} **āsyate**] J_{TV} P^E; āsyate 'tra P^E (ka, jha) V^E **vānenety**] P^E V^E; vā[tya] anenety J_{TV} **pādatale … bhadrāsanaṃ**] J_{TV}; *transposed to after* vīrāsana P^E V^E **dve**] J_{TV}; *om.* P^E V^E **-samīpe**] P^E V^E; samī[pa]⟨pe⟩ **etad**] J_{TV}; tad P^E V^E **bhadrāsanam**] P^E V^E; bhadrasanaṃ J_{TV} **sthitasyaikataraḥ**] P^E V^E; sthitaḥsyaikataraḥ J_{TV} **cākuñcitajānur bhūrdhvam**] *em.*; cākuñcitajānubhūrdhvam J_{TV}; cākuñcitajānor upari nyasta P^E V^E **kṣipet**] J_{TV}; nikṣipet V^E; *om.* P^E **cākuñcitaṃ**] J_{TV}; cākuñcitaṃ caraṇaṃ P^E V^E **vāmajaṅghorvantare**] J_{TV}; vāmajaṅghorvantare nikṣipet P^E V^E **tad**] J_{TV}; *om.* P^E V^E -jaṅghorupādau] **-jaṅghorū pādau**] J_{TV}; -jaṅghorupādau P^E V^E **daṇḍāsanam**] P^E; daṇḍāsa⟨na⟩m J_{TV}; caṇḍāsanam V^E **sopāśrayam**] P^E V^E; sāpāśrayaṃ J_{TV} **pārṣṇyagrapādābhyāṃ**] J_{TV} P^E; pārṣṇipādāgrābhyāṃ P^E (jha) V^E **-pīḍanam**] J_{TV}; saṃpīḍanam P^E V^E; **samasaṃsthānam**] P^E V^E; samasthānaṃ J_{TV} **sthairyaṃ**] J_{TV} P^E V^E; sthairya P^E (kha ja) **sukhaṃ**] J_{TV} P^E (kha ja jha); sukhaṃ ca P^E V^E **sthira**] P^E V^E sthiraṃ J_{TV} **prasrabdham**] J_{TV}; sukham V^E; mukham P^E **tatra**] J_{TV} P^E (ja); tad etat P^E; tat tatra P^E (ka jha); tad etat tatra V^E **bhagavataḥ**] P^E V^E; bhavataḥ J_{TV}

2.47 prabhyām] *em.*; prabhyam J_{TV}; prayatnaśaitilyānantasamāpattibhyām P^E V^E **sāṃsiddhiko**] J_{TV}; sa sāṃsiddhiko P^E V^E **yogāṅgasyopadeṣṭavyasyāsanasya**] J_{TV} V^E; yogāṅgasyopadeṣṭavyāsanasya P^E **kāraṇam tasya**] P^E V^E; *om.* J_{TV} (*ac*) **svarasata**] P^E V^E; svaraśata J_{TV} **viruddhaś**] J_{TV}; virodhī P^E V^E **tasya**] J_{TV}; tasya ca P^E V^E **upadiṣṭam āsanam**] J_{TV}; upadiṣṭaniyamāsanam P^E V^E **-śaithilyāya**] P^E; saithilyāya J_{TV}; śaitilyātmā P^E (kha ja) V^E **-śaithilyam**] P^E V^E; saithilyam J_{TV} **sthiratare**] J_{TV} P^E (kha ja); sthiratara P^E V^E **-sahasra-**] P^E V^E; sahśra J_{TV}

2.48 tataḥ] J_{TV}; tato dvaṃdvānabhighātaḥ P^E V^E **ekaṃ**] J_{TV}; evaṃ P^E V^E

References

Acharya, D. (2006). *Vācaspatimiśra's Tattvasamīkṣā: The Earliest Commentary on Maṇḍanamiśra's Brahmasiddhi. Critically Edited with an Introduction and Critical Notes.* Nepal Research Centre Publications 25. Stuttgart: Steiner.

Āgāśe, K. Ś. (Ed.). (1904). *VācaspatimiśraviracitaṭīkāsaṃvalitaVyāsabhāṣyasametāni Pātañjalayogasūtrāṇi tathā BhojadevaviracitaRājamārtaṇḍābhidhavṛttisametāni Pātañjalayogasūtrāṇi.* Ānandāśramasaṃskṛtagranthāvaliḥ 47. Puṇyākhyapattana: Ānandāśramamudraṇālaya.

Ahirbudhnyasaṃhitā
see Malaviya 2007.

Apte, V. S. A. (1957–1959). *Revised and Enlarged Edition of V. S. Apte's The Practical Sanskrit-English Dictionary*, ed. by P. K. Gode [...] and C. G. Karve [...] [et al.]. 3 vols. Poona: Prasad Prakashan.

Bahura, G. N. (1976). *Literary Heritage of the Rulers of Amber and Jaipur: With an Index to the Register of Manuscripts in the Pothikhana of Jaipur. <1. Khasmohor Collection.>* Maharaja Sawai Man Singh II Memorial Series 2. Jaipur: Maharaja Sawai Man Singh II Museum, City Palace Jaipur.

Bandini-König, D. (2003). Von Kranichen, Brachvögeln und 'Wildenten': Einige Anmerkungen zu ornithologischen Bestimmungen auf der Grundlage von Sanskrit-Texten. *Studien zur Indologie und Iranistik, 23*, 27–50.

Bhagavadgītā
see MBh.

Bhaskaran, T. (1984). *Alphabetical Index of Sanskrit Manuscripts in the Oriental Research Institute and Manuscript Library, Trivandrum.* Vol. 3: *ya to ṣa.* Trivandrum Sanskrit Series 254. Trivandrum: Oriental Research Institute and Manuscript Library, University of Kerala.

BHSD. F. Edgerton, *Buddhist Hybrid Sanskrit Grammar and Dictionary.* Vol. 2: *Dictionary.* William Dwight Whitney Linguistic Series. New Haven: Yale University Press, 1953.

Birch, J. (2011). The Meaning of haṭha in Early Haṭhayoga. *Journal of the American Oriental Society, 131*(4), 527–554.

Bryant, E. F. (2009). *The Yoga Sūtras of Patañjali: A New Edition, Translation and Commentary.* New York: North Point Press.

Buddhacarita
see Johnston 1936.

Bühler, G. (1896). *Indische Palaeographie von ca. 350 a. Chr. – ca. 1300 p. Chr.* Vol. 2: *Tafelband.* Grundriss der indo-arischen Philologie und Altertumskunde 1.11. Strassburg: Trübner.

Bühnemann, G. (1988). *Pūjā: A Study in Smārta Ritual.* Publications of the De Nobili Research Library 15. Vienna: Sammlung De Nobili.

Bühnemann, G. (2011). The Śāradātilakatantra on Yoga: A New Edition and Translation of Chapter 25. *Bulletin of the School of Oriental and African Studies, 74*(2), 205–235.

CPD. Det Kongelige Danske Videnskabernes Selskab (Ed.), A Critical Pāli Dictionary. Vol. 2: ā – ohīḷeti. Copenhagen: Munksgaard, 1990.

D. *Dīghanikāya. The Dīgha Nikāya*, vol. 1, ed. T. W. Rhys Davids & J. E. Carpenter. London: Luzac & Co, 1967.

Eimer, H. (2006). *Buddhistische Begriffsreihen als Skizzen des Erlösungsweges.* Grundlegende Neubearbeitung. Wien: Arbeitskreis für Tibetische und Buddhistische Studien, Universität Wien.

Filliozat, P.-S. (Trans). (2005). *Le Yogabhāṣya de Vyāsa sur le Yogasūtra de Patañjali.* Paris: Éd. Āgamāt.

Golzio, K.-H. (2008). Zur Datierung des Kuṣāṇa-Königs Kaniṣka I. In D. Dimitrov et al. (Eds.), *Bauddhasāhityastabakāvalī: Essays and Studies on Buddhist Sanskrit Literature Dedicated to Claus Vogel by Colleagues, Students, and Friends* (pp. 79–91). Indica et Tibetica 36. Marburg: Indica et Tibetica.

Gonda, J. (1980). *Vedic Ritual: The Non-Solemn Rites.* Handbuch der Orientalistik. Zweite Abteilung, Indien. Religionen 4.1. Leiden: Brill.

Goudriaan, T. & Gupta, S. (1981). *Hindu Tantric and Śākta Literature.* A History of Indian Literature 2.2. Wiesbaden: Harrassowitz.

Halbfass, W. (1991). *Tradition and Reflection: Explorations in Indian Thought.* New York: State University of New York Press.

Harimoto, K. (2014). *God, Reason, and Yoga: A Critical Edition and Translation of the Commentary Ascribed to Śaṅkara on Pātañjalayogaśāstra 1.23–28.* Indian and Tibetan Studies 1. Hamburg: Department of Indian and Tibetan Studies, University of Hamburg.

Hartmann, J.-U. (2006). Ein weiteres zentralasiatisches Fragment aus dem Buddhacarita. In U. Hüsken et al. (Eds.), *Jaina-itihāsa-ratna: Festschrift für Gustav Roth zum 90. Geburtstag* (pp. 259–264). Indica et Tibetica 47. Marburg: Indica et Tibetica.

Hiltebeitel, A. (2006). Aśvaghoṣa's Buddhacarita. The First Known Close and Critical Reading of the Brahmanical Sanskrit Epics. *Journal of Indian Philosophy*, 34(3), 229–286.

Hinüber, O. von (1997). *A Handbook of Pāli Literature.* First Indian ed. New Delhi: Munshiram Manohar.

Jambuvijaya, M. (2000). *A Catalogue of Manuscripts in Jaisalmer Jain Bhandaras. Jaisalmer ke prācīn jain graṃthbhaṃḍāroṃ kī sūcī.* Delhi & Jaisalmer: Motilal Banarsidass & Parshvanath Jain Shwetambar Trust.

Jambuvijaya, M. (Ed.). (2009). *Svopajñavṛttivibhūṣitam Yogaśāstram.* Part 3: *Caturthaprakāśataḥ ārabhya Dvādaśaprakāśam Yāvat.* Dilhī: Motīlāla Banārasīdāsa.

Johnston, E. H. (1936). *The Buddhacarita or Acts of the Buddha.* Part 1: *Sanskrit Text.* Part 2: *Cantos i–xiv Translated from the Original Sanskrit Supplemented by the Tibetan Version Together with an Introduction and Notes.* Lahore: University of the Panjab (repr. New Delhi: Oriental Books Reprint Corporation, 1972).

Kieffer-Pülz, P. (1992). *Die Sīmā: Vorschriften zur Regelung der buddhistischen Gemeindegrenze in älteren buddhistischen Texten.* Monographien zur indischen Archäologie, Kunst und Philologie 8. Berlin: Reimer.

Kooij, K. R. van (1972). *Worship of the Goddess According to the Kālikāpurāṇa.* Part 1: *A Translation with Introduction and Notes of Chapters 54–69.* Orientalia Rheno-Traiectina 1. Leiden: Brill.

Kuppuswami Sastri, S. & Subrahmanya Sastri, P. P. (1938). *An Alphabetical Index of Sanskrit Manuscripts in the Government Oriental Manuscripts Library, Madras.* Part 1 *(a–ma).* Madras: Superintendent Government Press.

Larson, G. J. (2008). Yogasūtras 1. Patañjali, Pātañjalayogaśāstra (Yogasūtras). In G. J. Larson – R. Sh. Bhattacharya (Eds.), *Yoga: India's Philosophy of Meditation* (pp. 161–183). Encyclopedia of Indian Philosophies 12. Delhi: Motilal Banarsidass.

Larson, G. J. & Bhattacharya, R. Sh. (Eds.). (1987). *Sāṃkhya: A Dualist Tradition in Indian Philosophy.* Encyclopedia of Indian Philosophies 4. Delhi: Motilal Banarsidass.

Leggett, T. (1990). *The Complete Commentary by Śaṅkara on the Yoga Sūtra-s: A Full Translation of the Newly Discovered Text.* London: Kegan Paul.

Leslie, J. (1998). A Bird Bereaved: The Identity and Significance of Vālmīki's Krauñca. *Journal of Indian Philosophy*, 26, 455–487.

Liṅgapurāṇa
Liṅgamahāpurāṇam Śivatoṣiṇīsaṃskṛtaṭīkopetam. Nāga Śaraṇa Siṃha-saṃpādita-Ślokānukramaṇyā sahitam, ed. Nāga-Śaraṇa Singh & Gaṇeśa Nātu. 3rd ed. Delhi: Nag Publishers, 2004.
Lüders, H. (1911). Das Śāriputraprakaraṇa, ein Drama des Aśvaghoṣa. *Sitzungsberichte der Königlich Preussischen Akademie der Wissenschaften, Philosophisch-historische Classe,* pp. 388–411.
Maas, Ph. A. (2006). *Samādhipāda: Das erste Kapitel des Pātañjalayogaśāstra zum ersten Mal kritisch ediert. The First Chapter of the Pātañjalayogaśāstra for the First Time Critically Edited.* Studia Indologica Universitatis Halensis. Geisteskultur Indiens. Texte und Studien 9. Aachen: Shaker.
Maas, Ph. A. (2008). 'Descent with Modification': The Opening of the Pātañjalayogaśāstra. In W. Slaje (Ed.), with a Preface by E. Gerow, *Śāstrārambha: Inquiries into the Preamble in Sanskrit* (pp. 97–119). Abhandlungen für die Kunde des Morgenlandes 62. Wiesbaden: Harrassowitz.
Maas, Ph. A. (2009). The So-called Yoga of Suppression in the Pātañjala Yogaśāstra. In E. Franco in collaboration with D. Eigner (Eds.), *Yogic Perception, Meditation, and Altered States of Consciousness* (pp. 263–282). Beiträge zur Kultur- und Geistesgeschichte Asiens 65. Wien: Verlag der Österreichischen Akademie der Wissenschaften.
Maas, Ph. A. (2010). On the Written Transmission of the Pātañjalayogaśāstra. In J. Bronkhorst & K. Preisendanz (Eds.), *From Vasubandhu to Caitanya: Studies in Indian Philosophy and its Textual History* (pp. 157–172). Papers of the 12th World Sanskrit Conference 10.1. Delhi: Motilal Banarsidass.
Maas, Ph. A. (2013). A Concise Historiography of Classical Yoga Philosophy. In E. Franco (Ed.), *Historiography and Periodization of Indian Philosophy* (pp. 53–90). Publications of the De Nobili Research Library 37. Vienna: Sammlung De Nobili.
Maas, Ph. A. (2014). Der Yogi und sein Heilsweg im Yoga des Patañjali. In K. Steiner (Ed.), *Wege zum Heil(igen)? Sakralität und Sakralisierung in hinduistischen Traditionen* (pp. 65–90). Wiesbaden: Otto Harrassowitz.
Mahajan, Sh. G. (1986). *Descriptive Catalogue of Manuscripts Available in the Jayakar Library, University of Poona.* Vol. 1, Part 1: Sanskrit Manuscripts. Pune: Jayakar Library, University of Poona.
Maheshananda et al. (2005). *Vasiṣṭha Saṃhitā (Yoga Kāṇḍa).* Rev. ed. Pune: Kaivalyadhama S. M. Y. M. Samiti.
Malaviya, S. (2007). *Ahirbudhnya-Saṃhitā of the Pañcarātrāgama With the Sarala Hindi Translation.* Vrajajivan Prachyabharati Granthamala 120. Delhi: Chaukhamba Sankrit Pratishthana.
Mallinson, J. (2004). *The Gheraṇḍa Saṃhitā: The Original Sanskrit and English Translation.* Woodstock, NY: Yogavidya.com.
Mallinson, J. & Singleton, M. (2017). *Roots of Yoga: Translated and Edited With an Introduction.* London: Penguin Books.
Marulasiddhaiah, G. (Ed.). (1984). *Descriptive Catalogue of Sanskrit Manuscripts.* Vol. 10: *Vyākaraṇa, Śilpa, Ratnaśāstra, Kāmaśāstra, Arthaśāstra, Sāṅkhya, Yoga, Pūrvamīmāmsā,* Nyāya. Oriental Research Institute Series 144. Mysore: Oriental Research Institute, University of Mysore.

MBh
The *Mahābhārata*, crit. ed. by V. S. Sukthankar, S. K. Belvalkar et al. 20 vols. Poona: Bhandarkar Oriental Research Institute, 1933(1927)–1966.
Mitra, R. (1883). *The Yoga Aphorisms of Patanjali With the commentary of Bhoja and an English Translation*. Bibliotheca Indica 93. Calcutta: Baptist Mission Press.
MW
M. Monier-Williams, *A Sanskrit-English Dictionary: Etymologically and Philologically Arranged with Special Reference to Cognate Indo-European Languages. New Edition Greatly Enlarged and Improved with the Collaboration of E. Leumann [...] C. Cappeller [...] [et al.]*. Oxford: Clarendon Press, 1899.
Nambiyar, R. (1942). *An Alphabetical List of Manuscripts in the Oriental Institute, Baroda*. Vol. 1. Gaekwad's Oriental Series 97. Baroda: Oriental Institute.
Nārāyaṇamiśra (1971). *Pātañjalayogadarśanam. Vācaspatimiśraviracita-Tattvavaiśāradī-Vijñānabhikṣukṛta-Yogavārtikavibhūṣita-Vyāsabhāṣyasametam. [...] Śrī[-]Nārāyaṇamiśreṇa ṭippaṇīpariśiṣṭādibhiḥ saha sampāditam*. Vārāṇasī: Bhāratīya Vidyā Prakāśan.
NGMPP
Nepal–German Manuscript Preservation Project
Olivelle, P. (2005). *Manu's Code of Law: A Critical Edition and Translation of the Mānava-Dharmaśāstra*. South Asia Research. New York: Oxford University Press.
Olivelle, P. (Trans.). (2008). *Life of the Buddha by Aśvaghoṣa*. The Clay Sanskrit Library 33. New York: New York University Press.
Pathak, M. N. (Ed.). (1999). *The Critical Edition of the Viṣṇupurāṇam*. Vol. 2 *(Aṃśas IV–VI & Pāda-Index)*. Vadodara: Oriental Institute.
Phillips, St. H. (2009). *Yoga, Karma, and Rebirth: A Brief History and Philosophy*. New York: Columbia University Press.
Pingree, D. E. (1981). *Census of the Exact Sciences in Sanskrit*. Series A, Vol. 4. Memoirs of the American Philosophical Society 146. Philadelphia: American Philosophical Society.
Plaeschke, H. & Plaeschke, I. (1988). *Frühe indische Plastik*. Leipzig: Koehler & Amelang.
Polakam Sri Rama Sastri & S. R. Krishnamurthi Sastri (Eds.). (1952). *Pātañjala-Yogasūtra-Bhāṣya-Vivaraṇa of Śaṅkara-Bhagavatpāda*. Madras Government Oriental Series 94. Madras: Government Oriental Manuscript Library.
Prasāda, R. (1910). *Patanjali's Yoga Sutras With the Commentary of Vyâsa and the Gloss of Vâchaspati Miśra. Translated by Râma Prasâda [...] With an Introduction from Rai Bahadur Śrīśa Chandra Vasu*. Sacred Books of the Hindus 4.7–9. Allahabad: Panini Office (2nd ed. = repr. Delhi: Oriental Books Reprint Corporation, 1978).
PYŚ. *Pātañjalayogaśāstra*
see Āgāśe 1904.
for PYŚ 2.46–48, see the critical edition presented in Appendix 1 of this chapter.
Ratnachandraji, Sh. (1930). *An Illustrated Ardha-Magadhi Dictionary. Literary, Philosophic and Scientific; with Sanskrit, Gujarati, Hindi and English Equivalents, References to the Texts and Copious Quotations*. Vol. 3. Indore: Kesarichand Bhandari (repr. Tokyo: Meicho-Fukyū-Kai, 1977).
Rhys Davids, Th. W. & Stede, W. (1921–1925). *The Pali Text Society's Pali-English Dictionary*. London: The Pali Text Society (repr. New Delhi: Munshiram Manohar, 1989).
RM. *Rājamārtaṇḍa* by Bhojadeva
see Āgāśe 1904.

Rukmani, T. S. (1983). *Yogavārttika of Vijñānabhikṣu: Text with English Translation of the Pātañjala Yogasūtra and Vyāsabhāṣya.* Vol. 2: *Sādhanapāda.* New Delhi: Munshiram Manoharlal.

Sahai Shastri, B. & Ram, L. (1941). *Catalogue of Manuscripts in the Panjab University Library.* Vol. 2. Lahore: University of the Panjab.

Sanderson, A. (1999). *Yoga in Śaivism: The Yoga Section of the Mṛgendratantra. An Annotated Translation with the Commentary of Bhaṭṭa Nārāyaṇakaṇṭha.* A draft published online at http://tinyurl.com/h8tv99w. Accessed 15 December 2016.

Sörensen, S. (1904–1925). *An Index to the Names in the Mahābhārata with Short Explanations and a Concordance to the Bombay and Calcutta Editions and P. C. Roy's Translation.* London: Williams & Norgate.

Ṭhakkura, N. (1934). *Tārābhaktisudhārṇava*, ed. P. Bhaṭṭācārya. Tantric Texts Series 21. Calcutta: Sanskrit Book Depot.

TVai. *Tattvavaiśāradī* by Vācaspatimiśra I
for the commentary on PYŚ 2.46–48, see the critical edition presented in Appendix 3 of this chapter.
for the complete text, see Nārāyaṇamiśra 1971.

Veda Bharati, S. (2001). *Yoga Sūtras of Patañjali With the Exposition of Vyāsa: A Translation and Commentary [...].* Vol. 2: *Sādhana-Pāda.* Delhi: Motilal Banarsidass (repr. 2004).

Visuddhimagga
see Warren & Kosambi 1950.

Vivaraṇa. Pātañjalayogaśāstravivaraṇa by Śaṅkara
for the commentary on PYŚ 2.46–48, see the critical edition presented in Appendix 2 of this chapter.
for the commentary on PYŚ 1.23–28, see Harimoto 2014.
for the complete text see Polakam Sri Rama Sastri & S. R. Krishnamurthi Sastri 1952.

Vogel, C. (1979). *Indian Lexicography.* A History of Indian Literature 5.4. Wiesbaden: Harrassowitz.

VS. *Vasiṣṭhasaṃhitā*
see Maheshananda et al. 2005.

Warren, H. C. & Kosambi, Dh. (Eds.). (1950). *Visuddhimagga of Buddhaghosâcariya.* Harvard Oriental Series 41. Cambridge: Harvard University Press (repr. Delhi: Motilal Banarsidass, 1989).

Woods, J. H. (1914). *The Yoga-System of Patañjali, Or the Ancient Hindu Doctrine of Concentration of Mind, Embracing the Mnemonic Rules, Called Yoga-Sūtras, of Patañjali and the Comment, Called Yoga-Bhāshya, Attributed to Veda-Vyāsa, and the Explanation, Called Tattva-Vaiçāradī, of Vāchaspati-Miçra.* Harvard Oriental Series 17. Cambridge: Harvard University Press (repr. Delhi: Motilal Banarsidass, 1992).

Wynne, A. (2007). *The Origin of Buddhist Meditation.* Routledge Critical Studies in Buddhism. London: Routledge.

YS. *Yogasūtra*
see Āgāśe 1904.

YŚ. *Yogaśāstra* by Hemacandra
see Jambuvijaya 2009.

YVā. *Yogavārttika* by Vijñānabhikṣu
see Nārāyaṇamiśra 1971.

Chapter 3

The Proliferation of *Āsana*-s in Late-Medieval Yoga Texts

Jason Birch

Contents

1. Introduction 103

2. The History of *Āsana* in Haṭha Yoga 105

3. Three Unpublished Manuscripts 110
3.1. The Ujjain Manuscript of the *Yogacintāmaṇi* 110
3.2. The *Haṭhapradīpikā-Siddhāntamuktāvalī* 127
3.3. The *Haṭhābhyāsapaddhati* 129

4. Chronology and Increments in the Number of *Āsana*-s in Medieval Yoga Texts 136

5. Connections between Medieval and Modern *Āsana*-s 137

6. Conclusion 142

Appendix 1: Descriptions of the Additional *Āsana*-s in the Ujjain Manuscript 143

Appendix 2: One Hundred and twelve Descriptions of *Āsana*-s in the *Haṭhābhyāsapaddhati* 148

Appendix 3: A Comparison of Medieval and Modern *Āsana*-s 169

Abbreviations (Primary Sources) 174

Other Abbreviations and Special Signs 174

References 175

Jason Birch

Chapter 3: The Proliferation of *Āsana*-s in Late-Medieval Yoga Texts*

1. Introduction

Some scholars have already noted that the number of postures (*āsana*) described in the better-known Sanskrit yoga texts is considerably smaller than the large number of *āsana*-s practised in twentieth-century yoga.[1] Relatively few *āsana*-s are mentioned in the *Pātañjalayogaśāstra,* its main commentaries and the three Haṭha Yoga texts which were widely published in the twentieth century, namely, the *Śivasaṃhitā* (ŚS), the *Haṭhapradīpikā* (HP) and the *Gheraṇḍasaṃhitā* (GS). Among these, the *Gheraṇḍasaṃhitā* teaches the most *āsana*-s, namely, thirty-two. On the basis of these sources, medieval yoga[2] appears to have little to do with

* The findings of this paper were first made public in the conference "Yoga in Transformation: Historical and Contemporary Perspectives on a Global Phenomenon" at the University of Vienna, 19–21 September 2013. Since then, my work on this paper has received funding from the European Research Council (ERC) under the European Union's Horizon 2020 research and innovation programme (grant agreement No. 647963). I wish to thank Jacqueline Hargreaves for her many suggestions and for proof-reading several drafts of this chapter. Thanks also to Mark Singleton, Beatrix Hauser and Seth Powell for their comments on an earlier draft and, in particular, to Philipp Maas and James Mallinson for their numerous comments and generous advice on specific matters. I am grateful to both Mallinson and Singleton for their help in transcribing, translating and suggesting emendations on the passages on *āsana* practice in Appendices 1 and 2. I am also grateful to Christina Ong and Fiona Tan of COMO Shambhala, Singapore, for providing me with periods of paid work, which has financed the preliminary research for this chapter, and the ERC-funded Haṭha Yoga Project for funding the work that has enabled me to complete this chapter.

1 For example, Dasgupta 1969: 205, Sjoman 1999: 39–40, Bühnemann 2007a: 20–21, Larson 2008: 148, Singleton 2010: 32–33, etc.

2 My periodisation of yoga's history is based on changes in its development. I take the beginning of the mediaeval period as the fifth or sixth century CE, which is the date of the earliest textual evidence for Tantric and Paurāṇic systems of yoga. I have extended the medieval period to the eighteenth century because the influence of modernity on yoga texts is evident only after this time. My designation of a late medieval period of the sixteenth to eighteenth century is based on distinct differences between the early corpus of Haṭha and Rāja Yoga, which culminated in the *Haṭhapradīpikā* (15th c.), and the yoga texts written after the fifteenth century, which tend to be more scholarly productions that either expound upon Haṭha and Rāja Yoga in greater

the proliferation of *āsana*-s in yoga texts written in the early twentieth century.[3] However, the lack of historical evidence on the practice of *āsana*-s has hampered scholarly efforts to reconstruct the modern history of yoga, as Joseph Alter has stated:[4]

> [...] there is virtually nothing that allows for the construction of a history of āsana practice. Clearly this signals the need for ongoing research. [...] the paucity of any clear history of practice in the eighteenth and nineteenth centuries should raise a red flag of sorts concerning the putative antiquity of everything that is now counted as Haṭha Yoga.

The writing of this chapter was prompted by the discovery of several manuscripts of medieval yoga texts which contain lists of more than eighty-four *āsana*-s, a canonical number mentioned in several yoga texts.[5] Until now, lists of eighty-four *āsana*-s have been found in only two recently published yoga texts, namely, the *Haṭharatnāvalī* (HR) and the *Jogapradīpyakā* (JP).[6] The manuscript evidence presented in this chapter indicates that these published texts are not isolated accounts of medieval yoga systems with many complex *āsana*-s. In fact, it is clear that more than eighty-four *āsana*-s were practised in some traditions of Haṭha Yoga before the British arrived in India. The majority of these *āsana*-s were not seated poses, but complex and physically-demanding postures, some of which involved repetitive movement, breath control and the use of ropes. When the *āsana*-s in the sources which I shall analyse in this chapter are considered in their totality, antecedents can be identified for many non-seated[7] and inverted postures in twentieth-century systems of Indian yoga.

When the above late-medieval yoga texts are taken into account within the broader history of Haṭha Yoga,[8] it becomes apparent that there was a substantial increase in the number of *āsana*-s after the sixteenth century and that, from the seventeenth century onwards, various lists of eighty-four or more *āsana*-s have been recorded. In contrast to this, very few *āsana*-s were mentioned or described

detail or attempt to synthesise teachings of Haṭha and Rāja Yoga with those of Brahmanical texts (including Pātañjalayoga).

3 One of the most extensive surveys of Indian *āsana*-s from both modern and pre-modern sources is Gharote et al. 2006.

4 Alter 2004: 23.

5 Bühnemann 2007a: 25–27.

6 Other yoga texts such as the *Yogāsanamālā* are mentioned in Gharote et al. 2006: lxxii and Kaivalyadhama Yoga Institute 2006: 13, but these texts have not yet been published.

7 Non-seated postures usually refer to those *āsana*-s performed in a standing, supine, prone, twisting, back-bending, forward-bending or arm-balancing position. The one exception to my comment above is that medieval yoga traditions provide very few antecedents to modern standing poses. See the Conclusion and Appendix 3 of the present chapter for more information on this.

8 For a chronology of published Haṭha texts, see Birch 2011: 528–529. The relevant unpublished material is described and dated in this paper.

in the early Haṭha texts, which can be dated from the twelfth to fifteenth centuries.

The present chapter consists of six sections. Following this Introduction, Section 2 is a general overview of the historical development of *āsana* in Haṭha Yoga. This should provide some context for the examination of three manuscripts in Section 3, which leads to questions concerning the chronology and increments of the number of *āsana*-s in medieval yoga discussed in Section 4. Section 5 investigates the relationship between medieval and modern *āsana* practices. There, I shall propose reasons for why these extensive lists of *āsana*-s occur only in sources which were written after the sixteenth century and I shall discuss whether these *āsana*-s influenced those gurus who led the revival of physical yoga in the twentieth century. Finally, Section 6 provides a summary of the main results of the present chapter as well as the prospects for future research.

2. The History of *Āsana* in Haṭha Yoga

In the fifteenth century, Svātmārāma compiled the *Haṭhapradīpikā* by borrowing verses from various medieval yoga texts, which taught either a system of Haṭha and Rāja Yoga or techniques that were incorporated into later traditions of Haṭha Yoga. Most of these earlier texts mention or describe only one or two *āsana*-s. In most cases, these are seated *āsana*-s such as the lotus pose (*padmāsana*). The names of these *āsana*-s are found in the *Pātañjalayogaśāstra*, except for *siddhāsana*, which may have been known to Patañjali by a different name.[9] The following table summarises the number of *āsana*-s in early Haṭha texts:[10]

9 The *Pātañjalayogaśāstra* contains the names of thirteen *āsana*-s but it does not describe them. Therefore, the postural shape of these *āsana*-s at the time of Patañjali is uncertain. The earliest descriptions of them are found in Śaṅkara's commentary on the *Pātañjalayogaśāstra* (see Maas' chapter in the present volume, p. 62) and none of these descriptions mention the penis being pressed by either one or both heels. *Siddhāsana* is referred to by other names in medieval yoga texts, such as the *Gorakṣaśataka* (15), which calls it *vajrāsana*. The *Haṭhapradīpikā* states that it was also known as *muktāsana* and *guptāsana*. As Philipp Maas has kindly pointed out to me (personal communication, 3 October 2013), the *Pātañjalayogaśāstra*'s list of thirteen *āsana*-s is not definitive because it ends with *ityevamādi* (i.e., "and so forth"). Nonetheless, there was no proliferation of *āsana*-s in the commentarial tradition of Pātañjalayoga, until the late medieval period when the seventeenth-century Nārāyaṇatīrtha listed and described thirty-eight *āsana*-s in his commentary the *Yogasiddhāntacandrikā* on *sūtra* 2.46. Most of these *āsana*-s are borrowed from earlier yoga texts, most notably the *Haṭhapradīpikā* (which Nārāyaṇatīrtha refers to as the *Yogapradīpa*), the *Vasiṣṭhasaṃhitā* and the *Dharmaputrikā* (for more information on the *Yogasiddhāntacandrikā*, see Birch 2013b: 414–415).

10 The *Yogatārāvalī*'s *terminus a quo* is the composition of the second chapter of the *Amanaska*

Text	Probable date CE	No. of *āsana*-s named but not described	No. of *āsana*-s named and described	Total
Amaraughaprabodha	14th c.	0	0	0
Amṛtasiddhi	12th c.	0	0	0
Khecarīvidyā	14th c.	0	0	0
Yogatārāvalī	14th c.	0	0	0
Yogabīja	14th c.	1	0	1
Dattātreyayogaśāstra	13th c.	1	1	2
Gorakṣaśataka	12–13th c.	0	2	2
Vivekamārtaṇḍa (Viv)	12–13th c.	0	2	2
Śivasaṃhitā	15th c.	2	4	6
Yogayājñavalkya	14th c.	0	8	8
Vasiṣṭhasaṃhitā	12th c.	0	10	10

Table 1: The number of *āsana*-s in early Haṭha texts.

Three of the above texts teach non-seated *āsana*-s, namely, the *Vasiṣṭhasaṃhitā,* the *Yogayājñavalkya* and the *Śivasaṃhitā.* The twelfth or thirteenth-century *Vasiṣṭhasaṃhitā* is the earliest extant textual source on Haṭha Yoga to include non-seated postures, which are *mayūrāsana* and *kukkuṭāsana.*[11] Eight of the *āsana*-s in the *Vasiṣṭhasaṃhitā,* including *mayūrāsana* but not *kukkuṭāsana,* were reproduced in the *Yogayājñavalkya,* which was probably written a century or two later and borrows extensively from the *Vasiṣṭhasaṃhitā.*[12] The fifteenth-

(11th–12th CE), on the basis of one parallel verse and the more general influence of the *Amanaska*'s Rāja Yoga (*Amanaska* 2.67 ≈ YTĀ 20; for my arguments on why this text would not predate the *Amanaska,* see Birch 2011: 528, n. 19). The *Yogatārāvalī*'s *terminus ad quem* is most probably the composition of the *Haṭhapradīpikā,* with which it shares one verse (HP 4.66 ≈ YTĀ 2), as well as the seamless combination of Haṭha and Rāja Yoga, which probably post-dates the hierarchy of four yogas (i. e., Mantra, Laya, Haṭha and Rāja). For a discussion of the date of the *Śivasaṃhitā,* see n. 13.

11 The Aṣṭāṅgayoga of Vasiṣṭha and Yājñavalkya is taught in these two texts. Their Aṣṭāṅgayoga is referred to as one of two types of Haṭha Yoga in DYŚ 26c–29: "That [described in the previous section] was Laya Yoga. Now listen to Haṭha Yoga. General observances, preliminary practices and, after that, postures, breath control is the fourth [auxiliary], sense withdrawal the fifth, then concentration is taught, meditaton is said to be the seventh and absorption, which bestows the rewards of all merit, is the eighth. Yājñavalkya and others know Aṣṭāṅgayoga thus. Siddhas, such as Kapila and so on, practise a Haṭha Yoga different to that" (*sa eva layayogaḥ syād dhaṭhayogaṃ tataḥ śṛṇu* || 26 || *yamaś ca niyamaś caiva āsanaṃ ca tataḥ param* | *prāṇāyāmaś caturthaḥ syāt pratyāhāras tu pañcamaḥ* || 27 || *tatas tu dhāraṇā proktā dhyānaṃ saptamam ucyate* | *samādhir aṣṭamaḥ proktaḥ sarvapuṇyaphalapradaḥ* || 28 || *evam aṣṭāṅgayogaṃ ca yājñavalkyādayo viduḥ* | *kapilādyās tu siddhāś ca haṭhaṃ kuryus tato 'nyathā*).

12 For the relevant references on dating the *Vasiṣṭhasaṃhitā* and the *Yogayājñavalkya,* see Birch 2011: 528.

century *Śivasaṃhitā* (3.109) teaches *paścimottānāsana*, a forward bending posture, and extols it as one of the foremost (*agrya*) *āsana*-s.[13] Nonetheless, these sources do not suggest that an early tradition of Haṭha Yoga incorporated the practice of numerous *āsana*-s. In fact, the emphasis of these texts is on *prāṇāyāma* and *mudrā* and, in most cases, only those *āsana*-s required for such practices were considered important.

Although the aforementioned texts of Haṭha Yoga's early traditions teach relatively few *āsana*-s, it would be a mistake to conclude that these were the only *āsana*-s known to their authors. Several of the early texts acknowledge the existence of eight million four hundred thousand *āsana*-s (*caturaśītilakṣa*) and assert that Śiva taught eighty-four of them. For example, the *Dattātreyayogaśāstra*, one of the earliest extant yoga texts to teach Haṭha Yoga (Mallinson 2011: 771), says:

> Among the eight million four hundred thousand *āsana*-s, listen to [my description of] the best one. In this system it is called lotus pose, [which] was taught by Śiva.[14]

A statement similar to the above is found in the *Vivekamārtaṇḍa* (8–10), a yoga text that may have been written close to the time of the *Dattātreyayogaśāstra*.[15] It does not mention Haṭha Yoga by name, but was one of the sources of the *Haṭhapradīpikā* (Mallinson 2014: 239):

> There are as many *āsana*-s as there are types of living beings. Śiva knows all the varieties of them. Every one of the eight million four hundred thousand *āsana*-s has been named by Śiva and, from among them, he taught eighty-four postures. From the aggregate of

13 The ŚS (3.108–109) may predate the *Haṭhapradīpikā* because the latter contains several verses of the former (see Mallinson 2014: 239–244). However, whether every chapter of the *Śivasaṃhitā* predates the *Haṭhapradīpikā* is, in my opinion, uncertain because the *Śivasaṃhitā* does not appear to be a cohesive text. The fifth chapter may have been written separately from the first four chapters because it contains some teachings that contradict statements in the earlier chapters. For example, in the third chapter (3.40–41), a list of twenty *niyama*-s is given. However, at 5.7, *niyama* is listed among the obstacles to yoga. Also, there are different lists of obstacles in the third and fifth chapters, and the fifth chapter teaches a tetrad of yogas (i. e., Mantra, Laya, Haṭha and Rāja), which is not mentioned as such in the earlier chapters. The dating of the *Śivasaṃhitā* is further complicated by the fact that it is a compilation containing verses of the *Dattātreyayogaśāstra* and the *Amṛtasiddhi* (Mallinson 2007b: x). Therefore, the *Haṭhapradīpikā* and the *Śivasaṃhitā* may have borrowed from a third source that is no longer extant. The composition of the *Yuktabhavadeva*, which contains a colophonic verse with the date 1623 CE, remains the most certain *terminus ad quem* of the *Śivasaṃhitā* in its current form because the *Yuktabhavadeva* (7.261–285) quotes with attribution passages from the third, fourth and fifth chapters of the *Śivasaṃhitā*.

14 DYŚ 34: *caturaśītilakṣeṣu āsaneṣūttamaṃ śṛṇu | ādināthena samproktaṃ padmāsanam ihocyate ||* .

15 Similar statements on eighty-four *āsana*-s also occur in the *Śivasaṃhitā* (3.96) and the *Haṭhapradīpikā* (1.35).

āsana-s, only these two are important; the first is called *siddhāsana* and the second *kamalāsana.*[16]

While such statements are partly rhetorical devices that assert the divine origin of all *āsana*-s, much like the so-called śāstric paradigm in various genres of Sanskrit literature,[17] the recognition of innumerable *āsana*-s in a culture accustomed to sitting on the ground should come as no surprise. Also, it is possible that many *āsana*-s were practised before the fifteenth century by other ascetic and martial traditions which have left no written record. References to *āsana* practice in the *Mallapurāṇa,* a late medieval text on wrestling, and *Kāmaśāstra* texts have been noted by Norman Sjoman[18] and Gudrun Bühnemann, respectively.[19] When one considers that the early traditions of Haṭha Yoga taught only a handful of *āsana*-s but were aware of many more, it suggests that these traditions dismissed the practice of many different *āsana*-s in favour of only those that facilitated other techniques, namely, *prāṇāyāma* and *mudrā.*

Christian Bouy[20] and Mallinson[21] have shown that the *Haṭhapradīpikā* is largely an anthology of earlier Haṭha and Rāja Yoga texts. By surreptitiously

16 Vivekamārtaṇḍa 8–10: *āsanāni ca tāvanti yāvatyo jīvajātayaḥ | eteṣām akhilān bhedān vijānāti maheśvaraḥ || 8 || caturāśītilakṣānām ekaikaṃ samudāhṛtam | tataḥ śivena pīṭhānāṃ ṣoḍaśonaṃ śataṃ kṛtam || 9 || āsanebhyaḥ samastebhyo dvayam eva viśiṣyate | ekaṃ siddhāsanaṃ proktaṃ dvitīyaṃ kamalāsanam || 10 ||* . 8a *ca*] Viv, VivB, VivN1, Gś : *tu* Gśk. 8a–b *tāvanti yāvatyo*] Viv : *tāvanti yāvato* VivN2 : *tāvanti yāvantyo* Gś, Gśl : *tāvanti yāvanto* VivB : *tāvanto yāvanto* VivN1. 8b *jīvajātayaḥ*] Viv, VivB, Gś, Gśk : *jīvajantavaḥ* VivN1, VivN2. 8c *akhilān bhedān*] Viv, VivB, Gś, Gśk, *akhilāb bhedān* VivN2 : *tulā bhedā yo* VivN1. 9b *ekaikaṃ samudāhṛtam*] VivB, VivN2, Gś : *caikaikaṃ samudrāhṛtaṃ* VivN1 : *ekaṃ ekam udāhṛtam* Viv, Gśk. 9c *pīṭhānāṃ*] ∑ : *pīṭhena* VivN1. 9d *ṣoḍaśonaṃ*] ∑ : *ṣoḍaśānāṃ* VivN1. 10b *eva viśiṣyate*] VivN1, Gśk : *eva praśasyate* Viv : *etad udāhṛtam* VivB, VivN2, Gś. 10c *proktaṃ*] Viv, VivB, VivN1, VivN2, Gśk : *tatra* Gś. For the abbreviations (e.g., Viv, VivB, etc.) in the apparatus, please see the list of abbreviations at the end of this chapter.

17 See Pollock 1985: 512 for his discussion of the śāstric paradigm. McComas Taylor (2007: 69) has defined it succinctly as follows: "This paradigm incorporates a set of common features, including claims of cosmogonic origins, divine authorship, and vast scope, which serve to empower and valorize śāstric texts."

18 Sjoman 1999: 56–57.

19 Bühnemann (2007a: 27, n. 62, 2007b: 158) cites a modern work called the *Saṅkhyāsaṅketakośa* by Haṇmaṃte, who lists eighty-four positions from the *Kokaśāstra.* However, my research on the *Kokaśāstra,* a Sanskrit text otherwise known as the *Ratirahasya* (Upadhyaya 1965) and generally ascribed to the twelfth century, has failed to confirm this. Chapter ten of the *Kokaśāstra* is on sexual positions (*bandha*), and it describes thirty-eight positions and mentions the names of another four. I was unable to find any mention of eighty-four positions in this work. Some manuscript catalogues indicate that there is a Persian translation of the *Kokaśāstra,* dated 1763–1764 and called *Khulāsat al-'aish-i 'Ālam Shāhī,* a Braj Bhāṣā translation called the *Kokamañjarī,* one manuscript of which is dated 1784 CE, and a Marathi one called the *Ratimañjarī.* I am yet to consult any of these eighteenth-century works, but it is possible that Haṇmaṃte took his list of *āsana*-s from one of them.

20 Bouy 1994.

21 Mallinson 2011: 772–773 and 2014: 239–244.

integrating a variety of sources, Svātmārāma described more postures in the *Haṭhapradīpikā* than did the earlier yoga texts, and he states that he knew more than the fifteen poses in his work:

> [Only] *some* of the *āsana*-s accepted by sages such as Vasiṣṭha and yogis such as Matsyendra are mentioned [in this text] by me.[22]

The reference to Vasiṣṭha points to the *āsana*-s of the *Vasiṣṭhasaṃhitā*, eight of which are reproduced verbatim in the *Haṭhapradīpikā*.[23] However, the exact nature of Matsyendra's association with Haṭha Yoga remains unclear because there is no earlier, extant Haṭha text attributed to him, and no earlier source for the pose called *matsyendrāsana*. Therefore, there is not enough textual evidence to determine how many postures Svātmārāma may have known beyond the fifteen he recorded in the *Haṭhapradīpikā*.

After the time of the *Haṭhapradīpikā*, a list of names of eighty-four *āsana*-s, thirty-six of which are described, was recorded in the *Haṭharatnāvalī*, which was probably written in the seventeenth century.[24] There are descriptions of eighty-four postures in the *Jogapradīpyakā* and one hundred and ten in the *Yogāsanamālā*.[25] Both of these texts can be dated to the eighteenth century on the basis of the oldest scribal dates in manuscripts of these texts (Kaivalyadhama Yoga Institute 2006: 11–13). The *Haṭharatnāvalī* and the *Jogapradīpyakā* have been published in India but are not widely available, though Bühnemann[26] has discussed them in her work on eighty-four *āsana*-s.

The three manuscripts that are the focus of this chapter, the *Yogacintāmaṇi* (YC) (Ujjain ms.), the *Haṭhapradīpikā-Siddhāntamuktāvalī* (SMĀ) and the *Haṭhābhyāsapaddhati* (HAP), corroborate the chronological increase in the number of *āsana*-s seen in published texts. The proliferation of *āsana*-s is shown in the following table:[27]

22 HP 1.18: *vasiṣṭhādyaiś ca munibhir matsyendrādyaiś ca yogibhiḥ | aṅgīkṛtāny āsanāni kathyante kāni cin mayā ||* .

23 These verses are identified in Mallinson 2014: 240.

24 Śrīnivāsabhaṭṭa's *Haṭharatnāvalī*'s *terminus a quo* is the composition of the fifteenth-century *Haṭhapradīpikā*, which is mentioned by name in the *Haṭharatnāvalī* at 1.12, 27–28, 50, 2.87, 141 and 3.23. The *Haṭharatnāvalī*'s *terminus ad quem* is the composition of the *Haṭhatattvakaumudī* of the eighteenth-century Sundaradeva who quotes the *Haṭharatnāvalī* with attribution at 8.3 and 13.

25 I have consulted one manuscript of the *Yogāsanamālā* (ms. no. 5450 Rajasthan Oriental Research Library, Jodhpur), which numbers its *āsana*-s up to one hundred and ten. However, folios 18, 24, 25, 26 and 27 are missing. Therefore, only one hundred and five *āsana*-s remain in this manuscript. All of these *āsana*-s have names and illustrations, and most of them are described.

26 Bühnemann 2007a: 27–29, 2007b: 159–160.

27 The numbers presented for the *Jogapradīpyakā* require specification: At JP v. 498, which is in the chapter on *prāṇāyāma*, *gorakha āsana* is mentioned but not described. In the third

Text	Probable date CE	No. of *āsana*-s named but not described	No. of *āsana*-s named and described	Total
Haṭhapradīpikā	15th c.	0	15	15
Yogacintāmaṇi	17th c.	0	34	34
Yogacintāmaṇi (Ujjain ms.)	1659	56	62	118
Haṭharatnāvalī	17th c.	48	36	84
Gheraṇḍasaṃhitā	18th c.	0	32	32
Haṭhapradīpikā-Siddhāntamuktāvalī	18th c.	0	96	96
Jogapradīpyakā	18th c.	1	89	90
Yogāsanamālā	18th c.	0	110	110
Haṭhābhyāsapaddhati	18th c.	0	112	112

Table 2: The proliferation of *āsana*-s.

Most of the texts listed in the above table repeat the statement that Śiva taught eighty-four *āsana*-s, which first occurs in the *Dattātreyayogaśāstra* and the *Vivekamārtaṇḍa*.[28] The significant difference is that they tend to add to this statement either lists of names or descriptions of eighty-four or more *āsana*-s.

3. Three Unpublished Manuscripts

3.1. The Ujjain Manuscript of the *Yogacintāmaṇi*

Two centuries after the *Haṭhapradīpikā*, several large yoga compilations which integrated teachings of Haṭha and Rāja Yoga with those of Pātañjalayoga and Brahmanical texts were written. One such work is the early seventeenth-century *Yogacintāmaṇi* of Śivānandasarasvatī, an Advaitavedāntin who probably resided in Vārāṇasī during the reigns of the Moghul rulers Shāh Jahān and his sons.[29] The

chapter of the *Jogapradīpyakā*, eighty-four *āsana*-s are described, but another four are described at various places in the chapter on *prāṇāyāma* (Kaivalyadhama Yoga Institute 2006: 73). Therefore, the *Jogapradīpyakā* contains just a single *āsana* that is mentioned but not described, whereas the total number of described *āsana*-s is 89.

28 The *Yogacintāmaṇi* (p. 157) quotes Viv 8cd–10 as Gorakṣa and HP 1.35 with attribution; HR 1.18, 3.7–8, 23; GS 2.1; SMĀ fol. 25v, ll. 4–5 (verse no. 2.31); JP vv. 360–361.

29 On the date of the *Yogacintāmaṇi*, see Birch 2013b: 421, n. 7. The hypothesis that Śivānanda was a resident of Vārāṇasī is supported by his reference to his devotion to Viśveśvara, a standard claim of Śaivas who resided there. I wish to thank Alexis Sanderson for pointing this out to me. Moreover, he also noted that similar references to Viśveśvara in works of Śaivas who resided in Vārāṇasī can be found in Jñānaśiva's *Jñānaratnāvalī* and Viśvanātha's *Siddhāntaśekhara*, which are both Saiddhāntika Paddhatis (personal communication, 24 April

latter half of this work is structured according to the standard eight auxiliaries of yoga. In the section on *āsana*, there are descriptions of thirty-four *āsana*-s from a wide selection of sources,[30] including the *Pātañjalayogaśāstra*, Vācaspatimiśra's commentary thereon, Bhojadeva's *Rājamārtaṇḍa*, several Purāṇas - the *Āgneya*, *Kūrma* and *Skandapurāṇa*, two Tantric Śaiva works - the *Mataṅgapārameśvara* and *Dharmaputrikā* - and six medieval yoga texts - the *Dattātreyayogaśāstra*, the *Vivekamārtaṇḍa*, the *Vasiṣṭhasaṃhitā*, the *Yogayājñavalkya*, the *Haṭhapradīpikā* and an unknown text called the *Pavanayogasaṅgraha*.[31] Śivānanda cited the names of all his sources, which makes the *Yogacintāmaṇi* a valuable resource for dating some yoga texts and for identifying others that are no longer extant.

Among the five manuscripts and one printed edition of the *Yogacintāmaṇi* that have been consulted for this chapter, one manuscript contains considerably more *āsana*-s than the others. The manuscript in question, which I refer to as the "Ujjain manuscript", is held at the Scindia Oriental Research Library in Ujjain. Its final colophon is the same as that of other manuscripts of the *Yogacintāmaṇi*.[32] After the final colophon, the scribe has written the date "1717 *jyeṣṭhe śuddha* 15 *bṛhaspatyāṃ*[33] *pūrṇaḥ*".[34]

Unfortunately, the era (i. e., *vikrama* or *śaka*) is not specified. However, the details concerning the bright half (*śuddha*) of the month named Jyaiṣṭha, the fifteenth *tithi* and the day, Thursday (*bṛhaspati*), confirm that the year was *vikramasaṃvat* 1717 (i. e., Thursday, 5 June 1659 CE), as long as one understands the 1717 as a current northern year, and not an expired one.[35] Therefore, this manuscript was written in the mid-seventeenth century. Some changes have been made to the numbers of folios and at least four folios have been added to the section on *āsana*.[36] However, the scribe's hand is consistent throughout the

2013). The reference to Śivānanda being a devotee of Viśveśvara occurs in a colophonic verse, which may have been written by Śivānanda himself, in ms. 6922, last folio, ll. 6–10 and ms. 9784 pp. 189–190.

30 The number thirty-four is achieved by counting different versions of the same pose separately.

31 For the list of the texts cited in the *Yogacintāmaṇi*, see Gode 1953: 472–473.

32 YC, ms. no. 3537, fol. 104v, ll. 7–8: *iti śrīmatparamahaṃsaparivrājakācāryaśrīrāmacandrasadānandasarasvatīśiṣyaśivānandasarasvatīviracitayogacintāmaṇau caturthaḥ paricchedaḥ samāptaś cāyaṃ grantho 'pi || rudrasūno[r] bālyagastino gargho* 1 *nāmn[o] 'yam granthas tenaiva likhitaḥ* [|||] .

33 Emend. *bṛhaspatyāṃ* : Codex *bṛhaspatyaṃ*.

34 YC, ms. no. 3537, fol. 104v, l. 8. Part of the date is in the left margin.

35 I wish to thank Philipp Maas for pointing out to me that the calculation of 1717 as a current northern year yields the right day (i. e., Thursday). The calculation of 1717 as an expired year in the *vikrama* era gives Wednesday and in the *śaka* era, Tuesday. Also, taking 1717 as a current year in the *śaka* era gives the wrong day (i. e., Friday). I have tested these calculations using both the Amānta and Pūrṇimānta schemes.

36 The changes made to the folio numbers begin at folio 43, which is well before the section on *āsana*. I can see no reason for the change at folio 43, other than, perhaps, to correct an error in

manuscript, so the date of its additional lists of *āsana*-s must be close to that of the manuscript. This means that it was probably written around the same time as the *Haṭharatnāvalī*. Seeing that the earliest date for a catalogued manuscript of the *Haṭharatnāvalī* is 1812 CE,[37] the Ujjain manuscript of the *Yogacintāmaṇi* is the earliest dated manuscript containing lists of more than eighty-four names of *āsana*-s.

The section on *āsana* in the Ujjain manuscript begins with the same introductory remarks as those in other manuscripts of the *Yogacintāmaṇi*. However, there is one small but significant variation in the opening comment, which reads:[38]

> *athāsanāni* 84 *tatra patañjaliḥ* || *sthirasukham āsanam* ||
> Now, the 84 *āsana*-s. On this [subject], Patañjali [said], "An *āsana* is steady and comfortable".

Other manuscripts do not mention the number eighty-four, but simply have *athāsanam*. The scribe of the Ujjain manuscript inserted the "84" with the intention of describing more than the thirty-four *āsana*-s that are usually found in the *Yogacintāmaṇi*.

Another significant difference between the Ujjain manuscript and other manuscripts of the *Yogacintāmaṇi* is that the scribe listed and numbered the *āsana*-s rather than just copying them as text. The number and the name of each pose are written on the left side of each folio and the description on the right side.[39] The change in format indicates that the scribe was compiling a list of *āsana*-s that went beyond the text of the *Yogacintāmaṇi*. After the thirty-fourth

---

the original numbering. Some of the changes were made by writing over the original numbers, but most by covering the original numbers with a yellow paste. The section on *āsana* begins on folio 58v, and the changes that have been made to folios 58–62 appear consistent with the changes made to the previous folios. However, the numbers of folios 63–66 have not been corrected, which indicates that these folios were probably added at a later time. These inserted folios contain most of the third list of *āsana*-s. The two folios following this inserted section have the same numbers as the previous two folios (i. e., 65–66) and, in this chapter, I refer to them as folios 65a and 66a. The verso side of the folio at the end of the section on *āsana* (i. e., 67v) has verses on yoga, which are not found in other manuscripts of the *Yogacintāmaṇi*. I have traced these verses to a chapter on yoga in the *Śārṅgarapaddhati* (4508–4516). On the next folio (i. e., 68), the second chapter of the *Yogacintāmaṇi* begins.

37 HR, reel No. A 990–19 (1), Kathmandu National Archives. See http://catalogue.ngmcp.uni-hamburg.de/wiki/A_990-19(1)_Haṭharatnāvalī (accessed 12 August 2014). The earliest dated manuscript used by M. L. Gharote (2009: xiii) for his critical edition of the *Haṭharatnāvalī* is ms. no. 4–39, dated *saṃvat* 1895, *mārgaśīrṣa śukla pañcamī bṛhaspativāre* (Thursday, 22 November 1838).

38 YC, ms. no. 3537, fol. 58v, l. 4.

39 There are actually two sets of numbers. The one on the right side of the name of each pose appears to be the original numbering because it excludes several *āsana*-s which were added in the margins and as interlinear comments at a later time.

āsana,[40] the scribe has inserted the colophon "*iti yogacintāmaṇāv āsanasaṅgrahaḥ*".[41]

This colophon marks the end of the collection of *āsana*-s as they appear in the other manuscripts of the *Yogacintāmaṇi*. An obscure scribal comment after the colophon seems to indicate that five *āsana*-s were added to this collection,[42] but the most important feature of the Ujjain manuscript is that its list of *āsana*-s continues beyond the colophon to add another twenty-one *āsana*-s, which are numbered thirty-five to fifty-four. Six of these additional *āsana*-s have the same names as *āsana*-s mentioned in the *bhāṣya* part of the *Pātañjalayogaśāstra* (2.46) and, apart from one exception, their descriptions derive from Vācaspatimiśra's *Tattvavaiśāradī*.[43] However, as far as I am aware, the remaining fifteen descriptions are not found in any yoga text that predates the sixteenth century.[44]

After the *āsana* numbered forty-nine, a table has been inserted at the bottom of folio 62v, as can be seen in Figure 1. It contains the names of eighty-one *āsana*-s in alphabetical order. Seeing that thirty-nine of these *āsana*-s are not found in the list above it, the contents of the table can be seen as a second, separate list. It is possible that the scribe intended to insert eighty-four *āsana*-s in the table but was prevented from doing so because of congestion within some of the cells, in particular, *ka* and *sa*.

On the folio following the table (i.e., 63r) begins an unnumbered list of one hundred and twelve names of *āsana*-s, which includes seventeen repetitions. This is a third separate list, in which the names of the *āsana*-s are placed vertically

40 This is numbered thirty-three on the left side of the name of the pose. The discrepancy in the numbering arises from the fact that the scribe has included two different types of *padmāsana* under one heading.

41 YC, ms. no. 3537, fol. 61v, l. 5.

42 The scribal comment after *iti yogacintāmaṇāv āsanasaṅgrahaḥ* is difficult to decipher but reads: *yatra puro 'ṅkaḥ* (29) *saḥ aṅkātiriktam* (7) *anyataḥ saṅgṛhītaṃ paścād aṅkaiḥ* || (note: the *ścā* of *paścād* is not clear). This comment, which has been corrected at another time, seems to be pointing out that the group of twenty-nine *āsana*-s (according to the manuscript's numbering on the left of each *āsana*'s name) above this colophon is from the *Yogacintāmaṇi*, whereas seven *āsana*-s were added from elsewhere. In actual fact, seven *āsana*-s have been added as marginal notes and interlinear comments to those usually found in the *Yogacintāmaṇi*. These are *kevalasvastika, ardha, garuḍa, markaṭa, garbhāsana, paryaṅka* and *vīrāsana*. Therefore, the scribal comment following the colophon is probably referring to those seven additional *āsana*-s which have been numbered. I wish to thank Péter-Dániel Szántó, Somdeva Vasudeva, Csaba Kiss, James Mallinson and Mark Singleton for their help in deciphering this comment.

43 These *āsana*-s are *daṇḍāsana, sopāśraya, krauñcaniṣadana, hastinaḥ* (= *hastiniṣadana*), *uṣṭrasya* (= *uṣṭraniṣadana*) and *samasthāna*. The descriptions of *daṇḍa, sopāśraya* and *samasthāna* are almost the same as those by Vācaspatimiśra, and the description of *sopāśraya* is followed by *iti vācaspati*. The descriptions of *krauñca* and *hastiniṣadana* do not vary much from earlier ones. However, the description of *uṣṭraniṣadana* may be unique (see Appendix 1).

44 These *āsana*-s are numbered 35, 38, 43–55 in Table 3, below.

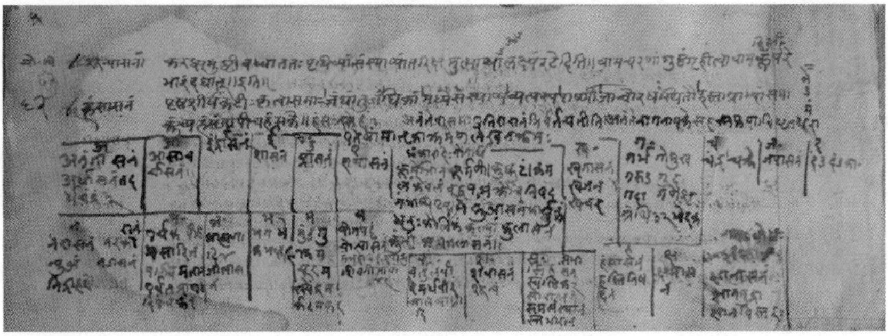

Figure 1: The Ujjain Manuscript of the *Yogacintāmaṇi*, fol. 62v (photograph: Jacqueline Hargreaves).

along the left side of each folio. The right side is blank, as though the scribe had intended to fill out descriptions for each *āsana*, but for some unknown reason never completed them. This hypothesis is supported by the fact that the very first *āsana* called *anantāsana* has its description included on the right side.[45] Several folios have names written upside down on the right side as well. The writing deteriorates as the list progresses. Most of the folios on which this list is written appear to have been inserted at a later time,[46] and the names of seventeen *āsana*-s have been repeated, which suggests that the scribe may have compiled this list from several unknown sources. Nonetheless, the scribe's hand remains consistent throughout the entire manuscript, though there are indications that he used a different pen at a later time to add corrections and marginal notes. Therefore, the third list can be dated reasonably close to the date of the manuscript.

The names of *āsana*-s in the Ujjain manuscript have been reproduced in Table 3, below. I have divided the first list into two parts called 1a and 1b, respectively. List 1a, which is written on folios 59r–61v, includes the *āsana*-s common to all manuscripts of the *Yogacintāmaṇi* and it ends with the colophon quoted above. In a few cases, I have inserted the number "2" or "3" in parentheses next to the name of an *āsana* in this list to indicate those instances in which two or three different descriptions are given for the same *āsana*. List 1b, which is written on folios 61v–62v and 67r, contains those *āsana*-s that have been added to list 1a by the scribe. The first seven were added as marginal and interlinear notes and the remaining twenty-one were written beneath the colophon (i. e., *iti yogacintāmaṇāv āsanasaṅgrahaḥ)*. A transcription of the descriptions of these twenty-eight *āsana*-s is presented in Appendix 1. List 2 has the names of the *āsana*-s in

45 For this description of *anantāsana*, see n. 50.

46 For further information on this, see n. 36.

the table on folio 62v (see Figure 1) and list 3 consists of the *āsana*-s listed on folios 63r–66bv. Please take note of the following symbols:

* = *āsana* in list 2 and not in lists 1a and 1b

• = *āsana* in list 3 and not in lists 1a, 1b and 2

(r) = a repetition of a name of an *āsana* in list 3

No.	List 1a	List 1b	List 2	List 3
1	mṛgasvastika	kevalasvastika	anaṅga*	ananta•
2	ardhacandra	ardha	ardha	ardhacandra
3	añjalikā	paryaṅka	ardhacandra	ardha
4	daṇḍa	vīra	āsāvarī	ardhodaya•
5	pīṭha	garuḍa	indra*	āsāvarī
6	paryaṅka	markaṭa	īśa*	indra
7	yogapaṭṭa	garbha	uṣṭra	īśakāmaka•
8	candrārdha	cakra	eṇa*	layodāsana•
9	prasārita	daṇḍa	kūrma	uṣṭra
10	kūrma	sopāśraya	uttānakūrma	eṇa
11	ardha	candra	kukkuṭa	kūrmottāna
12	svastika (2)	krauñca	kamalaṃ kevalam	kukkuṭa
13	gomukha	hasti	baddhapadma	padmaṃ kevalam
14	vīra	uṣṭra	krauñca	baddhapadma
15	siṃha	samasaṃsthāna	kubja	krauñca
16	bhadra	bhaga	kārmukadhanus*	kubja
17	mukta	kubja	kaulika*	kāmukadhanus
18	mayūra (2)	naḍa	kalpā*	kaulika
19	kukkuṭa	garbha	kula*	kalevara•
20	uttānakūrma	nyubja	kumbhīra*	kula
21	dhanus	stambha	kalā*	kumbhīra
22	matsysendra	śūnya	khaga*	khaga
23	paścimatāna	haṃsa	khañjana*	khañjana
24	śava	gaṇeśa	khecara*	khecara
25	naraka	guda	garbha	garuḍa
26	siddha (3)	pārvatī	gomukha	garbha
27	padmāsanaṃ baddham	āsāvarī	garuḍa	gomukha
28	kamala	nidrāhara	guda	guda
29	padmāsanaṃ kevalam (2)		gadā*	gaṇeśa

(Continued)

No.	List 1a	List 1b	List 2	List 3
30			gaṇeśa	granthibheda
31			granthibhedaka*	gadā
32			candra	kumbhīra (r)
33			cakra	matsya
34			japa*	kūrma
35			daṇḍa	makara
36			daṇḍakā*	siṃha
37			nara*	candra
38			naraka	cakra
39			nyubja*	japa
40			naḍa	daṇḍa
41			nidrāhara	daṇḍakā
42			paryaṅka	khecarakāraka•
43			pīṭha	kalpā
44			prasārita	siddha
45			paścimatāna	kālavaśakara•
46			parvata*	nara
47			prāṇādipañcaka*	naraka
48			brāhmaṇādi 4*	nyubja
49			bāla*	naḍa
50			bhaga	nidrāhara
51			bheka*	paryaṅka
52			bhakta*	granthibheda (r)
53			muṇḍa*	sarva•
54			mukta	jñāna
55			mayūra	kaulika (r)
56			matsyendra	khañjana (r)
57			markaṭa	pīṭha
58			makara*	prasārita
59			yogapaṭṭa	paścima
60			yoni*	parvata
61			mantradoṣahara-pātya*	prāṇādipañcaka
62			vartula*	śubha•
63			vīra	parvata (r)
64			ardhavīra*	prāṇādi 5 (r)

(Continued)

No.	List 1a	List 1b	List 2	List 3
65			vyāla*	brāhmaṇā-divarṇa 4•
66			vyāghrādi*	jāti 5•
67			śava	bhaga
68			śūnya	bheka
69			sabhā*	bhallūka•
70			siṃha	muṇḍa
71			svastika 2	mukta
72			sopāśraya	mayūra
73			samasaṃsthāna	matsyendra
74			stambha	markaṭa
75			haṃsa	yogapaṭta
76			hastiniṣadana	yoni
77			kṣamā*	jātya (r)
78			jñānabodha*	pāśava•
79			jñānāsana*	śavasādhanāni
80			jñānamudrā*	vartula
81			jñānavistara*	vīra
82				vīrārdha
83				vyāla
84				vyāghra
85				śava
86				śūnya
87				candra (r)
88				sūrya•
89				yoga•
90				gadā (r)
91				lakṣya•
92				kula (r)
93				brāhmaṇa (r)
94				sabhā
95				siṃha (r)
96				svastika
97				sopāśraya
98				samasaṃsthāna
99				stambha
100				haṃsa

(Continued)

No.	List 1a	List 1b	List 2	List 3
101				hasti
102				kṣamā
103				jñāna
104				jñānamudrā
105				jñānabodha
106				jñānavistara
107				haṃsa (r)
108				bhallūka (r)
109				vartula (r)
110				kṣemā (r)
111				divya•
112				ardhodaya (r)

Table 3: Names of *āsana*-s in the Ujjain manuscript.

As mentioned above (p. 111), list 1a is the compilation of thirty-four *āsana*-s common to all manuscripts of the *Yogacintāmaṇi.*[47] Its descriptions have been

47 The following additional remarks concern the names listed in column 1a of Table 3. Name no. 4: There is no description of *daṇḍāsana* next to the name. Its absence may be due to the fact that *daṇḍāsana* was included and described in list 1b. Name no. 11: In the list of names running down the left side of the folio, *ardhāsana* is an interlineal correction to the original name of *vīrāsana.* The description itself mentions *ardhāsana* (and not *vīrāsana*) and it is identical to the description of *ardhāsana* in the other manuscripts of the *Yogacintāmaṇi.* Name no. 12: Both types of *svastikāsana* are found in the *Yogayājñavalkya* and quoted with attribution in the *Yogacintāmaṇi.* In the Ujjain manuscript, both have been written, but the first has been crossed out by a single line. Name no. 18: All manuscripts of the *Yogacintāmaṇi* quote with attribution two descriptions of *mayūrāsana.* The first is from the *Yogayājñavalkya* and the second is from the *Haṭhapradīpikā.* Name no. 24: After the description of *śavāsana,* which is found in other manuscripts of the *Yogacintāmaṇi,* the Ujjain manuscript (fol. 61r) has inserted the following comment, which I have not traced to another text: "or [*śavāsana*] is as follows. Having lain supine on the ground, extending the legs and putting the hollowed hands on the chest and the gaze on the tip of the nose while visualising Śiva, the position in which [one is] on the back is *śavāsana.* This [*āsana*] is the destroyer of vitiated phlegm and the *vātagranthi*-disease in the chest, and it removes fatigue" (*yathā vā | uttānam urvyāṃ śayanaṃ vidhāya prasārya pādau karasaṃpuṭaṃ hṛdi | nāsāgram ādhāya dṛśaṃ smaran śivaṃ pṛṣṭhe sthitir yatra śavāsanaṃ hi tat || etad dhṛdikupitakaphavātagranthivibhedakaṃ śramaharaṃ ca ||* Conj. *urvyāṃ* : Codex *urvyā;* Corr. Preisendanz *etad dhṛdi* : Codex *etat hṛdi-).* Name no. 26: Three versions of *siddhāsana* are included in all manuscripts of the *Yogacintāmaṇi.* The first is quoted with attribution to the *Yogayājñavalkya* and the second to the *Pavanayogasaṅgraha,* though the latter version probably derives from the *Vivekamārtaṇḍa.* The third version is quoted without attribution and I am yet to trace it to another yoga text: "Having placed the left ankle on the penis and the other ankle on that, this is Siddhāsana" (*meḍhrād upari vinyasya savyaṃ gulphaṃ tathopari | gulphāntaraṃ tu vinyasya siddhāsanam idaṃ bhavet ||* Emend. *meḍhrād* : Codex *medrād*). Name no. 27: All

quoted and attributed to various Sanskrit texts written before the sixteenth century. The Ujjain manuscript extends our knowledge of *āsana*-s practised in the seventeenth century by providing lists 1b, 2 and 3. List 1b consists of the twenty-eight *āsana*-s that have been added to list 1a.[48] List 2 adds thirty-nine *āsana*-s to lists 1a and 1b.[49] List 3 adds another seventeen, which yields a total of one hundred and eighteen *āsana*-s in the Ujjain manuscript.[50] Therefore, the

manuscripts of the *Yogacintāmaṇi* quote with attribution this version of the bound lotus from the *Yogayājñavalkya*. However, the Ujjain manuscript is unique in using the name *padmāsanaṃ baddham*. Name no. 28: Quoted with attribution to the *Mataṅgaḥ*. Name no. 29: The *Yogacintāmaṇi* quotes these two versions of *padmāsana* and attributes the first to the *Haṭhayoga*, though this version of *padmāsana*, which involves holding the big toes with the hands, is found in the *Vivekamārtaṇḍa* and the *Haṭhapradīpikā*. The second, which does not involve holding the toes, is attributed to the *Dattātreyayogaśāstra*. The Ujjain manuscript is unique in using the name *padmāsanaṃ kevalam*.

48 In regard to list 1b, the name *nyubja* (no. 20 in column 1b of Table 3) is a conjecture. See n. 150.

49 A number of names in column 2 of Table 3 are in need of further explanations and comments. Name no. 14: The name *krauñcaniṣadana* is followed by *bhāṣyagranthane*, which refers to the inclusion of this posture in the commentary (*bhāṣya*) of the *Pātañjalayogaśāstra*. Name no. 20: Conj. *kumbhīra* : Codex *kumbhī+na*. The ligature following *bhī* appears to be crossed out. I have conjectured *kumbhī[rāsa]na* based on a similar name in the third list. Name no. 31: A pose by the name *granthibhedakāsana* is quite conceivable (i. e., "the *āsana* of piercing the knots"), and might be a precedent for *granthibhedanāsana* apparently reported in the *Sacitra Cauryaysin Asana*, the *Śrīyogakaustubha*, the *Kiraṇaṭīkā* and the *Yogamārgapradīpa* (Gharote et al. 2006: 117–118). However, the scribe of the Ujjain manuscript has inserted the number 32 between *granthi* and *bhedaka*, and I cannot see a reason for this. Name no. 39: Emend. *nyubja* : Codex *nyubhja*. Name no. 48: Emend. *brāhmaṇādi* : Codex *brahmaṇādi*. Name no. 61: The manuscript is unclear here. I can only be certain of the following ligatures: *++tradoṣaharapātya*. This could be a scribal comment, rather than the name of an *āsana* because it has *śivagītāyāṃ* (i. e., "in the *Śivagītā*") written underneath it. Name no. 71: The number "2" is written in the manuscript (see Fig. 1). Name no. 78: Diagnostic Conj. *jñānabodha* : Codex *++bodhaḥ*. I have conjectured *jñānabodhaḥ* on the basis that *++bodhaḥ* has been written in the table's cell for *āsana*-s beginning with *jña* and *jñānabodha* appears in the third list.

50 Several names listed in column 3 require further explanations: Name no. 1: *anantāsana* is the only *āsana* to be described. Folio 63r: "Patañjali's aphorism [states,] 'Or meditative absorption in Ananta brings about *āsana*.' From this statement, the cause of *āsana* is [said to be] *samādhi*, in which the mind is on one thing, fixed [in this case] only on Ananta the leader of snakes, on whom the earth is held by his one thousand hoods, [so that] *āsana* becomes what will be described as steady and a cause of comfort" (*anante vā samāpattir āsanaṃ nirvartayati iti patañjalisūtraṃ anante nāganāyake vidhṛtasahasraphaṇādharāmaṇḍala eva niścalaḥ samādhir ekacittaḥ sthiraṃ vakṣyamāṇam āsanaṃ sukhakaraṃ ca bhavati ity āsanakāraṇam ukteḥ* || Conj. *-phaṇādharāmaṇḍala eva* : Codex *-phaṇāsu dharāmaṇḍale iva*. Emend. *-kāraṇam* : Codex *-karaṇam*). This description appears to have been based on a comment in Vācaspatimiśra's *Tattvavaiśāradī* 2.47 ([...] *anante vā nāganāyake sthiratara-phaṇāsahasravidhṛtaviśvaṃbharāmaṇḍale samāpannaṃ cittam āsanaṃ nirvartayatīti*). Name no. 10: Beneath *eṇāsana*, there is an obscure comment, which has been slightly indented: *kādeḥ yogahitaṃ*. The first compound appears to point out that several *āsana*-s which have names beginning with *ka* follow at this point in the list. However, I am not sure what the second compound *yogahita* has to do with this. Name no. 11: Emend. *kūrmottā-*

Ujjain manuscript contains an additional eighty-four *āsana*-s to the thirty-four in other manuscripts of the *Yogacintāmaṇi* (i. e., list 1a). Eight of these have been taken from Vācaspatimiśra's *Tattvavaiśāradī*. However, I am yet to find the names of the other seventy-six additional *āsana*-s in any yoga text dated before the sixteenth century.

There are two more important pieces of information on *āsana* practice in the Ujjain manuscript. The first occurs in the description of *naḍāsana* (the "reed pose") in list 1b. Its initial comment indicates that the pose and, perhaps, those that follow it were taught by Mohanadāsa: *naḍāsanaṃ mohanadāsenokte*[51] | [...] ||.

A second similar comment is found on the folio on which this same list ends (i. e., 67r). At the centre top of the folio, as though it were a heading, is written the name of a yogi: *lakṣmaṇadāsasvarayogī*. Thus, it appears that the *āsana*-s numbered 44–49 have been attributed to Mohanadāsa and those numbered 50–54 to Lakṣmaṇadāsa. Also, a marginal comment at the beginning of the section

---

na : Codex *kūrmottāne*. Name no. 14: Emend. *baddhapadmaṃ* : Codex *paddhapadmaṃ*. Name no. 15: The entry for *krauñcaniṣadana* on folio 64r has been split in half, with *krauñcaniṣa* written above *danaṃ bhāṣye*. For an explanation of the word *bhāṣya* in a similar context, see note 48 on name no. 14 in column 2. Name no. 17: Monier-Williams (1899) cites *kāmuka* (s. v.) as a variant reading of *kārmuka*. Name no. 19: Diagnostic Conj. *kalevara* : Codex *kalera*. The word *kalera* (fol. 64r) is not found in any of the dictionaries. I have tentatively conjectured *kalevara*, but an *āsana* by this name is not attested elsewhere, as far as I am aware. Name no. 30: Under *granthibheda* (fol. 65r), three numbers separated by *daṇḍa*-s have been written: 21 | 7 | 4. Name no. 32: *kumbhīrāsana* and the four names following it have been written upside down on the right-hand side of folio 65r. Name no. 37: Emend. *candra*: Codex *cāndra*. Name no. 42: *khecarakāraka* and the four *āsana*-s following it have been written upside down on the right side of folio 65v. Name no. 45: Emend. *kālavaśakara* : Codex *kālavaśakera*. Name no. 52: *granthibhedāsanaṃ* 32 and the four *āsana*-s following it have been written upside down on the right side of folio 66r. Note that the number "32" written after *granthibhedāsanam* corresponds to the number written between *granthi* and *bhedaka* in name no. 31 in column 2. Name no. 64: The manuscript has *prāṇādyāsanāni* 5. The plural suggests that this may be referring to more than one *āsana*, perhaps, one for each of the five *prāṇa*-s. Name no. 65: The word *varṇa* and the number 4 indicate four *āsana*-s, one for each of the castes. Name no. 66: One must wonder whether this is a reference to a fifth caste (i. e., the untouchables). Name no. 76: There is a faint marginal comment under *yonyāsanaṃ* (fol. 65br): *śivahitāyāṃ pātha* [||]. Name no. 77: *jātyāsana* and the two *āsana*-s following it have been written upside down on the right side of folio 65bv. Name no. 82: The first ligature *vī* is unclear. In fact, this name appears to have been written over another word, which makes it difficult to read. Name no. 87: *candrāsana* and the six *āsana*-s following it have been written upside down on the right side of fol. 66br. Name no. 93: Emend. *brāhmaṇa* : Codex *brahmaṇa*. I presume that this is a repetition of *brāhmaṇādivarṇa* 4 (entry 65). Name no. 106: Diagnostic Conj. *jñānavistara* : Codex *vistara*. I have conjectured *jñānavistara* for *vistara* based on the fact that the poses preceding it begin with *jñāna* and the name *jñānavistara* is attested in list 2. The four entries below *vistara* appear to form a comment and may not be names of *āsana*: *evaṃ mā+trā++am lakṣanaṃ lekhyaṃ* [||]. I have excluded them from the list.

51 This comment is on fol. 62r.

on *āsana* quotes Lakṣmaṇadāsa, which suggests that his teachings may be connected in some way to the *āsana*-s that were added to the first list (i. e., list 1b).[52] The *dāsa* suffix indicates these two yogis were Vaiṣṇava. The fact that their *āsana*-s were added to a compilation on yoga authored by a Śaiva Advaitavedāntin demonstrates the willingness of yogis to combine yoga techniques from Śaiva and Vaiṣṇava traditions.[53] Also, apart from the attributions to mythical sages such as Vasiṣṭha and Yājñavalkya, the above attribution may be unique inasmuch as it ascribes specific *āsana*-s to what appears to be more recent yogis.

Though the additional *āsana*-s in the Ujjain manuscript are not found in earlier Sanskrit yoga texts, there are striking parallels in an illustrated manuscript of the *Baḥr al-Ḥayāt* held at the Chester Beatty Library.[54] This Persian manuscript has been dated to c 1600–1605 CE by art historians,[55] and its text is a Persian rendering of an Arabic translation of a supposed Sanskrit yoga text called the *Amṛtakuṇḍa*. Its fourth chapter describes and illustrates twenty-two yogic practices, some of which are *āsana*-s and others are *prāṇāyāma*-s performed in non-seated *āsana*-s.

The parallels occur with several of the *āsana*-s attributed to Mohanadāsa.[56] One example is *śūnyāsana*, which is depicted in the following detail of a painted folio in the Chester Beatty manuscript.

If one compares the image of Figure 2 to the description of *śūnyāsana* in the Ujjain manuscript, the similarities are clear:

> *Śūnyāsana*: Having clenched the fists of both hands and then having placed them on the ground, the yogi should raise [his body] up into the air and exclaim "alakṣya". Having

52 YC, ms. no. 3537, fol. 58v, bottom margin: "Lakṣmaṇasvarayogī says, 'By eating sea salt and pepper, success in all *āsana*-s [is obtained], but not by [eating] rock salt.' Because of this, itching is [also] cured" (*saindhavamarīcabhakṣaṇena sarvāsanasiddhir na tu lavaṇeneti lakṣmaṇasvarayogī || tena kaṇḍūnāśaḥ*).

53 An earlier example of this is the Śaiva-orientated *Haṭhapradīpikā*, which, as noted above, incorporated verses on *āsana*-s from the Vaiṣṇava *Vasiṣṭhasaṃhitā*.

54 I wish to thank James Mallinson for pointing out to me the parallels between the Ujjain manuscript and the illustrations in the Chester Beatty manuscript. Ernst (2003: 221, n. 47) has noted that this manuscript is not the only one with illustrations. He says: "Several manuscripts of the Persian translation contain miniature illustrations of the twenty-one asanas. One of these MSS is in the Chester Beatty Library in Dublin, another is in the Salar Jung Library in Hyderabad, a third is in the private collection of Simon Digby, and the fourth has recently been acquired by the University of North Carolina at Chapel Hill."

55 Leach 1995: 556.

56 Of the six *āsana*-s attributed to Mohanadāsa, the names of five correspond to names of yogic practices in the *Baḥr al-Ḥayāt*; i. e., *garbhāsana, stambhāsana, śūnyāsana, haṃsāsana* and *naulyāsana*. The last is called *bunawlī* in the Chester Beatty manuscript, but some of the other manuscripts of the *Baḥr al-Ḥayāt* call it *nauli* (personal communication Mallinson, 9 April 2014).

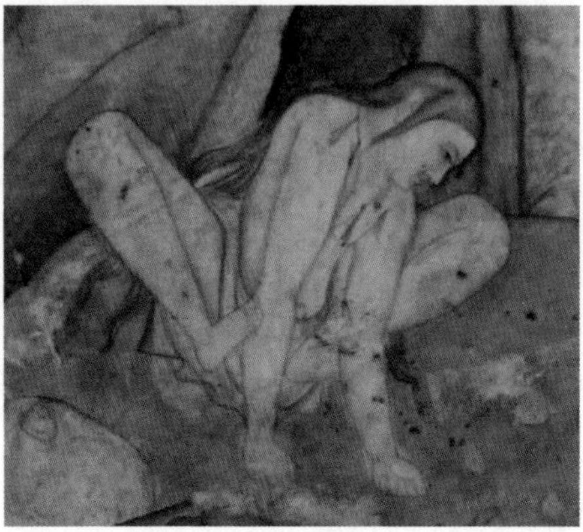

Figure 2: *Śūnyāsana* in the Chester Beatty manuscript of the *Baḥr al-Ḥayāt*, fol. 27v.

taken the big toe of the left foot on the left elbow [and the right big toe on the right elbow[57]], he should put the weight [of his body on the elbows].[58]

The fact that some of the poses of the Ujjain manuscript are in the *Baḥr al-Ḥayāt* confirms that these *āsana*-s existed in India in the seventeenth century. In many cases, the pictures of the Chester Beatty manuscript are invaluable for explaining the often obscure and corrupt Sanskrit descriptions of the *āsana*-s attributed to Mohanadāsa. A good example of this is *garbhāsana*. The Ujjain manuscript merely says:

The *garbhāsana*: Just as the shape of a foetus, so is [the shape of *garbhāsana*]. In it, one ought to do *nirañjanakriyā* and repetition [of a mantra] such as *so 'ham* and the like.[59]

The Ujjain manuscript does not explain the term *nirañjanakriyā*. This practice is, however, described at length in the *Baḥr al-Ḥayāt*, and *garbhāsana* is illustrated in the Chester Beatty manuscript.

The position of the yogi in *garbhāsana* is depicted in Figure 3. He is hunched over with his hands on his ears and his head between his knees. The following description is a translation of the Persian by Carl Ernst:[60]

---

57 It is clear from the illustration in the Chester Beatty manuscript as well as the description in the *Baḥr al-Ḥayāt* that the right elbow and leg are required for *śūnyāsana*.

58 Fol. 62v: *śūnyāsanam – karadvayamuṣṭī baddhvā tataḥ pṛthivyāṃ saṃsthāpyāntarikṣam utthāpyālakṣyaṃ raṭed iti || vāmacaraṇāṅguṣṭhaṃ gṛhītvā vāmakūrpare bhāraṃ dadyāt || iti ||*.

59 Fol. 62r: *garbhāsanam – garbhasaṃsthānaṃ yathā tathā tat | tatra nirañjanakriyā kartavyā | so 'ham ityāder japaḥ ||* Corr. Preisendanz *ityāder* : Codex *ityādeḥ*.

60 The Smithsonian Institute has posted on its website Ernst's translations of the yogic practices in the *Baḥr al-Ḥayāt*. His translation of *garbhāsana* is available at http://www.asia.si.edu/explore/yoga/chapter-4-bahr-al-hayat.asp#seven (accessed 15 July 2014).

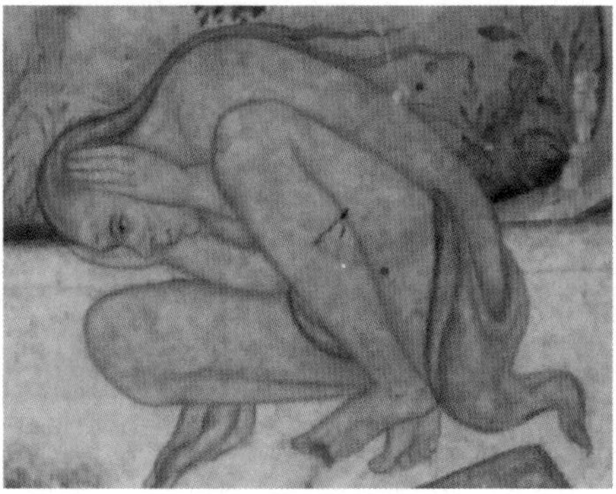

Figure 3: *Garbhāsana* in the Chester Beatty manuscript of the *Baḥr al-Ḥayāt*, fol. 18r.

> The word of recollection of *Niranjan*. When the seeker wishes to perform this activity, he should learn the *Gharba āsana*. They call it the *Gharba āsana* because when the child is in the womb of the mother it accomplishes it. One places the left foot on the right foot, holding the buttocks on both feet, holding the head evenly between the two knees, placing both elbows under the ribs, putting the hands over the ears, bringing the navel toward the spine. The breath of life (Ar. *ramq*) that appears from the navel they call *Niranjan*, which is an expression for the undifferentiated (*lā ta'ayyun*). One holds the breath; one brings it in the midst of the belly. One takes it above from below, and below from above, in this exercise to such a degree that the inner eye, winged imagination, wandering reflection, and incomparable thought - all four - emerge from their restrictions. They enter witnessing of the spiritual state and become one.

The fact that the Ujjain manuscript and the *Baḥr al-Ḥayāt* both connect *nirañjanakriyā* with *garbhāsana* strongly suggests that they were drawing from the same system of yoga, which must have been prominent enough in the seventeenth century to have come to the notice of the Moghul court. The Ujjain manuscript does not provide us with a clear description of these practices. However, a description is found in another unpublished eighteenth-century Sanskrit yoga text called the *Haṭhasaṅketacandrikā* (HSC). This voluminous work was composed by an erudite Brahman named Sundaradeva who lived in Vārāṇasī.[61] His description of *nirañjanakarma*[62] and *garbhāsana* has un-

61 The location of Sundaradeva, who was a Brahmin from the south, is confirmed by the final colophon of the HSC, ms. no. 2244, fol. 145v: "So ends the tenth chapter, called the explanation of the no-mind state, in the *Haṭhasaṅketacandrikā*, [which] was written by the physician Sundaradeva, the son of Govindadeva and the grandson of Viśvanāthadeva. Located in Kāśī, he was the ornament of southern Brahmins and sacred to the Kāśyapa clan" (*iti śrīkāśyapagotrapavitradākṣiṇātyadvijalalāmakāśisthaviśvanāthadevapautragovindadevasutasundaradevavaidyaviracitāyāṃ haṭhasaṅketacandrikāyāṃ amanaskatvavivecanaṃ nāmopadeśo daśamaḥ saṃpūrṇeyaṃ haṭhavidhicandrikā* [||] Corr. Preisendanz *-padeśo* : Codex *-padeśaḥ*; Emend. *daśamaḥ* : Codex *daśaḥ*).

62 Elsewhere in this chapter on *prāṇāyāma* in the *Haṭhasaṅketacandrikā*, other practices are

mistakable similarities to the descriptions and illustration of these practices in the *Baḥr al-Ḥayāt*. The parallels in the translation are set in bold:

> Now, the *āsana* in which the "spotless action" [is performed]. Just as a child curls up and remains in a **foetal position**, so the yogi should practise ***nirañjanakarma* in the foetal pose. Having put the left foot on the right,** he should cover the **buttocks with the heels** and then move *apānavāyu* forcefully upwards again and again. Gradually he should put his **head on his knees**, draw the **navel into the back** [of the body,] **cover the ears** and eyes **with the hands** and remain thus. Then, a faint sound rises directly up from his navel and a pure and subtle light shines in front of him. **The breath, having been restrained in the stomach, moves for a while in the abdomen. Having gone up again into the head, it goes [down] for a while into the stomach.** When this technique of meditation on the pure [light] is continually performed, the best of yogis sees the hidden Brahma revealed. Passions along with desires disappear because of the yogi's practice [of this technique]. So too, delusion and impurity, and the individual soul becomes one with Śiva.[63]

Not only is the posture the same, but also the cyclical movement of the breath between the abdomen and head. In the *Haṭhasaṅketacandrikā*, *nirañjanakarmāsana* is included in the section on *prāṇāyāma*, and there are further parallels between yogic practices in this section and those of the *Baḥr al-Ḥayāt*. These include *bhujaṅgakarmāsanakumbha* and *haṃsakarmāsanaprāṇāyāma* in the *Haṭhasaṅketacandrikā*, which are similar to *Bhuvangam* and *Hans* respectively in the *Baḥr al-Ḥayāt*. Sundaradeva describes *bhujaṅgakarmāsanakumbha* as follows:

> This has been taught in the scripture on [prognostication by means of the] breath [called] the *Svarodaya*: Having stood on both knees and having firmly closed the mouth, the wise man, [who] is very focused, should master the breath [flowing] through both

---

called *kriyā* (e.g., *pūrakakriyā*). So, *karma* (i.e., "action") is simply a synonym for *kriyā* in this context.

63 HSC, ms. no. R3239, fols. 167–168 and ms. no. 2244, fol. 84r: *atha nirañjanakarmāsanam* || *bālako garbhaśayyāyāṃ tiṣṭhet saṅkucito yathā* | *tathā garbhāsane yogī nirañjanavidhiṃ bhajet* || 124 || *dattvā dakṣāṅghrau vāmāṅghriṃ pārṣṇibhyāṃ rundhayet sphijau* | *apānam ūrdhvaṃ ca kuryād vāraṃ vāraṃ tato balāt* || 125 || *jānvante mastakaṃ dattvā nābhiṃ pṛṣṭhe vikarṣayet* | *pāṇibhyāṃ cchādayet karṇau netre tiṣṭhed iti kramāt* || 126 || *tadā nābheḥ sakāśāt tu śabdo 'syottiṣṭhate sa 'ṇuḥ* | *nirañjanaṃ jyotir agre sūkṣmaṃ cāsya parisphuret* || 127 || *ruddho 'ntar udare vāyur jaṭharāntar bhraman muhuḥ* | *ūrdhvaṃ gatvā mastakānte muhur yāty udarāntare* || 128 || *śaśvad vidhim imaṃ kṛtvā nirañjanavicintanam* | *labhate brahma yad guptaṃ prakaṭaṃ sādhakottamaḥ* || 129 || *naśyanti kāmabhiḥ kopā abhyāsenāsya yoginaḥ* | *moho malinatā naśyec chivajīvaikyatā bhavet* || 130 || *iti nirañjanakarmāsanam* ||. Variant readings: 125a–b *dakṣāṅghrau vāmāṅghriṃ pārṣṇibhyāṃ rundhayet sphijau*] 2244 : *datvā dakṣāṅghrivāmāṅghripārṣṇibhyāṃ rundhayet sinau* 3239. 126d *iti kramāt*] Diagnostic Conj. : *iti kramaiḥ* 2244 : *atikramaiḥ* 3239. 127a–b *sakāśāt tu śabdo 'syottiṣṭhate sa 'ṇuḥ* 2244 : *sakāśātva śabdo 'syottiṣṭhakonyaṇuḥ* 3239. 127d *cāsya parisphuret*] 2244 : *vāra ca parisphuret* 3239. 128a *ruddho 'ntar*] 2244 : *randhrātar* 3239. 128a *vāyur*] 2244 : *vāyu* 3239. 128b *jaṭharāntar bhraman muhuḥ*] emend. : *jaṭharāṃrbhraman muhuḥ* 2244 : *jaṭharābhramaran maruḥ* 3239.

nostrils. Having drawn the breath into the navel, he should practise in reverse. Having turned it upwards, the sage should repeatedly force it [further up]. When he knows [the breath] is situated at the tenth [door at the crown of the head], he should gradually release it. When the breath has gone below the navel, then, having again turned it upwards by that same action, he should draw it [further] upwards. If the disciplined ascetic does this technique repeatedly, he first balances nasal dominance (*svara*).[64] The practitioner should hold the breath according to his capacity, [doing so] gradually, not hurriedly. By this method, he should inhale deeply and gradually. Having given his mind to this action, the practitioner should accomplish it. When [this] action has been mastered, then, having held the breath for up to one day, he should remain comfortably [for longer] in order to increase his progress in the practice. As the yogi holds the breath, making it longer, so he should stop it from moving out for five or six days. By this [method] the practitioner certainly gains a long life. Thus, the retention in [this] practice is called the *āsana* whose action is like a serpent's.[65]

The Persian description of the "serpent" practice (*bhuvaṅga*) in the *Baḥr al-Ḥayāt* has clear parallels (marked in bold) with the above passage:

The word of recollection of *bhuvangam*. When one wishes to perform the bhuvangam practice - and bhuvangam is the expression for the serpent (*mār*) - just as the serpent inhales, the wayfarer must act according to this path and comprehend it. **He sits on both**

64 I am not sure of the meaning of *svaraṃ yāvat tu bibhṛyāt*. I have understood *svara* as nasal dominance according to its use in Svaraśāstra, in which this technique is supposedly taught. However, I am yet to find another instance of the verb *bhṛ* with this meaning in a yoga text.

65 HSC, ms. no. R3239, fols. 165–166 and ms. no. 2244, fol. 83r–83v: *tad uktaṃ svarodaye svaraśāstre || sthitvā jānudvaye vaktram ārudhya sudṛḍhaṃ sudhīḥ | nāsārandhrayugād vāyuṃ sādhayet susamāhitaḥ || 106 || ākṛṣya vāyuṃ nābhyantaṃ vidadhīta vilomataḥ | parāvṛtyordhvam ādadhyād balena satataṃ muniḥ || 107 || daśamāntagataṃ jñātvā śanair anu ca mocayet | yadā nābher adho yāto vāyus taṃ tu tadā punaḥ || 108 || amunā karmaṇaivordhvaṃ parāvṛtyordhvam āharet | amuṃ vidhiṃ yadi muhuḥ karoty abhyāsavān yatiḥ || 109 || svaraṃ tāvat tu bibhṛyād yāvacchakti samīraṇam | saṃrodhayet sādhako 'yaṃ śanair na tvarayā punaḥ || 110 || anena vidhinā bhūri gṛhṇīyāt pūrakaṃ śanaiḥ | asyām kriyāyāṃ hṛd dattvā sādhakaḥ sādhayet kriyām || 111 || yadā haste kriyā yātā tadā hy ekadināvadhi | ruddhvā tiṣṭhet sukhaṃ vāyum abhyāsakramaṃ vardhitum || 112 || yathādhikaṃ svaraṃ yogī kurvan saṃrodhayet tathā | vāyuṃ ṣaṭpañcadivasān rodhayed bahiścarāt || 113 || anena dīrgham āyuṣyaṃ sādhakasya bhaved dhruvam iti || bhujaṅgakarmāsanākhyo 'bhyāsakumbhakaḥ ||*. Variant readings: *svaraśāstre*] 3239 : *svaraśāstre bhujaṅgakarmāsanakuṃbhaḥ* 2244. 106b *ārudhya*] Conj. : *āmuḍya* 2244, 3239. 106d *sādhayet*] 3239 : *sādhayot* 2244. 107a *vāyuṃ*] 2244 : *vāyu* 3239. 107b *vidadhīta vilomataḥ*] Diagnostic Conj. Mallinson: *vidhāyāvilomataḥ* (hypometrical) 2244 : *vidhāyād avilomataḥ* 3239. 107d *muniḥ*] 2244 : *munā* 3239. 108a *daśamāntagataṃ*] 3239 : *daśamānte gataṃ* 2244. 108b *anu ca mocayat*] 2244 : *anu ca yācayet* 3239. 110a *tāvat tu bibhṛyād*] Conj. : *yāvat tu bibhṛyād* 2244 : *yāvad bibhṛyā* 3239. 111a *vidhinā bhūri*] Corr. : *vidhinād bhūri* 2244 : *vidhinā mūri* 3239. 111b *sādhakaḥ sādhayet*] 2244 : *sādhakās sādhaye* 3239. 112a *haste kriyā yātā*] 2244 : *hase kriyā mātā* 3239. 112b *tadā hy ekadināvadhi*] 2244 : *tadā ekadināvadhi* 3239. 112c *ruddhvā*] 2244 : *raddhvā* 3239. 112d *abhyāsakramaṃ vardhitum*] 3239 : *vāyuṃ krama 'bhyāsakramavardhitaṃ* (hypermetrical) 2244. 113b *kurvan*] 2244 : *kurvant* 3239. 113d *carāt*] 3239 : *caret* 2244. *bhujaṅgakarmāsanākhyo*] 2244 : *bhujaṅgakarmāsanābhyo* 3239.

> **knees, holding the mouth closed; he inhales by way of the nostrils, taking it beneath the navel, bringing it up from the navel by force to the base of the brain. From there, gradually one releases it, and it reaches below the navel. Again one brings up by force, and one repeats this in this manner, as long as one is able.** One holds the breath that was mentioned, not letting it go out by way of the nostril and mouth. When one is no longer able [to hold it], one lets out the breath by way of the nostrils with a loud voice, again from the top, and just as is mentioned, **one begins [again]. Some practitioners carry this subtle practice to such an extent that they remain for one or two days with a single breath, and some do more.**[66]

There are also loose parallels between *haṃsakarmāsanaprāṇāyāma* in the *Haṭhasaṅketacandrikā* and *Hans* in the *Baḥr al-Ḥayāt*. The former states:

> In his body, †[...]† the wise man should hold a *vajramallaka*. [With his senses] controlled, he should begin the practice of Haṃsa without attachment to the world. He should then hold his hips, back and upper limbs straight. [With his mind] focused, he should place one shin above the [other] shin. He should firmly place the heel of his left foot on the base of the right knee, and he should fix the heel of his right foot with the left knee. He should repeat the *ajapā* [mantra], while perceiving the nature of Haṃsa. Haṃsa is the self in the form of the breath. He should meditate on it as the self. By means of Haṃsa's *āsana*,[67] the sage who is constantly meditating on Haṃsa and repeating the mantra, "Haṃsa, Haṃsa," will obtain his own nature. [Such yogis] destroy impurity, dullness and diseases as well as [other] impurities. Thus, *prāṇāyāma* [performed] in *haṃsakarmāsana* is useful for purification of the channels [of vitality in the body.][68]

The relevant section of the description of *Hans* in the *Baḥr al-Ḥayāt* (parallels are in bold) is as follows:

> [...] The posture of this practice (*karma*) they call *sahaj āsana*; let it be unveiled! **One holds the head, waist, and back even, and one meditates, placing one shin over the other, holding the left ankle under the point of the right knee, and placing the right**

66 The translation by Ernst is available at http://www.asia.si.edu/explore/yoga/chapter-4-bahr-al-hayat.asp#fifteen (accessed 15 July 2014).

67 In this context, the term *pīṭha* is a synonym for *āsana*. Cf. HP 1.29, 32, 41 and 70.

68 HSC, ms. No. R3239, fols. 165–166 and ms. No. 2244, fol. 83r–83v: *aṅge †bhūtipurālāpya† dhārayed vajramallakam | vihāya lokasaṅgaṃ jño haṃsakarmārabhed vaśī || 119 || kaṭipṛṣṭhottamāṅgāni samāni bibhṛyāt tataḥ | samāhitas saṃvidadhyāt piṇḍikopari piṇḍikām || 120 || dakṣajānutale vāmapatpārṣṇiṃ sthāpayed dṛḍhaṃ | dakṣāṅghripārṣṇikaṃ vāmajānunā parikalpayet || 121 || ajapāṃ prajaped dhaṃsasvarūpaṃ sa samīkṣayan | svararūpo haṃsa ātmā tam ātmānaṃ vicintayet || 122 || anena haṃsapīṭhena haṃsaṃ dhyāyan japan manum | haṃsa haṃseti satataṃ svarūpaṃ munir āpnuyāt || 123 || mālinyajaḍatārogān naśyanti kaluṣāṇi ceti | iti haṃsakarmāsanaprāṇāyāmo nāḍīśuddhyupayogikaḥ ||*. Variant readings: 119c *lokasaṅgaṃ*] 2244 : *lokasaṅga* 3239. 120d *piṇḍikopari piṇḍakām*] 2244 : *piṇḍakopari piṇḍakīm* 3239. 121a *dakṣajānutale*] 2244 : *dakṣapādatale* 3239. 122a *-japed dhaṃsa-*] Corr. Preisendanz : *-japed haṃsa-* Codex. 123a *haṃsapīthena haṃsaṃ*] 2244 : *haṃsayogena hasan* 3239. 124b *mālinyajaḍatārogān naśyanti*] Corr. : *mālinyaḍajatārogān naśyanti* 3239 : *mālinyajaḍatārogān syanti* (hypometrical) 2244. I wish to thank James Mallinson for his comments on the above passages from the *Haṭhasaṅketacandrikā*.

> **ankle under the point of the left knee,** clasping both hands together. When exhaling, **one says hans, and hans** is an expression for "the spiritual Lord" (Ar. *rabb rūḥī*). When inhaling, one says *so ham*, and *so ham* is the expression for "Lord of Lords" (Ar. *rabb al-arbāb*) [...].[69]

These *kriyā*-s, which combine elaborate *prāṇāyāma* techniques with complex *āsana*-s, demonstrate the growing sophistication of Haṭha Yoga techniques after the sixteenth century, in addition to the proliferation of *āsana*-s evinced by the Ujjain manuscript. Far from falling into decline, the techniques of Haṭha Yoga evolved as they were appropriated by erudite Brahmins, such as Sundaradeva, whose work must have made Haṭha Yoga more accessible and appealing to a learned audience.

3.2. The *Haṭhapradīpikā-Siddhāntamuktāvalī*

The second unpublished manuscript discussed in the present chapter is an extended version of the *Haṭhapradīpikā*. This work is also called the *Siddhāntamuktāvalī* in its colophons. It has six chapters and a total of 1553 verses, which is over a thousand more than the number of verses in standard versions of the *Haṭhapradīpikā*. A scribal comment after the final colophon indicates clearly that the manuscript was completed in *saṃvat* 1765 (1708 CE).[70] Therefore, the extra verses of this text provide a window into the late seventeenth and early eighteenth centuries. The chapter on *āsana* describes more than eighty-two postures in addition to the fifteen in the standard *Haṭhapradīpikā*.[71] The names of the additional *āsana*-s are listed in Table 4. Those from the *Haṭhapradīpikā* are marked by an asterisk (*).[72]

---

69 The translation by Ernst is available at http://www.asia.si.edu/explore/yoga/chapter-4-bahr-al-hayat.asp#four (accessed 15 July 2014).

70 SMĀ fol. 171v, ll. 2–7: *iti śrīsahajanāthasiṣyeṇa śrīsvātmārāmayogīndreṇa viracitāyāṃ haṭhapradīpikāyāṃ siddhāntamuktāvalyāṃ ṣaṣṭhopadeśaḥ* || *iti* || *śrīmanmahārājādhirājajīśrījayasiṃhadevajīkasyājñayā likhitam idaṃ tulārāmeṇa* || *saṃvat* 1765 *varṣe caitre māse kṛṣṇe pakṣe* 10. The date corresponds to Sunday, 4 April 1708 in the *amānta* naming system.

71 For the descriptions of the *āsana*-s, see SMĀ, ms. no. 6756, fols. 26r, l. 6 – 49v, l. 7. The exact number of *āsana*-s in this manuscript cannot be calculated owing to a missing folio (i. e., fol. 31) which would have descriptions of another 3–4 postures.

72 On the names of *āsana*-s listed in Table 4 the following explanations and philological observations are necessary. No. 1: The first description of *svastikāsana* is that of the *Haṭhapradīpikā*. The second, which is quoted without attribution, is identical with that in the *Yogayājñavalkya*. No. 5: The first description of *gomukhāsana* is that of the *Haṭhapradīpikā*. The second, which is quoted without attribution, is identical with that in the *Yogayājñavalkya*. No. 18: The first description of *paścimatānāsana* is that of the *Haṭhapradīpikā*. A second follows, which is identical with the description in the *Śivasaṃhitā*. No. 19: The term *kandoraka* may be a wrong spelling for *kandūraka*. No. 28: This *āsana* is spelt *jaityāsana* in

No.	Name	No.	Name
1	svastika (2)*	48	prabhākara
2	vīra*	49	jarā
3	agnikuṇḍa	50	siṃhamukha
4	yoginī	51	nāgaphaṇa
5	gomukha (2)*	52	brahma
6	tūra	53	kurarī
7	kaṅkaṇa	54	cakravāka
8	gandharva	55	vaiśākhī
9	śiva	56	cakora
10	savitrīsamādhi	57	koka
11	maṇibandha	58	śukakīra
12	padmaprakāśa	59	ākāśatāna
13	padmaśaṅkha	60	kuhī
14	padmanābhabandha	61	kilakila
15	bhairava	62	daṃśa
16	matsyendra*	63	siddhamuktāvalī
17	matsyendrapīṭhabandha	64	kukkuṭa*
18	paścimatāna (2)*	65	mayūra*
19	kandoraka	66	mastaka
20	yoni	67	ātmārāma
†...†	(missing folio)	68	mṛttikābhañjaka
21	vibhūṣā	69	phoḍya
22	saptarṣi	70	bhagalabandha
23	kadalī	71	nidrānāśana
24	pūrva	72	[uttāna]kūrma*
25	tryambaka	73	vṛścika

the heading but *jityāsana* within the verse itself. No. 33: Also spelt *gorakṣajañjālaka* within the verse itself. No. 50: Diagnostic Conj. *siṃhamukhāsana* : Codex *sīhamurgāsana.* The name of this *āsana* is doubtful because the heading is *sīhamurgāsana,* but the name within the verse itself is *pakṣyāsana,* which is also the name of another *āsana* in this text (see No. 74). The word *sīha* is a Prakrit form of *siṃha* but I am not sure of *murga.* It might be a corruption of *mārga,* but *siṃhamukha* occurs in many texts and makes better sense in the context of *āsana.* No. 53: In the heading for the verse, this *āsana* is misspelt as *kurakalāsana.* In the verse itself, the name is *kuraryāsana.* No. 58: This *āsana* is referred to as *śukakīra* in the heading but as *śukāsana* within the verse itself. No. 62: Emend. *daṃśa* : Codex *ḍaṃsa.* No. 71: Emend. *nidrānāśanaṃ* : Codex *nidrānāsasanaṃ.* No. 72: The heading for this pose is *kūrmāsana,* but the verse following it is the *Haṭhapradīpikā*'s verse on *uttānakūrmāsana.* No. 77: *pāradhika* is spelt as *pāradhī āsana* in the heading and *pāradhika* in the verse itself. No. 79: The heading has *gohī āsana* but the verse describes *śiśumārāsana.* The former may be an alternate name for the latter. No. 81: The heading has *dṛkṣāsana* but the name in the verse is *nāsāgradṛkṣāsana.*

(Continued)

No.	Name	No.	Name
26	śoṣa	74	pakṣi
27	tīkṣṇa	75	abhika
28	jaityāsana	76	ājagara
29	bhaga	77	pāradhika
30	kūrma	78	ūrṇanābhi
31	paṅkaja	79	śiśumāra
32	pārvatī	80	kapālī
33	gorakṣajañjālī	81	nāsāgradṛkṣa
34	kapila	82	tapa
35	kāka	83	saṅgrāma
36	garuḍa	84	valījasya
37	aghora	85	vikaṭa
38	jāmā	86	karma
39	sārasa	87	nāgabodha
40	dhātra	88	haṃsa
41	liṅga	89	sarpa
42	pṛṣṭhabandha	90	madhupa
43	viṣṇu	91	siddha (2)*
44	gopī	92	padma (2)*
45	vaitālanāma	93	siṃha*
46	gaṇeśa	94	bhadra*
47	yogapadayoga	95	śava*

Table 4: The names of *āsana*-s taught in the *Siddhāntamuktāvalī*.

Over half of the additional poses are unique and some others resemble postures in other yoga texts, but have unique names. This extended version of the *Haṭhapradīpikā* is further proof of the continuing innovation and growth of *āsana* practice in Haṭha Yoga during the seventeenth century. Unfortunately, until another manuscript of it is found, it is unlikely to be published because the only available manuscript from Rajasthan is heavily tainted by scribal errors and is missing three folios.

3.3. The *Haṭhābhyāsapaddhati*

The third unpublished manuscript is of a text called the *Haṭhābhyāsapaddhati*. Its opening lines leave no question as to the name of the author and the work:

> For those afflicted by the pain of Samsara; those completely attached to sense objects; those obsessed with women; those fallen from their caste and [even] those who do rather egregious actions;[73] for their sake, this *Haṭhābhyāsapaddhati* was composed by Kapālakuraṇṭaka. Its topics and the techniques of the practice are written [here].[74]

In spite of the problems with the above Sanskrit sentence as it appears in the manuscript,[75] the name of the author and the title of the work are clear.[76] The

73 The meaning of *sāhasakarma* is not entirely clear here. As a broad category classifying actions, *sāhasa* can include various crimes of violence and cruelty, ranging from destruction of property and irrigation canals to adultery, rape and murder. For further examples, see the *sāhasaprakaraṇa* (p. 74) of the *Vyavahāramālā* (I wish to thank Shaman Hatley for this reference). However, in the context of Haṭha Yoga, the term can mean just "bold" or "rash". In the *Haṭhapradīpikā* (1.16), *sāhasa* is mentioned as a positive characteristic of the haṭhayogi. It is understood by Brahmānanda in his *Jyotsnā* as: "*sāhasa* is acting boldly, having not considered whether [the action] can or cannot be accomplished" (*sādhyatvāsādhyatve aparibhāvya sahasā pravṛttiḥ sāhasam*). The term *sāhasa* is also used in the *Haṭhābhyāsapaddhati*'s section on *vajrolīmudrā* (fol. 28r), which states, "It is sufficiently auspicious that by practising thus, by Īśvara's compassion, by being fit for the substances, by great fortitude and by understanding the teachings of the guru, [*vajrolī*] will be perfected [even] by those whose actions are egregrious" (*enam abhyāsena īśvarakṛpayā dravyānulyena atidhairyeṇa sāhasakarmāṇāṃ gurūktigrahaṇena siddhā bhaviṣyatīty alaṃ maṅgalam* || Emend. *evam* : Codex *enam*). In the context of *vajrolī*, *sāhasa* probably refers to those who do not practise celibacy (*brahmacarya*). However, in the opening lines of the *Haṭhābhyāsapaddhati* the more general meaning of *sāhasa* (i. e., egregious actions) seems to complete the range of people mentioned here, which starts with the most general category of person who needs salvation and ends with the most extreme.

74 HAP, fol. 1v, ll. 2–4: *saṃsāratāpataptānām* || *atyantaviṣayasaktānām* || *straiṇānāṃ jātibhraṣṭānām* || *atisāhasakarmakartṝṇām* || *tatkṛte* || *iyaṃ kapālakuraṇṭakakṛtahaṭhābhyāsapaddhatir* [||] *tadgatapadārthāḥ sādhanakarmāṇi ca likhyante* ||. I have made a number of corrections and conjectures. These are: Corr. *kartṝṇām* : Codex *kartṛṇām*. Corr. *tatkṛte* : Codex *tatkate*. Emend. *-paddhatir* : Codex *-paddhatar*. Conj. Dominic Goodall *tadgata-* : Codex *gata-*. Emend. *likhyante* : Codex *likhyate*.

75 The compounds *gatapadārthāḥ* and *sādhanakarmāṇi* are strange and incongruous with the singular verb. The *iyam* indicates that *-paddhatiḥ* was probably the subject. The reading *-haṭhābhyāsapaddhatigatapadārthāḥ* (i. e., "those subjects in the *Haṭhābhyāsapaddhati*") may have been intended but *iyam* and the singular verb seem to indicate otherwise. It is possible that *gatapadārthāḥ* and *sādhanakarmāṇi* are clumsy interpolations, which were made by the scribe to indicate that the text in the manuscript is only part of the *Haṭhābhyāsapaddhati* (personal communication Mallinson, 4 October 2013). The fact that the manuscript has no final colophon and finishes abruptly with an explanation of *viparītakaraṇī* (i. e., the last words of the text are *viparītakaraṇīmudrā bhavati* || *-karaṇī-*] Corr. Preisendanz : *karaṇi-* Codex) strongly suggests that it is incomplete. One would expect to find sections on *dhyāna* and *samādhi* at the end of a work like this.

76 The name Kapālakuraṇṭaka is not found in any other yoga text, as far as I am aware, but I am grateful to Mallinson for pointing out that *koraṇṭaka* is the name of one of the Siddhas known to have taught Haṭha Yoga according to HP 1.6c. The Kaivalyadhama edition (1998: 3) reports the alternate spellings of *kauraṇṭhaka* and *kauraṇṭaka* in its apparatus. The similar name of Korandaka for a Siddha of Haṭha Yoga is recorded in the *Haṭharatnāvalī* (1.81c), though many manuscripts of this text also have *gonandaka* (Gharote 2009: 35). In his edition of this text, Gharote speculates that the *Kapālakuraṇṭakahaṭhābhyāsapaddhati* may be ascribed to

manuscript appears to be incomplete because there is no final colophon, nor is there a scribal comment indicating the date.

The paper is unusually thin for a pre-twentieth century manuscript, which might suggest a more modern paper-making technology,[77] but it has the blemishes and uneven texture of hand-made paper. Unfortunately, the manuscript is undated. However, the text may date to the eighteenth century, based on a parallel in another text, which I shall discuss below.

A *paddhati* usually presents the "scattered instructions of a body of texts in an order that facilitates their practical application."[78] The *Haṭhābhyāsapaddhati* appears to be an exception to this inasmuch as it does not quote from earlier yoga texts. However, true to its designation as a *paddhati,* it does present the practice of Haṭha Yoga in a systematic way, beginning with *yama, niyama, āsana, ṣaṭkarma, prāṇāyāma* and finishing abruptly with *mudrā*. The text, as it is written in the manuscript, appears to be incomplete and may be a truncated form of an earlier work on yoga or an unfinished attempt to reorganise the contents of an earlier work into the form of a *paddhati.*[79]

The section on *āsana* practice has descriptions of one hundred and twelve postures and space for illustrations that were never made. Most of the *āsana*-s in the *Haṭhābhyāsapaddhati* are not found in earlier yoga texts, including the unpublished ones mentioned in this paper. The exceptions are a dozen or so *āsana*-s common in Haṭha texts such as the *Haṭhapradīpikā*. However, nearly all the names and descriptions of the *Haṭhābhyāsapaddhati*'s *āsana*-s are included in a more recent compendium called the *Śrītattvanidhi* (ŚTN) ascribed to a Mahārāja of Mysore who ruled from 1799 to 1868 (Mummaḍi Kṛṣṇarāja Woḍeyar III).[80] Therefore, the *Śrītattvanidhi* was probably written in the mid nineteenth century.

The table of contents in an early publication of the *Śrītattvanidhi* indicates that it is a digest of a number of wide-ranging topics.[81] Sjoman (1999) has worked on the *Śrītattvanidhi*'s chapter on *āsana* practice. Sjoman's book includes photographs of the illustrations of *āsana*-s from a manuscript of the *Śrītattvanidhi* held at a library in Mysore.[82] These illustrated folios, which include the Sanskrit

this Siddha. The name may also correspond to Koraṇḍa who is listed among Siddhas in *Ānandakanda* 1.3.49c (see White 1996: 83–86).

77 I wish to thank Dominik Wujastyk for pointing this out to me (personal communication, 10 September 2013).

78 Sanderson 2004: 356–357, n. 19.

79 On the incompleteness of the *Haṭhābhyāsapaddhati,* see n. 75.

80 This is according to the annals of the Mysore Palace (see Iyer & Nanjundayya 1935: 49).

81 Śrīkṛṣṇadāsa 1884: 1–44.

82 One photograph appears to be from a different manuscript. Sjoman (1999: 40) says that he photographed two manuscripts at the Sarasvati Bhandar Library in Mysore. One is of the

descriptions of each *āsana* in Telugu script, indicate that the *Śrītattvanidhi* has reproduced all except one of the *āsana*-s in the *Haṭhābhyāsapaddhati,* because their descriptions are identical. However, an important difference in the presentation of *āsana* practice in these texts is the order in which they appear. In the table below, the names of the *āsana*-s have been listed according to their order in the *Haṭhābhyāsapaddhati,* and their position in the *Śrītattvanidhi* is indicated by the number on the right. The one pose not in the *Śrītattvanidhi* is marked by an asterisk (*).[83]

No./HAP	Name	No./ŚTN	No./HAP	Name	No./ŚTN
1	vṛṣapādakṣepa	81	57	mālā	44
2	parigha	11	58	haṃsa	45
3	paraśvadha	16	59	vānara	37
4	ananta	1	60	parvata	43
5	aṅkuśa	3	61	pāśa	47
6	śvottāna	2	62	kādamba	91
7	mārjārottāna	82	63	kāñcī	92
8	vṛka	10	64	aṅgamoṭana	116
9	trikūṭa	21	65	ucchīrṣaka	48
10	markaṭa	83	66	(unnamed)	117
11	nauka	4	67	pādukā	41
12	tiryaṅnauka	84	68	graha	50
13	dhvaja	7	69	parpaṭa	93
14	naraka	8	70	aśva	73
15	lāṅgala	17	71	dviśīrṣa	46
16	paryaṅka	5	72	kubja	52

Śrītattvanidhi and the other is of the *Haṭhayogapradīpikā,* the text of which is different from the well-known *Haṭhapradīpikā.*

83 There are a number of differences between the names of *āsana*-s in the *Haṭhābhyāsapaddhati* and in the *Śrītattvanidhi.* These call for the following additional remarks: No. 6: This pose is called *uttāna* in the *Śrītattvanidhi.* No. 10: This pose is called *kāmapīṭhāsana* in the *Śrītattvanidhi.* No. 47: The description of this unnamed pose is the same as *nyubjāsana* in the *Śrītattvanidhi.* No. 48: The description of this unnamed pose is the same as *garbhāsana* in the *Śrītattvanidhi.* No. 51: The description of this unnamed pose is the same as *dhanurāsana* in the *Śrītattvanidhi.* No. 55: The description of this unnamed pose is the same as *pādahastasaṃyogāsana* in the *Śrītattvanidhi.* No. 64: This pose is called *hastāṅgulibaddha* in the *Śrītattvanidhi.* No. 66: The description of this unnamed pose is the same as *hṛjjānusaṃyogāsana* in the *Śrītattvanidhi.* No. 74: The description of this unnamed pose agrees with that of the *preṅkhāsana* in the *Śrītattvanidhi.* There are two poses by this name in the *Śrītattvanidhi* (see Sjoman 1999: 85). No. 76: This pose is called *vimalāsana* in the *Śrītattvanidhi.* No. 86: This pose is called *uḍḍānāsana* in the *Śrītattvanidhi.* No. 95: The description of this unnamed pose is the same as that of *daṇḍāsana* in the *Śrītattvanidhi.*

(Continued)

No./HAP	Name	No./ŚTN	No./HAP	Name	No./ŚTN
17	vetra	9	73	preṅkha	94
18	kanduka	6	74	(unnamed)	118
19	uttānakūrma	85	75	utpīḍa	53
20	virata	86	76	vimāna	51
21	dṛṣada	21	77	kapotapiṭaka	57
22	luṭhana	20	78	ardhacandra	95
23	saraṭa	12	79	śaṅku	22
24	matsya	14	80	tāṇḍava	55
25	gaja	13	81	trivikrama	62
26	tarakṣu	15	82	utthānotthāna	106
27	ṛkṣa	18	83	āliṅga	96
28	śaśa	24	84	bālāliṅgana	97
29	ratha	23	85	kaupīna	110
30	meṣa	87	86	dehalyullaṅghana	119
31	aja	25	87	hariṇa	69
32	caṭaka	26	88	musala	61
33	kāka	27	89	dhruva	56
34	tittira	29	90	kulālacakra	98
35	baka	30	91	uṣṭra	54
36	bhāradvāja	28	92	ākāśakapota	*
37	kukkuṭṭoddāna	88	93	garuḍa	39
38	araṇyacaṭaka	89	94	paroṣṇī	63
39	mayūra	32	95	(unnamed)	65
40	paṅgumayūra	111	96	bhāra	99
41	khaḍga	34	97	nārada	100
42	śūla	40	98	svarga	101
43	viparītanṛtya	90	99	ūrṇanābhi	49
44	śyena	38	100	śuka	71
45	kapāla	31	101	tṛṇajalāyukā	60
46	sarpa	42	102	vṛnta	72
47	(unnamed)	114	103	krauñca	67
48	(unnamed)	113	104	varāha	66
49	ardhapaścimatāna	107	105	matsyendra	102
50	ūrdhvapaści-matāna	108	106	yoni	103
51	(unnamed)	109	107	svastika	59
52	baddhapadma	33	108	vajra	68

(Continued)

No./HAP	Name	No./ŚTN	No./HAP	Name	No./ŚTN
53	kukkuṭa	36	109	utkaṭa	104
54	paṅgukukkuṭa	112	110	śukti	105
55	(unnamed)	115	111	śava	70
56	chatra	35	112	tāna	74[84]

Table 5: Names of *āsana*-s in the *Haṭhābhyāsapaddhati* and in the *Śrītattvanidhi.*

The order of the descriptions of the *āsana*-s in these texts is key to understanding how they are to be practised. In over a dozen instances, the description of one *āsana* relies on the description of the one directly before it. In other words, one must accomplish a "foundational" *āsana,* so to speak, in order to perform the next. Examples are *gajāsana* (26–31), *caṭakāsana* (32–34), *kukkuṭāsana* (53–54, 58), etc. (see Appendix 2). The order of the *āsana*-s in the *Haṭhābhyāsapaddhati* is correct in so far as the description of each foundational *āsana* is placed before the one that depends on it. However, in the *Śrītattvanidhi,* the *āsana*-s have been taken out of order, resulting in the foundational *āsana*-s being separated from those that depend on them. This means that one cannot understand many of the descriptions in the *Śrītattvanidhi* without reading ahead. More importantly, it suggests that the section on *āsana* practice in the *Haṭhābhyāsapaddhati* is in all probability the source of those in the *Śrītattvanidhi* because the latter has been compiled without retaining the correct textual order.

Furthermore, one would expect the *Śrītattvanidhi* to have borrowed its material from elsewhere because it is a digest which is not specifically about yoga. In contrast to this, the *Haṭhābhyāsapaddhati* is undoubtedly a yoga text, and is more likely to be the source, unless this material derives from a third, earlier work that remains unknown. Sjoman's hypothesis[85] that some of these *āsana*-s derive from Indian wrestling, gymnastics and so on, may still be true. However, the significance of the *Haṭhābhyāsapaddhati* is that it locates these *āsana*-s within Haṭha Yoga. Therefore, there is now evidence that haṭhayogis practised dynamic *āsana*-s, some of which required the use of rope and walls, and such yogis may have played an important role in the development of these *āsana*-s.

Though it is beyond the scope of this chapter to discuss fully the significance of the *Haṭhābhyāsapaddhati*'s *āsana*-s in the context of the historical development of Haṭha Yoga, two observations can be made. The first striking feature is the inclusion of moving *āsana*-s. Many *āsana*-s are combined with a movement that is to be repeated over and over. Examples include *vṛṣapādakṣepa* (1), *śvottāna* (6), *virata* (20), *luṭhana* (22), *matsya* (24), etc. (see Appendix 2).

84 This pose is called *uttānapādāsana* in the *Śrītattvanidhi.*

85 Sjoman 1999: 43ff.

The second feature, which is unique among medieval yoga texts, is that the *āsana*-s are arranged in six sequences, each with its own heading. The headings are as follows:

1. Supine *āsana*-s (*uttānāni āsanāni*)
2. Prone *āsana*-s (*nubjāsanāni*)
3. Stationary *āsana*-s (*sthānāsanāni*)
4. Standing *āsana*-s (*utthānāsanāni*)
5. Rope *āsana*-s (*rajjvāsanāni*)
6. *āsana*-s which pierce the sun and moon (*sūryacandrabhedanāny āsanāni*)[86]

It appears as though these *āsana*-s have been sequenced according to how they were practised because, in some instances, the foundational *āsana* does not resemble the *āsana* being described. For example, the description of the ball posture (*kandukāsana*) stipulates that one should do the reed posture (*vetrāsana*) beforehand.[87] However, the reed pose, in which the spine is extended, does not resemble the ball pose, in which the spine is flexed. Therefore, the instruction of positioning oneself in the reed pose is not simply a literary device employed by the scribe to assist in describing the ball pose. Such an instruction is intended to indicate the sequence of practice.[88]

Furthermore, the headings and sequences suggest that the postures were developed in groups. These groups appear to be antecedents to the modern categories of standing, seated and floor poses, which are also combined in some styles to form sequences.[89]

Though the one available manuscript of the *Haṭhābhyāsapaddhati* appears to be incomplete and the text itself may be a truncation of an earlier work, it significantly extends our knowledge of Haṭha Yoga in the eighteenth century. During this time, haṭhayogic *āsana*-s were adapted with a view to cultivating strength and fitness, through a comprehensive range of strenuous positions and continuous movements. Its section on *āsana* does not expatiate on the benefits of

86 These six headings correspond to *āsana*-s 1–22, 23–47, 48–74, 75–93, 94–103 and 104–122, respectively. Some of these headings are based on emendations. See Appendix 2. I do not know why there is a category called “piercing the sun and moon”. The sun and moon are not mentioned in the descriptions of the *āsana*-s that follow this heading, and these poses do not suggest concepts of the sun and moon as left and right sides of the body, nasal dominance, *prāṇāyāma*, head and abdomen, etc.

87 The ball posture is *āsana* 18 in Appendix 2.

88 I would like to thank Dominic Goodall for bringing this to my attention.

89 Iyengar’s subdividing of *āsana*-s into standing, sitting, supine, prone, etc., has been noted by Elizabeth De Michelis (2004: 234, n. 40). Swami Sivananda’s book, *Yoga Asanas* (1993, first published 1931) is without subdivisions, though Swami Satyananda’s book *Asana Pranayama Mudra Bandha* (1996, first published 1969) has subdivisions, including standing *āsana*-s. Other modern yoga books such as Shree Yogeshwaranand Paramahansa’s *First Steps to Higher Yoga* (2001, first published 1970) present *āsana*-s in various groups.

practising such *āsana*-s, other than to say they produce bodily strength (*śārīra-dārḍhya*). Another manuscript of this text or, more ideally, the source from which it may have been extracted, will most probably provide more information.

4. Chronology and Increments in the Number of *Āsana*-s in Medieval Yoga Texts

All the texts and manuscripts containing extensive lists of *āsana*-s date to after the sixteenth century. The chronology of medieval yoga texts indicates a steady increase in the number of *āsana*-s practised in Haṭha Yoga as it developed over time. A number of reasons seem probable here. Firstly, the increase may have resulted from competitive extension. In other words, one tradition tried to gain an advantage over another tradition by claiming to teach more *āsana*-s.

Secondly, if it ever comes to light that eighty-four *āsana*-s existed outside of Haṭha Yoga before the fifteenth century, then it would appear that haṭhayogis gradually adopted them over the course of several centuries, despite their initial view that most of these *āsana*-s were superfluous. Haṭha Yoga grew in popularity from the eleventh to the sixteenth centuries, as evinced by its transformation from an auxiliary practice in works such as the eleventh-century *Kālacakratantra* (Birch 2011: 535–538) and the thirteenth-century *Dattātreyayogaśāstra*, in which it is one of four yogas, to a tradition of yoga in its own right as seen in the *Haṭhapradīpikā*. It is reasonable to assume that, by the end of the fifteenth century, Haṭha Yoga must have been practised more widely and by a greater variety of people. Therefore, the growth in its popularity would have led to greater innovation, experimentation and the assimilation of practices from elsewhere, such as older traditions of asceticism and martial arts. This hypothesis is supported by the claim in some texts that Haṭha Yoga was practised by people of different religions and social backgrounds in India.[90]

A third possible reason for the incremental growth in the number of *āsana*-s in yoga texts has more to do with the development of the literature rather than the yoga systems themselves. The early Haṭha texts are short, pithy manuals that might have been written by and for practitioners. Over time, these yoga texts grew

90 For example, DYŚ 41–42ab: "Whether a Brahmin, renunciant, Buddhist, Jain, Kāpālika or follower of Cārvāka, the wise man who has confidence [in the efficacy of Haṭha Yoga] and who is always devoted to the practice of [Haṭha] yoga will attain all Siddhis" (*brāhmaṇaḥ śramaṇo vāpi bauddho vāpy ārhato 'thavā | kāpāliko vā cārvākaḥ śraddhayā sahitaḥ sudhīḥ || 41 || yogābhyāsarato nityaṃ sarvasiddhim avāpnuyāt*). For statements suggesting that all four castes and women practised Haṭha Yoga, see YY 6.12, 6.16–6.19ab and the *Yogacintāmaṇi* p. 57 (quoting without attribution *Viṣṇudharma* 98.16). The *Śivasaṃhitā* (4.79, 5.258–260) taught Haṭha Yoga for householders.

in size and became more scholarly in their language and style. Hence, lists and descriptions of eighty-four postures may have manifested because later compilers were concerned more with thoroughness than brevity. Large scholarly compilations like the *Yogacintāmaṇi* were written for a more learned audience and tended to include more techniques from a greater variety of sources.

These three proposed reasons are not mutually exclusive and may have combined to produce the proliferation of *āsana*-s seen in the later textual sources. Competitive extension and the growing popularity of Haṭha Yoga suggest a gradual process of accretion. The gathering of sources and the creation of lists of eighty-four or more *āsana*-s was probably the most recent stage, which was the result of scholarly activity.

5. Connections between Medieval and Modern *Āsana*-s

In light of the fact that Indian yoga systems of the early twentieth century incorporated large numbers of *āsana*-s, it is worth asking if their pioneers were influenced by any of the unpublished texts discussed in this chapter. I know of no citation of these texts in a modern book on yoga, apart from Dr. M. L. Gharote's work, which cites the last two manuscripts. Gharote was a disciple of Swāmī Kuvalayānanda, who founded the Kaivalyadhama Yoga Institute with a view to popularising physical yoga throughout India from the 1920s onwards.[91] However, I am yet to ascertain whether Swāmī Kuvalayānanda knew of these yoga compendiums. The early publications of the Institute do not cite them.

Nonetheless, the citation of the sources I have discussed is not a necessary condition for proving their influence on gurus in the twentieth century. These sources indicate that over eighty-four *āsana*-s were known to haṭhayogis from several areas in north and south India before the British opened the floodgates to European modernity,[92] and it is quite likely that knowledge of these *āsana*-s was

91 Alter 2004: 9, 86, 263, n. 22.

92 Various sources on the eighty-four *āsana*-s are ascribed to specific places. A scribal comment after the *Haṭharatnāvalī*'s first chapter colophon in a manuscript (no. 6715) held at the Tanjore Mahārāja Serfoji's Sarasvatī Mahāl Library, appears to identify the author, Śrīnivāsabhaṭṭa, as native to Tīrabhukta ([...] *pravartakatīrabhukte deśīya* [...]) (For the complete transcript, see Sastri 1931: 4918). Veṅkata Reddy (1982: 14–15) opines that Śrīnivāsa may have belonged to a Tīrabhukta in Andhra Pradesh, but this name may also refer to the Videha country which is in northern Bihar (Sircar 1971: 101). In the *Jogapradīpyakā* (v. 958), the author, Jayatarāma, says he was living in Vrindavan (i.e., near Mathura). Also, there are reports that libraries in Jodhpur and Jaipur hold several manuscripts which mention large numbers of *āsana*-s (e.g., the *Āsananāmāni, Āsanayogagrantha*, etc.; for details, see Gharote et al. 2006: lxiii). Also, eighty-four *āsana*-s are painted on the walls of the Mahāmandir in Jodhpur and one hundred miniatures are reportedly held at the Jaipur Central Museum

transmitted to twentieth-century gurus not only by textual sources which are unknown to modern scholars, but by Brahmins who may have inherited the knowledge from their families or teachers. Pioneering yoga gurus, such as Kṛṣṇamācārya, Swāmī Kuvalayānanda and Shree Yogendra, were all Brahmins who disapproved of the extreme asceticism and Kāpālika practices of some renunciants.[93] Therefore, it is more likely that they were influenced by the knowledge of Brahmins whose erudite forefathers had been appropriating Haṭha Yoga since the seventeenth century, as evinced by texts such as the *Yogacintāmaṇi,* the *Haṭhasaṅketacandrikā* and the so-called Yoga Upaniṣads.[94]

Generally speaking, most of the seated, forward, backward, twisting and arm-balancing poses in modern yoga have been anticipated by these seventeenth and eighteenth-century sources. This may not be so apparent in comparing the names of *āsana*-s from one tradition to another, because similar *āsana*-s can have different names.[95] This is true for both medieval and modern yoga. Such differences may reflect regional influences and attempts by gurus to distinguish their own repertoire of techniques. The main exceptions to this are the names of *āsana*-s in the well-known, principal texts such as the *Pātañjalayogaśāstra* and the *Haṭhapradīpikā.* Since these texts have been invoked to establish the traditional credentials, so to speak, of more recent lineages, the names of their *āsana*-s have endured.[96]

As far as I am aware, the prominent modern practices of *sūryanamaskāra* and *vinyāsa* are absent in medieval yoga texts.[97] Though moving *āsana*-s and se-

---

(Gharote et al. 2006: lxvi). These indicate that eighty-four *āsana*-s were known in Rajasthan in the eighteenth and nineteenth centuries. A comment in the *Haṭhābhyāsapaddhati* (fol. 26r) suggests the author was familiar with Maharashtra: "Similar to the Jāti sprout, the *haritaśara* by name is known in Mahārāṣṭra, etc. as the Lavālā" ([...] *jātyaṅkurasadṛśo haritaśaraḥ nāma lavālā iti mahārāṣṭrādau prasiddhaḥ* || Emend. *jāty-* : Codex *jānty-*. Emend. *dṛśo* : Codex *dṛśa*).

93 For more information on the disrepute of Haṭha Yoga in the nineteenth and early twentieth century, see Singleton 2010: 78. He also mentions the yogis' association with mercenary fighters and the "risible contortions of the mendicant fakir". Such views are also seen in the work of Indologists at this time (Birch 2011: 529–530).

94 My comments here are confined to the gurus whose names I have mentioned. Also, Swami Sivananda of Rishikesh, who is said to have been initiated into the Daśnāmī sect in 1924 (Satyananda 1996: v), must have been a Brahmin because the Sarasvatī lineage initiates only Brahmins (Clark 2006: 39). Nonetheless, one cannot rule out that there were non-Brahmanical channels of transmission of other types of modern Indian yoga.

95 See Appendix 3 for examples of this.

96 There are also textual variations in the names of *āsana*-s transmitted in different versions of the PYŚ. See Maas' chapter in the present volume.

97 In his biography of his teacher Kṛṣṇamācārya, A. G. Mohan (2010: 29) defines *vinyāsa* and states his belief that *vinyāsa* was Kṛṣṇamācārya's innovation: "A special feature of the asana system of Krishnamacharya was vinyasa. Many yoga students are no doubt familiar with this word – it is increasingly used now, often to describe the 'style' of a yoga class, as in 'hatha

quences are described in the *Haṭhābhyāsapaddhati,* this text does not provide general guidelines on how the postures were practised. In fact, Sanskrit yoga texts do not stipulate whether a specific *āsana* was held for a long or short period of time or whether manipulating the breath was important. The absence of such details suggests that there was no consensus on these matters, which may have been left to each guru's discretion.

The prostration-like movements of *sūryanamaskāra* may derive from older devotional practices of sun worship but its inclusion as a technique in a system of yoga is without any known precedent until the twentieth century. In fact, the one reference to *sūryanamaskāra* in a medieval text on Haṭha Yoga advises against its practice on the grounds that it might afflict the body (*kāyakleśa*) if performed many times.[98] This comment indicates that a rather strenuous form of *sūryanamaskāra* was known in the nineteenth century, but descriptions of such a practice are yet to be found.[99]

Both late medieval and modern yoga make use of inverted *āsana*-s. In early Haṭha Yoga, inversions are a *mudrā* called *viparītakaraṇī.* In late medieval sources, *viparītakaraṇī* is included among descriptions of *āsana*-s with names

---

vinyasa' or 'vinyasa flow'. Vinyasa is essential, and probably unique, to Krishnamacharya's teachings. As far as I know, he was the first yoga master in the last century to introduce the idea. A vinyasa, in essence, consists of moving from one asana, or body position, to another, combining breathing with the movement."

98 In his commentary on the *Haṭhapradīpikā* (1.61), the nineteenth-century Brahmānanda mentioned *sūryanamaskāra,* but he did so only in the context of providing an example of a practice that, in his opinion, would afflict the body (*kāyakleśa*) if performed many times: "A method of afflicting the body is a method that causes affliction to the body. [It is] an action in the form of many *sūryanamaskāra,* etc. and lifting great weights, etc." (*kāyakleśavidhiṃ kāyakleśakaraṃ vidhiṃ kriyāṃ bahusūryanamaskārādirūpāṃ bahubhārodvahanādirūpāṃ ca*). The physical act of prostrating the body in worship is mentioned in some classical and early medieval Sanskrit sources. Examples include references to an eight-limbed prostration (*aṣṭāṅgapraṇāma*), in which eight parts of the body touch the ground (*aṣṭāṅgapraṇipāta, aṣṭāṅgapraṇāma*). See the following etexts available at muktabodha.org: *Picumata/Brahmayāmala* 45.375; *Ciñcinīmatasārasamuccaya* 8.38; *Kulārṇavatantra* 17.98; etc. An *aṣṭāṅgapraṇāma* is described by Kṛṣṇānanda Āgamavāgīśa in his *Bṛhattantrasāra* 2.107–109. Chapter thirty-four of the *Aṃśumatitantra* is on "methods of prostration" (*namaskāravidhi*) and describes an eight-limbed prostration which destroys all diseases.

99 Polly O'Hanlon's article on "Military Sports and the History of the Martial Body in India" (2007: 511) refers to a letter written in 1759 by a trooper named Muzaffar Khan, who wrote to Nanasaheb Peshwa to inform him that a wound on his back was preventing him from practising his usual regime of *daṇḍa* and *sūryanamaskāra.* Also, a more recent reference to a physically demanding type of *sūryanamaskāra* can be found in *A Short History of Aryan Medical Science* by HH Sir Bhagvat Sinh Jee (1896: 61), who states, "There are various kinds of physical exercises, in-door and out-door. But some of the Hindoos set aside a portion of their daily worship for making salutations to the Sun by prostrations. This method of adoration affords them so much muscular activity that it takes to some extent the place of physical exercise."

such as *viparītakaraṇāsana,*[100] *narakāsana,*[101] *kapālāsana,*[102] etc. There is some ambiguity in the descriptions of *viparītakaraṇī* in early Haṭha texts as to whether this *mudrā* has only the top of the head on the ground as headstand (*śīrṣāsana*) in modern yoga or the back of the head and neck on the ground as shoulderstand (*sarvāṅgāsana*).[103] The descriptions of inverted *āsana*-s in texts such as the *Haṭhābhyāsapaddhati* and the *Jogapradīpyakā* are clear in this regard: *narakāsāna* and *viparītakaraṇāsana* are the equivalent of shoulderstand, and *kapālāsana,* headstand.[104] Apart from *viparītakaraṇī,* there are several other instances of early haṭhayogic *mudrā*-s becoming *āsana*-s in late medieval sources; for example, *mūlabandhāsana,*[105] *mahāmudrāsana*[106] and *yonimudrāsana.*[107] The deliberate application of haṭhayogic *mudrā*-s such as *uḍḍīyānabandha* to seated *āsana*-s is a salient feature of Haṭha Yoga.[108] However, the application of these *mudrā*-s in the practice of non-seated *āsana*-s is not mentioned in medieval sources and may be a modern development.

The extensive lists of *āsana*-s in medieval sources do not account for many of the standing poses in modern yoga. The similar shapes of these standing poses to exercises in European free-standing gymnastics and callisthenics is strong evidence for the influence of British physical culture on modern Indian yoga.[109] However, very little is known of the fighting stances and lunges of medieval Indian wrestling and martial traditions, which may also have inspired some of modern yoga's standing poses. It is possible that Indian yoga gurus may have viewed callisthenic and martial postures as an extension of older standing *āsana*-s in texts such as the *Haṭhābhyāsapaddhati.* Indeed, the ease with which these gurus integrated postures from outside yoga may well be the result of their knowledge of antecedents in earlier systems of Haṭha Yoga. The standing poses of modern yoga are prominent in the styles emanating from Kṛṣṇamācārya, who was familiar with one hundred and eleven *āsana*-s of the *Haṭhābhyāsapaddhati*

100 JP vv. 163–165.

101 YC p. 157.

102 *Haṭhābhyāsapaddhati* 45 (Appendix 2).

103 From the description of *viparītakaraṇī* in the *Haṭhapradīpikā* (3.81), one might infer that it is a headstand because it is supposed to be held for three hours every day, which seems more practicable for headstand (see Bernard 1958: 29–31) than shoulderstand.

104 In the *Yogacintāmaṇi* (p. 157), *narakāsana* is headstand.

105 HSC, ms. no. R3239, fols. 34–35.

106 JP vv. 103–106.

107 JP vv. 107–109.

108 For examples, see the definitions of *padmāsana* and *siddhāsana* in the *Haṭhapradīpikā* (1.35–36, 44–46). These and similar definitions occur in both earlier and later sources on Haṭha Yoga.

109 For the influence of physical culture on twentieth-century Indian yoga, see Singleton 2010.

because he had read the *Śrītattvanidhi*, which he cited in the introduction to his book called the *Yogamakaranda*.[110]

Kṛṣṇamācārya's knowledge of the *āsana*-s in the *Haṭhābhyāsapaddhati* via the *Śrītattvanidhi* raises the question of whether he knew their textual source(s). As mentioned above, the *Haṭhābhyāsapaddhati* appears to be an incomplete summary of another text,[111] and the *Śrītattvanidhi* is a compilation that must have borrowed its material on *āsana* practice from elsewhere. According to a biography[112] and Singleton's interviews with Pattabhi Jois,[113] some salient features of Kṛṣṇamācārya's teaching on *āsana* were derived from a Sanskrit yoga text called the *Yoga Kuruṇṭa*, which is also known to some of his students, including the Iyengars, Pattabhi Jois, Desikachar and his son, Kaustubh.[114] Despite the prominence of the *Yoga Kuruṇṭa* in this lineage, no one has produced a copy of it.[115] My research has not located a name similar to *Yoga Kuruṇṭa* in any catalogue of an Indian manuscript library.

Gītā Iyengar's book *Yoga: A Gem for Women*[116] has a section entitled, "Āsana: Yoga Kuruṇṭa", in which she states that these *āsana*-s involve the use of a rope. In a more recent article, she reveals that the inspiration behind the rope poses was Kṛṣṇamācārya's knowledge of the *Yoga Kuruṇṭa*.[117] The *Haṭhābhyāsapaddhati* has rope poses, which indicates that ropes were used in this way in Haṭha Yoga, possibly as early as the eighteenth century. None of the names of its rope poses correspond to those in Iyengar's book, but a connection between the *Haṭhābhyāsapaddhati* and the *Yoga Kuruṇṭa* seems probable given that the former is the only extant yoga text in which rope poses have been described. One must wonder whether the name "Yogakuruṇṭa" was derived from Kapālakuraṇṭaka, the author of the *Haṭhābhyāsapaddhati*.[118] Moreover, Kṛṣṇamācārya's knowl-

110 Singleton 2010: 222, n. 7.

111 See n. 75.

112 Mohan 2010: 45.

113 Singleton 2010: 184–186.

114 Singleton (2010: 185) was told of Kaustubh's knowledge of this text in an interview.

115 According to the official website for the K. Pattabhi Jois Ashtanga Yoga Institute, Kṛṣṇamācārya transcribed the *Yoga Kuruṇṭa* from a manuscript which may no longer be extant: "The method of Yoga taught at KPJAYI is that which has been told by the ancient Sage Vamana in his text called 'Yoga Korunta'. Although many books on Yoga have been written, Vamana is the only one who has delineated a complete practical method. In the 1920's, the Yogi and Sanskrit Scholar, T. Krishnamacharya traveled to Calcutta where he transcribed and recorded the Yoga Korunta, which was written on palm leaves and was in a bad state of decay, having been partially eaten by ants. Later, Krishnamacharya passed on these teachings to the late Pattabhi Jois, whose school continues to teach this method today" (http://kpjayi.org/the-practice/traditional-method. Accessed 4 August 2014).

116 Iyengar 1998: 252.

117 The relevant passage of this article is cited in Smith 2008: 157, n. 5.

118 The name *Yogakuraṇṭaka* might be understood as the *Yogayājñavalkya* (i.e., "Yājñavalkya on [the topic of] yoga"), but it might also be a play on the meaning of *kuraṇṭaka* as "yellow

edge of rope poses in the *Yoga Kuruṇṭa* and the reference to Kapālakuraṇṭaka in the *Haṭhābhyāsapaddhati* suggest a connection between these texts. It could be possible that *Yogakuruṇṭa* is another name for the *Haṭhābhyāsapaddhati* or the original work from which the incomplete manuscript of the *Haṭhābhyāsapaddhati* was extracted. Until the *Yoga Kuruṇṭa* is found, such hypotheses remain speculative, particularly in light of the inconsistencies in statements made about the contents of the *Yoga Kuruṇṭa* by various students within Kṛṣṇamācārya's lineage, as Singleton has noted:[119]

> Krishnamacharya's grandson, Kausthub Desikachar, refers to writings by his grandfather that "contradict the popularly held notion that the *Yoga Kuranta* [*sic*] was the basis for *Astanga Vinyasa Yoga*" (Desikachar 2005: 60). Since nobody has seen this text, such statements can be more profitably interpreted as an indication that the "content" of the work changed as Krishnamacharya's teaching changed (and perhaps also as another symptom of the struggles to manage the memory and heritage of Krishnamacharya). That is to say, during his time in Mysore with Pattabhi Jois, Krishnamacharya may have invoked the text to legitimize the sequences that became Ashtanga yoga, but in later life he used it to authorize a wider set of practices.

6. Conclusion

The manuscript evidence discussed in this paper will contribute toward a more nuanced history of *āsana* practice. Though the corpus of early Haṭha Yoga contains relatively few *āsana*-s, it is becoming clear as more textual evidence is found that after the sixteenth century Haṭha Yoga traditions gradually incorporated larger numbers of *āsana*-s to the point that some mention and describe more than eighty-four. The aggregate number of *āsana*-s in these late medieval sources is at least several hundred in addition to the dozen or so standard *āsana*-s which are found in earlier yoga texts.

Further research is required to determine the degree to which medieval *āsana*-s correspond to those taught in India in the modern period. As I mentioned above, it seems that certain types of *āsana*-s correspond whereas others do not. However, it is often very difficult to compare medieval and modern *āsana*-s because of the ambiguities and omissions in the Sanskrit descriptions of the former, the number of variations of the latter and the different names for the same *āsana* in both medieval and modern traditions. For example, as outlined in Appendix 3, a basic comparison between Pattabhi Jois' primary sequence of

---

amaranth" (Monier-Williams 1899, s. v.). One might understand *Yogakuraṇṭaka* as the "yellow amaranth of yoga", much like the title *Haṭhayogamañjarī*.

119 Singleton 2010: 185. Singleton's reference is to Desikachar's book *The Yoga of the Yogi: The Legacy of T. Krishnamacharya* (Chennai: Krishnamacharya Yoga Mandiram).

āsana-s and the sources consulted for this paper suggests that his floor and finishing poses are the types of modern *āsana*-s most similar to medieval ones. However, apart from iconic *āsana*-s such as *padmāsana,* few modern and medieval *āsana*-s have the same names or correspond in every detail.

Owing to the absence of citations of premodern texts that describe large numbers of *āsana*-s, such as the *Haṭharatnāvalī, Jogapradīpyakā* and *Haṭhābhyāsapaddhati,* in twentieth-century yoga books, such as Jois' *Yogamālā,* it is not possible to evaluate their influence on modern yoga in any definitive way. Nonetheless, these pre-modern works are important for reconstructing the history of yoga because their content indicates that Haṭha Yoga continued to evolve in the seventeenth and eighteenth centuries. During this time, the number and sophistication of its techniques grew not only in *āsana* practice, but also in the practice of *ṣaṭkarma, prāṇāyāma* and *mudrā.* Furthermore, some of these texts evince the integration of haṭhayogic teachings with mainstream Brahmanical traditions, which increases the likelihood that those Brahmins who taught physical yoga in the twentieth century knew of these relatively recent developments in Haṭha Yoga.

Appendix 1: Descriptions of the Additional *Āsana*-s in the Ujjain Manuscript

The following is a diplomatic transcription of the descriptions of *āsana*-s which appear in list 1b of the above chapter. These *āsana*-s and their descriptions do not occur in other manuscripts of the *Yogacintāmaṇi* and, apart from those few which are based on Vācaspatimiśra's *Tattvavaiśāradī* and three others which I have indicated in the footnotes, I am yet to find the majority of these descriptions in another text or manuscript. I have suggested some conjectures and emendations in the footnotes, and hope that this transcription may contribute to the critical editing of these descriptions. I have reproduced the numbering of these *āsana*-s in the Ujjain manuscript. The gaps in the numbering are those *āsana*-s in list 1a, descriptions of which occur in the edition and other manuscripts of the *Yogacintāmaṇi.*

[fol. 59r]
1. kevalasvastikam [||] jānūrvor antare samyak kṛtvā pādatale ubhe || ṛjukāyaḥ samāsīnaḥ svastikaṃ tat pracakṣate ||[120] anyac cāgre śīvanyā ātmana ityādi uttarapṛṣṭhe [||]

3. ardhāsanam[121] [||] ekapādam athaikasmin vinyasyoruṇi sattamaḥ || āsītārdhāsanam idaṃ yogasādhanam uttamam ||

8.[122] paryaṅkāsanam uktaṃ yogabhāṣyaṭīkāyāṃ vācaspatinā || jānuprasāritabāhvoḥ paryaṅka[123] iti || tattvaṃ tu paprāsanaḥ[124] [||] bhūmau śayitvopajānuhastadvayaṃ sthāpayet [||] tena catur sayakapādavad asya[125] jānudvayaskandhadvayarūpaṃ catuṣkaṃ bhātīti || 2 madīyaḥ ||[126]

[fol. 59v]
[no number][127] yathā vācyatyasyatalayor[128] ardhasaṃsparśād uccajaṅghayoḥ [||] pādayor jānudeśe vai vīrākhyaṃ yogapaṭṭataḥ || iti vīrāsanalakṣaṇāntaram [||]

20. garuḍāsanam [no description]

[fol. 60r]
28. markaṭaṃ [||] śavāsanasthau dvau pādau bhūmau mastakato [']nyataḥ [|] kuryād utthāya vegenādhasthitir markaṭaṃ[129] tu tat ||

29. garbhāsanaṃ [||] garbhāsane nirañjanakriyā tallakṣaṇaṃ tu ||

120 This is the same as *svastikāsana* in HP 1.21. The quotation following this (i. e., *śīvanyā ātmana*) refers to the description of *svastikāsana* in the *Yogayājñavalkya* (3.4–5ab), which is quoted on a subsequent page of this manuscript (i. e., as *āsana* no. 14).

121 This is the same as the description of *ardhāsana* in other manuscripts of the *Yogacintāmaṇi.*

122 The following descriptions of *paryaṅkāsana* are a marginal note in the lower margin of this folio (i. e., 59r).

123 One might consider the diagnostic conjecture *śayanaṃ paryaṅka iti.*

124 Consider *padmāsanaḥ* for *paprāsanaḥ.*

125 Consider *paryaṅkavad asya* for *sayakavad asya.* I wish to thank James Mallinson for this suggestion.

126 The first description of *paryaṅkāsana* is based on that in Vācaspatimiśra's *Tattvavaiśāradī.* I have not found the second description in another yoga text.

127 The following description of *vīrāsana* is a marginal note at the top of the folio.

128 Consider *vā vyatyasya* for *vācyatyasya.*

129 There are two numbers written as a fraction which divide this word in the Codex: *marka* 16/ 100 *ṭaṃ.* This is a reference to the word *caturaśīti*, which is in the line above.

[fol. 61v]
34. cakrāsanaṃ [||] śavāsanasthau dvau pādau kuryān mastakataḥ pari[130] || vyutkrameṇa tataḥ śīghram etat sarvasya sādhana[m] || sarvāsananidānaṃ[131] gulmaplīhāvātarogādināśanam ||[132]

35. daṇḍāsanaṃ [||] upaśliṣyāṅgulikau[133] bhūmiśliṣṭajaṅghorupādau prasārya daṇḍāsanam abhyased iti ||

36. sopāśrayaṃ [||] yogapaṭṭayogād idam evaṃ sopāśrayaṃ iti vācaspatiḥ ||

37. candrāsanaṃ [||] vāmaṃ vā dakṣiṇaṃ vāpi pādapārśvaṃ bhuvi nyaset || gulphe[134] tatrānyad āsthāpya saṃsthārdhenduprakīrtitam[135] ||

38. krauñcaniṣadanaṃ [||] krauñcaḥ pakṣiviśeṣaḥ tadvat yathā [||]

39. hastinaḥ [||] hastina iva sthitiḥ yathā [||]

40. uṣṭrasya [||] pādadvayatala[136] nitambau dhṛtvā karo talopari[137] karatalaṃ yuktaṃ liṅgāgre 'thavā muṣṭhidvaye[138] mastakaṃ[139] vā kṛtvoṣṭrasya sthitis tad āsanaṃ || nādaṃ śṛṇuyāt ||

41. samasaṃsthānaṃ [||] pārṣṇyāgrapādābhyāṃ[140] dvayor ākuñcitayor anyonyapīḍanaṃ yenāvasthitasya sthairyaṃ sukhaṃ ca jāyate sthirasukham āsanam iti yogasūtrāt ||

[fol. 62r]
42. bhagāsanaṃ [||] pādadvayasya pārṣṇyāgre liṅgabhūmyor[141] dṛḍhaṃ nyaset || śanair utthāya hastābhyāṃ dhṛtvā bhūmiṃ tataḥ punaḥ pādāgre pṛṣṭhataḥ kṛtvā

130 Consider *parau* for *pari.*
131 Consider *-nidhānaṃ* for *-nidānaṃ.*
132 This *āsana* is described in Nārāyaṇatīrtha's *Yogasiddhāntacandrikā* in the commentary on *sūtra* 2.46.
133 Correct *upaśliṣyāṅgulikau* to *upaśliṣṭāṅgulikau.*
134 Consider *gulphaṃ* for *gulphe.*
135 Correct *saṃsthārdhendu* to *saṃsthārdhenduṃ.*
136 Consider *-tale* for *-tala.*
137 Consider *karatalopari* for *karo talopari.*
138 Correct *muṣṭhi-* to *muṣṭi-.*
139 Consider *mastake* for *mastakaṃ.*
140 Consider *pārṣṇyagra* for *pārṣṇyāgra.*
141 Consider *liṅgaṃ bhūmyāṃ* for *liṅgabhūmyor.*

yuktau pārṣṇī puras tataḥ || pādayoḥ pṛṣṭhapārśve tu gudaṃ saṃsthāpya cāgrataḥ upasthapārśvayor[142] gulphau yat saṃsthāpyau bhagaṃ tu tat || phalam [||]

43. kubjāsanaṃ [||] vāmapādatalaṃ dakṣahastenākṛṣya vai balāt || vāmakakṣāṃ nyased dakṣaṃ dakṣakakṣe yathāvidhi || tattatpārṣṇer adhobhāge tattad +ūrparakāgrataḥ[143] dhārayet tiryagāsthānaṃ kubjāsanam idaṃ bhavet ||

44. naḍāsanaṃ [||] mohanadāsenokte | prathamaṃ jānudvaye sthitvā vāmakaramuṣṭiṃ baddhvā dakṣiṇajātuni[144] saṃsthāpya dakṣiṇajānunī[145] kim api saṃmardhya[146] dhārayet tena hastadvayam api bandhadvayaikībhūtena[147] nābhiṃ saṃmardayitvātrāntare [']dhaḥsthitapārṣṇibhyāṃ nitambau saṃmardhya[148] gudam ākuñcyāgrim[149] ūrdhvagataṃ kṛtvā līno bhaved iti || etenāghanāśaḥ alakṣyaprakāśaḥ ||

45. garbhāsanaṃ [||] garbhasaṃsthānaṃ yathā tathā tat || tatra nirañjanakriyā kartavyā || so [']ham ityādeḥ japaḥ ||

46. vūlyāsanaṃ[150] [||] ubhayapārṇiyugaṃ[151] jānvor ādhāya kaṭipṛṣṭhe same kṛtvā hastena nābhim utthāpya duttanyādbalena[152] gurudarśitena iḍāpiṅgale badhnīyāt yāvat granthidvayaṃ sthiraṃ patati tadā nānā sukhāni yatra tan naulīkarmopayuktam iti [||] ke cit tūtthāya jānudvaye hastadvayaṃ sthāpya tathā sthitvā jānudvaye kūrparadvayaṃ hastadvayena śaṅkhadvayam avalambya balena naulīṃ kurvanti ||

47. stambhāsanaṃ [||] nyubjaḥ jaṅghāmadhye karadvayaṃ kṛtvā karau bhūmau kṛtvāntarikṣo bhaved oṃkāraṃ raṭhed[153] iti || pṛthvīnīrāṃśanāśaḥ phalam ||

[fol. 62v]
48. śūnyāsanaṃ [||] karadvayamuṣṭī baddhvā tataḥ pṛthivyāṃ saṃsthāpyānta-

142 After *upasthapārśvayor*, there is a mark pointing to a definition of *upastha*, which has been written at the top of the folio: *upasthaṃ vakṣyamāṇayor bhagaliṅgayor ity amaraḥ.*
143 Consider *tattatkūrparakāgrataḥ* for *tattad+ūrparakāgrataḥ*.
144 Correct *dakṣiṇajātuni* to *dakṣiṇajānuni.*
145 Correct *-jānunī* to *-jānuni.*
146 Correct *saṃmardhya* to *saṃmardya.*
147 Consider *bandhayitvaikībhūtena* for *bandhadvayaikībhūtena.*
148 Correct *saṃmardhya* to *saṃmardya.*
149 Consider *ākuñcyāgnim* for *ākuñcyāgrim.*
150 The word *vūlyāsanam* is the result of a correction and the original reading is likely to have been *nyubjāsana.* The *ka* has been written over another ligature.
151 Correct *ubhayapārṇiyugaṃ* to *ubhayapārśṇiyugaṃ.*
152 The ligatures *-yādba-* are not clear. Consider *tūttanyād balena* for *duttanyādbalena.*
153 Correct *raṭhed* to *raṭed.*

rikṣam utthāpyālakṣyaṃ[154] raṭed iti || vāmacaraṇāṅguṣṭhaṃ gṛhītvā vāmakūrpare[155] bhāraṃ dadyāt || iti || dvi+unī[156] [||]

49. haṃsāsanaṃ [||] pṛṣṭhaśīrṣakaṭīḥ kṛtvā samāḥ jaṅghāṃ tu jaṅghikāṃ madhye saṃsthāpya vyatyasya pārṣṇī jānvor adhaḥ sthitau hastāgrābhyāṃ samākuñcya haṃsaṃ jāpī ca haṃsake || haṃsa so [']haṃ ||[157]

[fol. 67r]
|| lakṣmaṇadāsasvara yogī ||

50. gaṇeśāsanaṃ [||] gomukhe saṃsthitiṃ kṛtvā pārṣṇī vyatyasya yugmake || tatra sīvanikāṃ sthāpya gaṇeśāsanam īritaṃ [||] ālasyanidrākṣayam [||]

51. gudāsanaṃ [||] pādayoḥ pṛṣṭhake cobhe vyatyasya bhuvi saṃsthite || gudaṃ madhye tu saṃsthāpya gudāsanam iti smṛtam ||[158]

52. pārvatyāsanaṃ [||] dvau pādau melayitvā tu gudāgre ca pṛthak nyaset | bhūmau tadurdhvaṃ ca karau saṃpuṭau sthāpayet tataḥ || dakṣiṇānāmikāmadhye liṅgavad ūrdhvam ānayet | tatra dṛṣṭiṃ sthirāṃ kṛtvā prakāśo hṛdi jāyate ||

53. āsāvarī [||] madhyadaṇḍaṃ tiryagvyastagātraṃ kāṣṭhaṃ ca yogināṃ | āsāvarīti vikhyātaṃ āsanālambi tad viduḥ [||]

54. nidrāharaṃ [||] kṛtapadmāsano yogī tidvai[159] jānuparvaṇī[160] || āsāṃ ca svodare lagnāṃ kṛtvā saṃpuṭitau karau || muṣṭīkṛtau yojayet tu tarjanyau saṃprasāritau || ūrdhvaṃ vā nāsikāgraṃ lokayen mīlitekṣaṇaḥ madhukamūlikānasyaṃ[161] nasi kṣiptā[162] nidrā naśyati || yathā ||

---

154 Above *alakṣyam,* there is a small mark with the symbol of *oṃ* written next to it.

155 There is a marginal note above the word *kūrpare* but its first ligature is illegible to me: *+ihunī.*

156 This marginal note, which is very difficult to read, might be indicating that the position of the left foot and elbow should also be done on the right side.

157 There is a comment following the description of *haṃsāsana: anante vā samāpattir āsanaṃ nirvartayatīti | anante nāganāyake sahasraphaṇavidhṛtadharāmaṇḍale ||* . This comment appears to be derived from Vācaspatimiśra's commentary on *Yogasūtra* 2.47, and has little to do with *haṃsāsana.*

158 Following the description of *gudāsana,* there is a gap and then, in small and faint writing, what appears to be an interlinear comment: *bhāgāsanaṃ tūktam.*

159 Consider *tiṣṭhed vai* for *tidvai.*

160 Correct *jānuparvaṇī* to *jānuparvaṇi.*

161 Correct *madhuka-* to *mādhuka-.* Below the description of *nidrāhara* there is the following comment: *śuṇṭhāmarīcapippalī || samabhāgacūrṇa[ṃ] nasiprotaṃ san nidrābhaṅgi ||* .

162 Consider *kṣiptaṃ* for *kṣiptā.*

Appendix 2: One Hundred and twelve Descriptions of *Āsana*-s in the *Haṭhābhyāsapaddhati*[163]

Now, the Supine Poses.
athottānāni āsanāni

1. Having lain supinely, [the yogi] should bind the neck with the fingers, join the elbows, touch the buttocks on the ground, extend one leg and rotate [separately] the other leg to the left and right. [This] is "pawing the leg like a bull" [pose].
uttānaṃ śayanaṃ kṛtvā aṅgulibhiḥ kandharām baddhvā kūrparau militvā[164] *nitambena bhūmiṃ spṛṣṭvā ekaṃ pādaṃ prasārya ekaikena pādena savya-dakṣiṇaṃ bhrāmayet*[165] *vṛṣapādakṣepaṃ bhavati* || 1 ||

2. Having lain supinely, [the yogi] should join and extend the legs, touch the buttocks on the ground, clasp the neck with the hands and hold the breath and remain thus. [This] is the iron-bar pose.
uttānaṃ śayanaṃ kṛtvā pādau militvā prasārya nitambaṃ bhūmau spṛṣṭvā hastābhyāṃ[166] *kandharāṃ baddhvā kumbhakaṃ*[167] *kṛtvā tiṣṭhet parighāsanaṃ bhavati* || 2 ||

3. Lying supinely and having placed both elbows on the navel, [the yogi] should extend one hand at a time and hold the nose by the thumb, with the gaze on it, while supporting [the position] with the region of the hips. He should remain thus. [This] is the hatchet pose.
[fol. 3r] *uttānaśayanaṃ kūrparadvayaṃ*[168] *nābhau sthāpayitvā ekaikaṃ hastaṃ prasārya nāsikāyāṃ aṅguṣṭhapradeśena*[169] *dhṛtvā tallakṣyeṇa jaghanapradeśena dhṛtvā sthāpayet paraśvāsanaṃ bhavati* || 3 ||

4. Lying supinely and having fixed one foot on [the back of] the neck, [the yogi] should grasp the toes of [that] foot with the other hand, lengthen the other foot

163 The scribe of the manuscript has not applied the *sandhi* rules between two words that end and begin with vowels. I have retained this peculiarity in my edition. When this occurs between two words in a compound, I have indicated that this is a compound by linking the two words with an n-dash between square brackets (i.e., [–]).

164 Emend. *militvā* : Codex *mīlitvā*.

165 Emend *bhrāmayet* : Codex *bhrāmayitvā*.

166 Emend. *hastābhyāṃ* : Codex *hāstābhyāṃ*.

167 Emend. *kumbhakaṃ* : Codex *vumbhakaṃ*.

168 Emend. *kūrparadvayaṃ* : Codex *kūparadvayaṃ*.

169 Emend. *aṅguṣṭha-* : Codex *aguṣṭa-*.

and hand and remain thus. [He should then do the other side.[170] This] is Ananta's pose.
uttānaśayanaṃ ekaikaṃ pādaṃ grīvāyāṃ vinyasya itarahastena pādāgraṃ gṛhītvā itarapādahastau lambīkṛtya tiṣṭhet anantāsanaṃ bhavati || 4 ||

5. [The yogi] should lie supinely. Putting one foot on the [back of the] neck, he should place the other hand on the root of the ear. Having placed the elbow of this arm on the ground, while making the other hand and leg straight, he should remain thus [and then do the other side.[171] This] is the goad pose.
[fol. 3v] *uttānaṃ śayīta*[172] *ekaikaṃ pādaṃ grīvāyāṃ*[173] *kurvan itarahastaṃ*[174] *karṇamūle sthāpayet tasyaiva hastasya kūrparaṃ*[175] *bhūmau nidhāya itarahastapādau saralīkṛtya*[176] *tiṣṭhet aṅkuśāsanaṃ*[177] *bhavati* || 5 ||

6. Having placed the body [supinely] like a corpse, [the yogi] should join the knees together, bring [them] onto the navel, clasp the neck with the hands and rotate [the legs. This is] the up-turned dog [pose].
śavavac charīraṃ saṃsthāpya jānunī saṃmīlya nābhau ānīya[178] *hastābhyāṃ kandharāṃ*[179] *baddhvā bhrāmayet śvottānaṃ bhavati* || 6 ||[180]

7. Having positioned [himself] as in the up-turned dog [pose, the yogi] should touch both knees with his ears in turn. [This is] the up-turned cat [pose].
[fol. 4r] *śvottānavat saṃsthitiṃ*[181] *kṛtvā jānudvayaṃ paryāyeṇa karṇayoḥ saṃspṛśet mārjārottānaṃ*[182] *bhavati* || 7 ||

8. Then, having lain supinely and holding the earth with the soles of the feet, [the yogi] should stand up. [This] is the wolf pose.
atha uttānaṃ śayanaṃ kṛtvā pādatalābhyāṃ bhūmiṃ dhṛtvā uttiṣthet vṛkāsanaṃ bhavati || 8 ||

170 This is indicated by the use of *ekaikam*.
171 This is indicated by the use of *ekaikam*.
172 Emend. *śayīta* : Codex *śaḥ yīta*.
173 Emend. Preisendanz *grīvāyāṃ* : Codex *grivāyāṃ*.
174 Emend. *-hastaṃ* : Codex *hataṃ*.
175 Emend. *kūrparaṃ* : Codex *kūparaṃ*.
176 Emend. *saralī-* : Codex *sarali-*.
177 Emend. *aṅkuśāsanaṃ* : Codex *aṅkuśāsana*.
178 Emend. *ānīya* : Codex *aṃnīya*.
179 Emend. *kandharāṃ* : Codex *kadhārāṃ*.
180 At the bottom of this folio (3v) there is a marginal note: *dattātreyo gurur jayati* || .
181 Emend. *śvottānavat saṃsthitiṃ* : Codex *śvottānava saṃsthiti*.
182 Conj. *mārjārottānaṃ* : Codex *mārottānaṃ*.

9. Lying supinely, gripping the ground with the soles of both feet, [the yogi] should put the elbows on the ground and should raise up his back [from the ground. This] is the mount Trikūṭa [pose].
uttānaśayanaṃ pādatalābhyāṃ bhūmiṃ dhṛtvā kūrparau avanau nidhāya pṛṣṭhadeśam ūrdhvam unnamayet trikūṭaṃ bhavati || 9 ||

10. Lying supinely, [the yogi] should place the soles of the feet on the up-turned hands and raise the back part of the body from the ground. This] is the monkey's seat.
uttānaśayanaṃ pādatale uttānahastayoḥ sthāpayet pṛṣṭhabhāgaṃ unnamayet markaṭapīṭhaṃ bhavati || 10 ||

11. Lying supinely and having supported [himself] with both elbows on the ground and the hands on the buttocks, [the yogi] should hold his head, thighs, shanks and feet [straight] like a stick. [This] is the boat pose.
[fol. 4v] *uttānaśayanaṃ kūrparābhyām bhūmim avaṣṭabhya hastau nitambe nidhāya śiraḥ*[-]*ūrujaṅghāpādān daṇḍavat dhārayet naukāsanaṃ bhavati* || 11 ||

12. Having positioned [himself] like the boat, [the yogi] should take the toes of both feet upwards. This is the horizontal boat pose.
naukāvat[183] *sthitvā ūrdhvaṃ pādāgradvayaṃ nayet tiryaṅnaukāsanaṃ bhavati* || 12 ||

13. [Having positioned himself] like the horizontal boat and supporting [himself] with the neck, back and elbows on the ground, [the yogi] should take up the toes of both feet, pointing [them] toward the head. [This] is the banner pose.
[fol. 5r] *tiryaṅnaukāvat grīvāpṛṣṭhakūrparaiḥ bhūmim avaṣṭabhya mastakalakṣeṇa pādāgradvayaṃ ūrdhvaṃ nayet dhvajāsanaṃ*[184] *bhavati* || 13 ||

14. Having planted [firmly] the nape of the neck on the ground, [the yogi] should raise up the toes of both feet. [This] is the pose from hell.
grīvākaṇṭhena bhūmiṃ viṣṭabhya pādāgradvayam ūrdhvam unnayet narakāsanaṃ bhavati || 14 ||

15. Having remained in the pose from hell, [the yogi] should place the upper side of the feet on the ground near to the region of the nose and join both hands. [He] should make [the arms] long and "plough" the ground with the neck. [This] is the

183 Emend. *naukāvat* : Codex *naukāva*.
184 Emend. *dhvajāsanaṃ* : Codex *dhvajāsana*.

plough pose.
[fol. 5v] *narakāsane sthitvā ānāsikapradeśe*[185] *bhūmau pādapṛṣṭhe sthāpya hastadvayaṃ saṃmīlya lambīkuryāt*[186] *grīvapradeśena bhūmiṃ karṣayet lāṅgalāsanam bhavet* || 15 ||

16. Lying supinely and having placed the palms of both hands and the soles of both feet on the ground, [the yogi] should raise up the region of the navel. [This] is the sofa pose.
uttānaśayanaṃ hastatalābhyāṃ bhūmim avaṣṭabhya pādatalābhyāṃ bhūmiṃ dhṛtvā nābhipradeśaṃ ūrdhvaṃ kuryāt paryaṅkāsanaṃ bhavati || 16 ||

17. Having remained in the sofa pose, [the yogi] should join his hands and feet. [This] is the cane pose.
[fol. 6r] *paryaṅkāsane sthitvā hastapādau saṃmīlayet vetrāsanaṃ bhavati* || 17 ||

18. Having remained in the cane pose and pulling his hands and feet apart, [the yogi] should take [them] upwards and press the ground with his backbone. [This] is the ball pose.
vetrāsane sthitvā hastapādān niṣkṛṣya[-]*m*[187] *ūrdhvaṃ nayet pṛṣṭhavaṃśena*[188] *bhūmiṃ pīḍayet*[189] *kandukāsanaṃ bhavati* || 18 ||

19. Having placed one foot on one thigh and the other foot on the other thigh, [this] is the lotus pose. Having threaded the hands in between the thighs and knees, [the yogi] should clasp the neck [with the hands and remain up-turned. [This] is the up-turned turtle [pose].
ekasmin ūruṇi ekaṃ pādaṃ kṛtvā anyasmin ūruṇi anyaṃ pādaṃ kṛtvā padmāsanaṃ bhavati [||] *ūrujānvor antarayoḥ hastau praveśya*[190] *kandarām baddhvā uttānaṃ tiṣṭhet uttānakūrmaṃ bhavati* || 19 ||

20. Having placed the shanks and back on the ground and positioning the thighs on the calves, [the yogi] should touch his backbone [on the ground] again and again. [This] is the pose for one who has ceased [from worldly activities].

185 Conj. [Dominic Goodall] *ānāsika-* : Codex *nāsikā-*.
186 Emend. *saṃmīlya lambī-* : Codex *samīlya lambi-*.
187 Emend. *niṣkṛṣyam* : Codex *niṣkṣyam*. The final consonant appears to have been inserted to separate the preceding vowel from the following one.
188 Emend. *pṛṣṭhavaṃśena* : Codex *prāṣṭhavaṃśena*.
189 Diagnostic Conj. [Dominic Goodall] *pīḍayet* : Codex *pothayet*.
190 Emend. *praveśya* : Codex *praviśya*.

jaṅghāpṛṣṭhe[191] *bhūmau nidhāya jaṅghodarayoḥ ūruṇī*[192] *saṃsthāpya pṛṣṭha-vaṃśaṃ*[193] *vāraṃ vāraṃ spṛśyet*[194] *viratāsanaṃ bhavati* || 20 ||

21. Lying supinely, supporting the knees on [the region of] the heart and binding the hands on the thighs and shanks, [the yogi] should rock to the left and right. [This] is the stone pose.
[fol. 6v] *uttānaśayanaṃ jānunī hṛdaye 'vaṣṭabhya jaṅghāsahita*[-]*ūruṇi kara-dvaye baddhvā savyāpasavyaṃ loḍayet dṛṣadāsanaṃ bhavati* || 21 ||

22. Lying supinely, [the yogi] should pass the feet over the head, place them on the ground and lie prone. Having lain pronely, [the yogi] should place his back on the ground and do [this rolling movement] again and again, successively. [This] is the rolling pose.
uttānaśayanaṃ pādau śira ullaṅghya bhūmau sthāpayitvā[195] *nyubjaṃ bhūyate*[196] [||] *nyubjaṃ śayanaṃ pṛṣṭhe*[197] *bhūmau nidhāya punaḥ punaḥ paryāyeṇa*[198] *kartavyaṃ*[199] *luṭhanāsanaṃ*[200] *bhavati* || 22 ||

Now, the Prone Poses.
[fol. 7r] *atha nyubjāsanāni*[201]

23. Having lain pronely, placing the navel on the ground and supporting [himself on] the ground with the forearms like pillars, [the yogi] should join the lips, make the [sound] "sū" like a flute and remain thus. [This] is the lizard pose.
nyubjaśayanaṃ kṛtvā nābhiṃ bhūmau nidhāya stambhavat hastābhyāṃ[202] *bhūmim avaṣṭabhya oṣṭhau nimīlya*[203] *veṇuvat sūkṛtya tiṣṭhet saraṭāsanaṃ bhavati* || 23 ||

191 Emend. *jaṅghāpṛṣṭhe* : Codex *jaṅghāpṛṣṭhi.*
192 Emend. *ūruṇī* : Codex *ūruṇi.*
193 Emend. *pṛṣṭha-* : Codex *pṛṣṭhi-.*
194 Emend. *spṛśyet* : Codex *spṛyet.*
195 Emend. *sthāpayitvā* : Codex *sthāpayitvya.*
196 Emend. *bhūyate* : Codex *bhūyati.*
197 Emend. *pṛṣṭhe* : Codex *pṛṣṭhaṃ.*
198 Emend. *paryāyeṇa* : Codex *payāyeṇa.*
199 Emend. *kartavyaṃ* : Codex *katavyaṃ.*
200 Emend. *luṭhanāsanaṃ* : Codex *luṭanāsanaṃ.*
201 Emend. *atha nyubjāsanāni* : Codex *anyubjāsanāni.*
202 Conj. *stambhavat hastābhyāṃ* : Codex *staṃvatstābhyāṃ.*
203 Emend. *nimīlya* : Codex *nimilya.*

24. Lying pronely and having raised up the elbows by the sides [of the body, the yogi] should support [himself on] the ground with the palms of both hands and fly up again and again. [This] is the fish pose.
nyubjaṃ śayanaṃ kūrparau pārśvabhāgābhyāṃ ūrdhvīkṛtya[204] *hastatalābhyāṃ bhūmim avaṣṭabhya vāraṃ vāraṃ uḍḍānaṃ kuryāt matsyāsanaṃ bhavati* || 24 ||

25. [Lying] pronely, [the yogi] should put the toes on the ground, keep [the legs] long, place the palms of both hands at the top of the head and raise up the buttocks. Gazing at the navel and taking the nose onto the ground, [the yogi] should take [the nose forward] as far as the palms of his hands. He should do thus again and again. [This] is the elephant pose.
[fol. 7v] *nyubjaṃ pādāgre bhūmau kṛtvā lambībhūya mastakāgre hastatalau nidhāya nitambam ūrdhvam unnamayya nābhiṃ*[205] *lakṣya bhūmau nāsikām ānīya*[206] *hastatalaparyantaṃ*[207] *nayet itthaṃ punaḥ punaḥ kuryāt gajāsanaṃ bhavati* || 25 ||

26. Remaining as in the elephant pose, [the yogi] should take his head to the right armpit, [and then] to the left armpit, again and again.[208] [This] is the hyena pose.
gajāsanavat[209] *sthitvā mastakaṃ vāraṃ vāraṃ dakṣiṇakukṣiṃ savyakukṣiṃ nayet tarakṣvāsanaṃ bhavati* || 26 ||

27. Having bent one leg at a time, [the yogi] should do the elephant pose. [This] is the bear pose.
ekaikaṃ pādaṃ ākuñcya gajāsanaṃ kuryāt ṛkṣāsanaṃ bhavati || 27 ||

28. In the position of the elephant pose, [the yogi] should bend both knees and repeat it again and again. [This] is the hare pose.
[fol. 8r] *gajāsanasaṃsthitau jānudvayam ākuñcya vāraṃ vāraṃ kartavyaṃ śaśāsanaṃ bhavati* || 28 ||

29. In the position of the elephant pose, [the yogi] should rotate one leg at a time anteriorly and continue to do thus. [This] is the chariot pose.

---

204 Emend. *ūrdhvīkṛtya* : Codex *urdhvikṛtya.*
205 Emend. *nābhiṃ* : Codex *nābhi.*
206 Emend. *ānīya* : Codex *āniya.*
207 Emend. *hastatalaparyantaṃ* : Codex *hastatalāparyantaṃ.*
208 The practicalities of this pose suggest that the author is using the word *kukṣi* to refer to the armpit. This is supported by the use of this same word in the description of the *ucchīrṣakāsana* (no. 65), in which *kukṣi* clearly means the armpit.
209 Emend. *gajāsanavat* : Codex *gajāsanava.*

gajāsanasaṃsthitau ekaikaṃ pādaṃ purobhāgena bhrāmayitvā kartavyaṃ rathāsanaṃ bhavati || 29 ||

30. In the position of the elephant pose, [the yogi] should ram the ground with one arm at a time. [This] is the ram pose.
gajāsanasaṃsthitau ekaikaṃ bāhuṃ bhūmau tāḍayet meṣāsanaṃ bhavati || 30 ||

31. In the position of the elephant pose, having raised both legs into space, [the yogi] should touch the ground with the head. [This] is the goat pose.
gajāsanasaṃsthitau pādadvayam antarālekṛtya mastakena bhūmiṃ spṛśet ajāsanaṃ bhavati || 31 ||

32. Having supported [himself] with the forearms on the ground and bending the knees into the navel, [the yogi] should remain thus. [This] is the sparrow pose.
[fol. 8v] *kūrparaparyantau hastau dharām avaṣṭabhya jānunī nābhau saṃkuñcya tiṣṭhet caṭakāsanaṃ bhavati* || 32 ||

33. Having positioned [himself] on the hands like the sparrow pose, [the yogi] should touch the ears with the knees, place both shanks on the [upper] arms and remain thus. [This] is the crow pose.
hastau caṭakāsanavat saṃsthāpya jānudvayaṃ karṇau saṃspṛśya jaṅghādvayaṃ[210] *bāhvor nidhāya tiṣṭhet kākāsanaṃ bhavati* || 33 ||

34. In a position like the crow pose, [the yogi] should join the shanks on [each] thigh and raise up the back region [of his body]. [This] is the partridge pose.
kākāsanavat saṃsthitau jaṅghādvayam[211] *ūruṇi saṃmīlya pṛṣṭhapradeśe*[212] *ūrdhvaṃ nayet titiryāsanaṃ bhavati* || 34 ||

35. Having supported [himself] with both hands on the ground, joining both knees on the navel and supporting [in the air] the shanks and thighs, [the yogi] should remain thus. [This] is the heron pose.
hastābhyām avanim avaṣṭabhya jānudvayaṃ nābhau saṃmīlya jaṅghā[-]*ūruṇī*[213] *saṃstabhya tiṣṭhet bakāsanaṃ bhavati* || 35 ||

36. Having adopted the lotus pose, [the yogi] should support [himself] with the palms of both hands on the ground, lift posteriorly both feet, [which are] fastened

210 Emend. *-dvayaṃ* : Codex *-dvaye.*
211 Conj. Preisendanz *jaṅghādvayam* : Codex *jaṅghā.*
212 Emend. *pṛṣṭhapradeśe* : Codex *praṣṭapradeśe.*
213 Emend. *-ūruṇī* : Codex *-ūruṇi.*

in lotus pose, and remain thus. [This] is Bhāradvāja's pose.
[fol. 9r] *padmāsanaṃ saṃsthāpya hastatalābhyāṃ dharāṃ avaṣṭabhya padmāsanayuktacaraṇadvayaṃ pṛṣṭhabhāge nītvā tiṣṭhet bhāradvājāsanaṃ*[214] *bhavati* || 36 ||

37. Having put the palms of the hands on the ground, [the yogi] should make the soles of the feet fly upwards and [then] fall [down] to the ground. He should do thus again and again. [This] is the "flying up of the rooster" [pose].
hastatale bhūmau kṛtvā pādatale[215] *ca ūrdhvam uḍḍānaṃ kṛtvā bhūmau patet itthaṃ punaḥ punaḥ kuryāt kukkuṭoḍḍānaṃ*[216] *bhavati* || 37 ||

38. Having placed one foot on [the back of] the neck, [the yogi] should fix the second foot above it, support [the body] with the palms of both hands [on the ground][217] and remain thus. [This] is the wood-sparrow pose.
ekaṃ pādaṃ grīvāyāṃ saṃsthāpya dvitīyaṃ[218] *pādam upari vinyasya hastatalābhyāṃ avaṣṭabhya tiṣṭhet araṇyacaṭakāsanaṃ bhavati* || 38 ||

39. Having supported [himself] with the palms of both hands on the ground, fixing the elbows on the navel and holding the body [straight] like a stick, [the yogi] remains [thus. This] is the peacock pose.
hastatalābhyām avanim avaṣṭabhya kūrparau nābhau vinyasya daṇḍavac charīraṃ dhṛtvā tiṣṭhet mayūrāsanaṃ bhavati || 39 ||

40. Having positioned [himself] as in the peacock pose, [the yogi] should hold the wrist of one hand with the other. [This] is the lame peacock pose.
[fol. 9v] *mayūrāsanavat*[219] *saṃsthāpya ekena hastena ekasya hastasya maṇibandhaṃ dhārayet paṅgumayūrāsanaṃ bhavati* || 40 ||

41. Having adopted a prone, straight posture and having supported [himself] with the soles of both feet on the ground, [the yogi] should stand up. [This] is the sword pose.
nyubjaṃ saralam āsanaṃ kṛtvā pādatalābhyāṃ bhūmim avaṣṭabhya uttiṣṭhet khaḍgāsanaṃ bhavati || 41 ||

---

214 Emend. *bhāradvājāsanaṃ* : Codex *bhāsadvājāsanaṃ*.
215 Emend. Preisendanz *pādatale* : Codex *padatale*.
216 Emend. Preisendanz *kukkuṭo-* : Codex *kukkuṭṭo-*.
217 According to the picture of the *araṇyacaṭakāsana* in the *Śrītattvanidhi* (Sjoman 1999: pl. 15), the yogi's torso is upright and his hands on the ground. Thus, I suspect that the Sanskrit description of this pose in the *Haṭhābhyāsapaddhati* has omitted the word *bhūmau*.
218 Emend. *dvitīyaṃ* : Codex *dvītīyaṃ*.
219 Emend. *mayūrāsanavat* : Codex *mayūrāsanat*.

42. Having supported [himself] with both elbows on the ground and the jaw with the palms of both hands, [the yogi] should raise [himself] up.[220] [This] is the spear pose.
kūrparābhyāṃ avanim avaṣṭabhya hastatalābhyāṃ hanum avaṣṭabhya uttiṣṭhet śūlāsanaṃ bhavati || 42 ||

43. Having supported [himself] with the palms of both hands on the ground and lifting the toes up [into the air, the yogi] should dance on the palms of the hands. [This] is the "inverted dancing" [pose].
[fol. 10r] *hastatalābhyāṃ bhūmim avaṣṭabhya ūrdhvaṃ pādāgre kurvan hastatalābhyāṃ nartanaṃ kartavyaṃ viparītanṛtyaṃ bhavati* || 43 ||

44. In the position of inverted dancing, [the yogi] should touch the nose on the ground and take [it] up. He should touch [the ground] again [and again. This] is the hawk pose.
viparītanṛtyavat[221] *sthitau nāsikāṃ*[222] *bhūmau saṃspṛśya ūrdhvaṃ nītvā punaḥ saṃspṛśet śyenāsanaṃ bhavati* || 44 ||

45. Having placed the [top of the] skull on the ground, [the yogi] should lift up the feet. [This] is the skull pose.[223]
[fol. 10v] *kapālaṃ bhūmau nidhāya ūrdhvaṃ pādau nayet kapālāsanaṃ bhavati* || 45 ||

46. Having lain pronely, placing the hands on the buttocks, lengthening the legs and joining [them] together, [the yogi] should move with his chest. [This] is the snake pose.
nyubjaṃ śayanaṃ kṛtvā hastau nitambe saṃsthāpya pādau dīrghīkṛtya saṃmīlayan urasā[224] *gantavyaṃ sarpāsanaṃ bhavati* || 46 ||

47. Having lain pronely, [the yogi] should hold the big toes with the hands, with the heels crossed at the back, and should roll [around. This is the prone pose.[225]]

---

220 One might understand *uttiṣṭhet* to mean that the yogi should stand up. However, the picture of the *śūlāsana* in the *Śrītattvanidhi* (Sjoman 1999: pl. 7) clearly has the legs raised while the elbows are on the ground.

221 Emend. *viparīta-* : Codex *viparita-*.

222 Conj. *nāsikāṃ* : Codex *nāsikā.*

223 According to the picture of the *kapālāsana* in the *Śrītattvanidhi* (Sjoman 1999: pl. 6), the yogi is supporting himself with the palms on the ground, as in a three-point headstand. His arms are wide apart.

224 Emend. *urasā* : Codex *urasāṃ.*

225 The description of this pose matches the picture and description of the *nyubjāsana* in the *Śrītattvanidhi* (Sjoman 1999: pl. 19 and p. 84).

[fol. 11r] *nyubjaṃ śayanaṃ kṛtvā pṛṣṭhe pārṣṇivyutkrameṇa*[226] *hastābhyāṃ pādāṅguṣṭhau dhṛtvā loḍayet* || 47 ||

Now, the Stationary Poses.
atha sthānāsanāni[227]

48. Having extended the legs on the ground like a stick, [the yogi] should hold the big toes with the hands, fix the forehead on the knees and remain [thus. This is the "stretching the back" pose.[228]]
daṇḍavad bhūmau caraṇau prasārya hastābhyāṃ aṅguṣṭhau dhṛtvā jānūpari[229] *lalāṭaṃ vinyasya tiṣṭhet* || 48 ||

49. Having extended one leg, pressing the perineum with the heel of the [other] foot, holding the big toes of the extended leg with both hands, [the yogi] should fix his head on the knee. [This] is the "stretching half the back" [pose].
ekaṃ pādaṃ prasārya ekapādasya pārṣṇinā sīvanīṃ[230] *saṃpīḍya hastadvayena prasāritapādāṅguṣṭhaṃ dhṛtvā jānūpari*[231] *mastakaṃ nyaset ardhapaścimatānaṃ bhavati* || 49 ||

50. Having positioned [himself] as in the "stretching the back" [pose] and holding one foot on [the back of] the neck, [the yogi] should remain thus. [This] is the "stretching the upper back" [pose].
paścimatānavat saṃsthitiṃ kṛtvā ekaṃ pādaṃ grīvāyāṃ dhṛtvā tiṣṭhet ūrdhvapaścimatānaṃ[232] *bhavati* || 50 ||

51. Having grasped the toes of the feet with both hands, [the yogi] should touch the big toes, one at a time, on the ears. [This is the bow pose.[233]]

---

226 Emend. *pārṣṇi-* : Codex *pārṣṇī-*.

227 Conj. *sthānāsanāni* : Codex *sthānānyāsanāni.*

228 The description of this pose matches the picture and description of the *garbhāsana* in the *Śrītattvanidhi* (Sjoman 1999: pl. 19 and p. 84). However, it is quite probable that the name *garbhāsana* is a mistake in the *Śrītattvanidhi.* The sequence of *āsana*-s in the *Haṭhābhyāsapaddhati* indicates that this pose is the beginning of a series most probably based on *paścimatānāsana* because the name *paścimatāna* is mentioned in the description of the next pose called *ūrdhvapaścimatāna.* Furthermore, this pose is called *paścimatānāsana* or *paścimottānāsana* in earlier yoga texts (e.g., ŚS 3.109 and HP 1.30).

229 Emend. *jānūpari* : Codex *jānupari.*

230 Emend. *sīvanīṃ* : Codex *sīvani.*

231 Emend. *jānūpari* : Codex *jānupari.*

232 Emend. *ūrdhva-* : Codex *urdhva-*.

233 The description of this pose matches the picture and description of the *dhanurāsana* in the *Śrītattvanidhi* (Sjoman 1999: pl. 18 and p. 84).

[fol. 11v] *hastadvayena pādadvayāgre gṛhītvā ekaikaṃ pādāṅguṣṭhaṃ karṇayoḥ spṛśet* || 51 ||[234]

52. Having fixed [one] foot on the [opposite] thigh and the other foot on the other thigh, [the yogi] should hold the big toes with the hands crossed behind the back and remain thus. [This] is the bound lotus pose.
[fol. 12r] *ūruṇi pādaṃ vinyasya itarasmin ūruṇi itaraṃ pādaṃ nyasya pṛṣṭhibhāgena vyatyayena hastābhyāṃ pādaṅguṣṭhau dhṛtvā tiṣṭhet baddhapadmāsanaṃ bhavati* || 52 ||

53. Having adopted the lotus pose, [the yogi] should fix both arms inside the feet, thighs and shanks, support [himself] with the palms of both hands on the ground and remain [thus. This] is the rooster pose.
padmāsanaṃ kṛtvā caraṇa[-]*ūrujaṅghānām*[235] *antare bāhudvayaṃ nyasya hastatalābhyāṃ bhūmim avaṣṭabhya tiṣṭhet kukkuṭāsanaṃ bhavati* || 53 ||

54. Having remained as in the rooster pose, [the yogi] should hold the wrist of one hand with the other, support [himself firmly] with the palm of the [held] hand on the ground and remain [thus. This] is the lame rooster pose.
kukkuṭāsanavat[236] *sthitvā ekena hastena anyasya hastasya maṇibandhaṃ dhṛtvā hastatalena bhūmiṃ viṣṭabhya tiṣṭhet paṅgukukkuṭāsanaṃ bhavati* || 54 ||

55. Having lain pronely, [the yogi] should place both heels on the neck. Having held both ankles with the hands, [the yogi] should remain [thus. This is called the libation-bowl pose.[237]]
nyubjaṃ śayanaṃ kṛtvā pārṣṇidvayaṃ[238] *grīvāyāṃ sthāpayet hastadvayena gulphadvayaṃ dhṛtvā tiṣṭhet* || 55 ||

234 The following comment, which seems unrelated to the *āsana*-s in this section, has been written beneath the description of the *dhanurāsana* on fol. 11v: *doḥkuṭṭanaṃ* || *ūrukuṭṭanaṃ* || *pārśvakuṭṭanaṃ* || *ityādīni kuṭṭanāni muṣṭinā bāhunā pārṣṇinā bhittyā bhūminā kartavyāni* || Emend. Preisendanz *ityādīni* : Codex *ityādini*. "Beating of the arms, thighs, the sides and so on. [These] beatings should be done with a fist, arm, heel, wall [or] the ground."

235 Emend. *-jaṅghānām* : Codex *-jaghānām*.

236 Emend. *kukkuṭāsanavat* : Codex *kukkuṭāsanava*.

237 The name of this pose is given in the next description. However, the description of this pose matches the picture and description of the *pādahastasaṃyogāsana* in the *Śrītattvanidhi* (Sjoman 1999: pl. 19 and p. 84). The compound *pādahastasaṃyogāsana* appears to me to be a late improvisation, and the fact that the *arghyāsana* is mentioned (Sjoman 1999: 75) in the *Śrītattvanidhi*'s description of the *cakrāsana* but not described separately in its section on *āsana* practice, somewhat confirms this.

238 Emend. *pārṣṇidvayaṃ* : Codex *pārṣṇīdvayaṃ*.

56. Having remained as in the libation-bowl pose, [the yogi] should support [himself] with the palms of both hands on the ground. [This] is the parasol pose.[239]

[fol. 12v] *arghyāsanavat*[240] *sthitvā hastatalābhyāṃ bhūmim avaṣṭabhnuyāt chatrāsanaṃ bhavati* || 56 ||

57. Having supported [himself] with both hands on the ground, placing the knees on both shoulders and the heels on the chest, [the yogi] should remain thus. [This] is the garland pose.

hastābhyām avanim avaṣṭabhya skandhayor[241] *jānunī saṃsthāpya pārṣṇī*[242] *urasi nidhāya tiṣṭhet mālāsanaṃ bhavati* || 57 ||

58. Remaining in the rooster pose and taking the thighs as far as the shoulders, [the yogi] should remain [thus. This] is the Haṃsa-bird pose.

[fol. 13r] *kukkuṭāsanaṃ sthitvā skandhaparyantaṃ ūruṇī nītvā*[243] *tiṣṭhet haṃsāsanaṃ bhavati* || 58 ||

59. Having placed the knees on the ground, [the yogi] should hold with the hands both arms crossed over one another and remain upright. [This] is the monkey pose.

jānunī bhūmau saṃsthāpya hastābhyāṃ bāhū[244] *parasparaṃ dhṛtvā saralaṃ tiṣṭhet vānarāsanaṃ*[245] *bhavati* || 59 ||

60. [The yogi] should wrap both shanks one over the other, place them on the ground, put the thighs and buttocks on them and remain thus. [This] is the mountain pose.

jaṅghādvayaṃ parasparaṃ veṣṭayitvā bhūmau saṃsthāpya[246] *tadupari ūruṇī*[247] *nidhāya*[248] *tadupari nitambaṃ nidhāya tiṣṭhet parvatāsanaṃ bhavati* || 60 ||

61. Having placed the soles of the feet on the ground and the knees on the chest, [the yogi] should bind the shanks and thighs with the hands reversed and remain

239 The description of this pose matches the picture and description of the *cakrāsana* in the *Śrītattvanidhi* (Sjoman 1999: pl. 6 and p. 75).

240 Emend. *arghyāsanavat* : Codex *arghyāsanava.*

241 Emend. *skandhayor* : Codex *skandhayo.*

242 Emend. *pārṣṇī* : Codex *pārṣṇi.*

243 Emend. *ūruṇī nītvā* : Codex *ūruṇi nitvā.*

244 Emend. *bāhū* : Codex *bāhu.*

245 Conj. *vānarāsanaṃ* : Codex *vārāsanaṃ.*

246 Conj. *saṃsthāpya* : Codex *saṃsthā.*

247 Emend. *ūruṇī* : Codex *ūruṇi.*

248 Emend. *nidhāya* : Codex *nidhaya.*

thus. [This] is the noose pose.
pādatale bhūmau nidhāya jānunī[249] *urasi nidhāya viparītahastābhyām ūrusahitajaṅghe nibaddhvā*[250] *tiṣṭhet pāśāsanaṃ*[251] *bhavati* || 61 ||

62. Having supported [himself] with both heels on the ground and holding the ankles with both hands, [the yogi] should remain thus. [This] is the goose [pose].
[fol. 13v] *pārṣṇibhyāṃ bhūmim avaṣṭabhya hastadvayena gulphau dhṛtvā tiṣṭhet kādambaṃ bhavati* || 62 ||

63. Having inserted both hands through the thighs, [the yogi] should hold the buttocks, support [himself] with the soles of both feet on the ground and remain thus. [This] is the girdle pose.
ūrumadhyāt hastau niveśya nitambaṃ dhṛtvā pādatalābhyāṃ bhūmim avaṣṭabhya tiṣṭhet kāñcyāsanaṃ bhavati || 63 ||

64. Having bound the fingers of the hands, [the yogi] should make his whole body pass through the middle of the arms and remain thus. [This] is the "wringing the limbs" [pose].[252]
[fol. 14r] *hastayoḥ aṅgulīr baddhvā hastayor madhyāt sarvam aṅgaṃ niṣkāsayitvā tiṣṭhet aṅgamoṭanaṃ bhavati* || 64 ||

65. Having placed the soles of the feet, one at a time, in the armpits, [the yogi] should remain thus. [This] is the pillow [pose].
ekaikaṃ pādatalaṃ kukṣau nidhāya tiṣṭhet ucchīrṣakaṃ[253] *bhavati* || 65 ||

66. Having placed the knee on [one] side of the chest and the heel [of that leg] on the second side of the chest, [the yogi] should hold [the knee and heel] with both arms and remain thus. [This is the "union of the chest and knee" pose.[254]]
jānuṃ[255] *stanapradeśe nidhāya pārṣṇiṃ*[256] *dvitīyasthānapradeśe*[257] *nidhāya hastadvayena dhṛtvā tiṣṭhet* || 66 ||

---

249 Emend. *jānunī* : Codex *jānuni.*
250 Emend. *nibaddhvā* : Codex *nabaddhvā.*
251 Emend. *pāśāsanaṃ* : Codex *paśāsanaṃ.*
252 The description of this pose matches the picture and description of the *hastāṅgulibaddhāsana* in the *Śrītattvanidhi* (Sjoman 1999: pl. 19 and p. 84).
253 Emend. *ucchīrṣakaṃ* : Codex *ucchirṣakaṃ.*
254 The description of this pose matches the picture and description of the *hṛjjānusaṃyogāsana* in the *Śrītattvanidhi* (Sjoman 1999: pl. 19 and p. 85).
255 Emend. *jānuṃ* : Codex *jānu.*
256 Emend. *pārṣṇiṃ* : Codex *pārṣṇi.*
257 Conj. *dvitīya-* : Codex *dvitī-.*

67. Having put the soles of the feet on the palms of both hands, [the yogi] should remain thus and [then] walk around. [This] is the shoe pose.
hastatalayoḥ pādatale kṛtvā tiṣṭhet gacchet pādukāsanaṃ bhavati || 67 ||

68. [The yogi] should place the soles of both feet on the ground and the elbows on the insides of the [bent] knees and hold the region of the ankles with the hands. He should remain thus. [This] is the "snapping [at the heels]" pose.
[fol. 14v] *pādatale bhūmau saṃsthāpya jānumadhye kūrparau sthāpya hastābhyāṃ gulphapradeśe*[258] *dhṛtvā tiṣṭhet grāhāsanaṃ bhavati* || 68 ||

69. Having placed both fists on the ground and having extended the legs [straight] like a stick, [the yogi] should remain thus. [This] is the Parpaṭa-plant pose.
muṣṭī[259] *bhūmau saṃsthāpya pādau daṇḍavat prasārya tiṣṭhet parpaṭāsanaṃ bhavati* || 69 ||

70. Having placed on the ground the fists †on the little finger side† and placing the soles of the feet on [them, the yogi] should move his body like a horse. [This] is the horse pose. [Likewise,] the elephant's seat is [moving the body] like an elephant and the camel's seat is [moving the body] like a camel.
[fol. 15r] *muṣṭī*[260] †*kaniṣṭhikāpradeśena*† *bhūmau nidhāya upari pādatale saṃsthāpya aśvavat śarīraṃ calanīyam*[261] *aśvāsanaṃ bhavati gajavat gajasādanaṃ uṣṭravat uṣṭrāsādanaṃ bhavati* || 70 ||

71. Having taken the shoulders up to the head [while sitting, the yogi] should remain thus. [This] is the two-headed [pose].
skandhaṃ[262] *śiraḥparyantaṃ nītvā sthātavyaṃ dviśīrṣaṃ bhavati* || 71 ||

72. Having put his jaw on his navel, [the yogi] should remain thus. [This] is the humpbacked pose.
nābhau hanuṃ[263] *nidhāya tiṣṭhet kubjāsanaṃ bhavati* || 72 ||

73. Having placed the palms of both hands on the ground, [the yogi] should leave the ground [by lifting the body up] between the hands, make the legs [straight] like a stick and move the body around like a swing. [This] is the swing pose.

258 Emend. *gulphapradeśe* : Codex *gulpapradeśo.*
259 Emend. *muṣṭī* : Codex *muṣṭi.*
260 Emend. *muṣṭī-* : Codex *muṣṭi-.*
261 Emend. *calanīyam* : Codex *calaniyam.*
262 Emend. *skandhaṃ* : Codex *skandhaḥ.*
263 Emend. *hanuṃ* : Codex *hanaṃ.*

hastatale bhūmau nidhāya hastamadhyāt bhūmiṃ[264] *santyajya*[265] *daṇḍarūpau pādau kṛtvā preṅkhavac*[266] [fol. 15v] *charīraṃ cālanīyaṃ preṅkhāsanaṃ*[267] *bhavati* || 73 ||

74. Having remained as in the swing [pose, the yogi] should take the toes over the head, place the back [of the body] on the ground and remain thus.[268]
preṅkhavat sthitvā pādāgre mastakopari nītvā pṛṣṭhabhāgaṃ[269] *bhūmau nidhāya tiṣṭhet* || 74 ||

Now, the Standing Poses.
[fol. 16r] *atha utthānāsanāni*[270]

75. Having joined together both heels [while] standing, [the yogi] should take the buttocks to the level of the knees and remain thus. [This] is the pressure pose.
pārṣṇidvayaṃ[271] *saṃmīlya sthitvā nitambaṃ jānupradeśe ānīya*[272] *tiṣṭhet utpīḍāsanaṃ*[273] *bhavati* || 75 ||

76. Having placed one foot on the ground, [the yogi] should take the buttocks to the level of the knees, put the second foot on the knee and remain thus. [This] is the "flying chariot" pose.
ekaṃ pādaṃ bhūmau nidhāya nitambaṃ jānupradeśe ānīya dvitīyaṃ pādaṃ jānuni[274] *nidhāya tiṣṭhet vimānāsanaṃ*[275] *bhavati* || 76 ||

77. Having placed the soles of both feet on the ground and taking the hands [down] along the back [of the body] as far as the shanks, [this] is the pigeon's seat.

264 Emend. *bhūmiṃ* : Codex *bhūmi.*
265 Emend. *santyajya* : Codex *tyajya.*
266 Emend. *preṅkhavac* : Codex *prekhava.*
267 Emend. *preṅkhāsanaṃ* : Codex *prekhāsanaṃ.*
268 Unfortunately, the name of this pose is not recorded, and the *Śrītattvanidhi* (Sjoman 1999: pl. 19) simply repeats the name of the former pose (i.e., *preṅkhāsana*). One would expect something like *ūrdhvapreṅkhāsana* (cf. *ūrdhvapaścimatāna*, no. 50).
269 Emend. *pṛṣṭhabhāgaṃ* : Codex *pṛṣṭhibhāge.*
270 Emend. *utthānāsanāni* : Codex *uttāna āsanāni.*
271 Emend. *pārṣṇidvayaṃ* : Codex *pārṣṇidvaya.*
272 Emend. *ānīya* : Codex *aniya.*
273 Emend. *utpīḍāsanaṃ* : Codex *utpiṭāsanaṃ.*
274 Emend. *jānuni* : Codex *jānunī.*
275 Emend. *vimānāsanaṃ* : Codex *vimānasanaṃ.*

pādatale bhūmau nidhāya pṛṣṭhabhāgena[276] *hastau jaṅghāparyantaṃ*[277] *nītvā*[278] *kapotapīṭhakaṃ*[279] *bhavati* || 77 ||

78. Having supported [himself] with one foot on the ground and with the other foot on the thigh, [the yogi] should stand and sit. It should be done thus again and again. [This] is the half-moon [pose].
ekena pādena bhūmim avaṣṭabhya anyapādatalena ūrum[280] *avaṣṭabhya tiṣṭhet āsta*[281] *iti punaḥ punaḥ kartavyaṃ ardhacandraṃ bhavati* || 78 ||

79. While standing and pressing on the region of one hip[282] with the heel [of the other foot, the yogi] should stand [on one leg] and raise [the other. The yogi] should do thus again and again. [This] is the spike pose.
[fol. 16v] *tiṣṭhan san*[283] *pārṣṇinā itarajaghanapradeśe saṃpīḍya sthātavyam utthitavyam iti punaḥ punaḥ kartavyaṃ śaṅkvāsanaṃ bhavati* || 79 ||

80. [The yogi] should stand on one leg and raise [the other.[284] This] is [Śiva's] Tāṇḍava-dance pose.
ekena pādena sthātavyam utthātavyaṃ tāṇḍavāsanaṃ bhavati || 80 ||

81. Having placed one foot on the [back of the] neck, [the yogi] should sit [and then] stand up [with the leg on the neck. This] is Trivikrama's pose.
[fol. 17r] *grīvāyāṃ pādaṃ saṃsthāpya sthātavyam utthātavyaṃ trivikramāsanaṃ bhavati* || 81 ||

---

276 Emend. *pṛṣṭha-* : Codex *pṛṣṭhi-*.
277 Emend. *paryantaṃ* : Codex *parayantaṃ*.
278 Emend. *nītvā* : Codex *nitvā*.
279 Conj. *-pīṭhaka* : Codex *-niṭaka*. It is also possible that *niṭaka* is a corruption of *nāṭaka* (i.e., "pigeon-dancer" pose).
280 Emend. *ūrum* : Codex *ūru*.
281 Conj. *āsta* : Codex *āṣṭa*.
282 The usual meaning of *jaghana* is "hip" or "buttock", but it can also mean the genitals (Monier-Williams 1899, s.v.). The Sanskrit description somewhat contradicts the picture of *śaṅkvāsana* in the *Śrītattvanidhi* (Sjoman 1999: pl. 4), which depicts the yogi pressing the inner thigh with the heel of the other leg. The knee of the bent leg is in front of the body, so it could not press the buttock of the other leg in this position. Perhaps *jaghanapradeśa* (i.e., "the region of the hips/genitals") was believed to include the thighs.
283 Corr. Preisendanz *san* : Codex *saṃn*.
284 In the picture of the *tāṇḍavāsana* in the *Śrītattvanidhi* (Sjoman 1999: pl. 10), the yogi appears to have his right leg slightly raised to one side, so that his heel is off the ground.

82. Again and again, [the yogi] should stand up and sit down. [This] is the "standing up repeatedly" [pose].
punaḥ punaḥ utthātavyam āsitavyam[285] *utthānotthānaṃ bhavati* || 82 ||

83. At a distance of three cubits from a wall, [the yogi] should stand and having touched his chest on the wall and expanded [it,] he should touch it thus again [and again. This] is the "embracing [the wall]" pose.
hastatrayaṃ bhittiṃ parityajya sthātavyaṃ bhittau hṛdayaṃ saṃspṛśya niṣkāṣya punaḥ saṃspṛśet āliṅganāsanaṃ[286] *bhavati* || 83 ||

84. Hugging one knee to the chest, [the yogi] should stand. [This] is the "embracing the child" [pose].
ekaṃ jānum[287] *urasi āliṅgya sthātavyaṃ bālāliṅganaṃ bhavati* || 84 ||

85. Having held firmly the penis and scrotum between the thighs, [the yogi] should stand on the tips of the toes. [This] is the loincloth pose.
[fol. 17v] *vṛṣaṇasahitaliṅgam ūrumadhye gāḍhaṃ dhṛtvā caraṇāgrābhyāṃ sthātavyaṃ kaupīnāsanaṃ*[288] *bhavati* || 85 ||

86. Having clasped both hands [together], [the yogi] should jump both feet inside them, outside, and inside [again. This] is the "jumping over the threshold" [pose].[289]
hastadvayaṃ[290] *baddhvā*[291] *tanmadhye*[292] *caraṇadvayaṃ uḍḍānena bahir ānīya antaḥ*[293] *nayet dehalyullaṅghanaṃ bhavati* || 86 ||

87. Having jumped up, [the yogi] should strike his buttocks with both heels. [This] is the deer pose.
[fol. 18r] *uḍḍānaṃ kṛtvā pārṣṇibhyāṃ nitambaṃ tāḍayet hariṇāsanaṃ bhavati* || 87 ||

---

285 Conj. *utthātavyam āsitavyam* : Codex *utthātavya asitavyaṃ*.
286 Conj. *āliṅganāsanaṃ* : Codex *āliṅgāsanaṃ*.
287 Emend. *jānum* : Codex *jānu*.
288 Emend. *kaupīnāsanaṃ* : Codex *kaupinasanaṃ*.
289 In the *Śrītattvanidhi* (Sjoman 1999: pl. 19 and p. 119), this pose is called *uḍḍānāsana*. If this is the original name, it may be connected with the next pose because the latter begins with "jumping up" (i. e., *uḍḍānaṃ kṛtvā* [...]).
290 Emend. *hastadvayaṃ* : Codex *hastadvaye*.
291 Emend. *baddhvā* : Codex *vyadhvā*.
292 Emend. *tanmadhye* : Codex *tanmadhyā*.
293 Emend. *antaḥ* : Codex *ataḥ*.

88. Having stood straight, [the yogi] should take both arms up. Having jumped up again and again, he should take [them down. This] is the pestle pose.
saralaṃ sthitvā ūrdhvaṃ bāhū nayet vāraṃ vāraṃ uḍḍānaṃ kṛtvā nayet musalāsanaṃ bhavati || 88 ||

89. Holding with one hand the toes of one leg, which is [straight] like a stick, and placing the sole of the other foot on the ground, [the yogi] should spin around quickly. [This] is the pole star pose.
ekena hastena daṇḍarūpasya ekasya pādasyāgraṃ dhṛtvā itarapādatalaṃ bhūmau nidhāya tvarayā bhramaṇaṃ kartavyaṃ dhruvāsanaṃ bhavati || 89 ||

90. Having extended the hands [out to the sides, the yogi] should spin [them] around. [This] is the potter's disk pose.
hastau prasārya bhrāmaṇaṃ kartavyaṃ kulālacakrāsanaṃ bhavati || 90 ||

91. Having put the big toes of the feet on the ground and having raised up the arms, [the yogi] should remain thus. [This] is the camel pose.
[fol. 18v] *pādāṅguṣṭhābhyāṃ*[294] *bhūmiṃ dhṛtvā bāhū ūrdhvīkṛtya tiṣṭhet uṣṭrāsanaṃ*[295] *bhavati* || 91 ||

92. Remaining in camel pose, raising the feet from the ground and taking [them] above the head, [the yogi] should place his back on the ground. This is the "pigeon in space" [pose].[296]
uṣṭrāsane sthitvā caraṇau bhūmer utthāpya mastakopari nītvā[297] *pṛṣṭhapradeśena bhūmau sthāpayet ākāśakapotaṃ bhavati* || 92 ||

93. Having placed the ankle along with the little toe of one foot at the base of the [other] thigh, and having placed the knee [of the lotus leg] on the heel of the other foot, [the yogi] should remain thus and join his hands together. [This] is Garuḍa's pose.

294 Emend. *pādāṅguṣṭhābhyāṃ* : Codex *pādāṃ gulpābhyāṃ*.

295 Emend. *uṣṭrāsanaṃ* : Codex *uṣṭrasanaṃ*.

296 It is difficult to reconcile the description of the *uṣṭrāsana* with the instructions given for the *ākāśakapotāsana*. One might make sense of it by supplying; "Having stood in the camel pose, [bending forward to place the palms of both hands and the back of the head on the ground,] raising the feet from the ground and taking [them] above the head, [the yogi] should place his back on the ground. This is the 'pigeon in space' [pose]." This interpretation assumes that the *ākāśakapotāsana* is a forward rolling movement. Unfortunately, it is not illustrated or described in the *Śrītattvanidhi*.

297 Conj. *nītvā* : Codex *bhītvā*.

[fol. 19r] ūrumūle itarapādasya kaniṣṭhikāpradeśena[298] gulphaṃ[299] saṃsthāpya tad eva jānum[300] itarapādapārṣṇyāṃ[301] saṃsthāpya tiṣṭhet hastau saṃmīlayet garuḍāsanaṃ[302] bhavati || 93 ||

Now, the Poses with a Rope.
atha rajjvāsanāni[303]

94. Having clasped a rope [secured horizontally above the head[304]] with both hands, [the yogi] should hold both legs between the hands, above the head and [then] on the ground. He should throw [his legs up over his head in this manner] again and again. [This] is the cockroach pose.
[fol. 19v] *hastadvayena rajjuṃ dhṛtvā pādadvayaṃ hastamadhyāt*[305] *śirasopari bhūmau nidhāya punaḥ punaḥ saṃkṣipet paroṣṇyāsanaṃ bhavati* || 94 ||

95. Having supported the region of the navel on a rope, [the prone yogi should remain horizontal in the air,] rigid like a stick. [This] is the stick pose.[306]
nābhipradeśaṃ rajjau dhārayitvā daṇḍavat sthirībhavet daṇḍāsanaṃ bhavati[307] || 95 ||

96. Having placed the buttocks on a [horizontal] rope, [the supine yogi] should become rigid like a stick [horizontally in the air. This] is the weight pose.
[fol. 20r] *rajjau nitambaṃ sthāpayitvā daṇḍavat*[308] *sthirībhavet bhārāsanaṃ bhavati* || 96 ||

97. Having held a [vertical] rope with both hands, [the yogi] should climb up [it. This] is Nārada's pose.
hastābhyāṃ rajjuṃ dhṛtvā ūrdhvam ārohet nāradāsanaṃ bhavati || 97 ||

---

298 Conj. Preisendanz *-pradeśena* : Codex *-pradeśa-*.
299 Emend. *-gulphaṃ* : Codex *-gulphāṃ*.
300 Emend. *jānum* : Codex *jānu*.
301 Emend. *-pārṣṇyāṃ* : Codex *-pārṣṇyaṃ*.
302 Emend. *garuḍāsanaṃ* : Codex *gurūḍāsanaṃ*.
303 Diagnostic Conj. *rajjvāsanāni* : Codex *rajvānyāsanāni*.
304 This is depicted in the *Śrītattvanidhi*'s illustration of the *paroṣṇyāsana* (Sjoman 1999: pl. 11) and it makes sense of the Sanskrit description.
305 Emend. *madhyāt* : Codex *mādhyāt*.
306 The name of this pose has been omitted from this description, but it matches the description and illustration of the *daṇḍāsana* in the *Śrītattvanidhi* (Sjoman 1999: pl. 11 and p. 78).
307 Diagnostic Conj. *sthirībhavet daṇḍāsanaṃ bhavati* : Codex *sthiraṃ bhavati*.
308 Emend. *daṇḍavat* : Codex *daṇḍava*.

98. Having assumed the lotus pose and having held a [vertical] rope with both hands, [the yogi] should climb [up it. This] is the "[climbing up to] heaven" pose.
padmāsanaṃ kṛtvā hastābhyāṃ rajjuṃ dhṛtvā ārohet svargāsanaṃ bhavati || 98 ||

99. Having assumed the rooster pose and having held a [vertical] rope with the hands, [the inverted yogi] should climb [up it. This] is the spider pose.
kukkuṭāsanaṃ kṛtvā hastābhyāṃ rajjuṃ dhṛtvā ārohet ūrṇanābhyāsanaṃ bhavati[309] || 99 ||

100. Having held a [vertical] rope with both fists and having put the soles of the feet on the [fists, the yogi] should remain thus. [This] is the parrot pose.
[fol. 20v] *muṣṭibhyāṃ rajjuṃ dhṛtvā tadupari pādatale sthāpayitvā tiṣṭhet śukāsanaṃ bhavati* || 100 ||

101. Having held a [vertical] rope with the big toes above and the hands below, [the inverted yogi] should climb up [it. This] is the caterpillar [pose].
[fol. 21r] *pādāṅguṣṭhābhyām ūrdhvaṃ rajjuṃ dhṛtvā adhaḥ rajjuṃ hastābhyāṃ dhṛtvā ārohet tṛṇajalūkā*[310] *bhavati* || 101 ||

102. Having held a [vertical] rope with one fist, [the yogi] should climb up [it. This] is the grub pose.
ekayā muṣṭyā rajjuṃ[311] *dhṛtvā ārohet vṛntāsanaṃ bhavati* || 102 ||

103. Having pushed the fists through the thighs and knees, [the yogi] should hold two [vertical ropes] with them, while holding a [counter-]weight [such as a stone[312]] with the teeth, and should climb up. [This] is the curlew pose.
ūrujānvantarābhyāṃ muṣṭī[313] *niṣkāsya tābhyāṃ rajjudvayaṃ dhṛtvā dantaiḥ bhāraṃ dhṛtvā ārohet krauñcāsanaṃ*[314] *bhavati* || 103 ||

309 Diagnostic Conj. *ūrṇanābhyāsanaṃ bhavati* : Codex *ūrṇanābhyāsana.*
310 Emend. *tṛṇajalūkā* : Codex *traṇajalukaṃ.*
311 Emend. *rajjuṃ* : Codex *rañjjuṃ.*
312 This is depicted in the *Śrītattvanidhi*'s illustration of the *krauñcāsana* (Sjoman 1999: pl. 12).
313 Emend. *muṣṭī* : Codex *muṣṭīṃ.*
314 Emend. *krauñcāsanaṃ* : Codex *kraucāsanaṃ.*

Poses by which piercing of the sun and moon [occurs] are [now] taught.[315]
sūryacandrabhedanāny āsanāni[316] *kathyante* ||

104. Having placed both elbows on the ground, [the yogi] should support [himself] with the knees on the ground, place the hands on the head and heels on the buttocks and remain thus. [This] is the boar pose.
kūrparau bhūmau sthāpayitvā jānubhyāṃ avanim avaṣṭabhya hastau mastake saṃsthāpya parṣṇī[317] *nitambe saṃsthāpya tiṣṭhet vārāhāsanaṃ bhavati* || 104 ||

105. Having put the left heel on the navel [and] the other foot on the [opposite] thigh, [the yogi] should clasp the outside of the right knee with the left hand and hold the toes of the [right foot, which are] below the left knee. He should remain thus. [This] is Matsyendra's seat.
[fol. 21v] *vāmapārṣṇiṃ*[318] *nābhau itarapādaṃ ūruṇi saṃsthāpya vāmahastena dakṣiṇajānuṃ bahiḥpradeśena saṃveṣṭya vāmajānunaḥ adhaḥ pādāgraṃ dhṛtvā tiṣṭhet matsyendrapīṭhaṃ bhavati* || 105 ||

106. Having joined together the feet, [the yogi] should take the toes onto the pelvic floor and the heels below the penis and sit on the soles of the feet thus. [This] is the perineum pose.
pādau saṃmīlya pādāgre ādhāre[319] *pārṣṇī liṅgād adhaḥ ānīya pādatalayoḥ*[320] *saṃviśet yonyāsanaṃ bhavati* || 106 ||

107. Having placed the [upturned] sole of one foot on the [opposite] thigh and having fixed the other [foot] on the other thigh, [the yogi] should remain [sitting] upright. [This] is the "lucky mark" pose.[321]
[fol. 22r] *ūruṇi pādatalaṃ saṃsthāpya itara ūruṇi itaraṃ niveśya saralaṃ*[322] *tiṣṭhet svastikāsanaṃ bhavati* || 107 ||

---

315 I do not know why these poses have been classified as "sun" and "moon" poses. Whether one takes the sun and moon to mean *prāṇā* and *apāna*, the *piṅgalā* and *iḍā* channels, or the right and left sides of the body, such associations do not appear to characterise the following poses.

316 Emend. *sūryacandrabhedanāny āsanāni* : Codex *sūryaṃ candrabhedenāny āsanāni.*

317 Emend. *parṣṇī* : Codex *parṣṇi.*

318 Emend. *vāmapārṣṇiṃ* : Codex *vāmapārṣṇi.*

319 Conj. *ādhāre* : Codex *adhare.*

320 Emend. *-talayoḥ* : Codex *-talayo.*

321 In the *Haṭhābhyāsapaddhati, svastikāsana* is the same as the unbound version of *padmāsana* in other yoga texts (cf. HP 1.47–49). In the *Śrītattvanidhi,* a picture of the unbound lotus pose has been included under the name of *padmāsana* (Sjoman 1999: pl. 14), but the description of it is the same as that of the bound lotus pose (*baddhapadmāsana*).

322 Emend. *saralaṃ* : Codex *sasalaṃ.*

108. Having pressed the perineum with one heel and the penis with the heel of the other foot, [the yogi] should remain [sitting] upright. [This] is the thunderbolt pose.
ekayā pārṣṇyā sīvaniṃ saṃpīḍya itarapādapārṣṇyā[323] *liṅgaṃ niṣpīḍya saralaṃ tiṣṭhet vajrāsanaṃ bhavati* || 108 ||

109. Having placed the soles of the feet on the ground, [the yogi] should take his knees to the base of his ears. [This] is the difficult pose.
pādatalābhyāṃ bhūmim avaṣṭabhya jānunī karṇamūle nayet utkaṭāsanaṃ bhavati || 109 ||

110. Having placed both heels on the navel, [the yogi] should join the outer region of both shanks. [This] is the conch shell pose.
[fol. 22v] *pārṣṇī*[324] *nābhau saṃsthāpya jaṅghā bahiḥpradeśena saṃmīlayet śuktyāsanaṃ*[325] *bhavati* || 110 ||

111. [The yogi] should remain like a corpse on the ground. [This] is the corpse pose.
śavavad bhūmau tiṣṭhet śavāsanaṃ bhavati || 111 ||

112. Having stretched out both legs, [this] is the "stretching out [the legs]" pose.
pādadvayaṃ vitanyottānāsanaṃ[326] *bhavati* || 112 ||

Appendix 3: A Comparison of Medieval and Modern *Āsana*-s

The following table outlines a comparison between the shapes of the *āsana*-s of Pattabhi Jois' Aṣṭāṅgavinyāsa (PJAV) and those of medieval yoga texts. PJAV is only a small sample of the *āsana*-s taught in all modern Indian yoga schools. However, it provides a more representative sample of the *āsana*-s taught by Kṛṣṇamācārya and his students, whose yoga has been widely disseminated throughout the world.

When considering the results of this comparison, one should bear in mind the difficulties of comparing modern and medieval *āsana*-s, which I have mentioned in the conclusion of this chapter. These results neither prove nor disprove the direct influence of medieval texts on modern yoga traditions, but they suggest the

323 Conj. *itarapādapārṣṇyā* : Codex *itarapādārghyā.*
324 Conj. *pārṣṇī* : Codex *pārṣṇi.*
325 Conj. *śuktyāsanaṃ* : Codex *śukyāsanaṃ.*
326 Conj. *vitanyottānāsanaṃ* : Codex *vitanottānāsanaṃ.*

types of *āsana*-s which modern traditions have most probably adapted from premodern Haṭha Yoga. The number in round brackets indicates the number of *āsana*-s in a category such as standing poses. The names of the types of *āsana*-s (i. e., "standing", "floor" and "finishing") do not appear in Pattabhi Jois' book *Yoga Mala* but are generally used among practitioners: "standing" poses for those in which the body weight is supported by the legs, "floor poses" for those done close to the floor, and "finishing poses" for those which form a concluding sequence at the end of the practice. I have not counted separately variations in some of PJAV's *āsana*-s (e. g., *jānuśīrṣāsana* A, B, C, D, etc.) and have not included the names of PJAV's *āsana*-s which did not yield a correspondence.

There are further correspondences between the *āsana*-s in the above textual sources and those in the intermediate and advanced sequences of Pattabhi Jois' Aṣṭāṅgavinyāsa.

Type of *āsana* in PJAV's primary sequence	**Name of the PJAV *āsana***	**Name of the medieval *āsana***	**Textual source**
sūryanamaskāra		0	0
standing poses (10)	*utkaṭāsana*	*utkaṭāsana* (though this pose has the knees bent until the anus is on the heels)	GS 2.27
floor poses (20)	*daṇḍāsana*	*daṇḍāsana*	*Pātañjalayogaśāstravivaraṇa*, *Tattvavaiśāradī* on *sūtra* 2.46, etc.
	paścimatānāsana	*paścimatānāsana*	ŚS 3.109, HP 1.30, etc.
	ardhabaddhapadma-paścimottānāsana	a combination of *mahāmudrā* and *baddhapadmāsana*	The *Vivekamārtaṇḍa* (14, 81–82) is the earliest text to teach both these techniques.
	jānuśīrṣāśana	variations on *mahāmudrā; ardhapaścimatānāsana; mahāmudrāsana*	DYŚ 132–133; HAP 49; JP vv. 103–106
	navāsana	similar to *naukāsana* though *naukāsana* has the elbows on the ground	HAP 11
	bhujapīḍāsana	*mālāsana*	HAP 57
	kūrmāsana	similar to *bhiḍokāsana* (i. e., legs straight and parted with the head and shoulders on the ground), except for the position of the hands	JP vv. 183–187
	suptakūrmāsana	Variation on *phaṇīndrāsana* and *yoganidrāsana.* Balancing on the buttocks while the spine is upright and the legs are raised in various positions such as the soles of the feet together or behind the neck is seen in various *āsana*-s in the *Jogapradīpyakā* (e.g., *gopicandrāsana, bharatharyāsana*, etc.).	HR 3.65; HAP 70
	garbhapiṇḍāsana	*valgulyāsana*	HSC, ms. no 2244, fol. 18r, ll. 3–8
	kukkuṭāsana	*kukkuṭāsana*	VS 1.78, HP 1.25, etc.

(Continued)

Type of *āsana* in PJAV's primary sequence	**Name of the PJAV *āsana***	**Name of the medieval *āsana***	**Textual source**
	baddhakoṇāsana	*hālipāvāsana; jonāsana*	JP vv. 261–263; as illustrated in the *Yogāsanamālā* (Kaivalyadhama Yoga Institute 2006: 388)
	upaviṣṭakoṇāsana	a forward bending version of *uttānāsana; pakṣyāsana*	HAP 112; SMĀ fol. 43v, ll. 3–6
	suptakoṇāsana	This is a combination of *uttānāsana* (i. e., legs abducted) and *lāṅgalāsana; abhikāsana.*	HAP 15; SMĀ fol. 43v, ll. 6–8
	ūrdhvamukhapaścimottānāsana	*phodyāsana;* possibly, *śayitapaścimatānāsana*	JP vv. 120–122; HR 3.68
finishing poses (15)	*ūrdhvadhanurāsana*	*paryaṅkāsana*	HAP 16
	paścimatānāsana	*paścimatānāsana*	ŚS 3.109, HP 1.30, etc.
	sarvaṅgāsana	*narakāsana; viparītikaranāsana*	HAP 14; JP vv. 163–165
	halāsana	*lāṅgalāsana*	HAP 15
	karṇapīḍāsana	This is similar to *devāsana,* though the latter does not involve squeezing the ears.	JP vv. 166–169
	ūrdhvapadmāsana	Combination of *narakāsana* and *viparītikaranāsana* with *padmāsana.* The *Rudrayāmalottaratantra* (23.88) describes an *āsana* with the head and elbows on the ground and the legs in the air in *padmāsana.*	HAP 14; JP vv. 163–165
	piṇḍāsana	This is a variation of *uttānakūrmāsana,* in which the hips are raised and the arms wrapped around the legs rather than threaded through them.	HP 1.26
	matsyāsana	*nagrāsana*	JP vv. 351–353
	śīrṣāsana	*narakāsana; kapālyāsana*	YC p. 156; JP vv. 113–115, etc.

(Continued)

Type of *āsana* in PJAV's primary sequence	**Name of the PJAV *āsana***	**Name of the medieval *āsana***	**Textual source**
	baddhapadmāsana	*baddhapadmāsana*	Viv 14, etc.
	yogamudrā	bending forward in *padmāsana*	(see below)
	padmāsana	*padmāsana*	DYŚ 35–38, etc.
	utpluti	*lolāsana*	*Rudrayāmalottaratantra* 23.43–45
	śavāsana	*śavāsana*	HP 1.34, etc.

Table 6: A comparison of medieval and modern *āsana*-s.

Abbreviations (Primary Sources)

DYŚ.	*Dattātreyayogaśāstra.*
GS.	*Gheraṇḍasaṃhitā.*
Gś.	*Gorakṣaśataka,* ed. Fausta Nowotny. Köln: K. A. Nowotny, 1976.
Gśk.	*Gorakṣaśataka,* ed. Swāmī Kuvalayānanda and S. A. Shukla. Lonavla: Kaivalyadhama S. M. Y. M. Samiti, 2006.
HAP.	*Haṭhābhyāsapaddhati.*
HP.	*Haṭhapradīpikā.*
HR.	*Haṭharatnāvalī.*
HSC.	*Haṭhasaṅketacandrikā.*
JP.	*Jogapradīpyakā.*
SMĀ.	*Haṭhapradīpikā-Siddhāntamuktāvalī.*
ŚS.	*Śivasaṃhitā.*
ŚTN.	*Śrītattvanidhi.*
Viv.	*Vivekamārtaṇḍa.*
VivB.	*Vivekamārtaṇḍa,* ms. no. 4110, Central Library, Baroda.[327]
VivN1.	*Vivekamārtaṇḍa,* ms. no. C0060-03 (NS 919), National Archives of Kathmandu.
VivN2.	*Vivekamārtaṇḍa,* ms. no. G0058-15 (NS 858), National Archives of Kathmandu.
VS.	*Vasiṣṭhasaṃhitā.*
YC.	*Yogacintāmaṇi* (of Śivānandasarasvatī).
YTĀ.	*Yogatārāvalī.*
YY.	*Yogayājñavalkya.*

Other Abbreviations and Special Signs

[-]	Connects two words in a compound
Σ	All collated manuscripts except those listed after it
†yogaḥ†	The reading *yogaḥ* is spurious and the present editor has not been able to improve upon it.
ama+ska	One *akṣara* between "ma" and "ska" is illegible or missing
ca]	"ca" is the lemma (i.e., the word accepted in the edited text)
Conj.	A conjecture by the author
Conj. [Devadatta]	A conjecture by Devadatta
Corr.	A correction
Diagnostic Conj.	A diagnostic conjecture by the author
Diagnostic Conj. [Devadatta]	A diagnostic conjecture by Devadatta
ed.	editor
Emend.	An emendation
fol.	folio
fols.	folios

327 I wish to thank James Mallinson for providing me with a copy of this manuscript.

l.	line
ll.	lines
n.	note
ms. no.	manuscript number
r	recto
v	verso
v.	verse
Viv	The Gorakhnāth Mandir's edition of the *Vivekamārtaṇḍa*
vol.	volume
vv.	verses
[word]	Square brackets enclose a word supplied in the translation.

References

Primary Sources

Amanaska
see Birch 2013a.

Amaraughaprabodha
see Mallik 1954.

Amṛtasiddhi
Amṛtasiddhi, ms. no. H233-06. Kathmandu National Archives.

Aṃśumatitantra
Aṃśumadāgama, French Institute of Pondicherry transcript T0004, pp. 624–629. Available at muktabodha.org. Some chapters have been typed up as an etext by researchers at the École française d'Extrême-Orient.

Dattātreyayogaśāstra
Unpublished edition by J. Mallinson (with the help of Alexis Sanderson, Jason Birch and Péter Szántó), forthc.

Gheraṇḍasaṃhitā
see Mallinson 2004.

Gorakṣaśataka
Gorakṣaśataka, ms. no. R7874, Government Oriental Manuscripts Library, Madras University.

Haṭhābhyāsapaddhati
Āsanayoga, ms. no. 46/440, Bhārat Itihās Samśodhak Maṇḍal, Pune.

Haṭhapradīpikā
The Haṭhapradīpikā of Svātmārāma, ed. Swami Digambaraji & Pt. Raghunatha Shastri Kokaje. Lonavla: Kaivalyadhama S. M. Y. M. Samiti, 1998.

Haṭhapradīpikā-Siddhāntamuktāvalī
Haṭhayogapradīpikā, ms. no. 6756, Rajasthan Oriental Research Institute, Jodhpur.

Haṭharatnāvalī
Haṭharatnāvalī of Śrīnivāsayogī, ed. M. L. Gharote et al. Lonavla: Lonavla Yoga Institute, 2009.

Haṭhasaṅketacandrikā
(a) *Haṭhasaṅketacandrikā* of Sundaradeva, ms. no. R3239 (transcript), Government Oriental Manuscripts Library, Madras University.
(b) *Haṭhasaṅketacandrikā* of Sundaradeva, ms. no. 2244, Man Singh Pustak Prakash Library, Jodhpur.

Haṭhatattvakaumudī
Haṭhatattvakaumudī: A Treatise on Haṭhayoga by Sundaradeva, ed. M. L. Gharote et al. Lonavla: Lonavla Yoga Institute, 2007.

Jogapradīpyakā
see Kaivalyadhama Yoga Institute 2006.

Jyotsnā
see Kaivalyadhama Yoga Institute 2002.

Khecarīvidyā
see Mallinson 2007a.

Pātañjalayogaśāstra
Vācaspatimiśraviracitaṭīkāsaṃvalitavyāsabhāṣyasametāni pātañjalayogasūtrāṇi: tathā bhojadevaviracitarājamārtaṇḍābhidhavṛttisametāni pātañjaliyogasūtrāṇi. sūtrapāṭhasūtravarṇānukramasūcībhyāṃ ca sanāthīkṛtāni, ed. Kāśīnātha Śāstrī Āgāśe. Ānandāśramasaṃskṛtagranthāvaliḥ 47. Pune: Ānandāśramamudraṇālaya, 1904.

Rudrayāmalottaratantra
Rudrayāmalam (Uttaratantram), ed. Rāmakumāra Rāya. Varanasi: Kṛṣṇadāsa Akādamī, 2002.

Śārṅgarapaddhati
The Paddhati of Sarngadhara: A Sanskrit Anthology, ed. P. Peterson. Bombay Sanskrit Series 37. Bombay: Government Central Book Depot, 1888.

Śivasaṃhitā
see Mallinson 2007b.

Śrītattvanidhi
see Sjoman 1999.

Tattvavaiśāradī
see *Pātañjalayogaśāstra.*

Vasiṣṭhasaṃhitā
see Kaivalyadhama Yoga Institute 2005.

Vivekamārtaṇḍa
Vivekamārtaṇḍa (Praṇetā Śivagorakṣa Mahāyogī Gorakṣanātha), ed. Rāmlāl Śrīvāstav. Gorakhpur: Gorakhnāth Mandir, 1983.

Vyavahāramālā
Vyavahāramālā (nāma dharmaśāstragranthaḥ), ed. V. Veṅkaṭarāmaśarma. Ānandāśramasaṃkṛtagranthāvaliḥ 121. Pune: Ānandāśramamudraṇālaya, 1979.

Yogabīja
Yogabīja of Gorakhanātha, ed. Rāmalāla Śrīvāstava. Gorakhapur: Gorakhnāth Mandir, 1982.

Yogacintāmaṇi
(a) ed. Haridās Śarma. Calcutta: Calcutta Oriental Press (no date of publication).[328]
(b) unpublished ms. no. 3537, Scindia Oriental Institute, Ujjain. *Catalogue of Manuscripts preserved in the Oriental Manuscripts Library Ujjain.* Part 2 (collected from April 1935 to the end of May 1937). Gwalior: Alijar Darbar Press, 1941, p. 54.
(c) unpublished ms. no. 9784, Kaivalyadhama Yoga Institute Library, Lonavla.
(d) unpublished ms. no. 9785 (based on R635), Kaivalyadhama Yoga Institute Library, Lonavla.
(e) unpublished ms. no. 1-1337 (reel No. B39/5), National Archives Kathmandu.
(f) unpublished ms. no. M. a. I. 312, Universitätsbibliothek Tübingen.
Yogāsanamālā
see Kaivalyadhama Yoga Institute 2006.
Yogasūtra
see *Pātañjalayogaśāstra.*
Yogatārāvalī
Śrīmacchaṅkarābhagavatpādaviracitā Yogatārāvalī, ed. Swāmī Śrīdayānanda Śāstrī. Varanasi: Vārāṇaseya Saṃskṛta Saṃsthāna, 1982.
Yogayājñavalkya
Yoga-Yājñavalkyam: A Treatise on Yoga as Taught by Yogī Yājñavalkya, ed. P. C. Divanji. B. B. R. A. Society Monograph 3. Bombay: B. B. R. A. Society, 1954.
Yuktabhavadeva
Yuktabhavadeva of Bhavadeva Miśra, ed. M. L. Gharote & V. K. Jha. Lonavla: Lonavla Yoga Institute, 2002.

Secondary Sources

Alter, J. (2004). *Yoga in Modern India: The Body between Science and Philosophy.* Princeton, NJ: Princeton University Press.

Bernard, T. (1958). *Hatha Yoga: The Report of a Personal Experience.* London: Rider.

Birch, J. (2011). The Meaning of haṭha in Early Haṭhayoga. *Journal of the American Oriental Society, 131*(4), 527-554.

Birch, J. (2013a). *The Amanaska: King of All Yogas. A Critical Edition and Annotated Translation with a Monographic Introduction.* Unpublished Doctoral Thesis. University of Oxford.

Birch, J. (2013b). Rājayoga: The Reincarnations of the King of all Yogas. *International Journal of Hindu Studies, 17*(3), 401-444.

Bouy, C. (1994). *Les Nātha-Yogin et les Upaniṣads: étude d'histoire de la littérature hindoue.* Publications de l'Institut de Civilisation Indienne 62. Paris: Diffusion de Boccard.

Bühnemann, G. (2007a). *Eighty-Four Āsanas in Yoga: A Survey of Traditions (with Illustrations).* New Delhi: D. K. Printworld.

328 Citations which give page numbers of the *Yogacintāmaṇi* are from this edition, unless otherwise stated.

Bühnemann, G. (2007b). The Identification of an Illustrated Haṭhayoga Manuscript and Its Significance for Traditions of 84 Āsanas in Yoga. *Asian Medicine, Tradition and Modernity, 3*(1), 156–176.

Clark, M. (2006). *The Daśanāmī-Saṃnyāsīs: The Integration of Ascetic Lineages into an Order.* Leiden: Brill.

Dasgupta, S. (1969). *Obscure Religious Cults.* 3rd ed. Calcutta: Firma K. L. Mukhopadhyay.

De Michelis, E. (2004). *A History of Modern Yoga: Patañjali and Western Esotericism.* London: Continuum.

Ernst, C. (2003). The Islamization of Yoga in the Amrtakunda Translations. *Journal of the Royal Asiatic Society, Series 3, 13*(2), 199–226.

Gharote, M. L. (2009). See *Haṭharatnāvalī*

Gharote, M. L. et al. (2006). *Encyclopedia of Traditional Asanas.* Lonavla: Lonavla Yoga Institute.

Gode, P. K. (1953). *Studies in Indian Literary History.* Vol. 1. Bombay: Singhi Jain Śāstra Śikshāpīth Bhāratīya Vidyā Bhavan.

Iyengar, G. (1998). *Yoga: A Gem for Women.* New Delhi: Allied Publishers.

Iyer, L. K. A. & Nanjundayya, H. V. (1935). *The Mysore Tribes and Castes.* Vol. 2. Mysore: Mysore University.

Jois, P. (2002). *Yoga Mala: The Seminal Treatise and Guide from the Living Master of Ashtanga Yoga.* New York: North Point Press, a division of Farrar, Straus and Giroux.

Kaivalyadhama Yoga Institute (2002). *Brahmānandakṛtā Haṭhapradīpikā Jyotsnā,* ed. Maheśānand et al. Lonavla: Kaivalyadhama S. M. Y. M. Samiti.

Kaivalyadhama Yoga Institute (2005). *Vasiṣṭha Saṃhitā (Yoga Kāṇḍa),* ed. Philosophico-Literary Research Department. Revised ed. Lonavla: The Kaivalyadhama S. M. Y. M. Samiti.

Kaivalyadhama Yoga Institute (2006). *Jogapradīpyakā of Jayatarāma,* ed. Maheśānanda et. al. Lonavla: Kaivalyadhama S. M. Y. M. Samiti.

Larson, G. (2008). Introduction to the Philosophy of Yoga. In G. J. Larson & R. S. Bhattacharya (Eds.), *Yoga: India's Philosophy of Meditation* (pp. 21–159). Encyclopedia of Indian Philosophies 12. Delhi: Motilal Banarsidass.

Leach, L. (1995). *Mughal and other Indian Paintings from the Chester Beatty Library.* Vol. 2. London: Scorpion Cavendish.

Mallik, K. (Ed.). (1954). *Siddhasiddhāntapaddhati and Other Works of Nath Yogis.* Pune: Poona Oriental Book House.

Mallinson, J. (2004). *The Gheraṇḍa Saṃhitā: The Original Sanskrit and an English Translation.* Woodstock: YogaVidya.com.

Mallinson, J. (2007a). *The Khecarīvidyā of Ādinātha: A Critical Edition and Annotated Translation of an Early Text of Haṭhayoga.* Routledge Studies in Tantric Traditions. London: Routledge.

Mallinson, J. (2007b). *The Śiva Saṃhitā: A Critical Edition and an English Translation.* Woodstock: YogaVidya.com.

Mallinson, J. (2011). Haṭha Yoga. In K. A. Jacobsen (Ed.), *Brill's Encyclopedia of Hinduism.* Vol. 3 (p. 770–781). Leiden: Brill.

Mallinson, J. (2013). *Dattātreya's Discourse on Yoga* (a translation of the *Dattātreyayogaśāstra* circulated to those who supported the kickstarter campaign for "Roots of Yoga").

Mallinson, J. (2014). Haṭhayoga's Philosophy: A Fortuitous Union of Non-Dualities. *Journal of Indian Philosophy, 42*(1), 225–247.

Mohan, A. G. (2010). *Krishnamacharya: His Life and Teachings.* Boston: Shambhala Publications.

Monier-Williams, M. (1899). *A Sanskrit-English Dictionary: Etymologically and Philologically Arranged with Special Reference to Cognate Indo-European Languages by Sir Monier Monier-Williams M.A., K.C.I.E. New Edition, Greatly Enlarged and Improved with the Collaboration of Professor E. Leumann, Ph.D., Professor C. Cappeller, Ph.D. and other Scholars.* Oxford: Clarendon Press (repr. 1970).

O'Hanlon, P. (2007). Military Sports and the History of the Martial Body in India. *Journal of the Economic and Social History of the Orient, 50*(4), 490–523.

Pollock, S. (1985). The Theory of Practice and the Practice of Theory in Indian Intellectual History. *Journal of the American Oriental Society, 105*(3), 499–519.

Reddy, V. (1982). *Hatharatnavali of Srinivasabhatta Mahayogindra. With an Elaborate Introduction, Selected Text, English Translation, Critical Notes, Appendix and Word Index.* Sri Medapati Subireddy Memorial Yoga Series 1. Arthamuru, E. G. Dt.: Sri M. Ramakrishna Reddy.

Sanderson, A. (2004). The Śaiva Religion Among the Khmers. Part I. *Bulletin de l'Ecole Française d'Extrême-Orient, 90–91,* 349–462.

Sastri, P. P. S. (1931). *Descriptive Catalogue of the Sanskrit Manuscripts in the Tanjore Mahārāja Serfoji's Sarasvatī Mahāl Library, Tanjore.* Vol. 11. Srirangam: Sri Vani Vilas Press.

Satyananda, S. (1996). *Asana Pranayama Mudra Bandha.* Bihar: Yoga Publications Trust.

Singleton, M. (2010). *Yoga Body: The Origins of Modern Posture Practice.* Oxford: Oxford University Press.

Sinh Jee, HH Sir Bhagvat (1896). *A Short History of Aryan Medical Science.* London: Macmillan.

Sircar, D. C. (1971). *Studies in the Geography of Ancient and Medieval India.* Delhi: Motilal Banarsidass.

Sivananda, S. (1993). *Yoga Asanas.* Sivanandanagar: The Divine Life Society.

Sjoman, N. E. (1999). *The Yoga Tradition of the Mysore Palace.* New Delhi: Shakti Malik Abhinav Publications.

Śrīkṛṣṇadāsa K. (1884). *Śrītattvanidhigrantha.* Mumbai: Śrīveṅkaṭeśvara Steam Press.

Taylor, M. (2007). Perfumed by Golden Lotuses: Literary Place and Textual Authority in the Brahma- and Bhāgavatapurāṇas. *Acta Orientalia Vilnensia, 8*(1), 69–81.

Upadhyaya S. C. (1965). *Rati Rahasya of Pandit Kokkoka.* Bombay: Leaders Press.

White, D. (1996) *The Alchemical Body: Siddha Traditions in Medieval India.* Chicago: University of Chicago Press.

Yogeshwaranand S. (2001). *First Steps to Higher Yoga: An Exposition of First Five Constituents of Yoga.* New Delhi: Yoga Niketan Trust.

Chapter 4

Yoga and Sex: What is the Purpose of *Vajrolīmudrā*?

James Mallinson

Contents

1. Introduction 183

2. The Mechanics of *Vajrolī* 185

3. *Vajrolī* in Texts 186
3.1. *Vajrolī* and Haṭha Yoga 187
3.2. *Vajrolī* and Rāja Yoga 193
3.3. *Vajrolī* and Tantra 197

4. Conclusion 204

Appendix 1: Text Passages Which Teach or Mention *Vajrolīmudrā* 205

Appendix 2: Editions and Translations of the Descriptions of *Vajrolīmudrā* in the *Bṛhatkhecarīprakāśa* and the *Vajroliyoga* 206

References 217

James Mallinson

Chapter 4: Yoga and Sex: What is the Purpose of *Vajrolīmudrā*?[*]

1. Introduction

Predominant among the techniques which characterise the Haṭha method of yoga taught in Indic texts from at least the eleventh century CE onwards are its *mudrā*-s, physical methods for manipulating the vital energies. In the earliest systematic description of the *mudrā*-s of Haṭha Yoga, on which most subsequent teachings are based, the last and, by implication, the most important is *vajrolīmudrā*,[1] a method of drawing liquids up the urethra, which, through enabling *bindudhāraṇa*, the retention of semen, is said to lead directly to Rāja Yoga, the royal yoga.[2] In the course of fieldwork among male ascetic practitioners of Haṭha Yoga, I have met two exponents of *vajrolī*, both of whom are held in high esteem by their ascetic peers for their mastery of its practice.[3] Confirming the teachings of the texts, the two ascetics, who have been doggedly celibate all their

* Some of the research for this chapter was carried out as part of the Hatha Yoga Project (hyp.soas.ac.uk). This project has received funding from the European Research Council (ERC) under the European Union's Horizon 2020 research and innovation programme (grant agreement no. 647963). I thank Śrī Rām Bālak Dās Yogirāj, Rodo Pfister, Naren Singh, Ian Duncan, Richard Darmon, Sarkis Vermilyea and Timothy Bates for their help with this chapter, together with the organisers of the conference on "Yoga in Transformation: Historical and Contemporary Perspectives on a Global Phenomenon" held in Vienna on 19–21 September 2013, at which I presented an earlier draft. Particular thanks are due to Jason Birch, who provided me with scans and transcriptions of several of the manuscripts referred to herein and gave me useful comments and corrections on an earlier draft, Lubomír Ondračka whose insightful and tactfully critical remarks about the same earlier draft obliged me to rethink – and temper – many of my conclusions, and Philipp A. Maas whose comments and corrections during the editing process were invaluable. I thank also the chapter's two reviewers.

1 See n. 53 on p. 197f. for an analysis of the name *vajrolī*.

2 DYŚ 160. Cf. HR 2.104–105.

3 These are my guru, Śrī Rām Bālak Dās Jī Yogirāj (henceforth Rām Bālak Dās), a senior ascetic of the Terah Bhāī Tyāgī subdivision of the Rāmānandīs, with whom I have had extensive discussions about yoga practice since meeting him in 1992, and a Daśanāmī Nāgā Saṃnyāsī with whom I spent one afternoon in Gangotri in October 2006. I have also been in indirect communication with Naren Singh, a non-ascetic practitioner of *vajrolī* from Jammu.

lives – they were initiated as boys –, say that they practise *vajrolī* in order to prevent the loss of semen through involuntary ejaculation.[4]

By contrast, some editors and translators of Sanskrit manuals of Haṭha Yoga have chosen to omit the texts' treatments of *vajrolīmudrā*. Rai Bahadur Srisa Chandra Vasu does so because "it is an obscene practice indulged in by low class Tantrists".[5] Hans-Ulrich Rieker, in a translation of the *Haṭhapradīpikā* (HP) later approved by B. K. S. Iyengar,[6] concurs:

> In leaving out these passages, we merely bypass the description of a few obscure and repugnant practices that are followed by only those yogis who lack the will power *[sic]* to reach their goal otherwise. In these 20 slokas, we encounter a yoga that has nothing but its name in common with the yoga of a Patanjali or a Ramakrishna.[7]

Modern scholarship on yoga is in widespread agreement that Haṭha Yoga owes its origins to sexual rituals, in particular those of certain Kaula Śaiva tantric traditions.[8] For example,[9] Joseph Alter, drawing on the work of David Gordon White, writes (2011: 130) that

> there would seem to be no question but that hatha yoga developed between the ninth and fourteenth centuries as a form of practice directly linked to the subtle hydraulics and symbolic significance of ritualized sex.

This understanding of Haṭha Yoga's origins is necessarily explained with references to *vajrolīmudrā*, which is the only haṭhayogic practice that has any possible connection with sex. I myself have written that *vajrolīmudrā*'s "unorthodox 'left-hand' tantric origins are obvious" (2005a: 114). But, as shown by the statements of the two *vajrolī* practitioners I have met – neither of whom would ever consider himself a *tāntrika* – and the texts which teach it, *vajrolī*'s relationship with sex is

4 In recent fieldwork as part of the Hatha Yoga Project, Daniela Bevilacqua met three more ascetic practitioners of *vajrolīmudrā*, all of whom also say that its aim is *bindudhāraṇa*, the preservation of semen. Two popular modern Indian yoga gurus, Shri Yogeshvara and Swami Sivananda, say the same (Shri Yogeshwaranand Paramahansa 2011: 383, Sivananda 1998: 77).

5 Vasu 1914: 51.

6 Rieker's 1957 German translation was translated into English by Elsy Becherer in 1971. This English translation was republished in 1992 with a new foreword by B. K. S. Iyengar.

7 Rieker 1992: 127.

8 Claims by scholars that yoga's origins lie in sexual rituals allowed the prominent yoga journalist William Broad to write in the *New York Times* in 2012 that the many recent sexual scandals involving yoga gurus are not surprising since yoga "began as a sex cult" (http://www.nytimes.com/2012/02/28/health/nutrition/yoga-fans-sexual-flames-and-predictably-plenty-of-scandal.html, accessed 18 October 2017).

9 See also Muñoz 2011: 125: "probably sexual practices had always been an integral element of haṭha yoga, on account of the tantric origins of this system", and Lorenzen 2011: 36: "The rejection of ritual sexual activity was never complete among the Nath yogis, however, as is evident from the vajroli mudra, a technique of sexual control, described in the Haṭhayogapradīpikā."

not so straightforward. In this paper I shall draw on textual, ethnographic, experiential and anatomical data in order to determine the history, method and purpose of *vajrolīmudrā.* In doing so I shall show how the history of *vajrolī* epitomises the history of Haṭha Yoga as a whole.

2. The Mechanics of *Vajrolī*

I shall first explain the mechanics of the practice, my understanding of which has been helped considerably by conversations with Timothy Bates, a urologist. I shall restrict my comments to the practice of *vajrolī* by men. Several texts say that it is possible for women to practise it but they do not explain how and I have not heard of any modern female practitioners nor have I read of any in ethnographic reports.

Some scholars have suggested that it is not possible to suck liquids up through the penis,[10] but I have personally verified that it is. The method is fairly simple. A tube is inserted into the urethra as far as the bladder. Yogis have traditionally used a pipe made of copper, silver or gold, which is in an elongated s-shape.[11] The curves are necessary for the pipe to pass through the urethral sphincter, in the process of doing which the yogi rotates the tube through 180°. Inserting these rigid metal pipes into the urethra is at first quite painful, particularly during the preliminary stages in which pipes of progressively increasing diameters must be used. The two ascetic practitioners of *vajrolī* that I have met prefer to use these metal pipes, which they have specially made for them, but other modern practitioners of *vajrolī* of whom I am aware use latex catheters widely available from medical retailers.

In order to draw liquids up the urethra, after inserting the tube the yogi places the exposed end in a vessel of liquid, contracts his perineum and performs *madhyamā nauli,* in which the central abdominal muscles are contracted in isolation, making the lower abdomen stand forward in a column, thereby reducing the pressure in the lower intestine and bladder. The liquid in the vessel, propelled by the external atmospheric pressure, rises up into the bladder.[12]

The pipe or catheter is essential because the urethral sphincter must be open for liquids to pass through it. We have no voluntary muscular control over this

10 E.g., White 2003: 295–296, n. 88, misunderstanding Darmon 2002.

11 For illustrations see Ānandsvarūpjī 1937: 45.

12 Filliozat (1953: 32–33) is incorrect in his assumption that the yogi must somehow draw in air through the urethra before performing *vajrolī.*

sphincter and performing *nauli* would pull it tightly closed were there no pipe or catheter to keep it open.[13]

Corroborating this anatomical inference of the necessity of a pipe for the performance of *vajrolīmudrā* is the absence of experiential or ethnographic reports of it being done without one, and of texts saying that it is possible to do so.[14] Two scholar-practitioners who have written on *vajrolīmudrā*, Richard Darmon and Mat Rozmarynowski, both address the matter. Darmon (2002: 229), who did his fieldwork among tantric *sādhaka*-s at Tarapith in West Bengal, never heard of *vajrolī* being done without a catheter.[15] Rozmarynowski writes: "Supposedly the urethra is enlarged by this process to the point where it is possible to do Vajroli without any tube at all; this, however, I have not yet verified" (1979: 37). Rām Bālak Dās tells me that he cannot perform *vajrolī* without a pipe and nor could his guru.[16]

The reason for *vajrolī*'s notoriety is that it is said to confer the ability to absorb the commingled fluids produced in sexual intercourse. The first time I saw Rām Bālak Dās was at the Kumbh Mela festival in Ujjain in 1992. A fellow *sādhu* pointed at him as he walked through the camp, turned to a woman devotee and said: "Beware of that yogi: if he gets inside you he will suck out all your energy."

In the light of the apparent impossibility of performing *vajrolīmudrā* without a pipe in the urethra, however, this widespread understanding of the purpose of *vajrolī* must be reconsidered.

3. *Vajrolī* in Texts

I shall now turn to textual descriptions of *vajrolī*. I have identified passages which teach it in sixteen texts, but shall restrict myself here to analysing those which are most important for understanding *vajrolī*'s history and purpose.[17]

---

13 Richard Darmon (personal communication, 26 March 2014) suggested that *vajrolī* might be possible without a pipe if the urethra is stretched enough, but he thought it unlikely that anyone would have done it and added that "it would not be advisable".

14 A book on *vajrolī* published in Jodhpur in 1937 says that it is possible for advanced practitioners to practise *vajrolī* without a pipe and prescribes three methods of learning to do so, but they are only for the absorption of *vāyu*, air, not liquids (Ānandsvarūpjī 1937: 21–26).

15 Cf. Roşu 2002: 308.

16 Rām Bālak Dās told me that some Gorakhnāthīs in the Gorakhpur district may be able to perform *vajrolī* without a pipe, but he has not verified this himself. Swami Sivananda claims that *vajrolī* can be done without a pipe (1998: 77).

17 These sixteen passages (and passages from nine other texts containing information relevant to the study of *vajrolīmudrā*) are given in full in a document entitled "Textual Materials for the study of *Vajrolīmudrā*" available for download from http://www.academia.edu/4515911/Textual_Materials_for_the_study_of_Vajrolimudra (accessed 18 October 2017). An ap-

3.1. *Vajrolī* and Haṭha Yoga

The earliest mention of the practice of *vajrolī*[18] (although it is not named) is in verse 32 of the circa twelfth-century CE second chapter of the *Amanaska*. It is an oblique dismissal of those who "take upwards" (*ūrdhvaṃ nayanti*) "semen that is falling into/from a young woman's vagina" (*yuvatibhagapatadbindum*). The probable meaning is that these yogis are turning back their semen as it begins to fall during sexual intercourse, i. e., they are preventing ejaculation. As we have seen above, it is physiologically impossible to draw semen upwards once it has fallen into a vagina, but the verse may not refer to this: thanks to the ambiguity inherent in the case relationships of members of Sanskrit compounds, the yogis could be using pipes to draw semen upwards as it falls *from* young women's vaginas rather than into them. This possibility is supported by an instruction to do exactly this in the *Vajroliyoga* (c 1800) (on which see below, p. 192).[19]

The next text to mention *vajrolī*, and the first to mention it by name, is the circa thirteenth-century *Dattātreyayogaśāstra* (DYŚ), which is also the first text to teach a Haṭha Yoga named as such:[20]

pendix at the end of this paper lists the sixteen texts and gives transcriptions of the teachings on *vajrolī* from those of them which have not previously been published.

18 I omit here BĀU 6.4.10–11, which, in giving instructions for the resorption of sperm through the penis to avoid conception, is suggestive of *vajrolī*. The passage is cited in the prose section at the end of the *Vajroliyoga*, a transcription of a manuscript of which is given at the end of this chapter.

19 A parallel of sorts is found in the Buddhist *Caṇḍamahāroṣaṇatantra* (6.150–151) in which the male partner in a sexual ritual is instructed either to lick from his consort's vagina the combined products of intercourse or to inhale them into his nose through a pipe (*nāsayā nalikāyogāt pibet*).

20 DYŚ 150c–159b: *vajroliṃ kathayiṣyāmi gopitaṃ sarvayogibhiḥ* || 150 || *atīvaitad rahasyaṃ hi na deyaṃ yasya kasya cit* | *svaprāṇais tu samo yaḥ syāt tasmai ca kathayed dhruvam* || 151 || *svecchayā varttamāno 'pi yogoktaniyamair vinā* | *vajroliṃ yo vijānāti sa yogī siddhibhājanaḥ* || 152 || *tatra vastudvayaṃ vakṣye durlabhaṃ yena kena cit* | *labhyate yadi tasyaiva yogasiddhikaraṃ smṛtam* || 153 || *kṣīram āṅgirasaṃ ceti dvayor ādyaṃ tu labhyate* | *dvitīyaṃ durlabhaṃ puṃsāṃ strībhyaḥ sādhyam upāyataḥ* || 154 || *yogābhyāsaratāṃ strīṃ ca pumān yatnena sādhayet* | *pumān strī vā yad anyonyaṃ strītvapuṃstvānapekṣayā* || 155 || *svaprayojanamātraikasādhanāt siddhim āpnuyāt* | *calito yadi bindus tam ūrdhvam ākṛṣya rakṣayet* || 156 || *evaṃ ca rakṣito bindur mṛtyuṃ jayati tattvataḥ* | *maraṇaṃ bindupātena jīvanaṃ bindudhāraṇāt* || 157 || *bindurakṣāprasādena sarve sidhyanti yoginaḥ* | *amarolis tad yathā syāt sahajolis tato yathā* || 158 || *tadabhyāsakramaḥ śasyaḥ siddhānāṃ sampradāyataḥ* | . The conventions and symbols used in the apparatuses of this and other passages in this chapter edited from manuscripts are the same as those in my edition of the *Khecarīvidyā* (on which see Mallinson 2007: 62–64). Here I shall only indicate important features that are relevant. Where there are multiple witnesses, the apparatus is positive unless there is just one variant. Separate lemmata within the same *pāda* are separated by the symbol •. Crux marks (†...†) enclose passages which do not make sense to me and for which I cannot provide a suitable conjectural emendation. Square brackets ([...]) enclose material not found in the witnesses but supplied by me. The symbol ° indicates that a lemma or variant is part of a

I shall teach *vajrolī*, which is kept hidden by all yogis, (151) for it is a great secret, not to be given to all and sundry. But one certainly should teach it to him who is as dear to one as one's own life. (152) The yogi who knows *vajrolī* is worthy of success, even if he behaves self-indulgently, disregarding the rules taught in yoga. (153) I shall teach you a pair of items (necessary) for it which are hard for anyone to obtain, [and] which are said to bring about success in yoga for a [yogi] if he does obtain them: (154) *kṣīra* and *āṅgirasa*. For men, the first of the two may be obtained [easily but] the second is hard to get; they must use some stratagem to procure it from women. (155–156) A man should strive to find a woman devoted to the practice of yoga. Either a man or a woman can obtain success if they have no regard for one another's gender and practise with only their own ends in mind. If the semen moves then [the yogi] should draw it upwards and preserve it. (157) Semen preserved in this way truly overcomes death. Death [arises] through the fall of semen, life from its preservation. (158–159b) All yogis achieve success

---

longer word or compound. The symbols ⌈...⌉ indicate that a manuscript has supplied the enclosed material in a marginal reading (often indicated in the manuscript by a *kākapāda*). Raised small asterisks (*...*) enclose text which is unclear in a manuscript. A single large asterisk (✳) denotes an illegible syllable in a manuscript. The abbreviation *cett.* (i.e., *cetera*) means the remaining witnesses, i.e., those which have not yet been mentioned. The abbreviation *unm.* stands for unmetrical. The following abbreviations are used: *cod.* for *codex*, i.e., the only available witness; *codd.* for *codices*, i.e., all the available witnesses; *a.c.* for *ante correctionem*, i.e., "before correction"; *p.c.* for *post correctionem*, i.e., "after correction"; *corr.* for *correxit*, i.e., "[the editor] has corrected"; *em.* for *emendavit*, i.e., "[the editor] has emended"; *conj.* for *coniecit*, i.e., "[the editor] has conjectured". "fol. $103r^{11}$" means line 11 on folio 103 recto. I often do not report minor corrections or standardisations such as changing final *anusvāra* (*ṃ*) to *m*, the gemination or degemination of consonants (e.g., *tatva* > *tattva*, *arddha* > *ardha*), and the addition or removal of *avagraha*. Witnesses: *B* = *Dattātreyayogaśāstra* ed. Brahmamitra Avasthī, Svāmī Keśavānanda Yoga Saṃsthāna 1982 • J_1 = Mān Siṃh Pustak Prakāś 1936 • W_1 = Wai Prajñā Pāṭhaśālā 6–4/399 • V = Baroda Oriental Institute 4107 • M = Mysore Government Oriental Manuscripts Library 4369 • W_2 = Wai Prajñā Pāṭhaśālā 6163 • T = Thanjavur Palace Library B6390 • *U* = *Yogatattvopaniṣad*, ed. A. M. Śāstrī in *The Yoga Upaniṣads*, Madras, Adyar Library, 1920 • *H* = *Haṭhapradīpikā*. Readings: **150c** vajroliṃ] vajroli J_1 **150d** gopitaṃ] gopītaṃ J_1, yoṣitāṃ V **151a** atīvaitad] *B*W_2 V; atīvetad J_1, atīva tad W_1 **151c** yaḥ syāt] W_1W_2; yo syāt *B*, yasyā J_1, ya syāt V **151d** tasmai ca] tasmai va W_2, tasyaiva V • kathayed] *B*; kathaye J_1W_1, kathaye⌈t⌉ W_2V **152a** sve°] sva° J_1 **152b** °okta°] °oktair *H* **152c** vajroliṃ] vajroli J_1, vajrolī V • yo vijānāti] abhyased yas tu *U* **152d** °bhājanaḥ] °bhājanam *UH* **153b** yena kena cit] yasya kasya cit *H* **153d** yogasiddhikaraṃ smṛtam] yogasiddhiḥ kare sthitā *U* **154a** āṅgi°] āṅgī° V **154c** dvitīyaṃ durlabhaṃ] *B*W_1; dvayaṃ varṇanaṃ J_1, dvetīyaṃ varṇanaṃ W_2, dvitīyaṃ varṇanaṃ V **154d** strībhyaḥ] strībhiḥ W_1 **155a** °ratāṃ strīṃ] *conj.*; °ratā strī *codd.* **155b** pumān] J_1W_1V; puṃsā *B*, pumāṃn W_2 **155c** anyonyaṃ] anyoyaṃ J_1 **155d** strītvapuṃs°] W_1; strīpuṃs° *B* (*unm.*), strīttvaṃ pus° J_1, strītvapus° W_2, strīstvaṃ puṃs° V **156c** calito yadi bindus tam] *B*W_1; calito yadi padaṃs tadaṃs tam J_1 (*unm.*), calito yadi vipadas tam W_2 (*unm.*), calitaṃ tu svakaṃ bindum V, calitaṃ ca nijaṃ bindum *H* **157a** ca rakṣito] ca rakṣite W_2, saṃrakṣayed *H* • bindur] *B*W_1V; vimdu J_1, bindu W_2, binduṃ *H* **157b** tattvataḥ] yogavit *H* **157d** jīvanaṃ] jīvitaṃ W_1 • °dhāraṇāt] °rakṣaṇāt J_1 **158b** sarve sidhyanti] W_1W_2; sarvaṃ sidhyati *B*, sarva sidhyaṃti J_1, sarvaṃ sidhyaṃti V **158c** tad yathā syāt] *B*W_2V; tathā syāt yāt J_1, tad yathā sā W_1 **159a** °kramaḥ] *B*W_1; °kramo J_1W_2, °krame V • śasyaḥ] śasya $W_2^{p.c.}$ V, syaśasyaḥ $W_2^{a.c.}$ (*unm.*) **159b** siddhānāṃ] siddhināṃ J_1

through the preservation of semen. The method of practice by which *amaroli* and *sahajoli* arise is taught in the tradition of the Adepts.[21]

In the *Dattātreyayogaśāstra vajrolī* is one of nine *mudrā*-s, physical techniques which are the defining characteristics of early Haṭha Yoga, and which, in their earliest textual teachings, are for the control of the breath and semen, and hence the mind. *Vajrolīmudrā*'s purpose is the control of *bindu*, semen. Two substances are needed for its practice, *kṣīra* and *āṅgirasa*. The usual meaning of *kṣīra* is milk, but because the text says that it is hard for any person to obtain both substances (v. 153) it seems unlikely that this is its meaning here. In the light of Bengali tantric usage,[22] in which the names of dairy products are often used as an allusion to semen, the referent of *kṣīra* in this passage may also be semen.[23] The meaning of *āṅgirasa* is also obscure. Like *kṣīra*, it is not defined but must be procured from

21 *Amaroli* and *sahajoli* are taught as variants of *vajrolī* in several Haṭha texts. They are first explained in detail in the *Śivasaṃhitā* and *Haṭhapradīpikā* (but *vajrolī, amaroli* and *sahajoli* are perhaps obliquely referred to in *Amanaska* 2.32, which dates to the twelfth century. The two texts give different definitions, and it is one or other of these definitions which is usually adopted in subsequent works. In the *Śivasaṃhitā* (4.96; cf. *Yogamārgaprakāśikā* 147–154, YBhD 7.296ab, *Jogpradīpakā* 560) *amaroli* is another method of *bindudhāraṇa*, semen retention, for which the yogi trains by repeatedly checking the flow of urine when he urinates. The same contraction is then used to resorb semen should it start to flow. In the *Haṭhapradīpikā* (3.92–94; cf. *Haṭhatattvakaumudī* 16.17) *amaroli* is primarily the practice of drinking urine through the nose, but it is also said to be the massaging of the body with a mixture of ash and *cāndrī*. The latter is likely to be a bodily fluid but its identity is unclear. *Jogpradīpakā* 677–683 teaches the *varaṇak mudrā* which is also called *amaroli* and involves taking various herbal preparations to master *vajrolī*. In a verse near the end of the *Vajroliyoga amaroli* is said to be the absorption through a pipe of the mixed products of sexual intercourse. *Sahajoli* in the *Śivasaṃhitā* (4.97; cf. YBhD 7.296cd, *Yogamārgaprakāśikā* 145–146, *Vajroliyoga* [verse section near end]) is the contraction of the perineal region (using *yonimudrā*) in order to resorb semen. In the *Haṭhapradīpikā* (3.90a–91b = HR 2.113–115, cf. *Haṭhatattvakaumudī* 16.15–16) *sahajolī* is the smearing of the body with ash after intercourse using *vajrolī*.

22 I thank Lubomír Ondračka for this information (personal communication, 11 July 2014).

23 A commonplace of modern teachings on *vajrolī* is that in order to master it the yogi should practise by drawing up liquids of increasing density (e.g., water, milk, oil, honey, ghee and mercury). The earliest reference I have found to this is Ānandsvarūpjī 1937: 16–17 (later examples may be found at Rozmarynowski 1979: 39 and Svoboda 1986: 280). The only premodern text to mention the absorption of liquids other than water or milk is the *Bṛhatkhecarīprakāśa* (fol. 103v[6]), which prescribes milk then mercury. To draw mercury into the bladder as prescribed by Svoboda (1986: 280–281) would presumably be very dangerous because of mercury's toxicity and I prefer the inference of Rozmarynowski (1979: 39), namely that mercury is to be drawn only a short distance up the pipe in order to confirm the power of the vacuum created by the yogi. In textual sources for *vajrolī*'s preparatory practices from before the eighteenth century, no mention is made of the absorption of even water, although some texts do say that air is to be blown through the pipe in the urethra in order to purify it (HP 3.85, HR 2.85). The *Haṭhābhyāsapaddhati*, a late Haṭha text, instructs the yogi hoping to master *vajrolī* to absorb air, then water, and then water infused with various herbal preparations (fol. 26v, ll. 9–13); milk is to be drunk (otherwise the body will waste away, fol. 27r, ll. 10–11).

a woman "by means of some stratagem" (*upāyataḥ*, v. 154). The only definition of *āṅgirasa* that I have found is in a commentary on the *Khecarīvidyā* called the *Bṛhatkhecarīprakāśa,* which postdates the *Dattātreyayogaśāstra* by some 500 years but cites it frequently. *Āṅgirasa* is glossed by Ballāla, the commentator, with *rajas,* female generative fluid.[24] In the *Dattātreyayogaśāstra* women are said to be able to achieve *siddhi,* success, by means of *vajrolī.* There are no instructions for the yogi or yogini to have sex but it is implied (vv. 155–156). Nor are there instructions for either the yogi or yogini to draw up a mixture of *bindu* and *rajas*; the implication is rather that they are to conserve their own *bindu* or *rajas* and optionally draw up the other.

The next text that I shall mention is perhaps the most important for understanding the history - if not the true purpose - of *vajrolī.* It is the *Śivasaṃhitā* (ŚS), a work on yoga composed in the fourteenth or fifteenth centuries CE which is derivative of the Vaiṣṇava *Dattātreyayogaśāstra* but whose Haṭha Yoga is taught within a framework of Śrīvidyā Kaula Śaivism, a relatively tame form of Kaulism, some of whose practices are developments of the Love Magic of the earlier Nityā Tantras (Golovkova 2010). Unlike the *Dattātreyayogaśāstra,* the *Śivasaṃhitā* teaches that the purpose of the *mudrā*-s of Haṭha Yoga is the raising of Kuṇḍalinī (which is not mentioned in the *Dattātreyayogaśāstra*). In its teachings on *vajrolī* (4.78–104) the *Śivasaṃhitā* praises the technique's usefulness in bringing about *bindusiddhi,* mastery of semen, but its description of the practice starts with instructions for the yogi to draw up a woman's *rajas* from her vagina through his penis[25] (which, as we have seen, is physiologically impossible).[26] Should his semen fall during the process, he must draw that upwards too, and the mixing of the two substances within the yogi's body is the mixing of Śiva and Śakti. Unlike other early texts which teach *vajrolī,* the *Śivasaṃhitā* does not say that it can be practised by women. In keeping with its Love Magic heritage, however, the *Śivasaṃhitā* does say that the *bindu* of one who has mastered *vajrolī* will not fall even if he enjoys himself with a hundred women.

---

24 Fol. 103v, l. 5. On the possible identities of *rajas,* which in the texts of Haṭha Yoga seems to mean "women's generative fluid" but in other contexts, in particular Bengali tantric practice, means "menstrual blood", see Das 2003 (cf. Doniger 1980: 33–39).

25 ŚS 4.81: *liṅganālena.* One could take *liṅganālena* to mean "through a pipe in the penis" but that would be a rather forced interpretation, particularly as there is no mention anywhere in the text of inserting a *nāla* into the *liṅga* (and *liṅganāla* means urethra in the *Haṭhābhyāsapaddhati* [fol. 26r, ll. 13–14]).

26 There are other examples of impossible practices being taught in yogic texts. Perhaps the most unlikely is the *mūla śiśna śodhana* taught at *Jogpradīpakā* 838, in which water is to be drawn in through the anus and expelled through the urethra. *Gheraṇḍasaṃhitā* 1.22 teaches a practice in which the intestines are to be pulled out through the anus, washed and reinserted into the body. The durations of breath-retention taught in many texts are far beyond any that have ever been verified in clinical trials.

The next passage is from the fifteenth-century *Haṭhapradīpikā* (3.82–99), which is for the most part a compilation of extracts from earlier texts, including the three already cited. The *Haṭhapradīpikā*'s teachings on *vajrolī* borrow from the *Dattātreyayogaśāstra*[27] and repeat that text's extensive praise of the preservation of semen. At 3.86, the yogi is told to draw up *nārībhage patadbindum.* Unlike in the *Amanaska* passage cited earlier, here *-bhage* is the final member of a compound and so has a case ending, which is locative: the semen to be drawn up is falling into the vagina.[28] Women are yoginis, says HP 3.95, if they use *vajrolī* to preserve their *rajas,* and *vajrolī* and sex are explicitly linked in the description of *vajrolī*'s *sahajolī* variant, which is to be practised after sexual intercourse (HP 3.90).

Later texts, though more extensive in their treatment of the practical details of *vajrolī,* add little to our understanding of its purpose, with most teaching both the preservation of semen and, to a lesser extent, the absorption of mixed semen and generative fluid. Some give details about, for example, the shape and size of the pipe (e.g., *Haṭharatnāvalī* [HR] 2.91), but often it appears that the authors of the texts are not fully acquainted with the practice.[29] A curious omission from *all* textual teachings on the mechanics of *vajrolī* is any instruction to perform *nauli,* without which it is impossible to draw liquids into the body.[30] The terse teachings of earlier texts like the *Dattātreyayogaśāstra* clearly need to be elucidated by an expert guru, but some later works such as the *Bṛhatkhecarīprakāśa* and the *Haṭhābhyāsapaddhati* go into great detail about all the stages of the practice. Nevertheless, they teach that the drawing up of liquids through the penis is accomplished by clenching the perineal region or manipulating the *apāna*

---

27 HP 3.82a–83b = DYŚ 152a–153b (3.82b = ŚS 4.79ab); HP 3.86c–87d = DYŚ 156c–157d (3.87cd = ŚS 4.88ab).

28 In the passage as found in the Kaivalyadhama edition, one verse (3.96), which is not found in the majority of witnesses of the text and is said in Brahmānanda's nineteenth-century commentary (the *Haṭhapradīpikājyotsnā*) to be an interpolation, contains instructions for the yogi to draw up through his penis a woman's *rajas* or generative fluid.

29 Thus Brahmānanda says (*Haṭhapradīpikājyotsnā ad* 3.84) that the milk mentioned in the *Haṭhapradīpikā*'s description of *vajrolī* is for drinking, since if it were to be drawn up by the penis it would curdle and not come out again: *kṣīram iti | ekaṃ vastu kṣīraṃ dugdhaṃ pānārthaṃ, mehanānantaram indriyanairbalyāt tadbalārthaṃ kṣīrapānaṃ yuktam | ke cit tu abhyāsakāle ākarṣaṇārtham ity āhuḥ | tad ayuktam | tasyāntargatasya ghanībhāve nirgamanāsambhavāt |*. "*kṣīra:* one substance is *kṣīra,* which is milk, for drinking. After urinating, the senses are weakened, so one should drink [milk] to strengthen them. Some, however, say that the [milk] is for drawing up when practising [*vajrolī*]. That is wrong, because once it is in [the body] it curdles and cannot come out." This is not the case: Rām Bālak Dās regularly practises *vajrolī* with milk and it does not curdle while in his bladder.

30 Thus one can infer from mentions of *vajrolī* which predate the first textual mention of *nauli* (HP 2.34–35) that *nauli* was already being practised by yogis.

breath; that they make no mention of *nauli* suggests that their authors did not fully understand how *vajrolī* is to be carried out.

From these later texts I shall mention only those passages which add information relevant to this paper and not found elsewhere. The first is in the seventeenth-century *Haṭharatnāvalī* of Śrīnivāsa (2.80–117). By the time of the composition of the *Haṭharatnāvalī*, the awakening of the goddess Kuṇḍalinī, absent in early Haṭha works such as the *Amṛtasiddhi* (AS) and *Dattātreyayogaśāstra*, had become a key aim of the practices of Haṭha Yoga, and the *Haṭharatnāvalī* is the first text to state explicitly that *vajrolīmudrā* awakens her (2.82). Despite this apparent turn towards Kaula Śaivism (in whose texts yogic visualisations of Kuṇḍalinī first reached the form found in later haṭhayogic works), *vajrolī* is not taught as a method of absorbing the mixed products of sex (at least not by a man). The *Haṭharatnāvalī* gives instructions for a man to have sexual intercourse with a woman, but tells him to draw up only *bindu*, not *rajas* (2.97). This is followed by instructions for a woman to have sex with a man and to draw up both *bindu* and *rajas* (2.100).

In the instructions for male practitioners Śrīnivāsa includes HP 3.86, but there is an important variant in the *Haṭharatnāvalī*'s version of the verse (2.96). Instead of the *Haṭhapradīpikā*'s locative *-bhage*, "into the vagina", there is the ablative *-bhagāt* (which is not to be found in any of the manuscripts collated for the Lonavla edition of the *Haṭhapradīpikā*): the semen to be drawn up is falling "from the vagina". Here, as noted earlier, is the only possible way that *vajrolīmudrā* might be performed as part of sexual intercourse (by a man, at least): the fluid or fluids to be drawn up are collected (or perhaps left in the vagina) and the yogi uses *vajrolī* to absorb them through a pipe. A preference for the *Haṭharatnāvalī*'s reading over that of the *Haṭhapradīpikā* is supported by the fact that elsewhere Śrīnivāsa provides accurate practical details about yogic techniques not found in other texts; moreover he sometimes explicitly contradicts the *Haṭhapradīpikā*, voicing clear disapproval of the lack of practical knowledge of Svātmārāma, its author.[31]

A verse towards the end of the *Vajroliyoga* (c 1800) supports the notion that, whatever its purpose, *vajrolī* must be performed with a pipe. It identifies *amarolī*, a variant of *vajrolī*, as the combination of the sun and the moon (i. e., *bindu* and *rajas*) that occurs should the yogi happen to let his *bindu* fall, and that it should be sucked up "with a pipe" (*nālena*).[32]

31 E.g., HR 2.86–87 (in the section on *vajrolī*): *haṭhapradīpikākāramataṃ haṭhayogābhyāse 'jñānavilasitam ity upekṣaṇīyam.* "The teachings of the author of the *Haṭhapradīpikā* as regards the practice of Haṭha Yoga display his ignorance and should be disregarded." Cf. HR 1.27.

32 It is possible, as Lubomír Ondračka has pointed out to me (personal communication, 11 July

For the purposes of this chapter, the key points to be drawn from texts which include teachings on *vajrolīmudrā* are as follows. Sexual intercourse is always mentioned in textual teachings on *vajrolī*, whose main purpose is said to be *bindudhāraṇa*, the preservation of semen, or, when women are said to be able to perform it, *rajodhāraṇa*, the preservation of their generative fluid. Preservation of these vital principles defeats death. Some texts which postdate *vajrolī*'s earliest descriptions teach the absorption during sexual intercourse of a mixture of semen and menstrual fluid, but such instructions are fewer and given less prominence than the teachings on *bindudhāraṇa*. Some texts teach that the male yogi should suck up a woman's *rajas*, but after, not during, sexual intercourse, and by means of a pipe. No text giving practical details on how to perform the technique says that it can be done without a pipe.

3.2. *Vajrolī* and Rāja Yoga

Almost all the texts that teach *vajrolī* open their teachings with a declaration that it enables the yogi to succeed in yoga while flouting the *niyama*-s or regulations elsewhere said to be essential prerequisites for its practice. The regulation implied is that of *brahmacarya*, sexual continence.[33] One of the main aims of the *mudrā*-s that were the defining feature of Haṭha Yoga as taught in its early texts is *bindudhāraṇa*, the retention of semen. This would of course preclude ejaculatory sexual intercourse and many texts of Haṭha Yoga go as far as telling the aspiring male yogi to avoid the company of women altogether.[34]

But mastery of *vajrolīmudrā* will enable the yogi to indulge in ejaculatory sex, to have his cake and eat it, as it were, by, if necessary, resorbing his *bindu*. The method usually understood, however, namely the resorption of ejaculated semen into the penis during sexual intercourse, is, as I have shown above, anatomically impossible. It would be possible – albeit hard to imagine – for a yogi to make partial amends using a pipe, but I believe that *vajrolī*'s true purpose is otherwise and is in accordance with a hypothesis put forward by the andrologue, or spe-

2014), that in this case *nālena* means "through the urethra" (cf. n. 23), but in all other instances in yoga texts of *nāla* on its own, it always means "pipe" ("urethra" is *liṅganāla*).

33 Note that in the five-*yama*, five-*niyama* system of the *Pātañjalayogaśāstra*, *brahmacarya* is a *yama*, while in the ten-*yama*, ten-*niyama* system of the *Śāradātilaka* and several other texts (see Mallinson & Singleton 2017: 51), it is a *niyama*, so these passages on *vajrolī* in Haṭha Yoga texts appear to be referring to the latter systems, not that of the *Pātañjalayogaśāstra*. I am grateful to Philipp A. Maas for pointing this out to me.

34 E.g., AS 19.7; DYŚ 70, 86; *Amaraughaprabodha* 44; HP 1.61–62; ŚS 3.37; *Gheraṇḍasaṃhitā* 5.26. Cf. *Gorakhbāṇī pad* 68. The *pad*-s and *sakhī*-s found in the latter work are reproduced at Callewaert & Op de Beeck 1991: 489–510, whose verse numbering I have used.

cialist in male sexual health, Richard Darmon, in his article on *vajrolī*.[35] He suggests that passing a pipe through the urethra sensitises an erogenous region near the mouth of the bladder called the verumontanum, which is key to ejaculation. Through repeated practice the yogi develops a memory for the sensation, his verumontanum becomes desensitised and he gains control of the ejaculatory impulse.[36]

This concurs with what the two *vajrolī* practitioners I have met in India say about its purpose. Rām Bālak Dās, after describing the therapeutic benefits of rinsing out the bladder, says that *vajrolī* gives him control of his *svādhiṣṭhāna cakra*, which prevents him from ever shedding his semen. Thanks to his mastery of *vajrolī*, he says, he has never even had *svapn doṣ* (a "wet dream"). Similarly, a yogi I met in 2006 at Gangotri told me that mastery of *vajrolī* is essential when raising Kuṇḍalinī otherwise she will bring about involuntary ejaculation as she passes through the *svādhiṣṭhāna cakra*.[37]

As we have seen, rather than the ability to resorb semen, it is this ability to prevent it from falling in the first place with which *vajrolī* is most commonly associated in our textual sources. I know of only one mention of *vajrolī* in texts other than manuals of yoga and their commentaries. The passage, in Vidyāraṇya's *Śaṅkaradigvijaya* (9.90), says that desires cannot overcome one who is unattached, just as, thanks to *vajrolī*, Kṛṣṇa, the lover of 16,000 Gopīs, does not lose his seed.[38] Similar statements are found in Haṭha Yoga texts: ŚS 4.103 says that he who knows *vajrolī* will not shed his semen even after enjoying one hundred

35 Darmon 2002: 232 (cf. Roşu 2002: 309). Like Darmon, Andre van Lysebeth, in his treatment of *vajrolī* (1995: 326), says that its purpose is control of the ejaculatory impulse and that this is brought about "by desensitizing the nerves of the ejaculatory tract" through repeated insertion of a pipe or catheter.

36 When I asked Darmon if men who use latex urinary catheters for medical reasons experienced a desensitisation of the verumontanum he replied that medical research suggests that they do (personal communication, 26 March 2014) and added that in a similar fashion regular practice of *vajrolī* can eventually make the yogi unable to ejaculate. He also concurred with my suggestion that the rigid metal pipes used by ascetic yogis would be more efficacious than latex catheters in desensitising the verumontanum. The desensitisation of the verumontanum cannot be *vajrolī*'s sole purpose, however. Otherwise there would be no point in learning to draw liquids up the urethra. In addition to being a method of ensuring the preservation of semen, *vajrolī* is also taught as a method of cleansing the bladder (e.g., HR 1.62; the same has been said to me by Rām Bālak Dās) and perhaps this was the original purpose of drawing liquids up the urethra (cf. the haṭhayogic auto-enema, *basti* [e.g., HP 2.27–29] whose method is very similar to that of *vajrolī*).

37 See also Das 1992: 391, n. 23 on a *vajrolī*-type practice used by Bengali Bauls as part of *coitus reservatus*.

38 Cf. *Bindusiddhāntagrantha* verse 11: *solah sahaṃs gopī syūṃ gop, cāli jatī aisī bidhi jog*. I am grateful to Monika Horstmann for sending me her scan, transcription and translation of the *Bindusiddhāntagrantha* of Prīthināth (ms. 3190 of the Sri Sanjay Sarma Samgrahalay evam Sodh Samsthan, Jaipur, fol. 631 [r and v], dated VS 1671/1615 CE).

women, and the *Haṭhābhyāsapaddhati* says that once the practice of *vajrolī* is well established, the yogi can have sex with sixteen women a day (fol. 28r, ll. 6–9), adding that his continence, his *brahmacarya*, is firm and that he is dispassionate towards women.[39]

It is this ability that accounts for the connection between *vajrolī* and *rājayoga*, which, in the light of the modern understanding of *rājayoga* as meditation,[40] might be surprising to some. In the seventeenth-century Braj Bhasha *Sarvāṅgayogapradīpikā* of the Dādūpanthī Sundardās, *rājayoga* is the ability to sport like Śiva with Pārvatī and not be overcome by Kāma ("desire", i.e., the god of love). *Vajrolī* is not named in the passage but the yogi is to raise his semen having pierced the *nāḍī cakra* and the final verse says: "Rare are those who know the secrets of *rājayoga*; he who does not should shun the company of women" (2.24). In another Braj Bhasha text, the *Jogpradīpakā*, which was written in 1737, *vajrolīmudrā*, taught under the name of *vīrya mudrā*, i.e., "the semen *mudrā*", is said to bring about *rājayoga*, which is the ability to enjoy oneself with women without losing one's seed. A Braj Bhasha work which probably dates to a similar period, the *Jog Mañjarī*, equates *vajrolī* with *rāja joga* and says that the yogi who does not know it must not make love, adding that Śiva used it when sporting with Umā (71–72). Nor is this a late or localised development. The *Dattātreyayogaśāstra* follows its teachings on *vajrolī* by saying that the *mudrā*-s which have been taught are the only means of bringing about *rājayoga* (160), and the *Haṭharatnāvalī* (2.104) says that one becomes a *rājayogī* through control of semen.[41] The implication of the name *rājayoga* here is that to achieve success in yoga one need not renounce the world and become an ascetic; on the contrary, one can live like a king, indulging oneself in sensory pleasures, while also being a master yogi.[42] In a similar fashion, in tantric traditions kings may be given special

39 The *Haṭhapradīpikā* makes a similar claim about *khecarīmudrā*. By sealing it in his head with his tongue, the yogi's *bindu* will not fall even if he is embraced by an amorous woman (3.41). This verse is also found in the *Dhyānabindūpaniṣad* (83c–84b), commenting on which Upaniṣadbrahmayogin says that *khecarīmudrā* bestows *vajrolīsiddhi*. As taught in the *Niśvāsatattvasaṃhitā* (*mūlasūtra* 3.11), the ability to have sexual intercourse with large numbers of women results from a visualisation of Prajāpati.

40 On the now commonplace identification of *rājayoga* with the yoga of the *Pātañjalayogaśāstra*, see De Michelis 2004: 178–180.

41 See also the definition of *rājayoga* as the yoga of the Kaulas in the nineteenth-century Gujarati *Āgamaprakāśa* and the *Yogaśikhopaniṣad*'s definition of *rājayoga* as the union of *rajas* and *retas*, both noted by Bühnemann (2007: 15–16). Cf. Haṃsamiṭṭhu's designation of *rājayoga* as a *śākta* form of the *rāsalīlā* which involves sexual rites (Vasudeva 2011: 132).

42 The *Rājayogabhāṣya* says that *rājayoga* is yoga fit for a king (p. 1: *rājayogo rājña upayukto yogas tathocyate*) and Divākara, commenting on the *Bodhasāra*, says that *rājayoga* is so called because kings can accomplish it even while remaining in their position (section 14, verse 1: *rājayogo rājñāṃ nṛpāṇāṃ svasthāne sthitvāpi sādhayituṃ śakyatvāt*); see also Birch 2013: 70, n. 269.

initiations that do not require them to carry out the time-consuming rituals and restrictive observances of other initiates, while still receiving the same rewards.[43]

Here lies the key to understanding *vajrolīmudrā,* and to understanding the history of Haṭha Yoga as a whole. I have argued elsewhere that the physical practices of Haṭha Yoga developed within ascetic milieux, with records of some perhaps going back as far as the time of the Buddha.[44] The composition of the texts that make up the early Haṭha corpus during the course of the eleventh to fifteenth centuries CE brought these ascetic techniques, which had never previously been codified, to a householder audience.

There are no references to *vajrolī* in texts prior to the second millennium CE, but there are descriptions of a technique that appears to be part of the same ascetic and yogic paradigm. This is the *asidhārāvrata* or, as translated by Shaman Hatley (2016) in an article in which he presents the *Brahmayāmala*'s teachings on the subject, "the razor's edge observance". This practice, which involves a man either lying next to or having intercourse with a woman but not ejaculating, is attested from the early part of the first millennium, before the likely date of composition of the earliest tantric texts, and its practitioners probably included brahmin ascetics of the Śaiva Atimārga tradition.[45] The *asidhārāvrata* is subsequently taught in early tantric works, including the oldest known tantra, the *Niśvāsatattvasaṃhitā,* and is the first tantric ritual to involve sexual contact.[46] *Vajrolī* and the *asidhārāvrata* are never taught together (the latter is more or less obsolete by the time of the former's first mention in texts), but both involve sexual continence, and *vajrolī* would nicely complement the *asidhārāvrata* as a method of mastering it.[47]

43 Sanderson forthc.

44 Mallinson 2015.

45 Hatley 2016: 12–14. In the *Haṭhapradīpikā* the *amarolī* variant of *vajrolī* is said to be from the teachings of the Kāpālikas, an Atimārga ascetic tradition. The verse, which is found in most *Haṭhapradīpikā* manuscripts but, perhaps because of the reference to Kāpālikas, is not included in the Lonavla edition (in between whose verses 3.92 and 3.93 it falls) reads: "Leaving out the first and last parts of the flow of urine (because of an excess of *pitta* and a lack of essence respectively), the cool middle flow is to be used. In the teachings of [the siddha] Khaṇḍakāpālika, this is *amarolī*" (*pittolbaṇatvāt prathamāmbudhārāṃ vihāya niḥsāratayāntyadhārām | niṣevyate śītalamadhyadhārā kāpālike khaṇḍamate 'marolī ||*).

46 Hatley 2016: 4.

47 There are also parallels in the histories of *vajrolī* and the *asidhārāvrata.* Over the course of the first millennium the *asidhārāvrata* transformed from an Atimārga ascetic observance for the cultivation of sensory restraint into a Mantramārga method of attaining magical powers (Hatley 2016: 12). Likewise *vajrolī,* which in its earliest textual descriptions is an ascetic technique for preventing the loss of semen, is transformed (in texts if not in reality) into a means of both absorbing the combined products of sexual intercourse, the *siddhi*-bestowing *guhyāmṛta* or secret nectar of earlier tantric rites, and enabling the yogi to enjoy as much sex as he wants.

3.3. *Vajrolī* and Tantra

Like almost all of the central practices of Haṭha Yoga, *vajrolī* is not taught in tantric texts that predate the composition of the Haṭha corpus. Nor is it found in the early works of the Haṭha corpus associated with the tantric Siddha traditions, namely the *Amṛtasiddhi, Vivekamārtaṇḍa, Gorakṣaśataka* and *Jñāneśvarī,*[48] works, which do not call their yoga *haṭha.*[49] The Haṭha corpus is evidence of not only the popularisation of ancient and difficult ascetic practices (their difficulty accounting for the name *haṭha*) but also their appropriation by tantric traditions. It is this process of appropriation that brought about the superimposition of Kuṇḍalinī Yoga onto the ancient Haṭha techniques, together with the refashioning of *vajrolīmudrā.* It is seen most clearly in the *Śivasaṃhitā,* the first text to teach that the haṭhayogic *mudrā*-s are for the raising of Kuṇḍalinī rather than the control of breath and *bindu,* and the first text to teach that *vajrolī* is for the absorption of the combined products of sexual intercourse.

One reason for the widespread assumption of continuity between Tantra and Haṭha Yoga is their shared terminology.[50] What we in fact see in the Haṭha corpus is a reworking of tantric terminology. Words such as *mudrā, vedha, bindu* and *āsana* have meanings in the Haṭha corpus quite different from those which they have in earlier tantric works. It is a fruitless task to search tantric texts for Haṭha techniques under the names they are given in Haṭha texts. Tantric *mudrā*-s, for example, are physical attitudes, most commonly hand gestures, which are used for propitiating deities, while the *mudrā*-s taught in early Haṭha texts are methods of controlling the breath or semen. Similarly, semen is called *bindu* in Haṭha texts but in those of tantric Śaivism *bindu* is the first *tattva* (element) to evolve from Śiva, and/or a point on which to focus meditation.[51]

Vajrolī's use in Haṭha texts may also be a new application of an older tantric term. The etymology and meaning of the word *vajrolī* are unclear but a derivation from the compounds *vajrāvalī* (*vajra* + *āvalī*) or *vajrauvallī* (*vajra* + *ovallī*[52]), both of which mean "Vajra lineage", seems most likely.[53] I have found no in-

48 Kiehnle 2000: 270, n. 31: "Exercises like *vajrolī* that allow for keeping [*bindu* in the head], or taking it back, during sexual intercourse do not occur in the material handed down within the Jñānadeva tradition."

49 The *Amaraughaprabodha,* perhaps the first text of the Gorakṣa tradition to teach a Haṭha Yoga named as such, dismisses the physical practice of *vajrolīmudrā* (vv. 8–9).

50 Another reason for the assumption of continuity and a progression from Tantra to Haṭha Yoga is the chronology of their textual corpora. Some of the practices that the Haṭha Yoga corpus encodes, however, predate the texts of Śaivism (Mallinson 2015).

51 In the *Kaulajñānanirṇaya* we find references to *bindu* as a drop of fluid in the body (e.g., 5.23), but it is yet to be equated with semen.

52 On *ovallī* see Sanderson 2005: 122, n. 82.

53 Cf. the Marathi *Līlācaritra, uttarārdh* 475, which talks of the Nāths' cheating of death (*kā-*

stances of the word *vajrolī* in Śaiva texts, but a Buddhist tantric work called the *Avalokiteśvaravajroli* is found in a circa fourteenth-century manuscript.[54] The practices it teaches are obscure but have nothing to do with the haṭhayogic *vajrolīmudrā,* supporting the hypothesis that the name of the haṭhayogic *vajrolī,* like the names of other haṭhayogic practices and principles, was appropriated from a tantric practice of a completely different nature. In addition to this reference, a connection between *vajrolī* and specifically Buddhist tantric traditions is suggested by the *vajra* element in *vajrolī*'s name (and also by the *amara* and *sahaja* elements in *amaroli* and *sahajoli*) and further supported by the *Amṛtasiddhi,* a circa eleventh-century tantric Buddhist text which contains the earliest teachings on the practices and principles of Haṭha Yoga, and is the first text to assign many of their names (although it does not mention *vajrolī*).[55]

Certain aspects of *vajrolīmudrā* facilitated its appropriation and refashioning by tantric traditions. Some tantric texts teach rites in which the products of sexual intercourse (and other bodily fluids) are mixed with alcohol and consumed.[56] Tantric texts also speak of the union of male and female principles within the body of the yogi, most famously in Paścimāmnāya Kaula works in which the goddess Kuṇḍalinī rises from the base of the spine to union with Śiva in the head. Some, in particular Buddhist tantric works, also teach visualisations of the union of the products of sex and their rise up the body's central column. Despite assertions in secondary literature,[57] however, none of these Buddhist visualisations is accompanied by *vajrolī*-like physical techniques, nor are speculations

ḷavaṃcanā) and names their four *oḷī*-s or lineages: *vajroḷī* | *amaroḷī āti* | *siddhoḷī* | *divyoḷī* | *iyā cyāhī oḷī nāthāṃciyā* (of which only the first two are said to remain in this *kali yuga*); see also Feldhaus 1980: 104, n. 11. Because *vajrolī*'s meaning is uncertain, I am unsure whether to write *vajrolīmudrā* as a compound or as two words. By analogy with *khecarīmudrā,* "the *mudrā* of [the class of yoginis called] Khecarī", I have chosen to write it as a compound. The compound *khecarīmudrā* can be and sometimes is written as two words, however, with *khecarī* an adjective describing the *mudrā:* "the sky-roving *mudrā*". I see no possibility of taking *vajrolī* as an adjective in a similar fashion. Like the texts themselves (and yogis who speak modern Hindi), but contradicting my reasoning for writing *vajrolīmudrā* as a compound, for brevity I often write *vajrolī* rather than *vajrolīmudrā.* There is also some disagreement amongst our textual sources over whether the name is *vajroli* or *vajrolī.* The latter is more common and I have adopted it accordingly.

54 NGMPP C17/4. I thank Péter-Dániel Szántó for drawing this manuscript to my attention and providing me with his transcription of it, which may be found at http://www.academia.edu/4515911/Textual_Materials_for_the_study_of_Vajrolimudra.

55 See Mallinson forthc.

56 For references see Sanderson 2005: 113, n. 63. Such rites are still performed in Rajasthan by groups related to Nāth traditions (Khan 1994 and Gold 2002). Oort (2016) analyses St Augustine's descriptions of the Manichean eucharist in which a combination of semen and menstrual blood is consumed. Connections between Buddhism and Manicheism are well-known; perhaps this is another example.

57 E.g., Gray 2007: 120–121; White 1996: 63, 201–202.

that *vajrolī* was practised in first-millennium China corroborated by what is found in Chinese texts of that period.[58] Some modern tantric practitioners do believe that they can absorb their partner's *bindu* or *rajas* during sex by means of *vajrolī*.[59] Sexual practices in which men absorb (or at least imagine absorbing) their female partners' vital essences (but which do not involve *vajrolī*) have been used in China since at least the second century BCE[60] and a connection between such practices (as well as Chinese alchemical methods) and those of Indian tantric practitioners seems possible.

In an internalisation of earlier tantric rites involving the consumption of sexual fluids, two early Haṭha texts of the Siddha tradition (neither of which teaches *vajrolī*), the *Amṛtasiddhi*[61] and *Vivekamārtaṇḍa*,[62] say that both *rajas* and

58 *Pace* assertions by White (ibid.) et al., there is no evidence of *vajrolī* being part of Daoist or Buddhist sexual yoga in pre-modern Tibet, China or Japan. White cites Needham in the context of China, but the only physical practice for the retention or resorption of semen in the early Chinese texts discussed by Needham (1974: 198) very clearly involves pressing on the perineum and nothing more. Umekawa (2004) does not mention *vajrolī* in her analysis of Daoist and Buddhist sexual techniques in China and Japan in the early part of the second millennium, nor is it found in earlier Chinese texts (personal communication Rodo Pfister, 16 July 2014). I have found no references to *vajrolī* being practised in Tibet until the modern period (e.g., David-Neel [1931: 141] who reports how Tsang Yang Gyatso, the sixth Dalai Lama, is said to have publicly resorbed his urine in response to accusations of sexual incontinence).

59 Vaiṣṇava *tāntrika*-s in Bengal (whose tradition is distinct from that of the Tarapith *tāntrika*-s studied by Darmon, most of whom are *svātantrika*, i. e., not part of guru lineages [2002: 223]) claim to absorb the combined essences of sex by means of *vajrolī* (personal communication Lubomír Ondračka, 2 December 2013). Naren Singh says that through *vajrolī* and other means semen's downward movement may be reversed and it can be led back, through subtle channels, to "the *bindu cakra* near the *sahasrāra*" (personal communication via Ian Duncan, 8 December 2013). He adds that vaginal secretions may be absorbed into the "sperm sacks" and then raised through *ūrdhvagamana kriyā*. Svoboda (1986: 281) says that *vajrolī*'s main purpose is to prevent ejaculation during intercourse, but adds that it is used to suck up female secretions (and provides much additional detail on its practice by men and women). Das (1992: 391) says that Baul men draw up menstrual blood through the penis in sexual rituals, explaining this statement with a reference to the haṭhayogic *vajrolīmudrā*, but he adds that his understanding is unclear and remarks on how Bauls often mislead enquirers (Das 1992: 395).

60 I thank Rodo Pfister for this information (email communication, 16 July 2014, the purport of which is as follows). Absorption of *jing* "('essence', a life sap, in liquid form [which equals] female seed in many other Eurasian traditions, but having the same name as male seminal essence)" is mentioned in the **He yin yang* ("Uniting yin and yang", the title given it by modern editors), a bamboo text found in Mawangdui tomb three, which was sealed in 168 BCE. See also Pfister 2006 and 2013.

61 AS 7.8–13: *sa bindur dvividho jñeyaḥ pauruṣo vanitābhavaḥ | bījaṃ ca pauruṣaṃ proktaṃ rajaś ca strīsamudbhavam || 8 || anayor bāhyayogena sṛṣṭiḥ saṃjāyate nṛṇām | yadābhyantarato yogas tadā yogīti gīyate || 9 || kāmarūpe vased binduḥ kūṭāgārasya koṭare | pūrṇagiriṃ mudā sparśād vrajati madhyamāpathe || 10 || yonimadhye mahākṣetre javāsindūrasannibham | rajo vasati jantūnāṃ devītatvasamāśritam || 11 || binduś candramayo jñeyo rajaḥ sūryamayaṃ tathā | anayoḥ saṃgamaḥ sādhyaḥ kūṭāgāre 'tidurghaṭe || 12 ||*. Witnesses:

bindu exist within the body of the male yogi and that their union is the purpose of yoga.[63] When the Haṭha technique of *vajrolīmudrā* was adopted by tantric lineages, the idea – if not the actual practice – of uniting the external products of sex within the yogi's body would have been a natural development from these earlier teachings – which are then used in a later commentary to explain *vajrolī*[64] – despite its practice being alien to the milieu in which those texts were originally composed.

The absence of quintessential haṭhayogic techniques such as *vajrolī* and *khecarīmudrā* from the tantric corpus is symptomatic of the absence also of

---

C = China Nationalities Library of the Cultural Palace of Nationalities 005125 (21) • J_1 = Mān Siṃh Pustak Prakāś (MSPP) 1242 • J_2 = MSPP 1243 • K_1 = Nepal–German Manuscript Preservation Project (NGMPP) 655/39 • K_2 = NGMPP 1501/11 • K_5 = NGMPP 233/6 • M = Government Oriental Manuscripts Library Mysore AS4342 (folios 21b–40b). Readings: **8a** dvividho] $K_1K_2K_5$; dvivito C, vividho J_1J_2 **8d** °bhavam] °bhavaḥ C **9cd** yadābhyantarato yogas tadā yogīti gīyate] *Haṭhapradīpikājyotsnā ad* 4.100; yadā abhyantarato yogas tadā yogīti gīyate C (*unm.*), yadā tv abhyantare yogas tadā yogo hi bhaṇyate *cett.* **10a** kāmarūpe] C; kāmarūpo *cett.* • vased] dvased C **10b** kūṭāgārasya°] C; kūṭādhāraṇya J_1J_2, kūṭādhārasya $K_1K_2K_5$ **10c** pūrṇagiriṃ] C *(Tibetan transcription* only); pūrṇagiri *cett.* • mudā] C; sadā *cett.* **10d** vrajati] C; rājanti *cett.* • °pathā] C; °pathe *cett.* **11b** javā°] yavā° B, jāvā° K_5 • °sindūra°] $K_1K_2K_5$; °sindura ° C, °bindūra° J_1J_2, °bandhū✳ M • °jantūnām] °jantunāṃ B **11c** vasati] vasatiḥ K_2 **11d** ° samāśritaṃ] *conj.* SZANTO; °samādhṛtam C, °samāvṛtaṃ M, °samāvṛtaḥ *cett.* **12b** sūryamayaṃ smṛtaṃ] M; sūryamayaṃ tathā *Haṭhapradīpikājyotsnā ad* 4.100, sūryamayas tathā *cett.* "(8) Know that *bindu* to be of two kinds, male and female. Seed is said to be the male [*bindu*] and *rajas* is the *bindu* which is female. (9) As a result of their external union people are created. When they are united internally, one is declared a yogi. (10) *Bindu* resides in Kāmarūpa in the hollow of the multi-storeyed palace [in the head]. From contact, with delight it goes to Pūrṇagiri by way of the central channel. (11) *Rajas* resides in the great sacred field in the *yoni*. It is as red as a Javā flower and enveloped in the goddess element. (12) Know *bindu* to be lunar and *rajas* to be solar. Their union is to be brought about in the very inaccessible multi-storeyed palace."

62 *Vivekamārtaṇḍa*, Central Library, Baroda Acc. No. 4110 (dated 1534 *saṃvat*), with variants from Fausta Nowotny's edition of a later recension of the text called *Gorakṣaśataka* (GŚ = *Das Gorakṣaśataka*, Köln 1976, Dokumente der Geistesgeschichte): *sa eva dvividho binduḥ pāṇḍuro lohitas tathā* | (= GŚ 72ab) *pāṇḍuraṃ śukram ity āhur lohitākhyaṃ mahārajaḥ* || 54 || (= GŚ 72cd) *sindūradravasaṃkāśaṃ yonisthānasthitaṃ rajaḥ* | *śaśisthāne vased bindur dvayor ekyaṃ sudurlabham* || 55 || (= GŚ 73cd) *binduḥ śivo rajaḥ śaktir bindur indū rajo raviḥ* | (= GŚ 74ab) *ubhayoḥ saṃgamād eva prāpyate paramaṃ padam* || 56 || (= GŚ 74cd) *vāyunā śakticālena preritaṃ khe yadā rajaḥ* | (= GŚ 75ab) *bindor ekatvam āyāti yo jānāti sa yogavit* || 57 || (= GŚ 75cd). Readings: **55a** *bindur vidrumasaṃkāśo* ms. **55b** *ravisthāne sthitaḥ rajaḥ* GŚ **57cd** *bindunaiti sahaikatvaṃ bhaved divyaṃ vapus tathā* GŚ. "*Bindu* is of two kinds, white and red. White [*bindu*] is said to be semen, red the great *rajas* (female generative fluid). (55) *Rajas* resembles liquid vermilion and is situated at the *yoni*. *Bindu* resides in the place of the moon. It is very difficult to join the two. (56) *Bindu* is Śiva, *rajas* is Śakti. *Bindu* is the moon, *rajas* is the sun. It is only through uniting them both that the highest state is attained. (57) When *rajas* is propelled into the void [in the head] by means of the breath [and] the stimulation of Śakti, then it unites with *bindu*."

63 Cf. *Gorakhbāṇī pad* 12.5, *sabdī* 141b.

64 *Haṭhapradīpikājyotsnā ad* 4.100.

teachings on the preservation of semen. Despite popular notions of "tantric sex" as forsaking orgasm, a key purpose of tantric sexual rites is the production of fluids to be used as offerings to deities.[65] Some texts, particularly Buddhist tantric works, do teach that sexual bliss is to be prolonged, but orgasm is still required to produce the substances necessary in ritual.[66] The only tantric sexual rite not to end in orgasm is the *asidhārāvrata* mentioned earlier. The *asidhārāvrata* finds its last textual teaching in the seventh to eighth-century *Brahmayāmala.* By the eleventh century it has been sidelined by orgasmic sexual practices; Abhinavagupta "apparently viewed it as a form of penance (*tapas*) not specifically tantric in character".[67]

Like the *asidhārāvrata,* the haṭhayogic *vajrolīmudrā* most probably originated in a celibate ascetic milieu. The yoga traditions associated with the early Haṭha texts were all celibate, even those that developed out of Kaula lineages which had practised ritual sex.[68] The purpose of the composition of most of the texts of the Haṭha corpus seems to have been to bring the yogic techniques of these ascetic traditions to a non-celibate householder audience. *Vajrolīmudrā,* which was originally a method for ascetics to ensure their celibacy, was taught as a method for householders to remain sexually active while not losing the benefits of their yoga practice. It is difficult, however, to imagine normal householders learning *vajrolī,* and I know of only one example of this having happened.[69] I suspect that it was, as it still is, a technique practised by a very small number of ascetic yogis[70] which their householder disciples know of and might aspire to practising,[71] but

---

65 See Sanderson 1988: 680 and 2005: 113, n. 63, and *Brahmayāmala* ch. 22, 24, 25 on the *guhyāmṛta,* "the secret nectar of immortality", i. e., combined sexual fluids, which is "among the most important substances utilized in ritual" (Hatley 2016: 11).

66 Semen retention (*avagraha*) is prescribed in the *Brahmayāmala* during certain practices other than the *asidhārāvrata* but is to be abandoned in order to obtain the substance necessary for *siddhi.* The same text prescribes a *prāyaścitta* (expiatory rite) if the practitioner does not reach orgasm during a sexual rite (see *Tāntrikābhidhānakośa* III, s. v. *avagraha*).

67 Hatley 2016: 11.

68 See, e.g., *Gorakṣaśataka* 101 (Mallinson 2011).

69 Through a third party I have been in contact with Naren Singh of Jammu, a *vajrolī* practitioner who has not been initiated as an ascetic.

70 I know of only one premodern external reference to the practice of *vajrolī,* from the merchant Shushtarī, who travelled throughout India in the late eighteenth century. "When he interrogated one such jogi in Ḥaydarābād about the reasons for his success, he was told that behind all the legends is the practice of retention of semen as a means to perfect breath control. The jogi recommended that Shushtarī try practising breath control during sexual intercourse to prevent ejaculation, since loss of semen is the primary cause of aging. The jogi also claimed to have such control over breath as to be able to empty a cup of milk through vasicular *[sic]* suction" (Ernst 2007: 419).

71 Householder wrestlers in Kota, Rajasthan, for whom the refinement and preservation of *bindu* is an important part of their practice, speak highly of *vajrolī* but do not practise it (personal communication Norbert Peabody, 11 June 2010).

will never actually accomplish, in much the same way that a student of modern yoga might admire the advanced postures of a skilled yoga teacher.[72]

As noted above, many scholars have pointed to *vajrolī* as evidence that Haṭha Yoga developed from tantric practices of ritual sex. But Darmon has reported that the *vajrolī*-practising *tāntrika*-s of Tarapith do not use it as part of their sexual rites (or at least they do not go through the mechanics of its practice – they may of course reap its benefits). And when *vajrolī* is taught in texts as a means to sexual gratification it is not associated with ritual sex but with the more mundane variety. Just as the partner in the *asidhārāvrata* need not be a tantric initiate, the consort of the *vajrolī*-practitioner needs only to be a woman who is under one's control.[73] In the textual teachings on *vajrolī* that I have seen there is just one phrase which praises sex itself: the *Yuktabhavadeva* (YBhD) (7.239) says that *vajrolī* was taught by Gorakṣanātha for those householders who practise yoga but are devoted to the pleasure of sex because through it they obtain *brahmānanda*, the bliss of *brahman*.

Thus sex itself is not part of the practice of Haṭha Yoga, in which the preservation of semen or *rajas* is crucial to success. The techniques of Haṭha Yoga that help their preservation, of which *vajrolī* is the most efficacious, may be enlisted to ensure sexual continence, but sex itself is of no yogic benefit. Proclamations of *vajrolī*'s ability to allow yogis to have sex yet remain continent and to draw up the commingled products of sex did not sit well with those modern advocates of yoga who wanted to present it as a wholesome means to health and happiness, hence *vajrolī*'s removal from twentieth-century texts and translations.[74] Such an overtly censorious attitude towards *vajrolī* is nowhere to be found in premodern texts.[75]

---

72 Some of the teachings on *vajrolī* found in texts are enough to put off all but the most dedicated student. At the beginning of its teachings on *vajrolī* (fol. 25v, l. 14 – fol. 26r, l. 8), the *Haṭhābhyāsapaddhati* says that during its preliminary practice the yogi experiences such pain that he fears an imminent death. His skin erupts in boils, he becomes extremely thin and his attendants must do their utmost to keep him alive.

73 Some texts do say that the female partner should be expert in yoga: DYŚ 155 mentions a *yogābhyāsaratā strī*, "a woman well versed in yoga practice", as the source of *āṅgirasa*, i.e., women's generative fluid; the *Bṛhatkhecarīprakāśa* (fol. 103v) instructs the yogi to propitiate a "sixteen-year old virgin woman who is well versed in yoga practice" (*yogābhyāsaratām abhuktāṃ ṣoḍaśavarṣikīṃ striyam*) and then to have intercourse with her.

74 See page 184 for references; cf. Ānandsvarūpjī (1937: *u*) who says that *vajrolī* can be mastered without a woman and that those who say one is necessary for its practice are sinners.

75 Some texts do teach sanitised forms of *vajrolī*. Thus the circa fourteenth-century *Amaraughaprabodha*, which disparages other Haṭha techniques, says that *vajrolī* is the balanced state of mind which arises when the breath enters the central channel (v. 9) and the seventeenth or eighteenth-century *Gheraṇḍasaṃhitā* teaches a *vajrolīmudrā* which is a relatively simple *āsana*-type practice quite different from the *vajrolī* found in other texts (3.45–48). The *Gheraṇḍasaṃhitā*'s description might be considered a puritanical refashioning of the original *vajrolī* similar to those perpetrated in the twentieth century. However the

Western scholars, on the other hand, have viewed yoga and sex as inseparable.[76] This is based on the incorrect assumption that Haṭha Yoga is a direct development from tantra, in particular its sexual and alchemical rites. I have shown above how sexual rites are distinct from Haṭha Yoga; the same is true of alchemy. In the few instances in which texts on Haṭha Yoga mention alchemy, they do so disparagingly.[77] Nor is there anything in our textual sources to justify the claim found throughout Western scholarship (which perhaps results from drawing unwarranted parallels with Chinese sources) that Haṭha Yoga is itself a sexualised inner alchemy, in which, in an internalisation of orgasmic ejaculation, semen is raised from the base of the spine to its top and is sublimated into *amṛta*, the nectar of immortality, along the way.[78]

The distinction between the celibate ascetic milieu in which *vajrolī* originated and the tantric traditions which appropriated it should not, however, be seen as a simple distinction between puritanical ascetics and licentious libertines. Why, for example, should the *Dattātreyayogaśāstra*, a text that explicitly denigrates the tantric *sādhaka* and teaches a Haṭha Yoga full of practices for preserving semen, tell the aspiring *vajrolī*-practitioner that he needs to get hold of some female generative fluid (or semen if she is a woman)?[79] And Dattātreya may be the tutelary deity of an ancient lineage of celibate ascetics which flourishes to this day, but he is also the archetypal *avadhūta* yogi who can do what he wants. In the *Mārkaṇḍeyapurāṇa* he hides in a lake in order to avoid a group of young men seeking his tuition. When they do not go away even after a hundred years of the gods, he decides to put them off by openly drinking and making love with a beautiful woman, which, says the text, is all right, because as a master of yoga he is not at fault.[80] Kapila, meanwhile, is an ancient sage long associated with asceticism, celibacy and yoga. In the *Dattātreyayogaśāstra* he is said to be the first to have taught the haṭhayogic *mudrā*-s and in the *Haṭhatattvakaumudī* he is specifically said to have been the first to teach *vajrolī*. But Kapila is also associated with unorthodox practices and antinomian behaviour. The eleventh-century or

Gheraṇḍasaṃhitā adds that *vajrolī* leads to *bindusiddhi*, "mastery of semen", and that if one practises it while enjoying great indulgence, one will still attain complete perfection (*bhogena mahatā yukto yadi mudrāṃ samācaret | tathāpi sakalā siddhis tasya bhavati niścitam* || 3.48 ||). A more puritanical – and much more improbable – reworking of *vajrolī* can be found in Digambarji & Sahai 1969, in which with much linguistic casuistry they attempt to show that the teachings on *vajrolī* in Sanskrit texts have nothing to do with drawing liquids up the penis.

76 See page 184 for references.

77 See Mallinson 2014: 173, n. 32.

78 See, e.g., White 1996: 40–41.

79 The power and importance of *rajas* (female generative fluid) in the context of Baul practice are explained by Knight (2011: 73); such a notion may account for the *Dattātreyayogaśāstra*'s reference to *āṅgirasa*.

80 *Mārkaṇḍeyapurāṇa adhyāya* 17.

earlier *Bṛhatkathāślokasaṃgraha* says of Caṇḍasiṃha's city: "There the vices that usually terrify those who want to be liberated from the wheel of rebirth are prescribed by Kapila and others in treatises on liberation" (20.153).

4. Conclusion

I have drawn on all the verifiable textual, ethnographic and experiential data that I can find in my analysis of *vajrolī,* but my conclusions might require revision should new information come to light. As I have noted above, *vajrolī* is likely to have at least some roots in tantric Buddhist traditions and I think it probable that it is from these traditions that new information might be obtained. The vast majority of tantric Buddhist texts remain unstudied (Isaacson n. d.); among them are many Tibetan manuals of yogic practice. Some modern practitioners of Tibetan Buddhism claim that *vajrolī* has been used by Tibetan adepts to absorb the combined products of sexual intercourse as part of an unbroken yogic tradition that is more than a thousand years old.[81] Furthermore, the most advanced of these practitioners are said to be able to perform *vajrolī* without a pipe. Clinical studies of yogis have shown that they can control muscles that others cannot. Might it in fact be possible to hold open the urethral sphincter and draw up the combined products of sexual intercourse? And might my conclusion that *vajrolī* originated as a practice of celibate ascetics and was later appropriated by non-celibate tantric practitioners present too neat a historical progression? Might it in fact have evolved simultaneously among both types of practitioner? The information now at my disposal leads me to answer "no" to these questions. But my answer could change to a "yes" through the study of manuscripts of Sanskrit, Middle-Indic and Tibetan tantric Buddhist works,[82] or observation of the practices of living yogis. Many tantric Buddhist practices have remained secret for centuries, but recently, in part as a reaction to political circumstances in Tibet, some have been revealed.[83] If this revelation continues, perhaps we may learn of a Tibetan tradition of *vajrolī* practice that is still current.

81 Personal communication Sarkis Vermilyea, March 2015.

82 As Dan Martin has suggested to me (personal communication, 18 July 2016), study of the many references to *rdo rje chu 'thung,* "vajra-drinking," in Tibetan works may shed light on the practice of *vajrolī* in Vajrayāna Buddhism.

83 Thus the *Tibet's Secret Temple* exhibition at London's Wellcome Institute (November 2015 – February 2016) included a recreation of a previously secret temple from the Lukhang in Lhasa which was authorised by the present Dalai Lama, and at a presentation associated with the exhibition on 3 December 2015, a Tibetan rinpoche gave a demonstration of *rtsa rlung 'khrul 'khor* practices which have also been kept secret until very recently. The murals in the Lukhang temple include depictions of *'khrul 'khor,* some of which are reproduced in the chapter by Ian Baker in this volume.

With the caveats given above, my conclusions about the method, purpose and history of *vajrolīmudrā* are as follows. The history of *vajrolīmudrā*'s representation in textual sources epitomises the textual history of Haṭha Yoga as a whole. The physical practices which distinguish Haṭha Yoga from other forms of yoga developed within ancient ascetic traditions for which the preservation of semen was paramount. Texts composed from the beginning of the second millennium show how these practices were, firstly, opened up to an audience beyond their ascetic originators and, secondly, appropriated by Śaiva tantric traditions. Thus *vajrolīmudrā* was refashioned from a technique aimed at ensuring that an ascetic did not shed his semen into one that allowed a householder to enjoy the pleasures of sex and also be a yogi. It was then further remodelled in the light of two tantric concepts: an early notion of sexual fluids being the ultimate offering in ritual, and – as an interiorisation of the former – the visualisation of the combined products of sex being drawn up the central channel. As a result, certain tantric traditions made the fanciful but catchy claim that *vajrolī* allows one to absorb one's partner's sexual fluids during intercourse. Ethnography shows that among Haṭha Yoga-practising ascetics *vajrolī* remains one of a set of techniques used to prevent ejaculation, while tantric practitioners of ritual sex use *vajrolī* both to prevent ejaculation and, they believe, to absorb their partners' sexual fluids.

Appendix 1: Text Passages Which Teach or Mention *Vajrolīmudrā*

7th–6th century BCE	*Bṛhadāraṇyaka Upaniṣad* 6.4.10–11
12th century CE	*Amanaska* 2.32
13th century	*Dattātreyayogaśāstra* 150c–160d
14th century	*Amaraughaprabodha* 8–9 *Tirumantiram* 825–844 *Śaṅkaradigvijaya* 9.90
15th century	*Śivasaṃhitā* 4.78–104 *Haṭhapradīpikā* 3.82–99
17th century	*Yuktabhavadeva* 7.239–296 *Haṭharatnāvalī* 2.80–117 *Sarvāṅgayogapradīpikā* 3.13–24

(Continued)

18th century	*Haṭhatattvakaumudī udyota*-s 16 and 17 *Bṛhatkhecarīprakāśa* fol. 103r11 - fol. 104r6 *Yogamārgaprakāśikā* 3.138–154 *Siddhasiddhāntapaddhati* 2.13 *Gheraṇḍasaṃhitā* 3.45–48 *Jogpradīpakā* 552–561 and 677–684 *Vajroliyoga* *Haṭhābhyāsapaddhati* fol. 25v9 - fol. 28r15 *Jog Mañjarī* fols. 103–107, vv. 66–85
19th century	*Haṭhapradīpikājyotsnā* 3.83–103

Appendix 2: Editions and Translations of the Descriptions of *Vajrolīmudrā* in the *Bṛhatkhecarīprakāśa* and the *Vajroliyoga*

This appendix contains editions and translations (which are in many places tentative) of descriptions of *vajrolīmudrā* in two circa eighteenth-century unpublished sources. The first is a passage from the *Bṛhatkhecarīprakāśa* (a commentary on the *Khecarīvidyā*) and the second is the entire text of the *Vajroliyoga*. Each text has just one manuscript witness. Verse numbering and punctuation are as found in the manuscripts unless otherwise reported.

Bṛhatkhecarīprakāśa. Scindia Oriental Research Institute Library (Ujjain) ms. no. 14575, fol. 103r11 - fol. 104r6

atha vajrolī tadbhedau amarolīsahajolyau | vajram iva u vismayena na līyate kṣarati vīryam anayeti[84] | amara iva u na līyate 'nayā sahajā iva u na līyate 'nayeti ca tat[85] tanniruktеḥ |

(fol. 103v) tatrāntime haṭhapradīpikāyām[86] |

sahajoliś cāmarolir vajrolyā bheda ekata[87] iti |
amarolis tu

84 vismayena na līyate kṣarati vīryam anayeti] visma⌈ye⌉na na līyate ⌈kṣarati vīryam a⌉nayeti *cod.*

85 tat] ⌈ta⌉ t *cod.*

86 haṭhapradīpikāyām] haṭha°yām *cod.*

87 The manuscript reads *ekabhedataḥ*. At the suggestion of Philipp A. Maas, I have adopted *bheda ekataḥ* (which becomes *bheda ekata* before *iti* as a result of sandhi) from among the

jale bhasma vinihkṣipya dagdhagomayasaṃbhavam ||
vajrolīmaithunād ūrdhvaṃ strīpuṃsoḥ svāṅgalepanam iti |
āsīnayoḥ sukhenaiva muktavyāpārayoḥ kṣaṇāt ||
sahajolir iyaṃ proktā sevyate yogibhiḥ sadeti | [HP 3.90a–91b]

yadbhedau imau yā[88] vajrolī yathā | sā tu bhoge bhukte 'pi muktyarthaṃ sevyate | tatropāyaḥ | yogābhyāsaratām abhuktāṃ ṣoḍaśavarṣikīṃ sajātīyāṃ[89] striyaṃ dravyadānena sevādinā paramayatnena sādhayitvānyonyaṃ strītvapuṃstvānapekṣayā vidhim ārabhetām || yathā || prathamarajodarśane prathamaṃ dṛṣṭaṃ pittolbaṇaṃ rajo vihāya dvitīyadine rajasvalayā[90] tayā saha gupteṣṭiṃ[91] kṛtvā tasyāḥ strīyoner āṅgirasaṃ raja ākṛṣya[92] ṣaṇmāsam

svamūtrotsargakāle yo balād ākṛṣya vāyunā
stokaṃ stokaṃ tyajen mūtram ūrdhvam ākṛṣya vāyunā | [ŚS 4.101]

tataḥ dugdhākarṣaṇaṃ tataḥ pāradākarṣaṇaṃ | tena tattadākarṣaṇena pūrvaṃ †*pu†kīlapraveśena[93] sādhitaliṅganālena pūrvaṃ svaśarīre svareto bindum ākuñcanena saṃbodhya svaśarīre nābher adhobhāge tadraja ākṛṣya[94] praveśayet tasya nābhau granthau tu śatāṅganopabhoge 'pi tasya bindur na patati[95] naśyati |

yadi rajasa ākarṣaṇāt pūrvaṃ svabodhito bindur adhaḥ patati tadāṇḍakośād adhastanayonisthāne kṛtavāmahasto[96] madhyamānāmikāgrābhyāṃ[97] saṃmardya nirodhayet |

tatra svaliṅgavāmabhāge striyo yonau taddakṣiṇabhāge yady antaḥ spṛśati tadā taṃ liṅganiṣkāśanena vihāya svaliṅgadakṣiṇabhāge striyaś ca vāmabhāge yaḥ sa grāhya iti sūkṣmadṛśāvadheyam iti rajaḥsaṃprākarṣaṇaṃ tv apānavāyubalena[98] huṃ huṃ kṛtvā kāryam iti | rajasa ākarṣaṇānantaraṃ yonimadhye[99] liṅgacāla-

---

variant readings given in the Kaivalyadhama edition of the *Haṭhapradīpikā* (which has *eva bhedataḥ* in the *editio princeps*).

88 yā] *yā *cod.*
89 sajātīyāṃ] ⌈sajātīyāṃ⌉ *cod.*
90 rajasvalayā] *em.*; rajasvalāyā *cod.*
91 gupteṣṭiṃ] *conj.*; gupteṣṭaṃ *cod.*
92 āṅgirasaṃ raja ākṛṣya] *em.*; āṅg[i]rasaṃ rajaḥ ⌈ākṛṣya⌉ *cod.*
93 †*pu†kīlapraveśena] ⌈*pukīlapraveśena⌉ *cod.*
94 tadraja ākṛṣya] *em.*; tadrajaḥ ⌈ākṛṣya⌉ *cod.*
95 patati] *cod. p.c.*; naśyati *cod. a.c.*
96 °hasto] *em.*; °hasta *cod.*
97 prāṇaḥ *added in margin.*
98 apānavāyubalena] apānavāyu*⌈*liṃgena⌉ balena *cod.*
99 yonimadhye] *conj.*; yonitāye *cod.*

nam ācaret | etat sarvaṃ guruṃ saṃpūjya tadājñayā tatsmaraṇena ca gavyadugdhabhug eva kuryād iti |

bindur vidhuma(fol. 104r)yaḥ śivarūpaḥ | rajaḥ sūryamayaṃ śaktirūpam | ata ubhayor melanaṃ svanābher adhobhāge prayatnena kāryam [cf. ŚS 4.86] | tena tatrobhayasaṃmelanena granthau satyām anantalalanāsaṅge 'pi bindu[100]pātamaraṇe na syātām[101] | yadi rajaḥsaṃprākarṣaṇāt[102] striyo maraṇaprasaṅge varadānādināvairiṇīṃ kuryāt | nirvairaḥ sarvabhūteṣu yaḥ sa mām etīti gītokteḥ [*Bhagavadgītā* 11.55] | yadi ca tajjīvane samarthas tadauṣadhādinā svasāmarthyena gāyatrīhṛdayapāṭhapūrvakaṃ darbhaprokṣaṇena vilomasiddhamṛtyuṃjayena[103] ca jīvayed iti | idam uktam api gurusānnidhyādinaiva kāryam [|] anyathā yaḥ karoti tasya śivaśaktyor guroś ca pādānāṃ śapatha iti | atra pramāṇaṃ śivasaṃhitādayas tadadhikaṃ tu guruvacanāl likhitam anubhavād avagantavyam iti | †śivas tu† gataṃ svakaṃ binduṃ liṅganālenākarṣayed iti cāmarolī tathā tam eva yonimudrayā bandhayed iyaṃ sahajolīti tayoḥ saṃjñābhedena pṛthagbhedaḥ kārye tulyā gatir ity āha || iti vajrolyādayaḥ ||[104]

Bṛhatkhecarīprakāśa

Next *vajrolī* and its divisions *amarolī* and *sahajolī.* [*Vajrolī*] is like a *vajra,* by means of it semen (*vīrya*) is not dissolved by intense emotion [and] it does not melt; [*amarolī*] is like an immortal, by means of it [semen] is not dissolved; [*sahajolī*] is like the natural state, by means of it [semen] is not dissolved: that [analysis] is from etymological interpretation of those words.

At the end of the [passage on *vajrolī*] in the *Haṭhapradīpikā:*

Sahajoli and *amaroli* are each variations of *vajrolī. Amaroli* is when after sexual intercourse using *vajrolī* the woman and man smear their bodies with ashes made from burnt cowdung mixed with water. When they sit comfortably for a moment free from activity that is said to be *sahajoli*; it is regularly used by yogis. [HP 3.90a–91b]

100 'pi bindu°] *conj.*; 'bindu° *cod.*
101 na syātām] *conj.*; syātām *cod.*
102 rajaḥsaṃprākarṣaṇāt] *em.*; vrajasañprākarṣaṇā *cod.*
103 vilomasiddhamṛtyuṃjayena] ſvilomasiddhamṛtyuṃjayenal *cod.*
104 Along the bottom margin of fol. 103v is added in a later hand *Vivekamārtaṇḍa* 54–57 as found in Nowotny's edition of the *Gorakṣaśataka* and including the latter's verse 76, which is not found in the 1477 CE Baroda manuscript of the *Vivekamārtaṇḍa.*

The two variations are like *vajrolī*, which is used to achieve liberation even after enjoying pleasure. Their means is as follows. Having won over with great effort by means of gifts, service and so forth a sixteen-year old virgin woman of his own caste who is devoted to the practice of yoga, they should undertake the practice with no regard to each other's femininity or masculinity. Thus, for six months, at the first sight of *rajas*, having rejected the first menstrual fluid, in which there is an excess of *pitta*, on the second day he should perform the secret ritual with that menstruating woman and extract the *āṅgirasa rajas* from her vagina.

When urinating the yogi should forcefully use the [inner] breath to draw up urine and release it little by little after drawing it up by means of the [inner] breath. [ŚS 4.101]

Then there is the drawing up of milk, then of mercury. Through his urethra, which has been previously prepared by this drawing up of these [substances and] the insertion of a probe, the yogi should first, having awakened in his own body *bindu*, his own semen, by means of contraction, then draw up the *rajas* in the region below the navel in his own body, and make it enter the knot in his navel. Even if he makes love to a hundred women his *bindu* is not lost.

If his *bindu*, having been awakened by him, falls downwards before the drawing up of the *rajas*, he should stop it by rubbing the perineal region below the scrotum with the tips of the middle and ring fingers of the left hand. In that situation, if there is contact in the woman's vagina between the left side of the penis and the right side of the vagina then, leaving it by withdrawing the penis, it is to be taken on the right side of the penis and on the left side of the woman. This is to be concentrated upon with subtle sight. The extraction of *rajas* is to be performed using the power of the *apāna* breath while making the sound "*huṃ huṃ*". Immediately after extracting the *rajas* he should move his penis in the vagina. All this should be done after worshipping the guru, in accordance with his instruction and while rembering him, and while having a diet of nothing but cow's milk.

Bindu is lunar and takes the form of Śiva. *Rajas* is solar and has the form of Śakti. And their mixing is to be done carefully in the region below one's navel. When there is a knot there as a result of those two mixing, then even when there is desire for an endless number of women there will be neither the fall of *bindu* nor death. If as a result of the extraction of *rajas* the woman is close to death, then one should appease her with favours and so forth. As it is said in the *Gītā*: he who is without enemies among all living beings goes to me. And if he is capable of reviving her, then he should do so by means of herbs and other [medicines], his own best efforts, the sprinkling of *darbha* grass preceded by a recitation of the Gāyatrīhṛdaya[105] and the reverse perfected Mṛtyuṃjaya [mantra].

Even though this has been taught [here] it should only be performed in the presence of the guru. He who does otherwise insults the feet of Śiva and Śakti, and his guru. The authorities in this are texts such as the *Śivasaṃhitā* and, in addition to them, what is written from the teachings of the guru and that which must be understood from experience.

… [The yogi] should draw up his own *bindu* through the urethra when it has moved. This is *amarolī* and when he holds that same *bindu* by means of the *yonimudrā,* that is *sahajolī.* The two are differentiated by a difference in name [but] in effect their actions are said to be equal. Thus [are taught] *vajrolī* and the other [*mudrā*-s].

Vajroliyoga. Wai Prajñā Pāṭhaśālā ms. no. 6–4/399[106]

atha yogaśāstraprārambhaḥ || śrīḥ ||
śrīgaṇeśāya namaḥ || śrīkṛṣṇāya gurave namaḥ || ||
svecchayā vartamāno 'pi yogoktair niyamair vinā ||
vajrolīṃ yo vijānāti sa yogī siddhibhājanam || 1 ||
tatra vastudvayaṃ vakṣye durlabhaṃ yasya kasya cit ||
kṣīraṃ caikaṃ dvitīyaṃ tu nārī ca vaśavartinī || 2 ||
mehanena śanaiḥ samyag ūrdhvākuñcanam abhyaset ||
puruṣo vāpi nārī vā vajrolīsiddhim āpnuyāt || 3 || [3–5 = HP 3.82–84]
cittāyattaṃ[107] nṛṇāṃ śukraṃ śukrāyattaṃ[108] tu jīvitam ||
tasmāc chukraṃ manaś caiva rakṣaṇīyaṃ prayatnataḥ || 4 ||
nārīṃ ramyām avasthāpya rahasye tu digambarām |[109]
svayaṃ digambaro bhūtvā uttānāyās tathopari ||
aṅganyāsaṃ tataḥ kṛtvā mantratantravidhānataḥ || 5 ||
pādoruyoni[110]nābhīṣu stanayoś ca lalāṭake ||
śīrṣe nyāsaṃ vidhāyātha mūlamantreṇa tattvavit || 6 ||

105 A text called *Gāyatrīhṛdaya* is found in several manuscripts (e.g., Oriental Research Library, Srinagar Acc. Nos. 782 and 2315–99, NGMCP A1215–39, Berlin Staatsbibliothek 5882.5).
106 This manuscript contains several minor errors which I have corrected without reporting.
107 cittāyattaṃ] *corr.*; cittāyataṃ *cod.*
108 śukrāyattaṃ] *em.*; śukrāṃyataṃ *cod.*
109 5ab, which is needed to make sense of 5cd, is not found in the manuscript, but is found, together with 5cd, at YBhD 7.243ab and (with *adhaḥ sthāpya* for *avasthāpya*) HR 2.94ab.
110 °yoni°] *em.*; °ṇoni° *cod.*

māyāmūlaṃ samuccārya reto muñceti yugmakam ||
hrīṃ muñca muñca || 6 ||[111]
vāgbhavaṃ kāmabījaṃ ca samuccārya manuṃ[112] japet ||
aiṃ klīṃ svāhā ||
tataḥ śaktiṃ nijāṃ kṛtvā†kuñcaṃ dhṛtvā† manuṃ paṭhet || 7 ||
liṅge yonau tathā paścāt[113] prāṇāyāmān samabhyaset ||
śītalīkumbhakaṃ kuryāt vāmadakṣiṇayogataḥ || 8 ||
saṃketena svaraṃ pītvā nārī mandaṃ ca niḥśvaset ||
ayonau dṛḍham āliṅgya yonau liṅgaṃ na cārpayet || 9 ||
tatas tv adharapānaṃ ca parasparam athācaret ||
parasparam athāliṅget yāvat prasvedasaṃbhavaḥ[114] || 10 ||
yadi skhaled bahir vīryaṃ tadā svedena mardayet ||
yadi bindur na skhalati punar āliṅgya kāminīm || 11 ||
yonau liṅgaṃ cārpayed vā yathā binduḥ pated bahiḥ ||
patite ca punaḥ svedajalena parimardayet || 12 || [9–12 = YBhD 7.244-247]
sarvāṅgāni tataḥ paścāt tu liṅgavīryeṇa yatnataḥ ||
evaṃ dinatrayaṃ kṛtvā trivāraṃ[115] pratyahaṃ tataḥ || 13 || [13cd = YBhD 7.248cd]
iti śrāntiḥ ||
trivāraṃ pratyahaṃ kuryān nyāsam ekaṃ prayatnataḥ ||
jātaśramāṃ tatas tāṃ tu[116] viparītāṃ nijopari ||
kṛtvā kucau tu saṃpīḍya śītalī kārayet tataḥ ||
pāyayec ca svaraṃ tadvad vāmadakṣiṇayogataḥ ||[117]
śaranālena phūtkāraṃ vāyu[118]saṃcārakāraṇāt || 15 ||
kuryāc chanaiḥ śanair yogī yāvac chaktiḥ prajāyate ||
tato maithunakāle tu patadbinduṃ samunnayet || 16 ||
vajrakandaṃ[119] samāpīḍya kumbhayitvā tu mārutam ||
caladbinduṃ samākṛṣya manas tatraiva dhārayet || 17 ||
[15c–17d = YBhD 7.248c-250d]
jātīphalaṃ ca kṣīraṃ ca navanītaṃ tathaiva ca ||
bhakṣayed uttamaṃ vāsa[120]tāmbūlaṃ rasasaṃyutam || 18 ||
vāraṃ vāraṃ tato mantraṃ japed eva raman mudā ||
brahmākṣaraṃ lakārakāyeti śaktiḥ || bindunādasamanvitam || 19 ||

---

111 Verse numbering is as found in the manuscript.
112 manuṃ] *conj.*; bhe*ṭh*o *cod.*
113 paścāt] *em.*; paścā *cod.*
114 °saṃbhavaḥ] *em.*; °saṃbhava *cod.*
115 trivāraṃ] *corr.*; strivāraṃ *cod.*
116 jātaśramāṃ tatas tāṃ tu] *conj.*; jātaśramaṃ tataḥ stātuṃ *cod.*
117 This hemistich is added in the margin.
118 vāyu°] *em.* (cf. HP 3.85); vā yo *cod.*
119 vajrakandaṃ] *em.* (cf. YBhD 7.250a); vajrabandhaṃ *cod.*
120 vāsa°] *conj.*; vastra° *cod.*

bījam etat priyaṃ devyāḥ sarvaiśvaryapradāyakam ||
siddhidaṃ durlabhaṃ loke japet tataḥ[121] punaḥ punaḥ || 20 ||
evam abhyāsato bindur na yonau patati kva cit ||
itthaṃ maithunaśaktiḥ syād durmadām api kāminīm[122] ||
mardayed yogayuktātmā śataśo nātra saṃśayaḥ || 21 ||
evaṃ bindau sthire jāte mṛtyuṃ jayati sarvathā ||
maraṇaṃ bindupātena jīvanaṃ bindudhāraṇāt || 22 ||
[21–22 = YBhD 7.251a–253b]
evam abhyāsato nārī yadi retasam uddharet ||
dehe sthiratvam āyāti vajrolyābhyāsayogataḥ || 23 ||
abhyāsasya kramaṃ vakṣye nārīṇāṃ ca śanaiḥ śanaiḥ ||
bahiḥ śiśnagataṃ śukraṃ yadi skhalati kāmataḥ || 24 ||
ṭaṭikā[123]mukham ākuñcya maṇiṃ tatra praveśayet ||
tam uddharet[124] samākṛṣya vāyunā tena vartmanā || 25 ||
tadā reto[125] rajo nāśaṃ na gacchati kadā cana ||
mūlādhāre ca nārīṇāṃ sabinduṃ nādatāṃ vrajet || 26 ||
ayaṃ yogaḥ puṇyavatāṃ siddhaḥ saṃsāriṇāṃ na hi ||
[23a–27b = YBhD 7.254a–258b]
amunā siddhim āpnoti yogād yogaḥ pravartate[126] || 27 ||

ayaṃ bhāvo nirvāte vilāsamandire nānāprakāreṇa priyayā saha vilāsaṃ kurvan patadbindum apānena huṅkārasahitena balād ūrdhvam ākṛṣya śītalīṃ kuryāt ||[127] idam atra paryavasitaṃ yogī yadā ramyastriyaṃ gacchan yogaṃ ca vāñchaty ākṛṣya[128]māṇenāpānena retaḥ samānīyate[129] [|] garbham ādadhāmīty abhidhāya liṅgam yonau vinikṣipet || yadi tasyā garbhaṃ na vāñchati tadā †kriṣi†prāṇena vīryam ūrdhvam ākarṣayet || te retasā reta ādadāmīty[130] abhidhāya yogī jitaretā bhavati ||

tad uktaṃ bṛhadāraṇyake ||

121 japet tataḥ] *conj.*; japa tatra *cod.*
122 durmadām api kāminīm] YBhD; durmadāv api kāminī *cod.*
123 ṭaṭikā°] *cod.*; ṭiṇṭikā° YBhD.
124 tam uddharet] YBhD; samuddharet *cod.*
125 reto] YBhD; sṛtau *cod.*
126 This *pāda* may be a quotation of an unidentified quotation found at *Pātañjalayogaśāstra* 3.6 (as *yogo yogāt pravartate*). I am grateful to Philipp A. Maas for this suggestion.
127 Cf. YBhD 258–259.
128 ākṛṣya°] *corr.*; akṛṣya° *cod.*
129 samānīyate] *corr.*; samānīrayate *cod.*
130 ādadāmīty] *em.*; ādadhāmīty *cod.*

atha yām icchen na[131] garbhaṃ dadhīteti tasyām arthaṃ[132] niṣṭhāya mukhena mukhaṃ sandhāyābhiprāṇyāpānyād[133] indriyeṇa te retasā reta[134] ādada ity aretā bhavati ||
atha yām icched garbhaṃ[135] dadhīteti tasyām arthaṃ niṣṭhāya[136] mukhena mukhaṃ sandhāyāpānyā[137]bhiprāṇyād indriyeṇa te[138] retasā reta ādadhāmīti garbhiṇy eva bhavati || [= BĀU 6.4.10–11]

śivayoge ||
stokaṃ stokaṃ tyajen mūtram ūrdhvam ākṛṣya tat punaḥ ||
gurūpadeśamārgeṇa pratyahaṃ yaḥ samācaret ||
bindusiddhir bhavet tasya sarvasiddhipradāyinī ||

etasya ṣaṇmāsābhyāsena śatāṅganopabhoge 'pi na bindupātaḥ [||] anyac ca purīṣatyāga aṅgulibhir yonisthānaṃ svasya prapīḍayet || dvitīyahastena liṅgaṃ bandhayet || evaṃ mūtrarodho 'py abhyasanīyaḥ || evaṃ mūtratyāgakāle gudākuñcanena[139] purīṣarodhaḥ śanaiḥ śanaiḥ kāryaḥ [||] evaṃ tāvad abhyased[140] yāvat svayaṃ mūtrapurīṣakālabhedena[141] bhavataḥ || etadabhyāsato 'pi bindu-siddhir bhavati || [= YBhD 7.288–289]

prathamo 'yaṃ yogaḥ paścād vajrolīkāmukayogī †vāṃ† seyaṃ vajroly eva kiṃcidviśeṣavatī amarolī ca na bhidyate ||
yena kena prakāreṇa binduṃ yatnena dhārayet ||
daivāc ced bhavati bhage melanaṃ candrasūryayoḥ ||
amarolī samākhyātā enāṃ nālena śoṣayet ||
gataṃ[142] binduṃ svato yogī bandhayed yonimudrayā ||
sahajoli samākhyātā sarvatantreṣu gopitā ||
saṃjñābhedād bhaved bhedaḥ kārye tulyagatitrayam || [= ŚS 4.95c–98b]
tathā ca svabindor ūrdhvaṃ nayanaṃ vajrolī || bhage raktena saha mīlitasya

131 icchen na] BĀU; icched *cod.*
132 arthaṃ] BĀU; ardhaṃ liṅgaṃ *cod.*
133 °prāṇyāpānyād] BĀU; °prāṇāpānyād *cod.*
134 te retasā reta] BĀU; retasā retasyā reta *cod.*
135 garbhaṃ] *om.* BĀU.
136 niṣṭhāya] BĀU; niṣṭhā *cod.*
137 °pānyā°] BĀU; °prānyā° *cod.*
138 te] BĀU; *om. cod.*
139 gudākuñcanena] *conj.*; gudākuñcane *cod.*
140 abhyased] abhyaset || *cod.*
141 °purīṣakālabhedena] YBhD; °purīṣe kābheda *cod.*
142 gataṃ] *Śivasaṃhitā*; dattvā *cod.*

bindor ūrdhvaṃ nayanaṃ amarolī [||] svadehe saraktasya kevalasya svabindor ūrdhvaṃ nayanaṃ sahajolīti vivekaḥ ||[143] = YBhD 7.295–296.

Vajroliyoga

Now the beginning of the yoga treatise.

Homage to glorious Gaṇeśa! Homage to the guru, glorious Kṛṣṇa!

(1) Even though he behaves according to his desires without [observing] the rules taught in yoga, the yogi who knows vajrolī obtains success. (2) I shall teach two things for that which are hard for anyone to obtain. One is *kṣīra,* the second is a woman under one's control. (3) He should slowly and correctly practise upward suction by means of the penis. Either a man or a woman can master *vajrolī.* (4) In men, semen is dependent upon the mind and life is contingent upon semen, so semen and the mind should be carefully protected.

(5) [The yogi] should have a beautiful naked woman lie down on her back in a secret place, sit on her naked himself and perform an installation of mantras on her body according to the rules of mantra and tantra – (6) he who knows the levels of reality should perform the installation with the root mantra on her feet, thighs, vagina, navel, breasts, forehead and crown. He should recite the Māyā root mantra "Release semen!" (*reto muñca*) twice, [then] *hrīṃ muñca muñca.* (7) Having recited Vāgbhava (*aiṃ*) and the seed mantra of Kāma (*klīṃ*), he should repeat the mantra *aiṃ klīṃ svāhā.*

Then he should make her his own *śakti,* †embrace her† and repeat the mantra. (8) He should next perform repeated breath controls in the penis and vagina; he should practise *śītalī kumbhaka* through the left and right [nostrils]. (9) At a signal the woman should inhale and slowly exhale. The yogi should press tightly against her but not her vagina: he should not put his penis in her vagina. (10) Then they should kiss one another; then they should embrace one another until sweat arises. (11) If semen should be emitted then he should rub [his body] with sweat. If semen is not emitted, he should embrace the woman again (12) and put his penis in her vagina so that semen is emitted. When it has fallen he should

143 After the teachings on *vajrolī,* the manuscript has the following before it ends: *ikṣabhikṣutilavaṅgamāraṇaṃ tālakābhraviṣasūtaṭaṃkaṇam* || *bhānuvajriyayasānumarditambho narendrakutāraparvatam* || || || *cha* || || .

again rub with sweat (13) all his body and then carefully with his semen. He should do this for three days, three times a day. [Practising] thus, fatigue [arises].

(14)[144] [The yogi] should carefully perform one mantra-installation three times a day. When [the woman] is exhausted he should turn her over, put her on top of him, squeeze her breasts and then practise *śītalī* [*kumbhaka*]. (15) He should make her breathe in the same way [as before] through the left and right [nostrils] or blow through a reed pipe to make the breath flow [in those nostrils]. (16) The yogi should do this very gently until energy (*śakti*) arises [again]. Then during sexual intercourse he should draw up the falling *bindu.* (17) [The yogi] should squeeze the *vajrakanda,*[145] hold the breath, draw up the moving *bindu* and hold the mind in that very place.

(18) [The yogi] should eat nutmeg, milk, and ghee, and the finest scented betel together with liquid (*rasa*?). (19) Then while happily making love he should recite over and over again the mantra, the syllable of *brahman,* Śakti containing the syllable *la,* together with the dot (*bindu*) and the resonance (*nāda*). (20) This is the seed syllable beloved of the goddess, which gives complete sovereignty. It bestows success and is hard to obtain in the world, so [the yogi] should recite it over and over again. (21) As a result of practising in this way *bindu* never falls into the vagina. Thus sexual power arises and he who is engaged in yoga may penetrate (*mardayet*?) even an insatiable lover hundreds of times. In this there is no doubt. (22) When bindu has thus become steady, [the yogi] completely conquers death. Death comes from the fall of *bindu,* life from holding on to it.

(23) By practising in this way a woman may extract semen [and] attain steadiness of the body through the practice of *vajrolī.* (24) I shall very carefully teach the sequence of practice for women. If through passion the semen in the penis should be emitted, (25) then [the woman] should contract the aperture of the *ṭaṭikā* (?) and insert the jewel [i. e., semen] there. Pulling it with the breath, she should draw it upwards along that passage. (26) Then [neither] semen [nor] *rajas* is ever lost, and *rajas* together with *bindu* becomes *nāda* in the *mūlādhāra* of women. This yoga is successful for those who have religious merit, not for worldly people. By means of that one obtains success. Yoga results from yoga.

This is what is intended. In a pleasure pavilion out of the wind, while making love with his sweetheart in various different ways, the yogi should perform *śītalī*

144 The number 14 is not given in the manuscript.

145 The location of the *vajrakanda* is unclear. In the *Khecarīvidyā* it is situated in the head (*Khecarīvidyā* 2.26 and Mallinson 2007: 215, n. 293), which does not fit the context here.

kumbhaka and forcefully draw up his falling *bindu* using the *apāna* breath together with the syllable *huṃ*. On this matter, the following has been settled: when a yogi wants to achieve yoga while having sex with a lovely woman, by means of the *apāna* breath being drawn up the semen should be drawn up. He should insert his penis in her vagina and say "I deposit the embryo". If he does not want her to become pregnant, then he should draw up his semen using the *kriṣi* (?) breath. Saying "I take your semen with semen" the yogi conquers his semen.

In the *Bṛhadāraṇyakopaniṣad* the following is said:
If he does not want her to become pregnant, then he should put his penis in her, join [her] mouth with his, breathe [into her mouth] and then breathe out, saying "with my penis I take your semen by means of semen". She becomes free from semen.
And if he wants her to become pregnant then he should put his penis in her, join [her] mouth with his, breathe out and then breathe into her, saying "with [my] penis I deposit semen in you by means of semen". She is certain to become pregnant. [BĀU 6.4.10–11]

In the *Śivayoga* [it is said]:
[The yogi] should emit urine little by little having drawn it upwards again. He who does this every day in the manner taught by his guru gains mastery of *bindu*, which bestows all powers. [= ŚS 4.101a–102b, YBhD 7.286a–287b]

By practising this for six months *bindu* should not fall even when sex is had with one hundred women. And another thing: when defecating, the yogi should press his perineum with his fingers and lock (*bandhayet*?) his penis with his other hand. In this way restraint of urine should be practised. In the same way, when urinating faeces should be very gently restrained by contracting the anus. [The yogi] should practise thus until both happen automatically when urinating and defecating. Practising thus is another way of achieving mastery of *bindu*.

This is the first yoga. Afterwards [the yogi becomes] the amorous *vajrolī* yogi. It is this that is *vajrolī*. *Amarolī* has some particularities, [but in practice] is not different.

[The yogi] should carefully hold his *bindu* by any possible method. If it happens to go into the vagina and there is mixing of the moon and sun, then what he sucks up with a pipe is called *amarolī*. If his *bindu* moves [out] from him, the yogi should bind it by means of *yonimudrā*. [This] is called *sahajolī*, which is kept secret in all the tantras. The difference is in name; in effect the three are equal.

Thus the drawing upwards of one's own *bindu* is *vajrolī*. The drawing upwards of *bindu* mixed with blood in the vagina is *amarolī*. *Sahajolī* has been determined to be the drawing upwards of one's own *bindu* alone together with blood [i. e., *rajas*] from one's own body.

References

Primary Sources

Amanaska
see Birch 2013

Amaraughaprabodha
Amaraughaprabodha of Gorakṣanātha. In K. Mallik (Ed.), *The Siddha Siddhānta Paddhati and Other Works of Nath Yogis* (pp. 48–55). Poona: Poona Oriental Book House, 1954.

AS. *Amṛtasiddhi*
Unpublished edition by J. Mallinson.

BĀU. *Bṛhadāraṇyaka Upaniṣad*
In P. Olivelle, *The Early Upaniṣads: Annotated Text and Translation* (pp. 29–165). New York: Oxford University Press, 1998.

Bhagavadgītā
Buitenen, J. A. B. van (1981). *The Bhagavadgītā in the Mahābhārata: Text and Translation.* Chicago: University of Chicago Press, 1981.

Bodhasāra
Cover, J. & Cover, G. (Trans.). (2010). *Bodhasāra: An Eighteenth Century Sanskrit Treasure by Narahari.* Charleston: CreateSpace, 2010.

Brahmayāmala/Picumata
Unpublished edition by S. Hatley.

Bṛhatkathāślokasaṃgraha
see Mallinson 2005b

Bṛhatkhecarīprakāśa
Bṛhatkhecarīprakāśa. Scindia Oriental Research Institute Library (Ujjain) ms. no. 14575.

Caṇḍamahāroṣaṇatantra
George, Ch. S. (1974). *The Caṇḍamahāroṣaṇatantra: Chapters 1–8. A Critical Edition and English Translation.* New Haven, Connecticut: American Oriental Society.

Dhyānabindūpaniṣad
In A. M. Śāstrī (Ed.), *The Yoga Upanishads with the Commentary of Sri Upanishad-brahma-yogin* (pp. 186–213). Madras: Adyar Library, 1920.

DYŚ. *Dattātreyayogaśāstra*
Unpublished critical edition by J. Mallinson.

Gheraṇḍasaṃhitā
Mallinson, J. (2004). *The Gheranda Samhita: The Original Sanskrit and an English Translation*. New York: YogaVidya.com.
Gorakhbānī
Gorakhbānī, ed. P. D. Baḍathvāl. Prayāg: Hindī Sāhity Sammelan, 1960.
Gorakṣaśataka
Unpublished edition by J. Mallinson.
Haṭhābhyāsapaddhati
Unpublished manuscript. Bhārat Itihās Saṃśodhak Maṇḍal (Pune) ms. 46/440 (catalogued as *Āsanabandhāḥ*).
Haṭhapradīpikājyotsnā
Brahmānandakṛtā Haṭhapradīpikā Jyotsnā: Ālocanātmaka saṃskaraṇa, ed. Svāmī Maheśānand et al. Lonavla: Kaivalyadhama S. M. Y. M. Samiti, 2002.
Haṭhatattvakaumudī
Haṭhatattvakaumudī: A Treatise on Haṭhayoga, ed. M. L. Gharote et al. Lonavla: Lonavla Yoga Institute, 2007.
HP. *Haṭhapradīpikā*
Haṭhapradīpikā of Svātmārāma, ed. Svāmī Digambarjī & Pītambar Jhā. Lonavla: Kaivalyadhama S. M. Y. M. Samiti, 1970.
HR. *Haṭharatnāvalī*
Haṭharatnāvalī: A Treatise on Haṭhayoga of Śrīnivāsayogī, crit. ed. M. L. Gharote et al. Lonavla: Lonavla Yoga Institute, 2002.
Jog Mañjarī
Jog Mañjarī. Rajasthan Prācya Vidyā Pratiṣṭhān, Bikaner, Acc. No. 6543, *vajrolī* section (folios 103–107) as transcribed in M. M. Gharote et al. (Eds.), *Therapeutic References in Traditional Yoga Texts* (p. 258). Lonavla: Lonavla Yoga Institute, 2010.
Jogpradīpakā
Jogpradīpakā of Jayatarāma, ed. M. L. Gharote. Jodhpur: Rajasthan Oriental Research Institute, 1999.
Kaulajñānanirṇaya
Unpublished edition by S. Hatley.
Līḷācaritra by Mhāiṃbhaṭa
Līḷācaritra, ed. V. Bh. Kolte. Muṃbaī: Mahārāṣṭra Rājya Sāhitya Saṃskṛti Maṃḍala, 1978.
Mārkaṇḍeyapurāṇa
The Márcaṇḍeya Purána in the Original Sanscrit, ed. K. M. Banerjea. Calcutta: Bishop's College Press, 1862.
Niśvāsatattvasaṃhitā
The Niśvāsatattvasaṃhitā: The Earliest Surviving Śaiva Tantra. Vol. 1: *A Critical Edition and Annotated Translation of the Mūlasūtra, Uttarasūtra, and Nayasūtra*, ed. D. Goodall et al. Collection Indologie 128. Early Tantra Series 1. Pondicherry: Institut Français d'Indologie / École française d'Extrême-Orient, 2015.
Rājayogabhāṣya
Maṇḍalabrāhmaṇopaniṣad with a Commentary (Rājayogabhaṣya), ed. Mahādeva Śāstrī. Government Oriental Library Series. Mysore: The Government Branch Press, 1896.

Śaṅkaradigvijaya
Śrī-Vidyāraṇya viracitaḥ śrīmac-Chaṅkaradigvijayaḥ Advaitarājyalakṣmī ṭīkāntargataviśeṣavibhāgaṭippaṇībhis tathā Dhanapati-Sūri-kṛta-Diṇḍimākhya-ṭīkayā ca sametaḥ, ed. Ānandāśramasthapaṇḍita-s. Ānandāśramasaṃskṛtagranthāvali 22. Pune: M. C. Apte, 1891.

Sarvāṅgayogapradīpikā
In *Sundargranthāvalī*, ed. R. C. Mishra (pp. 80–115). New Delhi: Kitab Ghar, 1992.

Siddhasiddhāntapaddhati
Siddhasiddhāntapaddhatiḥ: A Treatise on the Nātha Philosophy by Gorakṣanātha, eds. M. L. Gharote & G. K. Pai. Lonavla: Lonavla Yoga Institute, 2005.

ŚS. *Śivasaṃhitā*
Mallinson, J. (2007). *The Śivasaṃhitā. A Critical Edition and English Translation.* New York: YogaVidya.com.

Tirumantiram
Natarajan, T. B. (1991). *Tirumantiram: A Tamil Scriptural Classic. Tamil Text with English Translation and Notes.* Madras: Sri Ramakrishna Math.

Vajroliyoga
Unpublished manuscript. Wai Prajñā Pāṭhaśālā ms. no. 6–4/399.

Vivekamārtaṇḍa
Unpublished manuscript. Oriental Institute of Baroda Library Acc. No. 4110.

YBhD. *Yuktabhavadeva*
Yuktabhavadeva of Bhavadevamiśra: A Treatise on Yoga, ed. M. L. Gharote & V. K. Jha. Lonavla: Lonavla Yoga Institute, 2002.

Yogamārgaprakāśikā
Yogamārgaprakāśikā arthāt yogarahasyagranthabhāṣāṭīkāsametā Śrīmahāntayugaladāsanirmitā, ed. Giridhara Śāstrī. Bombay: Khemarāj Śrīkṛṣṇadās, Śrīveṅkaṭeśvara Steam Press, 1904.

Secondary Sources

Alter, J. (2011). *Moral Materialism: Sex and Masculinity in Modern India.* Delhi: Penguin.

Ānandsvarūpjī, N. B. M. (1937). *BindYog: arthāt vajrolī mudrā dvārā vīry vijay.* Jodhpur: Marudhar Prakāśan Mandir.

Birch, J. (2013). *The Amanaska: King of All Yogas. A Critical Edition and Annotated Translation with a Monographic Introduction.* Unpublished Doctoral Thesis. University of Oxford.

Bühnemann, G. (2007). *Eighty-four Āsanas in Yoga: A Survey of Traditions (with Illustrations).* Delhi: D. K. Printworld.

Callewaert, W. M. & Op de Beeck, B. (Eds.). (1991). *Devotional Hindī Literature: A Critical Edition of the Pañc-Vāṇī or Five Works of Dādū, Kabīr, Nāmdev, Rāidās, Hardās with the Hindī Songs of Gorakhnāth and Sundardās, and a Complete Word-Index.* 2 vols. New Delhi: Manohar.

Darmon, R. A. (2002). Vajrolī Mudrā: La rétention séminale chez les yogis vāmācāri. In V. Bouillier & G. Tarabout (Eds.), *Images du corps dans le monde hindou* (pp. 213–240). Paris: CNRS Éditions.

Das, R. P. (1992). Problematic Aspects of the Sexual Rituals of the Bauls of Bengal. *Journal of the American Oriental Society, 112*(3), 388–432.

Das, R. P. (2003). *The Origin of the Life of a Human Being: Conception and the Female According to Ancient Indian Medical and Sexological Literature.* New Delhi: Motilal Banarsidass.

David-Neel, A. (1931). *Initiations and Initiates in Tibet,* trans. F. Rothwell. London: Rider and Co.

De Michelis, E. (2004). *A History of Modern Yoga.* London: Continuum.

Digambarji, S. & Sahai, M. (1969). Vajroli, Amaroli and Sahajoli. *Yoga Mimamsa, 11*(4), 15–24.

Doniger, W. (1980). *Women, Androgynes and Other Mythical Beasts.* Chicago: University of Chicago Press.

Ernst, C. (2007). Accounts of Yogis in Arabic and Persian Historical and Travel Texts. *Jerusalem Studies in Arabic and Islam, 33,* 409–426.

Feldhaus, A. (1980). The "Devatācakra" of the Mahānubhavas. *Bulletin of the School of Oriental and African Studies, 43,* 101–109.

Filliozat, J. (1953). Les limites de pouvoirs humains dans l'Inde. In Ch. Baudoin (Ed.), *Limites de l'humain. Études carmélitaines* (pp. 23–38). Paris: Desclée de Brouwer.

Gharote, M. M. et. al. (2010). *Therapeutic References in Traditional Yoga Texts.* Lonavla: The Lonavla Yoga Institute.

Gold, D. (2002). Kabīr's Secrets for Householders: Truths and Rumours among Rajasthani Nāths. In M. Horstmann (Ed.), *Images of Kabir* (pp. 143–156). Delhi: Manohar.

Golovkova, A. (2010). The Cult of the Goddess Tripurasundarī in the Vāmakeśvarīmata. Unpublished Master Thesis. University of Oxford.

Gray, D. B. (2007). *The Cakrasamvara Tantra (The Discourse of Śrī Heruka). (Śrīherukābhidhāna): A Study and Annotated Translation.* Treasury of the Buddhist Sciences Series. New York: The American Institute of Buddhist Studies at Columbia University in New York & Columbia University's Center for Buddhist Studies and Tibet House US.

Hatley, S. (2016). Erotic Asceticism: The Razor's Edge Observance (asidhārāvrata) and the Early History of Tantric Coital Ritual. *Bulletin of the School of Oriental and African Studies, 79*(2), 1–17.

Isaacson, H. (n. d.). Tantric Buddhism in India. Revised paper of a lecture given at Hamburg University in 1997. Unpublished.

Khan, D.-S. (1994). Deux rites tantriques dans une communauté d'intouchables au Rajasthan. *Revue de l'histoire des religions, 211*(4), 443–462.

Kiehnle, C. (2000). Love and Bhakti in the Early Nāth Tradition of Mahārāṣṭra: The Lotus of the Heart. In M. K. Gautam & G. H. Schokker (Eds.), *Bhakti Literature in South Asia* (pp. 255–276). Leiden: Kern Institute.

Knight, L. (2011). *Contradictory Lives: Baul Women in India and Bangladesh.* New York: Oxford University Press.

Lorenzen, D. N. (2011). Religious Identity in Gorakhnath and Kabir: Hindus, Muslims, Yogis, and Sants. In D. N. Lorenzen & A. Muñoz (Eds.), *Yogi Heroes and Poets: Histories and Legends of the Nāths* (pp. 19–50). New York: State University of New York Press.

Lysebeth, A. van (1995). *Tantra: The Cult of the Feminine.* Maine: Samuel Weiser.

Mallinson, J. (2005a). Rāmānandī Tyāgīs and Haṭha Yoga. *Journal of Vaishnava Studies 14*(1), 107–121.

Mallinson, J. (Ed., Trans.). (2005b). *The Emperor of the Sorcerers by Budhasvāmin.* 2 vols. New York: Princeton University Press.

Mallinson, J. (2007). *The Khecarīvidyā of Ādinātha: A Critical Edition and Annotated Translation.* London: Routledge.

Mallinson, J. (2011). The Original Gorakṣaśataka. In D. G. White (Ed.), *Yoga in Practice* (pp. 257–272). Princeton: Princeton University Press.

Mallinson, J. (2014). The Yogīs' Latest Trick. *Journal of the Royal Asiatic Society, 24*(1), 165–180.

Mallinson, J. (2015). Śāktism and Haṭhayoga. In B. W. Olesen (Ed.), *Goddess Traditions in Tantric Hinduism* (pp. 109–140). London: Routledge.

Mallinson, J. (forthc.). The Amṛtasiddhi, haṭhayoga's Tantric Buddhist Source Text. In D. Goodall et al. (Eds.), *Śaivism and the Tantric Traditions, a festschrift for Alexis Sanderson.* Leiden: Brill.

Mallinson, J. & Singleton, M. (2017). *Roots of Yoga.* London: Penguin Classics.

Muñoz, A. (2011). Matsyendra's "Golden Legend": Yogi Tales and Nath Ideology. In D. N. Lorenzen & A. Muñoz (Eds.), *Yogi Heroes and Poets: Histories and Legends of the Nāths* (pp. 109–128). New York: State University of New York Press.

Needham, J. (1974). *Science and Civilisation in China.* Vol. 5, pt. 5. Cambridge: Cambridge University Press.

Oort, J. van (2016). "Human Semen Eucharist" Among the Manichaeans? The Testimony of Augustine Reconsidered in Context. *Vigiliae Christianae, 70*(2), 193–216.

Pfister, R. (2006). The Jade Spring as a Source of Pleasure and Pain: The Prostatic Experience in Ancient and Medieval Medical and Daoist Texts. In H. U. Vogel et al. (Eds.), *Studies On Ancient Chinese Scientific and Technical Texts, Proceedings of the 3rd ISACBRST* (pp. 88–106). Zhengzhou: Elephant Press.

Pfister, R. (2013). Gendering Sexual Pleasures in Early and Medieval China. *Asian Medicine, 7,* 34–64.

Rieker, H.-U. (1992). *Hatha Yoga Pradipika: Translation and Commentary.* London: Aquarian Press.

Roşu, A. (2002). Pratiques tantriques au regard de l'andrologie médicale. *Journal Asiatique, 290*(1), 293–313.

Rozmarynowski, M. (1979). Experiments with Vajroli. *Yoga Mimamsa, 19*(4), 36–45.

Sanderson, A. (1988). Śaivism and the Tantric Traditions. In S. Sutherland et al. (Eds.), *The World's Religions* (pp. 660–704). London: Routledge.

Sanderson, A. (2005). A Commentary on the Opening Verses of the Tantrasāra of Abhinavagupta. In S. Das & E. Fürlinger (Eds.), *Sāmarasya: Studies in Indian Arts, Philosophy, and Interreligious Dialogue in Honour of Bettina Bäumer* (pp. 89–148). New Delhi: D. K. Printworld.

Sanderson, A. (forthc.). *Religion and the State: Initiating the Monarch in Śaivism and the Buddhist Way of Mantras.* Heidelberg Studies in South Asian Rituals 2. Wiesbaden: Harrassowitz.

Shri Yogeshwaranand Paramahansa (2011). *First Steps to Higher Yoga.* New Delhi: Yoga Niketan Trust.

Sivananda, S. (1998). *Yoga Asana.* Rishikesh: Divine Life Society.

Svoboda, R. (1986). *Aghora: At the Left Hand of God.* Albuquerque: Brotherhood of Life.

Tāntrikābhidhānakośa III, ed. D. Goodall and M. Rastelli. Wien: Verlag der Österreichischen Akademie der Wissenschaften, 2013.

Umekawa, S. (2004). *Sex and Immortality: A Study of Chinese Sexual Techniques for Better-Being.* Unpublished Doctoral Thesis. School of Oriental and African Studies, University of London.

Vasu, R. B. S. Ch. (1914). *The Siva Samhita.* Allahabad: Panini Office.

Vasudeva, S. (2011). Haṃsamiṭṭhu: "Pātañjalayoga is Nonsense." *Journal of Indian Philosophy, 39*(2), 123–145.

White, D. G. (1996). *The Alchemical Body.* Chicago: University of Chicago Press, 1996.

White, D. G. (2003). *Kiss of the Yoginī: "Tantric Sex" in its South Asian Contexts.* Chicago: University of Chicago Press.

Chapter 5

Yoga in the Daily Routine of the Pāñcarātrins

Marion Rastelli

Contents

1. Introduction 225

2. The Time for Practising Yoga 227

3. The Nature of Yoga in the Context of the Five Time Periods 236
3.1. Mental Visualisation of God 236
3.2. Identifying Meditation 237

4. *Yogāṅga*-s 239

5. Tattva Yoga 241

6. Veṅkaṭanātha 246

7. Conclusion 252

References 252

Marion Rastelli

Chapter 5: Yoga in the Daily Routine of the Pāñcarātrins*

1. Introduction

In the Vaiṣṇava tradition of Pāñcarātra, yoga and yogic techniques – which may assume many different forms as we will see in this chapter – are utilised in various contexts and for manifold purposes. For example, yogic techniques are used in rituals in order to purify certain objects of worship as well as the worshipper himself.[1] Yoga is also practised independently from these ritual contexts in order to reach the two classical goals of a Pāñcarātrin, i.e., liberation (*mukti*) from transmigration and worldly pleasure (*bhukti*).[2]

One characteristic feature of the Pāñcarātra, however, is the practice of yoga in a special context, namely, within the framework of the religious rites of the "five time periods" (*pañca kāla*). The five time periods are a daily routine that is already described in relatively early *saṃhitā*-s such as the *Jayākhyasaṃhitā* (JS) and the *Pauṣkarasaṃhitā* (PauṣS) and that has been presented as obligatory for Pāñcarātrins by the tradition's authoritative texts at least from the twelfth century CE onwards.[3] These five time periods structure a Pāñcarātrin's entire day; they consist of the following parts: "approaching" (*abhigamana*), "appropriating" (*upādāna*), worship (*ijyā*), studying (*svādhyāya*), and yoga.

* I would like to thank the editors of this volume for their valuable comments and suggestions to improve this chapter and Katharine Apostle for suggesting various stylistic corrections of the English manuscript.

1 Examples for this are the purifying preparations for the daily ritual such as the "purification of the elements" (*bhūtaśuddhi*) (e.g., in JS 10; cf. Rastelli 1999: 210–238) and the mental purification of the *maṇḍala* and the *arghya* vessel (JS 13.87d–90b; cf. Rastelli 1999: 278f.).

2 An example for this can be found in JS 33 (Rastelli 1999: 323–366 and 405–412). Rastelli 2009 also examines various forms of yoga described in the *saṃhitā*-s of Pāñcarātra.

3 For a description of the *pañca kāla* rituals and their role at the time of the earlier extant *saṃhitā*-s, see Rastelli 2000; for their development into a characteristic of all Pāñcarātrins, see Rastelli 2006: 63–91.

"Approaching" (*abhigamana*) includes all morning rites from getting up to the morning toilet and the rituals at dawn (*sandhyā*).[4] These rites are called "approaching" because they are considered a way to approach God.[5] "Appropriating" (*upādāna*) means acquiring all substances that are necessary to perform a ritual of worship such as flowers, fruits or lamps.[6] "Worship" (*ijyā*) means the ritual worship of God, the daily *pūjā*.[7] "Studying" (*svādhyāya*) means to study and recite the authoritative texts of the tradition.[8] "Yoga", the final time period of the day, which is the object of our investigation, completes the day and is practised before falling asleep and/or at midnight after waking up again.

In the following part of this chapter (sections 2–7), I will examine the prescriptions for this yoga practice as found in Pāñcarātra texts, such as the *saṃhitā*-s and Veṅkaṭanātha's *Pāñcarātrarakṣā* (PRR), focusing on the particular nature of this type of yoga and, as a first step, on the time that is prescribed for practising it.

Descriptions of the rituals of the "five time periods" can be found in many *saṃhitā*-s of the Pāñcarātra, although by no means in all of them. In addition, there are a few passages in the *saṃhitā*-s that describe the nocturnal practice of yoga in other contexts than the *pañca kāla*-s. These passages will also be taken into consideration here. Altogether, passages describing this kind of yoga will be examined from the following texts: *Jayākhyasaṃhitā* (22.73–74b), *Sāttvatasaṃhitā* (SS) (6.191c–215, non-*pañca kāla* context), *Pauṣkarasaṃhitā* (38.289–292, 41.62–63a, 34.1–6b, the last two passages in non-*pañca kāla* contexts), *Sanatkumārasaṃhitā* (SanS) (*ṛṣirātra* 1.13c–14), *Lakṣmītantra* (LT) (40.102–103b), *Pādmasaṃhitā* (PādS) (*caryāpāda* 13.72c–77), *Nāradīyasaṃhitā* (NārS) (30.8c–21), *Pārameśvarasaṃhitā* (PārS) (7.438–495b), *Īśvarasaṃhitā* (ĪS) (6.81–89b), *Śrīpraśnasaṃhitā* (ŚrīprśS) (17.61–68), *Bhārgavatantra* (BhT) (25.11c–23), *Parāśarasaṃhitā* (ParāśaraS) (4.154c–157b). Two texts not strictly belonging to the *saṃhitā*-s of the Pāñcarātra will also be investigated, as they contain descriptions of the *pañca kāla* rituals, namely, the *Viṣṇudharmottarapurāṇa* (VDhP) (1.64.7–1.65.38) and the *Śāṇḍilyasmṛti* (ŚSmṛ) (ch. 5). The *Pāñcarātrarakṣā* was written by Veṅkaṭanātha, a famous Viśiṣṭādvaita Vedānta theolo-

4 See, e.g., *Pāñcarātrarakṣā* (PRR) p. 87, l. 17 – p. 127, l. 3.

5 Cf. JS 22.68–69b: "During the first day in the morning, from the *brāhma muhūrta* (cf. n. 46) onwards, oh sage, he should approach the source of the world (i.e., God) with recitations, visualisations, homages and hymns of praise in deeds, words and thoughts; and this is known as 'approaching'" (*brāhmān muhūrtād ārabhya prāgaṃśaṃ vipra vāsare | japadhyānārcanastotraiḥ karmavākcittasaṃyutaiḥ* || 68 || *abhigacchej jagadyoniṃ tac cābhigamanaṃ smṛtam* |).

6 See, e.g., PRR p. 127, l. 4 – p. 137, l. 13.

7 See, e.g., JS 22.71, PauṣS 38.287c–288b, PādS *caryāpāda* 13.34–66b. The main part of the PRR's description of *ijyā* is lost.

8 See, e.g., PRR p. 147, l. 12 – p. 149, l. 16.

gian of the thirteenth/fourteenth centuries and also a follower of the Pāñcarātra. The aim of his *Pāñcarātrarakṣā* was to defend the tradition of Pāñcarātra. Two of its three extensive chapters deal with the *pañca kāla* rituals. Veṅkaṭanātha quotes and comments on various passages from the *saṃhitā*-s with the aim of reconciling divergent statements. This work is thus an immensely valuable source of information about the history of the tradition of the Pāñcarātra in Veṅkaṭanātha's time.

2. The Time for Practising Yoga

I would like to start my exposition of Pāñcarātra yoga by addressing the topic of the proper time for yoga practice. First, I will describe the evening routine, the sequence of acts that are performed before and after yoga practice, and then I will discuss the prescribed time for this yoga practice.

Almost all examined texts agree that, having studied in the afternoon, the devotee should perform the *sandhyā* rituals, the rituals at dusk, as these are the duties that, for example, the Gṛhya- and Dharmasūtras prescribe for all twice-borns.[9] Some of the texts offer details - with a few variations - of what the *sandhyā* rituals consist of: a purifying bath, ritual worship of God with offerings of flowers and *arghya* water, oblations with fire (*homa*), and the recitation (*japa*) of mantras.[10] Usually, the *sandhyā* rituals start when the sun is about to set and last until the stars appear.[11]

After the *sandhyā* rituals, the devotee has dinner, which is also called the "final sacrifice" (*anuyāga*), as it is considered an oblation to the fire of the vital breaths (*prāṇa*-s) (*prāṇāgnihavana,* JS 22.80ab).[12] Then he goes to bed.[13]

9 A few texts even state explicitly that the *sandhyā* rituals should be performed according to the prescriptions of "one's *sūtra*" (ŚrīprśS 17.59, ParāśaraS 4.154c–155a, PRR p. 150, l. 1). For the *sandhyā* rituals according to the Gṛhya- and Dharmasūtras and other dharma texts see Kane 1974: 312–321.

10 JS 22.73ab: *pūjā;* SS 6.190–191c ≈ PārS 7.436c–438a ≈ ĪS 6.81–83a: bathing or washing the lower part of the body, dressing, worshipping God and the fire, recitation; PauṣS 38.289c–290b: worshipping, reciting and visualising the mantra; LT 40.102a: worship; PādS *caryāpāda* 13.72c–73: recitation, oblations with fire, worship of God; ŚrīprśS 17.59–60b: oblations with fire, worship of God; VDhP 1.64.3–5b: sipping water (*ācamana*), worship of God in the temple; BhT 25.11–12a; bathing, acquiring *arghya* water, recitation, oblations with fire, worshipping and praising God; ParāśaraS 4.154c–155a: worship of God, etc.; ŚSmṛ 5.2–7b: purification of the body, dressing, sprinkling (*prokṣaṇa*) and sipping water, offering of *arghya* water, visualisation of God, either in silence or while reciting, worship of God, oblations with fire, recitations and praises of God; PRR p. 150, ll. 1–2: worship of God, oblations with fire.

11 Kane 1974: 313. See also ŚSmṛ 5.3d: *yāvan nakṣatradarśanam,* "until one sees the stars".

12 PādS *caryāpāda* 13.74a, ŚrīprśS 17.60c, VDhP 1.64.5c, BhT 25.12a, ParāśaraS 4.155b, ŚSmṛ

In bed, according to most of the examined *saṃhitā*-s, the devotee should think of God till he falls asleep.[14] This already could be considered yoga, and indeed a few *saṃhitā*-s explicitly prescribe yoga for this time of day and do not only mean reflecting upon God, but yoga in a technical sense, including, e. g., breath control and mental dissolution of the *tattva*-s, which constitute the body of the devotee.[15]

Later at night, usually at midnight,[16] the devotee has to get up again and practise yoga, according to most of the sources. Some *saṃhitā*-s prescribe a few preparatory rites before the proper yoga practice such as purification of the feet, sipping water (*ācamana*), worshipping the teacher and God or placing mantras on one's body.[17] Then the devotee assumes a seated position[18] and practises yoga in one way or another. I will address this topic below (p. 236 ff.). After that the devotee goes back to bed and sleeps. At a particular time in the morning called *brāhma muhūrta*, a certain period before sunrise,[19] he gets up[20] and his daily practice of the *pañca kāla* rites starts again.

5.7c–12, PRR p. 150, ll. 2–11 (according to Veṅkaṭanātha, the *prāṇāgnihotramantra*-s should be recited if dinner is skipped; for the *prāṇāgnihotramantra*-s cf. *Mahānārāyaṇa Upaniṣad* 479–486 and Varenne 1960: 2/92).

13 SS 6.191d (≈ PārS 7.438b ≈ ĪS 6.83b), PauṣS 38.290c, PādS *caryāpāda* 13.74a, ŚrīprśS 17.61a, ParāśaraS 4.155c.

14 SS 6.192–193b (≈ PārS 7.438c–439 ≈ ĪS 6.83c–84), PauṣS 38.290d, 41.62ab, ŚrīprśS 17.61b, ParāśaraS 4.155c, ŚSmṛ 5.48cd (the devotee should mentally recite mantras till he falls asleep). PādS *caryāpāda* 13.74ab, which does not mention sleep explicitly, only says that one should go to bed. This probably implies that the devotee should sleep. ŚrīprśS 17.61c–62 gives additional instructions of how to proceed in case the devotee has sexual intercourse with his wife.

15 JS 22.73: "[…] he should practise yoga […]" ([…] *samabhyaset | yogam* […]), VDhP 1.64.7: "Afterwards, having noticed [that] the time for yoga [has come], he should dissolve [the *tattva*-s constituting his body]. Having dissolved [the *tattva*-s], he should unwearily remain concentrated (*yukta*) for three hours" (*yogakālam upādāya paścāt kuryād visarjanam | kṛtvā visarjanaṃ yuktas tiṣṭhed yāmam atandritaḥ* ||) and 1.65.1–38, BhT 25.12b–19 (purification of the bodily tubes by means of breath control [*prāṇāyāma*], dissolution of the *tattva*-s, meditation on the *brahman*). For the *tattva*-s see n. 78.

16 SS 6.193c (= PārS 7.440a = ĪS 6.85a), PauṣS 38.291ab, PādS *caryāpāda* 13.74b, ŚrīprśS 17.63a, BhT 25.15a. The *Jayākhyāsaṃhitā* phrases it differently: it is not sleep that is interrupted by yoga practice, but yoga practice that is interrupted by sleep: "He should practise yoga, which is interrupted by rests at the end of the night" (JS 22.73bcd: […] *samabhyaset | yogaṃ niśāvasāne ca viśramair antarīkṛtam* ||). Midnight should probably not be taken too literally here. It probably means a time at night when one wakes up; see p. 229 f. on segmented sleep.

17 SS 6.193d–197b: sipping water, worship of teacher and God, placing mantras on the body; PādS *caryāpāda* 13.74cd: sipping water, a kind of mental preparation (*prayato bhūtvā*), visualisation of God; ŚrīprśS 17.63cd: purification of the feet, sipping water; BhT 25.15ab: bathing at a bathing place (?, this prescription sounds strange, especially as such bathing is not only requested at midnight, but also at night and at daybreak: *rātrau niśīthe vimale snātvā tirthe 'nvahaṃ sudhiḥ* |, which does not seem realistic); PārS 7.440cd (= SS 6.194ab): sipping water; ĪS 6.85d–86b (≈ SS 6.193d–194): sipping water, worship of teacher and God.

18 SS 6.197c–201, PādS *caryāpāda* 13.75a, ŚrīprśS 17.64ab, BhT 25.15c.

19 Cf. n. 46.

In order to give a general overview, I have drawn a harmonised picture of what goes on in the evening and at night. However, I have to emphasise that the prescriptions of the *saṃhitā*-s differ quite a bit from each other. Some prescribe yoga practice only at night before falling asleep (PauṣS 41, VDhP 1.64.7–8, *Parāśarasaṃhitā*), one only at midnight (*Pādmasaṃhitā*), some at night and at midnight (*Jayākhyasaṃhitā, Sāttvatasaṃhitā*, PauṣS 38, *Pārameśvarasaṃhitā, Īśvarasaṃhitā, Śrīpraśnasaṃhitā*), one at night and in the morning (*Lakṣmītantra*), one at night, at midnight, and in the morning (*Bhārgavatantra*), and one even for the whole night without sleep (PauṣS 34)[21]. Two *saṃhitā*-s (*Sanatkumārasaṃhitā, Nāradīyasaṃhitā*) do not specify a time for yoga practice.

These differences are not surprising at all if one takes into consideration that for the most part the various *saṃhitā*-s are not unified in any aspect, although they all belong to the same tradition called Pāñcarātra. Concerning their ritual prescriptions and theological doctrines, there are almost always variations. For a very long time and perhaps till today, there existed various traditions centred on particular *saṃhitā*-s within the Pāñcarātra rather than a single unified tradition of Pāñcarātra.[22] For our specific case we can thus conclude that various Pāñcarātrins in different places and times practised yoga at different times of the night (and in different ways, as we will see), before and/or after sleeping and often between two phases of sleep at midnight.

From our modern Western perspective, getting up at midnight in order to practise yoga seems to be very hard or even inhuman. However, historical and medical research has shown that our pattern of seamless slumber is quite a modern phenomenon and that segmented sleep, often consisting of a "first sleep" and a "second" or "morning sleep", is and actually was the natural sleep pattern up to the early modern era.[23] These two phases of sleep lasted about the same length of time, sometimes with a waking period around midnight, of course, depending on what time a person went to bed.[24] In this waking period, some people stayed in bed, reflecting or talking with their bedfellow, some got up for various activities before going to bed again to have their second sleep; probably very few remained awake.[25] There is early evidence for this segmented sleep, for example, in the history of Rome by the Roman historian Livy (Titus

20 SS 6.215c–216b, PauṣS 38.292, PādS *caryāpāda* 13.77ab, BhT 25.20ab. According to PārS 7.495cff., a bed and other items are offered to the image of Viṣṇu after yoga practice but nothing is said about the devotee going back to bed.

21 It is unclear whether the prescriptions for nocturnal yoga without sleeping in PauṣS 34.1–12 are really intended for daily practice but according to Veṅkaṭanātha, such prescriptions, aimed only at particular persons, existed; see n. 31.

22 Cf. on this topic the illuminating study of Leach (2012).

23 See Ekirch 2005: 300–323.

24 Ekirch 2005: 300f.

25 Ekirch 2005: 305f.

Livius) who lived around the beginning of the Common Era.[26] In a religious context, we may mention, for example, the regulations of the Benedictine order by St. Benedict requiring "that monks rise after midnight for the recital of verses and psalms" or the morning prayers and night vigils prescribed by the Catholic Church in the High Middle Ages and later.[27] Thus, segmented sleep with possibly getting up at midnight is not as unusual as it might seem.

Let us now see what Veṅkaṭanātha said on this issue. In his *Pāñcarātrarakṣā*, Veṅkaṭanātha aimed at defending the tradition of Pāñcarātra as a whole and not that of particular *saṃhitā*-s. Thus he tried to reconcile the varying prescriptions of the *saṃhitā*-s and explain the meanings of their variations. Further, he tried to accommodate these prescriptions with Smṛti[28] texts of the Vedic orthodoxy in order to show that the Pāñcarātra did not contradict the prescriptions of the latter but that both formed a unit.

With regard to the diverging prescriptions on the time of yoga practice within the *pañca kāla* rites, Veṅkaṭanātha pursued the following strategy.

Generally, according to his aim of reconciliation, Veṅkaṭanātha did not strictly insist on a particular rule, but was flexible and considered diverging prescriptions as equally valid depending on different situations. This is a very pragmatic solution because it gives many more persons the possibility to follow the rules in a valid manner than a strict interpretation would allow. Thus the Pāñcarātra becomes attractive for more people than it would be otherwise.

To begin with, the most radical interpretation of Veṅkaṭanātha's is that it is not even necessary to practise yoga in the context of the *pañca kāla* rites, if one is not able to do so.[29] Generally, a prescription needs only be followed if one has the

---

26 Ekirch 2005: 303 and 2001: 367, n. 78.

27 Ekirch 2005: 302, 307f.

28 The term *smṛti* designates "a group of texts whose authority derives from the Veda, but that, unlike the Veda, have been transmitted and not directly heard by the ancient seers". By contrast, *śruti* refers to "sacred texts, believed to have been heard (root *śru*-) by the ancient seers (ṛṣi-s), Veda" (Freschi 2012: 384f.).

29 PRR p. 76, ll. 1–5: "If, however, later [in *Dakṣasmṛti* (DakṣSmṛ) 2.54 the following] is said: 'He should spend the two night watches after the evening with the study of the Veda, since one who sleeps for two night watches effects identity with the *brahman*', there is no contradiction between the two teachings (i.e., that of the *Dakṣasmṛti* and that of the Pāñcarātra) that both enjoin these two [rituals (i.e., study of the Veda and yoga practice)] at the same time because here study, which is a subsidiary component (*śeṣa*) of [yoga], is for a person who is not able [to practise] yoga. Yoga, however, is for a person who is able [to do so]" (*yat tu paścād uktam – "pradoṣapaścimau yāmau vedābhyāsena yāpayet | yāmadvayaṃ śayāno hi brahmabhūyāya kalpate ||" iti. atra yogāsamarthasya taccheṣabhūtaḥ svādhyāyaḥ, samarthasya tu yoga eveti na samānakālatadubhayavidhāyakaśāstradvayavirodhaḥ*). Veṅkaṭanātha produced this argument in order to show that the *Dakṣasmṛti*, which prescribes a daily ritual consisting of eight parts that do not include yoga practice, does not contradict the prescriptions of the Pāñcarātra scriptures.

appropriate ability to do so.[30] Thus, unsurprisingly, texts that prescribe, for example, yoga practice for the whole night without sleeping are meant only for particular persons who are very advanced in yoga practice.[31] Similarly, getting up at midnight is meant only for persons who are followers of the particular *saṃhitā* that gives that prescription or, alternatively, does not literally mean yoga practice at midnight, but yoga practice at a silent time that is especially suitable.[32] On the other hand, if one has the ability to practise yoga, one has to do so according to one's abilities.[33]

Yoga can also be practised at a different time of the day, even if another constituent of the *pañca kāla* rites, such as studying (*svādhyāya*), is then left out. The only precondition that is set for the time of yoga is that it must be adequate

30 PRR p. 81, l. 17f.: "Since all teachings that deal with regular [rituals], [rituals] that must be accomplished on certain occasions, and [rituals] for the fulfillment of desires, hold good only in accordance with the power of the respective person" (*tattatpuruṣaśaktyanusāreṇaiva hi nityanaimittikakāmyaviṣayāṇāṃ sarveṣāṃ śāstrāṇāṃ pravṛttiḥ*).

31 PRR p. 81, ll. 15–17: "And the yoga treatises that teach staying awake in order to [practise] uninterrupted yoga the whole night long in order to avoid agitation, etc., of the senses that is effected on the occasion of sleep, concern particular persons who are altogether healthy and have reached a yoga state which is independent of repose" (*yeṣu ca yogagrantheṣu kṛtsnāyāṃ rātrau niśchidrayogārthaṃ svapnasamayasambhāvitendriyakṣobhādiparihārāya ca jāgaraḥ pratipādyate, te viśramanirapekṣayogadaśāpannapūrṇārogyapuruṣaviśeṣaviṣayāḥ*).

32 PRR p. 82, ll. 11–18: "What is explained in detail as to be performed before the *brāhma muhūrta* in the Sāttvata- and other [*saṃhitā*-s, namely:] 'Then he should get up at midnight, overcome sleep and fatigue, sip water from a waterpot, do homage to [his] teachers [and] the deities, [and] sit down on a seat made of the skin of a black antelope [...]' (SS 6.193c–194), etc., this is a restriction for the time for yoga [practice] for those who follow these *saṃhitā*-s. [Or another interpretation of this passage could be (cf. PRR_1 p. 343, n. 2: *pakṣāntaram āha niśśabde iti*):] The prescription for [yoga practice at midnight applies] to a silent time during which everybody is in deep sleep and because [it] is excellently adequate for the intentness on a single object. And because it accords with the power, etc., of the respective person there is no contradiction to a prescription for this and that time [other than midnight]. Thus this is explained" (*ya eṣa sāttvatādiṣu brāhmamuhūrtāt pūrvam eva kartavyatvena prapañcyate – "samutthāyārdharātre 'tha jitanidro jitaśramaḥ | kamaṇḍalusthitenaiva samācamya tu vāriṇā | gurūn devān namaskṛtya hy upaviśyājināsane ||" ityādinā etatsaṃhitāniṣṭhānām eṣa yogakālaniyamaḥ. niḥśabde sarvasuṣuptikāle ca aikāgryātiśayasambhāvanayā ca tadvidhiḥ. tattatpuruṣaśaktyādyanusārāc ca tattatkālavidher avirodha ity uktam*).

33 PRR p. 165, l. 9 – p. 166, l. 1: "And the uninterrupted contemplation of the Venerable One must not be omitted, thinking: 'This which has to be learned from [sages such as] Sanaka, etc., cannot be practised by people like us' because tasting it according to [one's] ability must not be given up just as eating according to [one's] health [must not be given up]. [...] Therefore, just as the Venerable One showed Arjuna, who said: '[...] [quotation of *Bhagavadgītā* (BhG) 11.3c–4]', His Self that wears all forms, so also here (i.e., at yoga practice) the most illustrious Venerable One Himself makes those who hope for an own experience to experience His Self according to His wish" (*na caitan nirantarabhagavadanusandhānaṃ sanakādisādhyam asmadādibhir duḥśakam iti matvodāsitavyam. yathārogyaṃ bhojanavad yathāśakti tadāsvādasyāparityājyatvāt. [...] ato yathā vā [...] ityetāvadvādino 'rjunasya bhagavān viśvarūpaṃ svātmānaṃ darśayāmāsa; evam atrāpi svānubhavasāpekṣān yathāmanorathaṃ paramodāro bhagavān eva svātmānam anubhāvayati*).

for obtaining concentration (literally "intentness on a single object", *aikāgrya, ekāgratā*).[34] It is especially *svādhyāya,* the rite preceding yoga in the daily *pañca kāla* routine, with which yoga can merge,[35] as the boundaries between the respective natures of these two practices are fluid: both may include elements of recitation and concentration. And both are also constituents of other rituals, which means that they are practised also in many other ritual contexts of the daily routine.[36]

Veṅkaṭanātha admitted that night is an especially appropriate time for yoga practice,[37] but actually he preferred the time before going to bed.[38]

Furthermore, Veṅkaṭanātha emphasised the great importance of sleep. Sleep is necessary to keep body and mind healthy in order to remain able to fulfill ritual duties.[39] For this purpose sleep is also a service to and a means of worshipping God. Veṅkaṭanātha presents a series of rules for how to fall asleep. These rules

34 PRR p. 76, ll. 11–13: "In the manner that is asserted by the *Brahmasūtra* [BSū] [with the words]: 'As no peculiarity [with regard to the place or time of meditation is prescribed, meditation should be practised] where and when intentness on a single object [is possible]' [BSū 4.1.11], it is suitable to practise yoga also at another time that is suitable for intentness on a single object, even if studying, which is [actually] appropriate, is canceled" (*'yatraikāgratā tatrāviśeṣāt' iti śārīrakasamarthitaprakāreṇa ekāgratānuguṇakālāntare 'pi svaguṇabhūta-svādhyāyādinirodhenāpi yogo 'nuṣṭhātuṃ yuktam.*); PRR p. 162, l. 6: "Since there is no restriction on the time for yoga, it [may] take place also at any other time that is adequate for intentness on a single object" (*yogakālāniyamād aikāgryānurūpe kālāntare 'pi kadācid bhavati.*); PRR p. 167, l. 1f.: "It was already taught that [yoga practice] also on another occasion that is adequate for intentness on a single object by abridgment of another rite has to be admitted" (*avasarāntare 'py aikāgryasambhave karmāntarasaṅkocena svīkārya iti prāg evoktam*).

35 PRR p. 152, l. 5f.: "And in a few particular *saṃhitā*-s, studying and yoga are prescribed [to be practised] simultaneously just before the daily final sacrifice (i.e., dinner)" (*etau ca svādhyāyayogau āhnikānuyāgāt pūrvam eva keṣucit saṃhitāviśeṣeṣu samāhṛtyopadiśyete*); PRR p. 168, ll. 6–8: "On the occasions for which there is a prohibition with [the words] 'the couple of equinox and solstice and the fifteenth [lunar day]', etc., studying in the form of Veda recitation is canceled. Then for [the devotee] who is devoted to no other [God], yoga, which is the most important, occupies the time of [studying]" (*'viṣuvāyanadvitayapañcadaśī' ityādinā pratiṣiddheṣv avasareṣu vedābhyāsarūpasvādhyāyo lupyate. tadā tatkālam apy ananyaparasya pradhānatamo yogaḥ samāskandati*).

36 PRR p. 158, l. 10f.: "And it was already shown that studying and yoga are moderately contained everywhere according to the occasion" (*svādhyāyayogayoś ca yathāvasaraṃ mātrayā sarvatrānupraveśaḥ prāg eva darśitaḥ*).

37 PRR p. 162, ll. 7–9: "The excellence of the pureness of the meditation on the Venerable One in the night is declared by the transmitted authoritative text (*smṛti*): 'Both one who has committed a minor misdeed and one who has committed a heinous crime should practise meditation on the *brahman* for a quarter of the night' [source unidentified]" (*yāminyāṃ bhagavaddhyānāsya tu pāvanatvātiśayaḥ smaryate – 'upapātakayukto 'pi mahāpātakavān api | yāminyāḥ pādam ekaṃ tu brahmadhyānaṃ samācaret || ' iti*).

38 PRR p. 166, ll. 1–5 (see below, n. 45).

39 Cf. also PādS *caryāpāda* 13.77ab and ŚrīprśS 17.68ab, according to which sleep removes mental afflictions (*kleśa*-s).

refer to the devotee's physical condition, such as cleanliness, not being naked, or holding one's head in the correct direction, but more than that they concern the thoughts the devotee should have while falling asleep.

The devotee should make himself aware of the place to which his self (*ātman*) moves while he is in deep sleep. Various passages in the Upaniṣads teach that this place consists of the bodily tubes (*nāḍī*), the heart sac, and the *brahman*. In order to solve this contradiction of teachings naming different places, Rāmānuja, Veṅkaṭanātha's great predecessor, whom he follows here and in many other contexts, taught that these various places should be understood in the same way that a palace, a bedframe, and a bed (i. e., mattress, etc.) relate to each other, with the bodily tubes representing the palace, the heart sac representing the bedframe, and the *brahman* representing the proper bed.[40]

Further, the devotee should consider deep sleep as an embrace of the supreme self (*paramātman*), i. e., God, in which he is oblivious to everything just as he would be in the arms of a beloved woman. He should make himself aware of the fact that just like everything else he does in his life sleep is also a form of worshiping God. He should think only of God, praise only him in chants, and fall asleep. Whenever he awakes, he should think only of God and chant the names of God until he falls asleep again:

> Thereafter, when he thinks that he has reached his aim on account of the great bliss in experiencing the Venerable One, which was attained without any effort, he should comfortably sit as long as it is agreeable for his body and his sense organs. Then he should not suppress sleep that occurs by itself for the sake of the repose of the sense organs, which are exerted by the manifold activities [and] which are the instruments for the yoga that will be practised [in the future], since [the *Bhagavadgītā*] transmits: "for one who is attentive with regard to sleep and wakefulness" (BhG 6.17c]. It is this very sleep that is then [his] service. And according to the principle of palace, bedframe and bed, which the Śārīrakasūtra teaches [with the words] "[Deep sleep, which is] the absence of [dreams, takes place] in the bodily tubes (*nāḍī*-s) and in the self (*ātman*), as this is taught by the sacred texts (*śruti*)" [BSū 3.2.7], he should think of the bedstead of his self (*ātman*) in the bodily tubes, the heart sac and the *brahman*. Chanting the word "Mādhava", which indicates an embrace of Lakṣmī, for the Venerable One, he should reflect upon the distinctiveness of the embrace of the supreme self (*paramātman*) in the manner that was taught by the sacred texts (*śruti*) [with the words]: "As a man embraced by a woman he loves [...] [so this person] embraced by the self (*ātman*) consisting of knowledge is oblivious to everything within or without."[41]. Considering also sleep as worship according to the method [taught with the words:] "What you do"[42], etc., he

40 See *Śrībhāṣya ad* BSū 3.2.7.

41 *Bṛhadāraṇyaka Upaniṣad* 4.3.21, translation by Patrick Olivelle (1998: 115).

42 Here, Veṅkaṭanātha refers to BhG 9.27: "What you do, what you enjoy, what you sacrifice, what you give, what you practise as austerities, Kaunteya, this offer to me" (*yat karoṣi yad aśnāsi yaj juhoṣi dadāsi yat | yat tapasyasi kaunteya tat kuruṣva madarpaṇam ||*).

> [should take] to a bed that is in accordance with the teachings at a place that suits the manner that is taught by the teachings, with clean and dry feet, his head directed at the enjoined direction, following the rules regarding cleanliness and not-nakedness. Placing his head on the lotus feet of the Venerable One, who is to be worshipped by him, in the manner that was taught by the Venerable Śāṇḍilyasmṛti,[43] etc., he should meditate in his heart only on Him, Mādhava, on account of the prescription "while sleeping, sitting, going, etc.",[44] praising in chants only Him and sleep well. And whenever sleep is interrupted, he should meditate only on Him. And he should chant the names [of God] again until he falls asleep.[45]

The next day, the devotee should get up at the *brāhma muhūrta,* at about three hours before sunrise[46].[47] This is the time that is generally recommended for

43 See ŚSmṛ 5.30c–31a: "When the mind organ remains at the lotus feet of the Venerable One, thinking stops motionlessly" (*yadā tu bhagavatpādasarasīruhayor manaḥ || niścalaṃ ramate cittaṃ*).

44 This is a variant of JS 4.47a; see PRR p. 72, l. 5f.

45 PRR p. 166, ll. 1–17: *ato niryatnalabdhena bhagavadanubhavānandasandohena kṛtārtho 'smīti manyamānaḥ karaṇakalebarānuguṇyāvadhi sukham āsīno vividhavyāpārāyas tasya kariṣyamāṇayogopakaraṇabhūtasya karaṇavargasya viśrāntaye svayam upanamantīṃ nidrāṃ na nivārayet. "yuktasvapnāvabodhasya" iti smaraṇāt. nidraiva tadā kaiṅkaryam. suṣuptau ca "tadabhāvo nāḍīṣu tacchruter ātmani ca" iti śārīrakasūtroktena prāsādakhaṭvāparyaṅkanyāyena nāḍīpurītadbrahmasu svātmanaḥ śayanam anusandhāya, lakṣmīpariṣvaṅgavyañjakena mādhavaśabdena bhagavantaṃ saṃkīrtayan, "yathā priyayā sampariṣvaktaḥ" ity ārabhya, "prājñenātmanā sampariṣvakto na bāhyaṃ kiṃcana veda nāntaram" ityāmnātaprakriyayā paramātmapariṣvaṅgaviśeṣaṃ ca parāmṛśya, "yat karoṣi" ityādiprasthānena nidrām api samārādhanatvena manyamānaḥ, saṃśuddhaśuṣkapādaḥ, śāstroktaprakāreṇa samucite sthāne śāstrīye śayanīye coditadikchirāḥ, śuddhatvānagnatvādiniyamayuktaḥ, śrīśāṇḍilyasmṛtyādyuktaprakāreṇa svārādhyasya bhagavataś caraṇāravindayor vinyastaśiraskaḥ, "śayanāsanayānādau" ityādividhānāt tam eva mādhavaṃ hṛdaye dhyāyan tam eva kīrtayan sukhaṃ śayīta. yadā yadā ca nidrāvicchedas tadā tadā tam eva dhyāyet. saṃkīrtayec ca tāni nāmāni punar ānidrāgamāt.*

46 It seems that there are different opinions about the time of the *brāhma muhūrta.* Cf. Rastelli 2006: 77f. where, based on Vijñāneśvara's commentary on the *Yājñavalkyasmṛti,* I concluded that the *brāhma muhūrta* is half a night watch long, i. e., one and a half hours, before sunrise. However, this does not fit the details Veṅkaṭanātha gives: According to DakṣSmṛ 2.54 (quoted in n. 29), a night consists of four night watches (*yāma*), each lasting three hours. A person should sleep for two night watches (ibid. and PRR p. 81, l. 10 – p. 82, l. 7, partly quoted in nn. 30, 31, 47, and 50) and get up when the last night watch has come (PRR p. 81, l. 12f., see n. 47). Thus we can conclude that for Veṅkaṭanātha, the *brāhma muhūrta* was about three hours before sunrise.

47 PRR p. 81, ll. 11–13: "First he should go to sleep at the proper time in order to repose. When the last night watch (*yāma*) of the night has come he should attentively give up sleep, as the transmitted authoritative texts (*smṛti*) teach: 'sleeping, however, for two night watches' (DakṣSmṛ 2.54c), 'for one who is attentive with regard to sleep and wakefulness' (BhG 6.17c), etc." (*pūrvam eva yathākālaṃ viśrāntyai nidrāṃ nirviśya prāpte yāminyāḥ paścime yāme sāvadhānena nidrā parityājyā "yāmadvayaṃ śayānas tu", "yuktasvapnāvabodhasya" ityādiṣu smaraṇāt*).

getting up in the Dharmaśāstra and also in medical texts,[48] and according to Veṅkaṭanātha it has special qualities. During the night, while being in deep sleep, the devotee has experienced the *brahman*, as was described just above, lying in its embrace, oblivious to everything else. Getting up at the early time of the *brāhma muhūrta* seems to make it possible to prolong this experience a little. The devotee is characterised by goodness (*sattva*), the highest of the three constituents (*guṇa*) of the material world, and has a clear mind, as Veṅkaṭanātha says, and thus possessing sattvic knowledge metaphorically functioning as a lamp, he can light up the darkness of sleep and experience the *brahman*. Such an early morning meditation has positive effects also on the success of the yoga practice in the next night.[49]

However, Veṅkaṭanātha is also liberal with regard to the time of getting up. The crucial factor is again the individual ability of a person. If one cannot get up that early for health reasons or if one is tired after practising yoga at the *brāhma muhūrta*, one is allowed to sleep even after the *brāhma muhūrta*.[50]

---

48 For example, *Baudhāyanadharmasūtra* 2.10.17.22, *Manusmṛti* 4.92, *Yājñavalkyasmṛti* 1.115, *Viṣṇusmṛti* 60.1, *Aṣṭāṅgahṛdaya sūtrasthāna* 2.1.

49 PRR p. 82, ll. 7–11: "In this way, having removed the darkness of sleep at the proper time, one becomes characterised by goodness (*sattva*) and clear-minded. Thereby the [*brahman*], which is to be meditated on, that, being characterised by manifold auspicious meditation objects (*śubhāśraya*)*, has been explored on the painted wall of the internal organ in the previous night watch, can be reflected upon, even if it is concealed by the darkness of sleep, in a proper manner by means of the light of a lamp having the form of sattvic knowledge, which has been inflamed by goodness (*sattva*) and was eclipsed at that time (i.e., in the night). And only thus the yoga (i.e., the union with the *brahman*) in the following night is effected" (*evaṃ prāptakālam apanītanidrātamaskatvena sattvasthaḥ prasannadhīś ca bhavati. tena pūrvayāmānusaṃhitam antaḥkaraṇacitrabhittigataṃ vicitraśubhāśrayaviśiṣṭaṃ dhyeyaṃ nidrātamo 'ntaritam api tatkālasamunmuṣitasattvasandhukṣitasāttvikajñānarūpapradīpaprakāśena samyag avalokyeta. tata eva cāpararātrayogo niṣpadyate*). * "Being characterised by manifold auspicious meditation objects" means that the *brahman* can be meditated upon by being imagined or visualised in the form of various meditation objects, such as a Vyūha or an idol. Cf. PRR p. 162, ll. 15–17: "Further, among the supports of the mind such as the Supreme One, the Vyūhas, etc., persons solely devoted to self-surrender, such as Nāthamuni, support themselves only on [God's] descent into an idol (*arcāvatāra*) as the mind's auspicious meditation object, which is to be contemplated also by persons, whose minds are absorbed (i.e., successful yogis) because [its] easy accessibility does not lead to a difference [of this form from the other forms] with regard to perfectness" (*eṣu ca paravyūhaprabhṛtiṣu cittālambaneṣu prapattyekaniṣṭhā nāthamuniprabhṛtayaḥ sulabhatamatvena paripūrṇatvāviśeṣāc ca samāhitacittānām apy anusandheyam arcāvatāram eva cetasaḥ śubhāśrayam ālambanta*). For a description of the *arcāvatāra* as a *śubhāśraya*, cf. also Srinivasa Chari 1994: 226.

50 PRR p. 81, l. 18 – p. 82, l. 4: "For this very reason, the Āyurveda, which is a sub-veda of the Atharvaveda according to [the statement:] 'Brahmā, having remembered the Āyurveda, which is a sub-veda of the Atharvaveda', the purpose of which is to protect the body, which is the most important instrument [for the fulfillment] of the Dharma, says: 'At the *brāhma muhūrta* he should get up, investigating if [he] has digested or not' and prescribes to sleep again till

3. The Nature of Yoga in the Context of the Five Time Periods

Let us now turn to the nature of yoga in the context of the five time periods, to the actual meaning of the term yoga and to the manner in which yoga is practised.

Generally, when the *saṃhitā*-s prescribe yoga in the context of the five time periods, they mean one of four things, which are, as we will see, not altogether different from each other: (1) mental visualisation of God, (2) meditation by which the devotee identifies himself with God, (3) the practice of several yogic techniques called *yogāṅga*-s, and (4) a technique that can be called *tattvayoga* (cf. PauṣS 33.90), by which the *tattva*-s that constitute the body are dissolved into each other up to their supreme source, which is God. The last two items also include the visualisation of God.

3.1. Mental Visualisation of God

Yoga before falling asleep very often means mere meditation on God. How this should be done is usually not described in detail. The verbs used for this meditation are √*dhyai, sam ā* √*dhā* and √*smṛ*, which are probably synonyms here.[51]

In the *saṃhitā*-s, the verb √*dhyai* and the noun *dhyāna* are usually used for a mental process in which an object is "mentally constructed" or "created"[52]. When successfully conducted, this object becomes subjectively present to the devotee, and in ritual, for example, he can mentally perform actions with regard to this object. This kind of "mental construction" usually has a strong visual com-

dawn if one has not yet digested" (*ata eva hi dharmasādhaneṣu pradhānatamaṃ śarīraṃ rakṣituṃ pravṛtte "brahmā smṛtvāyuṣo vedam upavedam atharvaṇāṃ" ity atharvaṇavedopavedabhūtāyurvede "brāhme muhūrta uttiṣṭhej jīrṇājīrṇe nirūpayan" ity abhidhāya, ajīrṇe punar āsandhyāgamanāt svāpo vidhīyate*) (The sources of the two Āyurveda quotations are unknown) and PRR p. 87, l. 13f.: "In the same way, provided that the one who has practised yoga properly is tired, another repose is allowed after the *brāhma muhūrta*" (*evaṃ yathāvadanuṣṭhitayogasya śrāntisambhāvanāyāṃ brāhmamuhūrtāt punar viśramo 'nujñāpyate*).

51 PauṣS 38.290d: "He should think of the Lord of the mantras within the heart" (*smaren mantreśvaraṃ hṛdi*), PauṣS 41.62ab: "Then he should concentrate on the interior part of the lotus of his heart" (*ācartavyaṃ samādhānaṃ svahṛtpadmāntare tataḥ* |), SS 6.192–193b: "He should concentrate on God being in [His] independent abode outside [of his body], with an unrestrained mind without any effort, till sleep properly comes together with Him" (*samādhāya bahir devaṃ nirālambapade sthitam* | *aprayatnena vai tāvad aniruddhena cetasā* [emendation based on PārS 7.439b, ĪS 6.84b, PRR p. 164, l. 9 and SSBh p. 116, l. 8; the edition reads *tejasā*) || 192 || *saha tenaiva vai nidrā yāvad abhyeti sāmpratam* |), PādS *caryāpāda* 13.74d: "having visualised the supreme person" (*dhyātvā paramapuruṣam*) (this is the only example adduced in this footnote that refers to midnight and not to the time before falling asleep), ŚrīprśS 17.61b: "visualising the all-pervading Nārāyaṇa" (*dhyāyan nārāyaṇaṃ vibhum*), ParāśaraS 4.155c: "having visualised Hari" (*hariṃ dhyātvā*).

52 Cf. Brunner 1994: 442.

ponent.[53] When the *saṃhitā*-s describe the *dhyāna* of a deity, they give a visual image, for example, the anthropomorphic form of Viṣṇu, his attributes, his garments, etc.[54]

Thus it is quite probable that *dhyāna* before falling asleep also means mental visualisation. The *Pauṣkarasaṃhitā* particularises that God should be visualised within the devotee's heart. The *Sāttvatasaṃhitā,* on the contrary, prescribes that God should be visualised outside of the devotee's body, in His supreme, transcendent abode. Further, the *Sāttvatasaṃhitā* says that this meditation before falling asleep should be conducted without effort because otherwise, during yoga practice with great effort, it would be hard to fall asleep, as the commentator of the *Sāttvatasaṃhitā* explains.[55]

3.2. Identifying Meditation

The object or process that is contemplated in yogic meditation depends on the view the yogi's tradition has on God, the world and the relationship between the two, or, vice versa, the philosophy and theology of a religious system coins the meditation object of a yogi. This fact is clearly visible in a passage that is an original part of the *Sāttvatasaṃhitā* and was reshaped and reinterpreted in other texts.

The *Sāttvatasaṃhitā* prescribes the following yogic practice to be performed at midnight: After sipping water, doing homage to his teachers and the deities, and sitting down on a seat made of the skin of a black antelope, the devotee should place the mantras of four manifestations of Viṣṇu, the so-called Vyūhas bearing the names Aniruddha, Pradyumna, Saṃkarṣaṇa, and Vāsudeva, on his body (SS 6.193c–198b).

This ritual is called *mantranyāsa,* "placing of mantras". It is very common in the Tantric traditions and usually performed before ritual worship. Through this ritual, particular aspects of God, which are expressed by the mantras, are made present on the devotee's body, by which the devotee becomes identical with God. In addition, the devotee also mentally identifies himself with God. The *man-*

53 Cf. TAK 3 s.v. *dhyāna.*

54 For examples see Rastelli 1999: 129–136.

55 Cf. *Sāttvatasaṃhitābhāṣya* (SSBh) p. 116, ll. 6–8: "If visualisation would be performed with an effortfully restrained mind here, sleep would not be possible. If there is no [sleep], a sound state of mind in order to practise yoga is not possible. With this intention, [the text] says: with an unrestrained mind without any effort" (*iha prayatnapūrvakaṃ cittanirodhaṃ kṛtvā dhyāne kṛte nidrā na sambhavati. tadabhāve yogaṃ kartuṃ cittasvāsthyaṃ na jāyata ity āśayenāprayatnenāniruddhena cetasety uktam*).

tranyāsa is thus a method for becoming identical with God, which is a necessary precondition for worshipping Him.[56]

Then, supported by a particular technique of breath control, the devotee should withdraw his mind[57] from all objects, dissolve the mind in the intellect (*buddhi*), and dissolve the intellect in God[58].[59] Then the devotee should draw his attention to one of the Vyūhamantras – at the beginning of his practice, this is the Aniruddhamantra, the lowest of the four – and mentally repeat it one hundred times. While meditating on this mantra, which is a manifestation of Aniruddha, the devotee should make himself aware that he is identical with Aniruddha, that he himself is Aniruddha, without any difference. Having successfully practised this, after a year or so the devotee starts to practise with the next mantra expressing Pradyumna and, in addition, increases the number of mental recitations. Later, he switches to the next mantra and so on, till he has reached complete identification with the supreme *brahman*.[60]

The relationship between the individual soul and God described in this passage of the *Sāttvatasaṃhitā* is clearly one of identity. God and the soul are completely identical, without any difference. The usages of terms like *abhinna*, "not different", *advaita*, "not dual", and *dhyātṛdhyeyāvibhāga*, "non-difference between meditating subject and meditation object" (SS 6.206d, 209b, 213c) do not leave any room for doubt about this.

This means that there are Advaitic concepts in the *Sāttvatasaṃhitā*, which is one of the early Pāñcarātra *saṃhitā*-s. If we consider this in the context of the whole tradition of Pāñcarātra, this is quite unusual. Normally, the *saṃhitā*-s do not teach complete non-difference between God and the soul. The usual concept is that the soul and God are identical in certain aspects, but in other aspects they are different. This is taught either in terms of a *bhedābhedavāda*, a doctrine that compares the relationship between God and the soul, for example, with that of the ocean and its waves – the waves are not identical with the ocean but also not different from it –,[61] or under the influence of Viśiṣṭādvaita Vedānta, the philosophical tradition to which the Pāñcarātra became most closely related.[62]

56 Cf., e.g., Rastelli 2009: 313.

57 The term used in this passage (SS 6.203) is *citta*, but it is meant in the sense of the *tattva manas*.

58 SS 6.203 gives *svagocare*, which Alaśiṅga Bhaṭṭa renders with *bhagavati* (SSBh p. 118, l. 13).

59 We will treat the dissolution of *tattva*-s on p. 241 ff. below.

60 SS 6.202–214. For a translation of SS 6.194c–214 into German and a detailed analysis of this and parallel passages, see Rastelli 2006: 507–516.

61 For examples from the *Jayākhyasaṃhitā* see Rastelli 1999: 49 f., 99, 115, 189 f.

62 Explicit examples of the usage of Viśiṣṭādvaitic key terms in the *saṃhitā*-s are rare, but see *śeṣa* and *śeṣin*, e.g., in *Ahirbudhnyasaṃhitā* 36.49 and 52.7, BhT 24.11 and *Bṛhadbrahmasaṃhitā* 2.2.47.

There is clear evidence that these Advaitic views were difficult to accept for later Pāñcarātrins. The *Pārameśvarasaṃhitā* uses the beginning and the end of the prescription for nocturnal yoga of the *Sāttvatasaṃhitā* but omits the part describing the devotee's identification with the Vyūhas and ultimately the *brahman.*[63] The same is true for the *Īśvarasaṃhitā*. In addition, this text changes the expression *dhyātṛdhyeyāvibhāga,* "non-difference between meditating subject and meditation object", to *dhyātṛjñeyavibhāga,* "difference between meditating subject and the object that has to be recognized".[64] Veṅkaṭanātha commented on this passage from the *Sāttvatasaṃhitā* and explained in great detail that it is not to be understood in the sense of an identity, but in the sense of a nondualism qualified by difference (*viśiṣṭādvaita*).[65] Alaśiṅga Bhaṭṭa, the commentator of the *Sāttvatasaṃhitā* from the nineteenth century, follows Veṅkaṭanātha's opinion (*Sāttvatasaṃhitābhāṣya* [SSBh] p. 119, l. 17 - p. 121, l. 14).

With regard to the topic of this chapter, yoga in the context of the *pañca kāla*-s, we can conclude that although the *saṃhitā*-s agree that yoga should at least include meditation on God, the form He is meditated on depends on the concept of God and his relation to the soul. This concept can differ in the various *saṃhitā*-s but in our particular example we see that the Pāñcarātric authors were eager to eliminate deviations from the mainstream.

4. *Yogāṅga*-s

A few *saṃhitā*-s understand yoga in the context of the *pañca kāla*-s as the form of yoga consisting of several yogic techniques generally known as *yogāṅga*-s. Mostly six or eight *yogāṅga*-s are listed, but sometimes their number is seven.

If they are six, they are usually listed as breath control (*prāṇāyāma*), withdrawal (*pratyāhāra*), visualisation (*dhyāna*), fixation (*dhāraṇā*), judgement (*tarka, ūha*), and absorption (*samādhi*). *Japa,* the recitation of mantras, is sometimes added between *dhāraṇā* and *tarka* as item number seven.[66]

63 PārS 7.438–440 ≈ SS 6.191c–194b, PārS 7.493–494 ≈ SS 6.213–214. See also Rastelli 2006: 507–512.

64 ĪS 6.83–86b ≈ SS 6.191c–194, ĪS 6.87–88 ≈ SS 6.213–214. See also Rastelli 2006: 512f.

65 PRR p. 84, l. 13 - p. 86, l. 9. For a translation into German and a detailed analysis of this passage see Rastelli 2006: 513–516.

66 In the context of the *pañca kāla*-s, SanS *ṛṣirātra* 1.13c–14 prescribes yoga with six limbs without listing these in detail: "Hari himself, the Lord of the deities, should be worshipped by the yoga that the yogis who are the best experts in yoga call yoga. This yoga comprising six limbs was indeed taught in the Padmodbhava" (*yo yoga iti samprokto yogibhir yogavittamaiḥ* || 13 || *tena yogena deveśaḥ pūjitaḥ syāt svayaṃ hariḥ* | *ṣaḍaṅgayukto yogaḥ sa uktaḥ padmodbhave kila* || 14 ||). The subsequent, long passage deals with breath control; for a detailed study on this see Rastelli forthc. PārS 7.441–477, a passage deriving from JS 33.1–37,

If eight *yogāṅga*-s are listed, these are: restraint (*yama*), observances (*niyama*), posture (*āsana*), breath control, withdrawal, fixation, visualisation, and absorption,[67] like the eight *yogāṅga*-s of classical yoga.[68]

As the list of six or seven limbs has been examined in detail elsewhere (Rastelli 1999: 323–342), I will focus here on the Aṣṭāṅga Yoga according to the *Nāradīyasaṃhitā,* the only place where this type of yoga is described in the context of the *pañca kāla*-s.[69]

The *Nāradīyasaṃhitā* lists ten *yama*-s: benevolence (*ānṛśaṃsya*), patience (*kṣamā*), truth (*satya*), non-violence (*ahiṃsā*), self-restraint (*dama*), rectitude (*ārjava*), giving (*dāna*), calmness (*prasāda*), loveliness (*mādhurya*), leniency (*mārdava*), and ten *niyama*-s: purity (*śauca*), worship (*ijyā*), austerities (*tapas*), truth (*satya*) (!), study (*svādhyāya*), restraint of sexual desire (*upasthanigraha*), religious observances (*vrata*), fasting (*upavāsa*), silence (*mauna*), meditation (*dhyāna*).[70] *Āsana* means the posture of the yogi, but the *Nāradīyasaṃhitā* does not describe particular details.[71] *Prāṇāyāma* is breath control, controlled inhaling, exhaling and retention of air and fixing the mind on this process.[72] *Pratyāhāra* means to withdraw the senses from their objects and direct them toward the mind.[73] *Dhāraṇā* means fixing the mind on an appropriate object.[74] If

describes yoga with six or seven limbs (on the unsolved question of six or seven see Rastelli 1999: 326 and Vasudeva 2004: 370, n. 4). The sequence given above is that from this passage but principally also other sequences of the six limbs are possible; see, e.g., Vasudeva 2004: 368.

67 This list is from the *pañca kāla* prescription in NārS 30.8c–21.

68 See *Pātañjalayogaśāstra* (PYŚ) 2.29–3.3.

69 In other contexts, eight-limbed and other forms of yoga are described also in other *saṃhitā*-s (e.g., *Ahirbudhnyasaṃhitā* 31–32, PādS *yogapāda*), but these cannot be dealt with here.

70 The lists of *yama*-s and *niyama*-s vary in the *saṃhitā*-s; cf. Rastelli 1999: 178–182.

71 NārS 30.12c–13b: "The posture of yogis that causes the complete accomplishment of yoga is taught as having the right measure (?), being immovable, [and] giving pleasure according to one's liking" (*pramāṇayuktam acalaṃ yathāruci sukhapradam* || *yogināṃ āsanaṃ proktaṃ yogasaṃsiddhikāraṇam* |).

72 NārS 30.13c–16b: "The effort of people to breathe, which results from inhaling, exhaling or retaining the air, is called breath control. First, one should fill the bodily tube (*nāḍī*) with air, then one should emit [the air]. Then one should retain the air. This sequence is taught. These, which are nothing but cessations, are known to possess the quality of [being mental] support. Another fourth [method] connected with [mental] support is known as that connected with an exterior or interior object" (*pūraṇād recanād vāyoḥ rodhanād vāpi* [emendation based on ParS 4.8; the edition reads *vā ca*] *yaḥ śramaḥ* || 13 || *bhavet prāṇakṛtaḥ puṃsāṃ prāṇāyāmaḥ sa ucyate* | *prathamaṃ pūrayen nāḍīṃ vāyunā recayet tataḥ* || 14 || *tatas tu stambhayed vāyuṃ kramo hy eṣaḥ prakīrtitaḥ* | *ete nirodhamātrās tu ālambanaguṇāḥ smṛtāḥ* || 15 || *sālambanaś caturtho 'nyo bāhyāntarviṣayaḥ smṛtaḥ* |). NārS 30.13c–14b is practically identical with ParS 4.8c–9b.

73 NārS 30.16c–17b: "The yoga expert should restrain the senses, which are attached to [their object such as] sound, etc., and make them follow the mind. [This is] called withdrawal" (*śabdādiṣv anuraktāni nigṛhyākṣāṇi* [emendation based on GherS 4.8; the edition reads *grāhyāṇy akṣāṇi*] *yogavit* || 16 || *kuryāc cittānukārīṇi pratyāhāraḥ prakīrtitaḥ* |) (≈ GherS 4.8).

this *dhāraṇā* is prolonged, it becomes *dhyāna,* visualisation.[75] *Samādhi* is an effect of prolonged *dhyāna,* in which the yogi grasps the pure nature of his object, without having any images or thoughts of his own.[76]

If we consider the functions of these *aṅga*-s, which altogether are means of ultimately reaching complete concentration on, or absorption into, an object, it becomes clear that also the other prescriptions for yoga or meditation in the context of the *pañca kāla*-s that do not use the structure or terminology of the *yogāṅga*-s nevertheless imply these techniques. Certain postures, breath control, and techniques for concentration are always necessary for yoga practice and sometimes also explicitly mentioned.[77] This means that prescriptions for Ṣaḍaṅga or Aṣṭāṅga Yoga actually do not necessarily differ from prescriptions that are not structured in the sense of *yogāṅga*-s.

5. Tattva Yoga

The fourth yogic technique can be called Tattva Yoga. In this kind of yoga, the principles (*tattva*) that constitute the yogi's body[78] are mentally dissolved into each other and finally into God himself who is their ultimate source. Then God is visualised and meditated on. In the end, the *tattva*-s are mentally recreated again.

A very clear and short description of this process is given in the *Bhārgavatantra:*

> He should cause earth to enter into water, water into fire, fire into air, and air into ether, ether into the individual soul, [and] the individual soul into the stainless, supreme *brahman.* (14) Every day, in the night, at midnight, during the ritual of yoga, an intelligent initiated person should bathe at a clean bathing place, sit down on a neat seat in the correct manner and, with a pure mind, visualise the supreme *brahman* in the following way: It is the consciousness in the centre of the lotus of the heart, the im-

74 NārS 30.17c–18b: "Fixing the mind immovably on a single auspicious object by lords of yogis is taught as fixation" (*śubhe hy ekatra viṣaye cetaso yac ca dhāraṇam* || 17 || *niścalena tu yogīndrair dhāraṇā tu samīritā* |).

75 NārS 30.18c–19b: "Repeated fixation on an object is always called visualisation by twice-born Bhāgavatas, oh Brahmin" (*paunaḥpunyena yatraiva viṣaye saiva dhāraṇā* || 18 || *dhyānam ity ucyate brahman sadā bhāgavatair dvijaiḥ* |).

76 NārS 30.19c–20b: "Mentally grasping the essential nature of the [object] without an image, which is to be effected by visualisation, is called absorption" (*tasyaiva kalpanāhīnaṃ svarūpagrahaṇaṃ hi yat* || 19 || *manasā dhyānaniṣpādyaṃ samādhis so 'bhidhīyate* |).

77 For descriptions or mentions of posture see SS 6.198c–201, PādS *caryāpāda* 13.75a, VDhP 1.65.1–15, of breath control see VDhP 1.65.16, BhT 25.12c–13.

78 The principles that are actually mentioned vary. In the examples quoted below, these are the five elements, i. e., earth, water, fire, air, and ether, and the individual soul (BhT), or the five elements, the mind organ (*manas*), the intellect (*buddhi*), and the individual soul (VDhP).

perishable light, (15–16) that has the shape of a *kadamba* bud,[79] that is eternally satisfied, free from illness, endless, made of bliss and thought, shining, all-pervading, (17) that resembles a lamp that is sheltered from wind, that shines like a real gem. An expert in yoga knowledge should spend his time visualising [the *brahman*] in this way. (18) At the end of yoga, he should create [the *tattva*-s] from the individual soul up to earth again in the sequence opposite of that of destruction, and he should satisfy God. (19)[80]

This process imitates the recurring process of creation and destruction of the world. The *tattva*-s, which constitute not only the yogi's body but also the whole world, are destroyed and recreated in the same sequence as they are destroyed and recreated at the time of the world's destruction and creation. The function of this process in the context of yoga practice is to eliminate the material world in order to reach its ultimate source, namely, God.[81]

A more detailed example of this yoga practice can be found in the *Viṣṇudharmottarapurāṇa:*

Having blocked his sense organs, a wise man should conquer breath by means of continued practice. Having conquered breath according to his ability, the intelligent man should practise yoga. (16)[82]

At the beginning, he should think of the gross [element] earth together with the five qualities [of the elements]. When the great yogi has reached this goal, he should give up

79 God being present as the individual soul in the lotus of the heart is compared with a flower of the *kadamba* tree also in other *saṃhitā*-s, see, e.g., JS 12.38 (cf. Rastelli 1999: 138). The *kadamba* flower is globular and orange-coloured (Syed 1990: 153).

80 BhT 25.14–19: *pṛthivīm apsu tā* [emendation; the edition reads *tāṃ*] *vahnau taṃ vāyāv ambare ca tam* | *taj* [reading of the manuscript from Tirupati that was used for the edition; the edition reads *taṃ*] *jīve taṃ pare brahmaṇy amale viniveśayet* || 14 || *rātrau niśīthe vimale snātvā tīrthe 'nvahaṃ sudhīḥ* | *āsane samyagāsīnaḥ vivikte 'malamānasaḥ* || 15 || *evaṃ dhyāyet paraṃ brahma yogakarmaṇi dīkṣitaḥ* | *hṛtpuṇḍarīkamadhyasthaṃ caitanyaṃ jyotir avyayam* || 16 || *kadambamukulākāraṃ nityatṛptaṃ nirāmayam* | *anantam ānandamayaṃ cinmayaṃ bhāsvaraṃ vibhum* || 17 || *nivātadīpasadṛśam akṛtrimamaṇiprabham* | *evaṃ dhyāyan nayet kālaṃ yogavidyāviśāradaḥ* || 18 || *yogāvasāne bhūyo 'pi layakramaviparyayāt* | *jīvādivasumatyantaṃ sṛṣṭvā devāya tarpayet* || 19 ||. For other prescriptions for this kind of yoga in the framework of the *pañca kāla*-s, see PādS *caryāpāda* 13.76–77b > ŚrīprśS 17.66–68b, PārS 7.484–494 (translated into German and discussed in Rastelli 2006: 491–502), and VDhP 1.65.16–37b (see below); see also PauṣS 34.3 and 33.90c–130.

81 A similar process appears in the so-called "purification of elements" (*bhūtaśuddhi*), which is performed before ritually worshipping God (see, e.g., JS 10; cf. Rastelli 1999: 210–238). Although also in the *bhūtaśuddhi* the supreme God is reached after the destruction of the material constituents of the body, the main aim of this mental ritual is a purification of the body, which is reached by recreating its constituents. One would expect such a purifying function also in the context of the yoga practice described previously, but I could not find any passage that explicitly says this. According to PādS *caryāpāda* 13.77ab (≈ ŚrīprśS 17.68ab), the sleep following yoga practice removes all mental afflictions (*kleśa*) but there is no statement about the function of yoga practice itself in these contexts.

82 VDhP 1.65.16: *sa baddhakaraṇo vidvān abhyāsāt pavanaṃ jayet* | *jitvā vāyuṃ yathāśakti yogaṃ yuñjīta buddhimā* ||.

[his] concentration on the [element] earth. (17)[83]
Then the visualisation endowed with four qualities with regard to water should be performed, oh Twice-born. When the man who practises concentration on water has reached his goal he should give up [his] concentration on water. (18)[84]
Then he should practise yoga endowed with three qualities with regards to fire, oh Twice-born. And when he has reached his goal also with regard to this, he should give up concentration on fire. (19)[85]
Then he should practise yoga endowed with two qualities with regards to air, oh Twice-born. And when he has reached his goal also with regard to this, he should give up air yoga. (20)[86]
Then the wise man should practise yoga endowed with one quality with regard to ether. And when he has reached his goal also with regard to this, he should obtain access to concentration on the mind. (21) A moon is taught [to represent] the mind organ.[87] Having taken aim above [himself] (?) at the lunar disc first, he should take as his goal the *puruṣa* with the length of a thumb in the centre of the lunar disc, which is as bright as a hundred moons and is adorned with all ornaments. (22–23)[88]
And when he has reached his goal also with regard to this, he obtains access to concentration on the intellect (*buddhiyoga*). And the intellect is the Venerable as sun. By means of visualisation (*dhyānayogena*), the intelligent man should at first behold everything [as being] in the solar disc. Restrained, exclusively devoted to this [meditation], well concentrated he should think of the *puruṣa* having the length of a thumb in the centre of the solar disc, which shines like a hundred suns and is adorned with all ornaments. (24–26)[89]
And when he has reached his goal also with regard to this, he himself should behold his eternal self that is present in himself by means of visualisation, oh Bhārgava. (27) Just as he should behold the *puruṣa* having the length of a thumb in the solar disc by means of visualisation, he should behold [the *puruṣa*] in himself, (28) in the receptacle of the lotus of the heart turned downwards, oh Best of the Bhṛgus.[90]

---

83 VDhP 1.65.17: *ādau tu cintayet sthūlāṃ bhūmiṃ pañcaguṇānvitām | labdhalakṣo mahāyogī bhūmiyogaṃ samutsṛjet* ||.

84 VDhP 1.65.18: *tataś caturguṇaṃ dhyānaṃ kartavyam udake dvija | labdhalakṣa apāṃ yogī jalayogaṃ samutsṛjet* ||.

85 VDhP 1.65.19: *tatas tu yogaṃ yuñjīta triguṇaṃ dvija tejasi | labdhalakṣaś ca tatrāpi vahniyogaṃ samutsṛjet* ||.

86 VDhP 1.65.20: *tatas tu yogaṃ yuñjīta pavane dviguṇaṃ dvija | labdhalakṣaś ca tatrāpi vāyuyogaṃ samutsṛjet* ||.

87 That is, the mind organ should be visualised in the form of a moon.

88 VDhP 1.65.21–23: *tatas tu ekaguṇaṃ yogaṃ yuñjīta gagane budhaḥ | labdhalakṣaś ca tatrāpi manoyogagatir bhavet* || 21 || *manasaś candramāḥ proktaḥ prathamaṃ candramaṇḍale | ūrdhvalakṣaṃ budhaḥ kṛtvā candramaṇḍalamadhyage* || 22 || *aṅguṣṭhamātre puruṣe lakṣabandhaṃ tu kārayet | śaśāṅkaśatasaṃkāśe sarvālaṅkārabhūṣite* || 23 ||.

89 VDhP 1.65.24–26: *labdhalakṣaś ca tatrāpi buddhiyogagatir bhavet | buddhiś ca bhagavān sūryaḥ prathamaṃ sūryamaṇḍale* || 24 || *samagram eva sampaśyed dhyānayogena buddhimān | sūryamaṇḍalamadhyasthaṃ śatasūryasamaprabham* || 25 || *aṅguṣṭhamātraṃ puruṣaṃ sarvābharaṇabhūṣitam | cintayet prayato nāma tatparaḥ susamāhitaḥ* || 26 ||.

90 VDhP 1.65.27–29b: *labdhalakṣaś ca tatrāpi nityam ātmānam ātmanā | ātmastham eva sampaśyed dhyānayogena bhārgava* || 27 || *aṅguṣṭhamātraṃ puruṣaṃ sūryabimbagataṃ*

And when he has reached his goal also with regard to this, he should think of the non-manifest state. (29) With regard to this he should think of [it] as light everywhere, outwards and inwards, not as sun, not as moon, [but] as entirely all-pervading [light]. (30)[91]

And when he has reached his goal also with regard to this, he should think of the supreme *puruṣa*. The sages declare the empty (*śūnya*) *puruṣa* for visualisation (?). (31) [Only] a man who has fixed his goal with regard to [an object] having a form is able to think of an empty [object]. Otherwise, thinking of an [object] without any support would be very difficult. (32) For cessation of mental activities seems very difficult to me. Effort should always be made at this and at conquering breath. (33) Fruitlessness is effected by the cessation of mental activities, conquest of breath, and devotional meditation[92] on the empty [*puruṣa*]. (34) Oh Rāma, a visualisation is called empty if one visualises the *puruṣa*, who possesses all qualities [perceivable] by the senses, who is omnipresent and all-pervading, as free from visibility, scent, taste, sound, and touch. A man who devotionally meditates on the empty [*puruṣa*] after having recognised His essential nature, oh Rāma, (35–36) attains fruitlessness when he is freed from all bonds.[93]

In the process described here, the first meditation objects are the five elements in sequence. Earth is imagined as being endowed with all five qualities: scent, taste, visibility, touch, and sound. The next element, water, is imagined to be endowed with the last four of these, fire with the last three, air with the last two, and ether with only its own quality, i. e., sound.[94] The next two principles that are visualised are the mind organ (*manas*) and intellect (*buddhi*). Like everything in the ma-

---

yathā | dhyānayogena sampaśyet tathā paśyet tathātmani || 28 || adhomukhe hṛtkamale karṇikāyāṃ bhṛguttama ||.

91 VDhP 1.65.29c–30: *labdhalakṣaś ca tatrāpi avyaktaṃ cintayet padam || 29 || bahir antaś ca sarvatra tejasā tatra cintayet | naivārkeṇa na candreṇa sarvaṃ vyāptam aśeṣataḥ || 30 ||.*

92 I understand the term *upāsanā* in the sense it is used by Rāmānuja; see, e. g., Srinivasa Chari 1994: 101–103.

93 VDhP 1.65.31–37b: *labdhalakṣaś ca tatrāpi puruṣaṃ cintayet param || śūnyaṃ tu puruṣaṃ dhyāne* [?] [emendation; the edition reads *dhyānaṃ*] *pravadanti manīṣiṇaḥ || 31 || sākāre baddhalakṣas tu śūnyaṃ śaknoti cintitum | anyathā tu sukaṣṭaṃ syān nirālambasya cintanam || 32 || cittavṛttinirodho hi duṣkaraḥ pratibhāti me | tatra yatnaḥ sadā kāryo vijaye pavanasya ca || 33 || cittavṛttinirodhena pavanasya jayena ca | upāsanayā* [emendation; the edition reads *upāsanāyā*] *śūnyasya niṣphalatvaṃ vidhīyate || 34 || arūpagandham arasaṃ* [emendation; the edition reads *anasaṃ*] *śabdasparśavivarjitam | sarvendriyaguṇaṃ rāma sarvasthaṃ sarvagaṃ ca yat || 35 || (taṃ dhyāyan puruṣaṃ tasya dhyānaṃ śūnyaṃ prakīrtitam |) tasya svarūpaṃ vijñāya rāma śūnyam upāsataḥ || 36 || sarvabandhanamuktasya niṣphalatvaṃ vidhīyate |.*

94 Usually, the five elements are also envisioned in a particular visual form; for an example see JS 10.26–57 (translated into German and discussed in Rastelli 1999: 216–223). The described distribution of the qualities was called "accumulation theory" (*Akkumulationstheorie*) by Erich Frauwallner. It is already found in natural philosophy passages of the *Mahābhārata* (e. g., MBh 12.224.35–40, see Frauwallner 1953: 113–123), furthermore in classical Yoga and Sāṃkhya (e. g., PYŚ 2.19 and *Yuktidīpikā* p. 225, ll. 14–19; I thank Philipp A. Maas for this information), and, with some modifications, in Vaiśeṣika (Frauwallner 1956: 32f., 43f., 123).

terial world, they are manifestations of God himself.[95] The *manas* is visualised as God having the form of the *puruṣa* with the length of a thumb[96] present in a lunar disc. The intellect is visualised as God having the form of the *puruṣa* with the length of a thumb present in a solar disc. Then the *puruṣa* with the length of a thumb in a solar disc is visualised within the devotee's heart, that is, his individual soul. Then God's "non-manifest state" (*avyakta pada*) is meditated on. While the three forms of the *aṅguṣṭamātra puruṣa* were visualised as light in a limited size, the "non-manifest state" is visualised as unlimited, all-pervading light.

The final aim is the supreme *puruṣa* (*parama puruṣa*). The supreme *puruṣa* should be meditated on as "empty" (*śūnya*), which means, as lacking all qualities. The *Viṣṇudharmottarapurāṇa* admits that this is a very difficult task and has to be practised for a while but the consecutive meditation on the elements with reduced qualities in each case was already a preliminary exercise for the meditation on the *śūnya puruṣa*. The qualities of the elements are the objects of sense organs: scent, the quality of earth, is perceived with the nose, taste, the quality of water, with the tongue, visibility, the quality of fire, with the eyes, touch, the quality of air, with the skin and sound, the quality of ether, with the ears. If, while meditating on various objects, step by step one quality, that is, one sensation, is reduced, one finally arrives at an object without any qualities, that is, without experiencing any sensation. This is what meditation on the *śūnya puruṣa* means: the realisation of the omnipresent and all-pervading *puruṣa* that does not possess any quality that can be perceived by sense organs. The final aim that is promised as a result of this practice is "fruitlessness" (*niṣphalatva*). This is not meant as negatively as it may appear, but rather means "fruitlessness" of the deeds (*karman*) one performs so that one is no longer bound by them and liberation from transmigration can be reached soon.[97]

Both examples of Tattva Yoga make clear that the mental destruction of the *tattva*-s is only a means of reaching the final meditation object, i.e., God. How God is meditated on can differ. It can be the supreme *brahman* as in the *Bhārgavatantra*, the empty *puruṣa* as in the *Viṣṇudharmottarapurāṇa*, God Vāsudeva in an anthropomorphic form,[98] or any other form in which God may appear.[99]

95 Cf. Rastelli 1999: 98f.

96 The *puruṣa* with the length of a thumb (*aṅguṣṭhamātra puruṣa*), a concept derived from the Upaniṣads (see *Kaṭha Upaniṣad* 4.12–13, 6.17; *Śvetāśvatara Upaniṣad* 3.13, 5.8), is God in the form of the individual soul that is present in the human being's heart in the Pāñcarātra texts (see JS 12.26, *Agnipurāṇa* 60.22, PādS *caryāpāda* 24.95).

97 Cf. VDhP 1.65.38: "Oh strong-armed man, when a century and a third have passed, the eternal supreme abode occurs as fruitlessness, oh Bhārgava" (*saṃvatsaraśate pūrṇe satribhāge mahābhuja | niṣphalatvaṃ paraṃ sthānaṃ dhruvaṃ bhavati bhārgava ||*).

98 See the example from the *Śrīpraśnasaṃhitā*. Here the anthropomorphic Vāsudeva is visualised first, then the *tattva*-s are mentally destroyed in order to reach this Vāsudeva: "[Supported] by breath control, the wise one should practise yoga by visualising the *puruṣa*

6. Veṅkaṭanātha

Let us now look at what Veṅkaṭanātha taught concerning the nature of yoga practice. Generally, Veṅkaṭanātha agreed with the prescriptions of the *saṃhitā*-s – as long as they did not contradict his own doctrines. And, by definition, they "never contradicted" his doctrines, as he is eager to show, for example, with regard to the *Sāttvatasaṃhitā*. As I have already mentioned (p. 239 above), the yoga exercise in this *saṃhitā* is characterised by Advaitic ideas but Veṅkaṭanātha invested a lot of energy in order to show that it has to be understood in a Viśiṣṭādvaitic sense.[100]

So according to Veṅkaṭanātha, yoga practice must involve considering the relationship between the individual soul and God as one of nondualism qualified by difference (*viśiṣṭādvaita*). But what does this mean in concrete terms?

Veṅkaṭanātha had a particular kind of devotee in mind: the so-called *prapanna*, "the one who has taken refuge".

In Viśiṣṭādvaita Vedānta, there are two important means to achieve liberation from transmigration: Bhakti Yoga and Prapatti Yoga. Among these two alternatives, Viśiṣṭādvaita Vedānta attaches much more importance to *prapatti* ("self-surrender"). While Bhakti Yoga is a "rigourous discipline and is restricted to a certain class of individuals", *prapatti* is a "much easier path intendend for all without any restriction of caste, creed and status of individuals".[101] Bhakti Yoga requires the acquisition of philosophical knowledge, strict observance of the religious rituals (known as Karma Yoga), and constant meditation on the in-

---

bearing a conch, a discus and a mace, wearing yellow garments, being of white colour, adorned with a garland of forest flowers and other [ornaments], the supreme Vāsudeva. He should withdraw the *tattva*-s into his self in the sequence of destruction. He should join his self with Vāsudeva who is present in the heart. Having visualised [him] in that way for a while, he should create [his] body out of [his] self [again]" (ŚrīprśS 17.64c–67b: *prāṇāyāmena puruṣaṃ śaṅkhacakragadādharam* || 64 || *pītāmbaraṃ śvetavarṇaṃ vanamālādibhūṣitam* | *vāsudevaṃ paraṃ dhyāyan yogaṃ kṛtvā vicakṣaṇaḥ* || 65 || *saṃhārakramam āśritya tattvāny ātmani saṃharet* | *hṛdi sthite vāsudeve svātmānam api yojayet* || 66 || *kaṃcit kālaṃ tathā dhyātvā sṛjed dehāt* [conj. *dehaṃ*] *tam ātmanaḥ* |).

99 See, for example, PārS 7.478c–483 (translated into German and discussed in Rastelli 2006: 481–491).

100 Cf. also PRR p. 158, ll. 12–15: "Now we will discuss yoga. With regard to this, the specific characteristic of the yoga with which a person without another goal (*ananyaprayojana*) is to be entrusted and which was taught by the Venerable Śāṇḍilyasmṛti [with the words]: 'Endowed with such qualitites is the supreme self', etc., has been explained already above. And the fact that [this] does not contradict the modes of yoga that are taught in the Venerable Sāttvata[saṃhitā], etc., is well established. [...]" (*atha yogaṃ vyākhyāsyāmaḥ. tatra, ananyaprayojanādhikartavyo yogaviśeṣaḥ "īdṛśaḥ paramātmāyam" ityādinā śrīśāṇḍilyasmṛtyuktaḥ prāg eva darśitaḥ. śrīsāttvatādyupadiṣṭayogaprakārāṇām avirodhaś ca samyak samarthitaḥ*).

101 Srinivasa Chari 1994: 261.

dividual self (known as Jñāna Yoga). When a devotee is successful in these three fields, he can practise Bhakti Yoga, which means "unceasing meditation on God until the person is able to perfect it to the extent of reaching a stage of God-realisation similar to the perceptual vision of God", in this and in all future lives until all *prārabdhakarman,* i. e., the karma which has already begun to show results, is erased.[102] In comparison, *prapatti* is much easier to perform. "It is to be observed only once in the form of absolute self-surrender at the feet of God, with all humility, faith and the realisation of one's utter incapacity to adopt any other means of *mokṣa.*"[103] Liberation from transmigration can be achieved already in this life "as soon as the *prārabdha-karma* [...] is eradicated by enduring it".[104]

If sole self-surrender that is observed only once is enough in order to achieve liberation from transmigration, then basically the performance of the rites of the five time periods, which also include yoga practice, would not be necessary. However, Veṅkaṭanātha devoted a huge part of his *Pāñcarātrarakṣā* (p. 55, l. 5 – p. 79, l. 4) to establish that this is not the case. According to him, even a *prapanna* must perform the *pañca kāla* rites and thus he also must practise yoga. Just as he still has to perform worship rituals, not in order to gain personal benefit, but as an end in itself,[105] he has to practise yoga as an end in itself, in order to experience bliss through its practice – just as one also enjoys the bliss of being God's servant while ritually worshipping Him –, but not in order to achieve any other end.[106]

102 Srinivasa Chari 1994: 266 and 355.

103 Srinivasa Chari 1994: 266.

104 Ibid.

105 Cf. Rastelli 2007.

106 PRR p. 55, ll. 9–13: "The opposing view is: [The rites of the five time periods] are to be given up [by one who has taken refuge] [...] and because, if yoga, which is a part of these, was effective, one would have to accept the conclusion that the [rites of the five time periods] alone would be a means [for achieving liberation from transmigration]" ([...] *tadekadeśabhūtayogaśaktau ca tasyaivopāyatvasvīkāraprāpter* [...] *parityājya iti pūrvaḥ pakṣaḥ*) and p. 59, ll. 1–8: "If moreover it is said: 'If yoga was effective, one would assent that the [rites of the five time periods] alone would be a means [for achieving liberation from transmigration]', this is also stupid because it is generally known that those who perceived the three *tattva*-s (i. e., the *brahman,* the individual soul, and the material universe; cf. Srinivasa Chari 1994: xxix) by means of the power of their yoga, such as Nāthamuni and Kurukeśvara, who were exclusively devoted to the means of self-surrender that [they] had adopted before, also afterwards enjoyed the bliss of the Venerable One that derives from yoga [and] is obtained by the Venerable One's grace; [and] because otherwise, if the worship, etc., taught by the author of the [Śrī]bhāṣya, which is preceded by contemplation of such a kind (i. e., that is similar to yoga), was effective there would be the undesirable consequence of assenting that also this would be a means [for achieving liberation from transmigration]. Consequently, if 'having the form of service for the Lord'* is accepted as an end in itself on account of the great sweetness [of worship], also in the case of absorption, which has the nature of an abundance of happiness that is deprived of something that is equal or superior, this is the same justification" (*yac cānyad uktaṃ yogaśaktau tasyaivopāyatvasvīkāraḥ prāpnotīti tad api mandam. svayogamahimapratyakṣitatattvatrayāṇāṃ nāthamunikuru-*

Veṅkaṭanātha compares the devotee practising yoga with a hungry person who eats food. Just as eating food is necessary in order to sustain one's life, yoga practice is necessary in order to nourish the soul and keep it alive.[107]

Veṅkaṭanātha's prescriptions of how to practise yoga are strongly based on the *Vaikuṇṭhagadya* (VaiG). The *Vaikuṇṭhagadya* is a text belonging to a group of three Gadyas, the others being *Śaraṇāgatigadya* and *Śrīraṅgagadya*. These are short texts dealing with *prapatti* and the manner in which to perform *prapatti*. The tradition, and thus also Veṅkaṭanātha, attributes them to Rāmānuja.[108]

Among the three Gadyas, Veṅkaṭanātha considers the contents of the *Vaikuṇṭhagadya* as especially appropriate for the practice of yoga.[109] Consequently,

---

keśvaraprabhṛtīnāṃ prākparigṛhītaprapattyupāyaikaniṣṭhānām eva paścād api bhagavatprasādalabdhayaugikabhagavadānandāsvādasya prasiddhatvāt; anyathā tathāvidhānusandhānapūrvakabhāṣyakāroktasamārādhanādiśaktau tasyāpy upāyatvasvīkāraprasaṅgāt. tac cet svāmikaiṅkaryarūpam iti svādutamatayā svayamprayojanatvenopādīyeta samādhāv apy ayaṃ samādhikadaridrasukhasandohātmani samaḥ samādhiḥ*). * This expression could refer to *Nityagrantha* p. 182, l. 5f.: *tatas tadanubhavajanitātimātraprītikāritaparipūrṇakaiṅkaryarūpapūjām ārabheta*, "Then he should start [to perform] the complete ritual worship that causes measureless pleasure produced by experiencing that [God is his master]."

107 PRR p. 159, l. 11 – p. 160, l. 5: "In the Śrīvaikuṇṭhagadya, however, only self-surrender has been prescribed as the means for liberation for a person without another refuge. For the same [person], the peculiarity of yoga consisting in visualisation (*dhyānayoga*) as being only an end in itself just as a hungry healthy person consumes milk and food, etc., and the peculiarities of the contemplation connected with [yoga] have been fully described. [...] Having prescribed only choosing refuge as the means for liberation [with the words]: 'His whole being focussed on Him, which nourishes the soul that has no other [end], he should take refuge with [His] pair of lotus feet' [VaiG p. 189, l. 13], [and] having prescribed the peculiarity of the recollection in order to nourish the soul of the very person devoted to independent self-surrender according to the principle of eating, etc., daily in order to protect [one's] life [with the words]: 'And thereafter he should recollect in this manner in order to nourish the soul daily' [VaiG p. 189, l. 14] [...]" (*śrīvaikuṇṭhagadye tu ananyagateḥ prapattim evāpavargopāyaṃ vidhāya, tasyaiva kṣudhitasyārogasya kṣīrānnabhojanādivat svayamprayojanatayaiva dhyānayogaviśeṣaḥ tadanubandhyanusandhānaviśeṣāś ca prapañcitāḥ.* [...] *"caraṇāravindayugalam ananyātmasaṃjīvanena tadgatasarvabhāvena śaraṇam anuvrajet" iti śaraṇavaraṇam eva mokṣopāyatvena vidhāya, "tataś ca pratyaham ātmojjīvanāyaivam anusmaret" iti svatantraprapattiniṣṭhasyaiva pratyahaṃ prāṇarakṣaṇārthabhojanādinyāyena ātmojjīvanārtham anusmaraṇaviśeṣaṃ vidhāya*). Independent self-surrender (*svatantraprapatti*) means to apply the means of self-surrender alone without practising Bhakti Yoga in addition; cf., e.g., Srinivasa Chari 1994: 264f.

108 Some modern scholars doubt that the three Gadyas are authentic works of Rāmānuja, but the actual authorship of these texts is not important in our context. For a short summary of the discussion of the authorship and content of the Gadyas, see Raman 2007: 40–47.

109 PRR p. 161, l. 9 – p. 162, l. 1: "Moreover, with regard to this [subject] (i.e., yoga), among the three Gadyas, which have the form of a commentary on the *dvaya*[*mantra*], the brief Gadya's (i.e., the Śrīraṅgagadya's) contemplation is appropriate for the matutinal approaching, because it deals mainly with despondency and because service is one of its eminent topics. The long Gadya (i.e., the Śaraṇāgatigadya) in turn is enjoined by the author of the [Śrī]bhāṣya himself for the beginning and the end of ritual worship by saying 'Having

his description of the *prapanna*'s yoga practice in the *Pāñcarātrarakṣā* is a kind of commentary on this text.[110]

The procedure starts with the devotee's taking refuge in God. Veṅkaṭanātha emphasises various components of this act of taking refuge: the devotee mentally determines[111] that God Nārāyaṇa, that is, Viṣṇu, is both the means and the goal; he realises that there is no other end than the wish to obtain God and that there is no other means for obtaining God than taking refuge in Him:

> That is to say, by saying "having comprehended the one who controls the variety of essential nature, existence, and activity of the three sentient and the three non-sentient [entities][112] [...] as master, friend and teacher" (VaiG p. 189, ll. 5–7), he expresses the conviction that the one who grants refuge is both the goal to be achieved and the one leading to the goal. Afterwards, by saying "only wishing to serve [Him] exclusively and permanently" [VaiG p. 189, l. 8], he establishes that there is no other aim than the wish to

---

contemplated the specifications of [His] essential nature, form, qualities, manifestation of power (*vibhūti*), and instruments of sport as they are in reality, he should take refuge only in Him by [saying] *akhila*, etc.' [*Nityagrantha* p. 182, l. 3], as [this Gadya] is the cause for the correct contemplation of [His] essential nature, form, qualities, manifestation of power (*vibhūti*), goddess, ornaments, weapons, attendants, entourage, doorkeeper, companions, etc., which are to be contemplated especially at the time of ritual worship. The Śrīvaikuṇṭhagadya in turn is to be contemplated especially at the time reserved for the purpose of yoga, because it starts with 'Having immersed myself in the noble ocean of nectar of Yāmuna to the best of my knowledge and having acquired the jewel called Bhakti Yoga, I will present [this Bhakti Yoga]' [VaiG p. 189, l. 3f.], because it later says: 'by means of visualisation he should see' [VaiG p. 190, l. 29], because it prescribes various contemplations that differ [from each other] on account of the form of [their] result, and because it says specifically: 'He should continue looking [only at the Venerable One] by means of a gaze in form of an uninterrupted stream' [VaiG p. 191, l. 18f.]. Thus the intention of the author of the [Śrī]bhāṣya can be ascertained" (*api cātra dvayavyākhyānarūpe gadyatraye nirvedabhūyastayā kaiṅkaryatvātiśayāc* [corrected for *kaiṅkaryatvarātiśayāc*] *ca prābhātike 'bhigamane mitagadyānusandhānam ucitam. bṛhadgadyaṃ tu samārādhanākāle viśeṣato 'nusandheyānāṃ svarūparūpaguṇavibhūtidevībhūṣaṇāyudhaparijanaparicchadadvārapālapārṣadādīnāṃ yathāvadanusandhānahetutayā "yathāvasthitasvarūparūpaguṇavibhūtilīlopakaraṇavistāram anusandhāya tam eva śaraṇam upagacched akhiletyādinā" iti samārādhanasyādāv ante ca bhāṣyakārair eva viniyuktam. śrīvaikuṇṭhagadyaṃ tu, "yāmunāryasudhāmbhodhim avagāhya yathāmati | ādāya bhaktiyogākhyaṃ ratnaṃ sandarśayāmy aham ||" iti prārambhāt, paścād api "dhyānayogena dṛṣṭvā" ity abhidhānāt, phalarūpavilakṣaṇānusandhānabhedānāṃ vidhānāt, "avicchinnasrotorūpeṇāvalokanenāvalokayann āsīta" iti kaṇṭhokteś ca, yogārthakalpite kāle viśeṣato 'nusandheyam iti bhāṣyakārāśayaḥ pratīyate*). Cf. also PRR p. 57, ll. 9–16.

110 Apart from this passage in the *Pāñcarātrarakṣā*, Veṅkaṭanātha also wrote a commentary on the *Vaikuṇṭhagadya* in his *Gadyatrayabhāṣya*.

111 On the term *adhyavasāya*, "mental determination", cf. Raman 2007: 153f.

112 The three sentient entities are the bound (*baddha*), liberated (*mukta*), and eternally free (*nitya*) souls. The non-sentient entities are primary matter (*prakṛti*), time (*kāla*), and the "transcendental universe" (*nityavibhūti*; for the concept of *nityavibhūti* see Srinivasa Chari 1994: 233–243) (*Rahasyatrayasāra* p. 140, ll. 1–3). I would like to thank Marcus Schmücker for finding this passage for me.

achieve this specific goal of life (*puruṣārtha*). Then, by saying: "Thinking that even for a thousand crores of ages there is no other means for me than self-surrender (*prapatti*) to His pair of lotus feet in order to achieve Him" [VaiG p. 189, l. 8 f.], he speaks about the contemplation that there is no other means. After that, by saying "of just this Venerable One, [...] of the one who possesses the great realm manifesting His rule,[113] the illustrious one" [VaiG p. 189, ll. 9–13], he designates the forms in which He can grant refuge, etc. Subsequently, by saying: "His whole being directed at Him, a person who nourishes his soul that is directed at nobody else, he should take refuge to His pair of lotus feet" [VaiG p. 189, l. 13], he declares that only choosing refuge is a means for liberation.[114]

After this mental act of taking refuge, the devotee should remember Nārāyaṇa daily, in order to nourish his soul, as mentioned above,[115] in a particular way: He should visualise God together with his consort Śrī in the heavenly world Vaikuṇṭha:

Having extensively depicted the supreme abode, which is in the One who is to be achieved, he describes the complete visualisation by saying: "By means of visualisation he should see the Venerable Nārāyaṇa, [...] seated together with Śrī on the great serpent Ananta, who is the divine yoga couch. As His loveliness [Śrī] makes the universe prosper, [the universe] which includes the divine world such as the sovereignty, etc., of the splendid Vaikuṇṭha,[116] she commands the entire entourage such as Śeṣa, Śeṣāśana, etc., to worship Him [in a manner that is] appropriate to His respective states, [and] she corresponds to Himself on account of [her] virtue, form, qualities, play, etc." [VaiG p. 190, ll. 7–9 and p. 190, l. 28 f.].[117]

---

113 The term *mahāvibhūti* is difficult to translate. This translation is based on Carman 1974: 143; for the meaning of *vibhūti*, see Carman 1974: 140–146.

114 PRR p. 159, l. 14 – p. 160, l. 3: *tathā hi – "svādhīnatrividhacetanācetanasvarūpasthitipravṛttibhedam" ity ārabhya "svāmitvena suhṛttvena gurutvena ca parigṛhya" ityantena prāpyaprāpakabhūtaśaraṇyādhyavasāyam uktvā, anantaram "aikāntikātyantikaparicaryaikamanorathaḥ" iti puruṣārthaviśeṣalipsāyā ananyaprayojanatāṃ pratipādya, "tatprāptaye ca tatpādāmbujadvayaprapatter anyan na me kalpakoṭisahasreṇāpi sādhanam astīti manvānaḥ" ity ananyopāyatānusandhānam abhidhāya, "tasyaiva bhagavataḥ" ityādinā "mahāvibhūteḥ śrīmataḥ" ityantena śaraṇyatvādyupayuktākārān abhidhāya, "caraṇāravindayugalam ananyātmasaṃjīvanena tadgatasarvabhāvena śaraṇam anuvrajet" iti śaraṇavaraṇam eva mokṣopāyatvena vidhāya.*

115 PRR p. 160, ll. 3–5; see n. 107.

116 The expression *śrīmadvaikuṇṭhaiśvaryādidivyalokam* is problematic because Vaikuṇṭha is the divine world (*divyaloka*) itself and not a part of it (cf. Rastelli 2003: 428, based on the *Nityagrantha* and *Vaikuṇṭhagadya*). In his commentary on this passage, Veṅkaṭanātha tries to solve the problem in the following way: "In the passage *śrīmadvaikuṇṭhaiśvaryādidivyalokam,* however, the word *vaikuṇṭha* means a place situated within [it] such as a town. This very [place] is metaphorically designated with the word *aiśvarya* [power, might] since [it] has the form of an excellent manifestation of power (*vibhūti*)" (*Gadyatrayabhāṣya* p. 192, l. 11 f.: *śrīmadvaikuṇṭhaiśvaryādidivyalokam ity atra tu vaikuṇṭhaśabdena nagarādyavāntarapradeśo vivakṣitaḥ; sa eva praśastavibhūtirūpatvād aiśvaryaśabdenopacaryate*).

117 PRR p. 160, ll. 5-10: *vistareṇa prāpyāntargataṃ paramapadaṃ varṇayitvā, "mahati divyayogaparyaṅke 'nantabhogini śrīmadvaikuṇṭhaiśvaryādidivyalokam ātmakāntyā viśvam āpyāyayantyā śeṣaśeṣāśanādikaṃ sarvaṃ parijanaṃ bhagavatas tattadavasthocitaparica-*

After this visualisation, the devotee intensifies his wish to obtain God:

> Further, by saying "[...] of the Venerable One, [...] having strengthened the wish to worship the Venerable One" VaiG p. 190, l. 29 – p. 191, l. 7], he teaches the types of wishes for the achievement of the objects of men such as "If Kākutstha leads me away, this will be worthy of him" [*Rāmāyaṇa* 5.37.29cd] [and] "When will the Lord see me?" [*Rāmāyaṇa* 5.35.6d].[118]

Through this wish, which is strengthened by God's grace, the devotee approaches Him, bows down again and again, reciting a mantra devoted to Nārāyaṇa:

> Then he speaks about approaching the Venerable One by means of this wish, which is strengthened by His grace,[119] bowing from afar to the Venerable One and His retinue [while reciting] the mantra "[Homage to the illustrious Nārāyaṇa] with His entire retinue" [VaiG p. 191, l. 9], standing up and bowing again and again.[120]

He comes even closer to God and offers himself to Him. God, with a gaze full of love, accepts him and permits him to worship Him. The devotee worships Him, serving Him fearfully and modestly. He experiences unsurpassable joy that makes him unable to do, see or remember anything else, and remains immersed in an ocean of bliss, his self (*ātman*) being nourished by gazing at God:

> Immediately afterwards he teaches contemplation in the following way: "Bent down by excessive fear and modesty, beheld by a gaze of compassion filled with affection of the Venerable One's retinue, leaders of the attendants [and] doorkeepers, saluted respectfully [by them] in the correct manner, approved by these various [divine beings], he should approach the Venerable One [while reciting] the illustrious *mūlamantra*. He should bow, begging 'Accept me for serving [You] exclusively and permanently', and offer himself to the Venerable One. Then, taken into possession and assented by a gaze full of excessive love of the Venerable One, whose virtues are without limits, in order to be [His] permanent subordinate who is suitable for all places, all times, and all circumstances, he should worship the Venerable One, bent down by excessive fear and modesty, serving [Him] joining the palms of his hands for obeisance. And then, characterised by a state that is experienced, on account of unsurpassed pleasure being unable to do, see [or] think anything else, he should ask again for being [His] subordinate and continue looking only at the Venerable One by means of a gaze in the form

---

ryāyām ājñāpayantyā śīlarūpaguṇavilāsādibhir ātmānurūpayā śriyā sahāsīnam" ityādinā "bhagavantaṃ nārāyaṇaṃ dhyānayogena dṛṣṭvā" ityantena paripūrṇadhyānam uktvā. On Vaikuṇṭha see Rastelli 2003 (with a translation of the *Vaikuṇṭhagadya*'s description of Vaikuṇṭha on p. 428f.).

118 PRR p. 160, ll. 10–13: *punaḥ "bhagavataḥ" ity ārabhya "bhagavatparicaryāyām āśāṃ vardhayitvā" ityantena "māṃ nayed yadi kākutsthas tat tasya sadṛśaṃ bhavet", "kadā drakṣyati māṃ patir" ityādivat puruṣārthaprāptimanorathaprakārān pratipādya.*

119 *Tayaivāśayā tatprasādopabṛṃhitayā* is an expression that appears in VaiG p. 191, l. 7f.

120 PRR p. 160, ll. 13–16: *tayaivāśayā tatprasādopabṛṃhitayā bhagavadabhigamanaṃ dūrāt saparivārasya bhagavato nārāyaṇasya "samastaparivārāya" ityādinā mantreṇa praṇamya, utthāya punaḥ punaḥ praṇāmaṃ cābhidhāya.*

of an uninterrupted stream. Then, having looked [at Him] by means of the gaze that nourishes the self (*ātman*) on account of the Venerable One Himself, he should invite [Him] with a smile and, visualising that the pair of lotus feet of the Illustrious One, which removes all mental afflictions (*kleśa*), confers unsurpassed pleasure [and] belongs to himself (?) (*ātmīya*), is placed on [his] head, he should sit comfortably, all limbs immersed in an ocean of immortality" [VaiG p. 191, ll. 10–22].[121]

7. Conclusion

What can we conclude from all these details? We have seen that yoga is an essential component of the life of a Pāñcarātrin, not only as yogic techniques used in ritual, but also as an independent, autonomous practice. It is practised daily before sleep, between two phases of sleep, and/or after sleep, and in many different forms. Its function is not only to train the mind, but to make the devotee aware of the nature of God and of his relation to God. When practised before falling asleep (and this is also the case if practised between two phases of sleep), it is especially effectful, because the insights gained in yoga practice can be deepened in sleep. The contents of these insights, however, depend on the theology of the tradition or sub-tradition the devotee belongs to.

References

Primary Sources

Agnipurāṇa
Agnipurāṇa of Maharṣi Vedavyāsa, ed. Bāladeva Upādhyāya. Kashi Sanskrit Series 174. Varanasi: Chowkhamba Sanskrit Series Office, 1966.

121 PRR p. 160, l. 16 – p. 161, l. 8: *anantaram evam anusandhānam uktam – "atyantasādhvasavinayāvanato bhūtvā bhagavatpārṣadagaṇanāyakair dvārapālakaiḥ kṛpayā snehagarbhayā dṛśāvalokitaḥ samyagabhivanditas tais tair evānumato bhagavantam upetya śrīmatā mūlamantreṇa mām aikāntikātyantikaparicaryākaraṇāya parigṛhṇīṣveti yācamānaḥ praṇamya, ātmānaṃ bhagavate nivedayet. tato bhagavatā amaryādaśīlavatā atipremānvitenāvalokanena sarvadeśasarvakālasarvāvasthocitātyantaśeṣabhāvāya svīkṛto 'nujñātaś ca atyantasādhvasavinayāvanataḥ kiṃkurvāṇaḥ kṛtāñjalipuṭo bhagavantam upāsīta. tataś cānubhūyamānabhāvaviśeṣo niratiśayaprītyā anyat kiṃcit kartuṃ draṣṭuṃ smartum aśaktaḥ punar api śeṣabhāvam eva yācamāno bhagavantam evāvicchinnasrotorūpeṇa avalokanenāvalokayann āsīta. tato bhagavatā svayam evātmasaṃjīvanenāvalokanenāvalokya sasmitam āhūya samastakleśāpahaṃ niratiśayasukhāvaham ātmīyaṃ śrīmatpādāravindayugalaṃ śirasi kṛtaṃ dhyātvā amṛtasāgarāntarnirmagnasarvāvayavaḥ sukham āsīta" iti.*

Ahirbudhnyasaṃhitā
Ahirbudhnya-Saṃhitā of the Pāñcarātrāgama, ed. M. D. Ramanujacharya under the Supervision of F. O. Schrader. 2 vols. 2nd rev. ed. V. Krishnamacharya. The Adyar Library Series 4. Madras: The Adyar Library and Research Centre, 1916 (repr. 1966).

Aṣṭāṅgahṛdaya
Aṣṭāṅgahṛdaya (A Compendium of the Āyurvedic System) of Vāgbhaṭa With the Commentaries 'Sarvāṅgasundarā' of Aruṇadatta and 'Āyurvedarasāyana' of Hemadri, ed. Hari Sadāśiva Śāstrī Parāḍakara. Kashi Sanskrit Series 315. 6th ed. Bombay: Nirnayasagara Press, 1939 (repr. Varanasi: Chaukhamba Sanskrit Sansthan, 2010).

Baudhāyanadharmasūtra
Das Baudhāyanadharmasūtra, ed. W. Hultzsch. 2nd ed. Abhandlungen für die Kunde des Morgenlandes 16.2. Leipzig: Brockhaus, 1922 (repr. Nendeln, Liechtenstein: Kraus, 1966).

BhG. *Bhagavadgītā*
In *Gītārthasaṃgraharakṣā, Gītābhāṣyatātparyacandrikā ca. paryavekṣakaḥ pariṣkārakaś ca Aṇṇaṅgarācāryaḥ.* Śrīmadvedāntadeśikagranthamālā vyākhyāvavibhāga 2. Kāñjīvaram: n.p., 1941.

BhT. *Bhargavatantra*
Bhargava Tantram (A Pancaratragama Text), ed. Raghava Prasad Chaudhary. Ganganath Jha Kendriya Sanskrit Vidyapeetha Text Series 8. Allahabad: Gaṅgānātha Jhā Kendrīya Saṃskṛta Vidyāpīṭham, 1981.

Bṛhadāraṇyakopaniṣad
In V. P. Limaye & R. D. Vadekar (Eds.), *Eighteen Principal Upaniṣads: Upaniṣadic Text with Parallels from extant Vedic Literature, Exegetical and Grammatical Notes.* Vol. 1 (pp. 174–282). Poona: Vaidika Saṃśodhana Maṇḍala, 1958.

Bṛhadbrahmasaṃhitā
Nāradapañcarātrāntargatā Bṛhadbrahmasaṃhitā. etat pustakaṃ Ś. Veṇegāvakarabhiḥ saṃśodhitam. Ānandāśramasaṃskṛtagranthāvaliḥ 68. Poona: Ānandāśramamudraṇālaya, 1912.

BSū. *Brahmasūtra*
see *Śrībhāṣya.*

DakṣSmṛ. *Dakṣasmṛti*
Dakṣa-Smṛti. Introduction, Critical edition, Translation and Appendices by Irma Piovano. Corpus Juris Sanscriticum 1. Torino: Comitato Promotore per la Pubblicazione del Corpus Juris Sanscriticum, 2002.

Gadyatrayabhāṣya
In *Srimad Vedanta Desika's Chatusslokibhashyam, Sthothraratnabhashyam, and Gadyatrayabhashyam*, ed. V. Srivatsankacharyar (pp. 125–193). Madras: Sri Vedanta Desika Seventh Centenary Trust, n. d.

Gheraṇḍasaṃhitā
P. Thomi, *Das indische Yoga-Lehrbuch Gheraṇḍa-Saṃhitā. Aus dem Sanskrit übersetzt, kommentiert und herausgegeben.* Wichtrach; Institut für Indologie, 1993.

ĪS. *Īśvarasaṃhitā*
Īśvarasaṃhitā, ed. P. Bh. Anantācārya. Śāstramuktāvaḷī 45. Kāñcī: Sudarśana, 1923.

JS. *Jayākhyasaṁhitā*
Jayākhyasaṁhitā. Critical Edition With an Introduction in Sanskrit, Indices etc., ed. E. Krishnamacharya. Gaekwad's Oriental Series 54. Baroda: Oriental Institute, 1931.
Kaṭha Upaniṣad
Kaṭhopaniṣad. In V. P. Limaye & R. D. Vadekar (Eds.), *Eighteen Principal Upaniṣads: Upaniṣadic Text with Parallels from extant Vedic Literature, Exegetical and Grammatical Notes.* Vol. 1 (pp. 11–27). Poona: Vaidika Saṃśodhana Maṇḍala, 1958.
LT. *Lakṣmītantra*
Lakṣmī-Tantra: A Pāñcarātra Āgama. Edited with Sanskrit Gloss and Introduction by V. Krishnamacharya. The Adyar Library Series 87. Madras: The Adyar Library and Research Centre, 1959 (repr. 1975).
Mahānārāyaṇopaniṣad
see Varenne 1960.
Manusmṛti
Mânava Dharma-Śâstra: The Code of Manu. Original Sanskrit Text Critically Edited According to the Standard Sanskrit Commentaries by J. Jolly. Trübner's Oriental Series. London: Trübner, 1887.
MBh. *Mahābhārata*
The Mahābhārata, crit. ed. V. S. Sukthankar et al. 20 vols. Poona: Bhandarkar Oriental Research Institute, 1933(1927)–1966.
NārS. *Nāradīyasaṃhitā*
Nāradīya Saṁhitā, ed. Rāghava Prasāda Chaudhary. Kendriya Sanskrita Vidyapeetha Series 15. Tirupati: Kendriya Sanskrit Vidyapeetha, 1971.
Nityagrantha
In *Sri Bhagavad Ramanuja Granthamala,* ed. P. B. Annangaracharya (pp. 181–188). Kancheepuram: Granthamala Office, 1956.
PādS. *Pādmasaṃhitā*
Padma Samhita, crit. ed. Seetha Padmanabhan & R. N. Sampath (part I), Seetha Padmanabhan & V. Varadachari (part II). Pāñcarātra Parisodhanā Pariṣad Series 3, 4. Madras: Pāñcarātra Parisodhanā Pariṣad, 1974, 1982.
ParāśaraS. *Parāśarasaṃhitā*
Parāśara Saṃhitā (With Sanskrit Text & Tamil Translation). Transliteration From Telugu to Devanagari Done by Thirukkannapuram Satakopachar and Translation From Sanskrit to Tamil Done by E. S. V. Narasimhachariar. Srirangam: Sri Pancharatra Agama Samrakshana Trust, 2000.
PārS. *Pārameśvarasaṃhitā*
Pārameśvarasaṃhitā Govindācāryaiḥ saṃskṛtā, anekavidhādarśādibhiḥ saṃyojitā ca. Śrīraṅgam: Kodaṇḍarāmasannidhi, 1953.
PauṣS. *Pauṣkarasaṃhitā*
Sree Poushkara Samhita: One of the Three Gems in Pancharatra, ed. Sampathkumara Ramanuja Muni. Bangalore: Aiyangar and Thirumalachariar, 1934.
PRR. *Pāñcarātrarakṣā*
Śrī Pāñcarātra Rakṣā of Śrī Vedānta Deśika. Critical Edition with Notes and Variant Readings by M. Duraiswami Aiyangar and T. Venugopalacharya with an Introduction in English by G. Srinivasa Murti. The Adyar Library Series 36. Madras: Adyar Library and Research Centre, 1942.

PRR$_1$. *Pāñcarātrarakṣā*
In *Veṅkaṭanātha-Vedāntadeśika-viracitāḥ Rakṣāgranthāḥ ṭippaṇādisaṃyojanena pariṣkṛtya mudritāḥ* (pp. 279–459). [Madras]: Ubhayavedāntagranthamālā, 1969.
PYŚ. *Pātañjalayogaśāstra*
In *Pātañjala-Yogasūtra-Bhāṣya-Vivaraṇam of Śaṅkara-Bhagavatpāda,* crit. ed. Polakam Sri Rama Sastri & S. R. Krishnamurthi Sastri. Madras Government Oriental Series 94. Madras: Government Oriental Manuscript Library, 1952.
Rahasyatrayasāra
Śrīmad Rahasyatrasāra of Vedānta Deśika with Sāravistara by Uttamur T. Viraraghavaccharya. 2 vols. Madras: Ubhayavedāntagranthamālā, 1980.
Rāmāyaṇa
The Vālmīki-Rāmāyaṇa, crit. ed. G. H. Bhatt et al. 7 vols. Baroda: Oriental Institute, 1960–1975.
SanS. *Sanatkumārasaṃhitā*
Sanatkumāra-Saṃhitā of the Pāñcarātrāgam, ed. V. Krishnamacharya. The Adyar Library Series 95. Adyar: The Adyar Library and Research Centre, 1969.
Śrībhāṣya
Bādarāyaṇapraṇītabrahmasūtrākhyaśārīrakamīmāṃsābhāṣyam Rāmānujaviracitaṃ Śrībhāṣyaṃ Sudarśanasūriviracitaśrutaprakāśikākhyavyākhyāsamudbhāsitam Uttamūr T. Vīrarāghavācāryeṇa pariṣkṛtya mudritam. 2 vols. Madras: Ubhayavedāntagranthamālā, 1967.
ŚrīpraśS. *Śrīpraśnasaṃhitā*
Śrīpraśna Saṃhitā. Edited by Seetha Padmanabhan with the Foreword of V. Raghavan. Kendriya Sanskrit Vidyapeetha Series 12. Tirupati: Kendriya Sanskrit Vidyapeetha, 1969.
SS. *Sāttvatasaṃhitā*
Sātvata-Saṁhitā With Commentary by Alaśiṅga Bhaṭṭa, ed. Vraja Vallabha Dwivedi. Library Rare Texts Publication Series 6. Varanasi: Sarasvati Bhavana Library, Sampurnanand Sanskrit Vishvavidyalaya, 1982.
SSBh. *Sāttvatasaṃhitābhāṣya*
see SS.
ŚSmṛ. *Śāṇḍilyasmṛti*
In *The Smriti Sandarbha: Collection of Ten Dharmashastric Texts by Maharshis.* Vol. 5 (pp. 2793–2859). Delhi: Nag Publishers, 1988.
Śvetāśvataropaniṣad
In V. P. Limaye & R. D. Vadekar (Eds.), *Eighteen Principal Upaniṣads (Upaniṣadic Text with Parallels from extant Vedic Literature, Exegetical and Grammatical Notes).* Vol. 1 (pp. 283–300). Poona: Vaidika Saṃśodhana Maṇḍala, 1958.
VaiG. *Vaikuṇṭhagadya*
In *Srimad Vedanta Desika's Chatusslokibhashyam, Sthothraratnabhashyam, and Gadyatrayabhashyam,* ed. V. Srivatsankacharyar (pp. 189–191). Madras: Sri Vedanta Desika Seventh Centenary Trust, n. d.
VDhP. *Viṣṇudharmottarapurāṇa*
Viṣṇudharmottarapurāṇam. Bombay: Shri Venkateshwar Steam Press, 1912.
ViṣṇuP. *Viṣṇupurāṇa*
Śrīparāśaramaharṣipraṇītam purāṇaratnaṃ nāma Śrīviṣṇupurāṇam (Śrīviṣṇucittīyā-

khyayā) vyākhyayā sanātham Aṇṇaṅgarācāryaiḥ paryavekṣitaṃ saṃpāditaṃ ca Saṃpatkumārācāryaiḥ pariśodhitam. Kāñcīpuram: Granthamala Office, 1972.

Viṣṇusmṛti

Patrick Olivelle, *Viṣṇusmṛti: The Law Code of Viṣṇu. A Critical Edition and Annotated Translation of the Vaiṣṇava-Dharmaśāstra.* Harvard Oriental Series 73. Cambridge, MA: Department of Sanskrit and Indian Studies, 2009.

Yājñavalkyasmṛti

Yājñavalkya Smṛti With 'Viramitrodaya' Commentary of Mitra Mishra and 'Mitakshara' Commentary of Vijnaneshwara, ed. Narayana Shastri Khiste & Jagannatha Shastri Hoshinga. Chowkhamba Sanskrit Series 62. Varanasi: Chowkhamba Sanskrit Series Office, 1997.

Yuktidīpikā

Yuktidīpikā: The Most Significant Commentary on the Sāṅkhyakārikā, crit. ed. Albrecht Wezler & Shujun Motegi. Vol. 1. Alt- und Neu-Indische Studien 44. Stuttgart: Franz Steiner Verlag, 1998.

Secondary Sources

Brunner, H. (1994). The Place of Yoga in the Śaivāgamas. In P.-S. Filliozat et al. (Eds.), *Pandit N. R. Bhatt Felicitation Volume* (pp. 425–461). Delhi: Motilal Banarsidass, 1994.

Carman, J. B. (1974). *The Theology of Rāmānuja: An Essay in Interreligious Understanding.* Yale Publications in Religion 18. New Haven: Yale University Press (repr. Bombay: Ananthacharya Indological Research Institute, 1981).

Ekirch, A. R. (2001). Sleep We Have Lost: Pre-industrial Slumber in the British Isles. *American Historical Review, 106*(2), 343–386.

Ekirch, A. R. (2005). *At Day's Close: Night in Times Past.* New York: W. W. Norton.

Frauwallner, E. (1953). *Geschichte der indischen Philosophie.* Vol. 1. Salzburg: Otto Müller Verlag.

Frauwallner, E. (1956). *Geschichte der indischen Philosophie.* Vol. 2. Salzburg: Otto Müller Verlag.

Freschi, E. (2012). *Duty, Language and Exegesis in Prābhākara Mīmāṃsā: Including an Edition and Translation of Rāmānujācārya's Tantrarahasya, Śāstraprameyapariccheda.* Jerusalem Studies in Religion and Culture 17. Leiden: Brill.

Kane, P. V. (1974). *History of Dharmaśāstra (Ancient and Mediæval Religious and Civil Law).* Vol. II, Part 1. 2nd ed. Government Oriental Series Class B, No. 6. Poona: Bhandarkar Oriental Research Institute.

Leach, R. (2012). *Textual Traditions and Religious Identities in the Pāñcarātra.* Unpublished Doctoral Thesis. University of Edinburgh.

Olivelle, P. (1998). *The Early Upaniṣads. Annotated Text and Translation.* South Asia Research. New York: Oxford University Press.

Raman, S. (2007). *Self-Surrender (prapatti) to God in Śrīvaiṣṇavism: Tamil Cats and Sanskrit Monkeys.* Routledge Hindu Studies Series. London: Routledge.

Rastelli, M. (1999). *Philosophisch-theologische Grundanschauungen der Jayākhyasaṃhitā: Mit einer Darstellung des täglichen Rituals*. Beiträge zur Kultur- und Geistesgeschichte Asiens 33. Wien: Verlag der Österreichischen Akademie der Wissenschaften.

Rastelli, M. (2000). Die fünf Zeiten (pañca kālas) in den ältesten Pāñcarātra-Saṃhitās. *Wiener Zeitschrift für die Kunde Südasiens, 44,* 101–134.

Rastelli, M. (2003). On the Concept of Vaikuṇṭha in Viśiṣṭādvaitavedānta and Pāñcarātra. In R. Czekalska & H. Marlewicz (Eds.), *2nd International Conference on Indian Studies: Proceedings* (pp. 427–447). Cracow Indological Studies 4–5. Cracow: The Enigma Press.

Rastelli, M. (2006). *Die Tradition des Pāñcarātra im Spiegel der Pārameśvarasaṃhitā*. Beiträge zur Kultur- und Geistesgeschichte Asiens 51. Wien: Verlag der Österreichischen Akademie der Wissenschaften.

Rastelli, M. (2007). Service as an End in Itself: Viśiṣṭādvaitic Modifications of Pāñcarātra Ritual. In G. Oberhammer & M. Rastelli (Eds.), *Studies in Hinduism IV: On the Mutual Influences and Relationship of Viśiṣṭādvaitavedānta and Pāñcarātra* (pp. 287–314). Beiträge zur Kultur- und Geistesgeschichte Asiens 54. Wien: Verlag der Österreichischen Akademie der Wissenschaften.

Rastelli, M. (2009). Perceiving God and Becoming Like Him: Yogic Perception and Its Implications in the Viṣṇuitic Tradition of Pāñcarātra. In E. Franco (Ed.) in collaboration with D. Eigner, *Yogic Perception, Meditation and Altered States of Consciousness* (pp. 299–317). Beiträge zur Kultur- und Geistesgeschichte Asiens 65. Wien: Verlag der Österreichischen Akademie der Wissenschaften.

Rastelli, M. (forthc.). nāḍīs, prāṇas, and prāṇāyāma: A Yogic Text Crossing the Boundaries of Tradition. In P.-S. Filliozat & D. Goodall (Eds.), *Mélanges à la mémoire de N. Ramachandra Bhatt.*

Srinivasa Chari, S. M. (1994). *Vaiṣṇavism: Its Philosophy, Theology and Religious Discipline.* Delhi: Motilal Banarsidass (repr. 2000).

Syed, R. (1990). *Die Flora Altindiens in Literatur und Kunst.* Unpublished Doctoral Thesis. Ludwig-Maximilians-Universität zu München.

TAK 3

Tāntrikābhidhānakośa III: Ṭ-PH. Dictionnaire des termes techniques de la littérature hindoue tantrique. Ed. M. Rastelli & D. Goodall. Beiträge zur Kultur- und Geistesgeschichte Asiens 76. Wien: Verlag der Österreichischen Akademie der Wissenschaften.

Varenne, J. (1960). *La Mahā Nārāyaṇa Upaniṣad. Édition critique, avec une traduction française, une étude, des notes et, en annexe, la Prāṇāgnihotra Upaniṣad par Jean Varenne.* 2 vols. Publications de l'institut de civilisation indienne, série in-8°, fasc. 11, 13. Paris: E. de Boccard.

Vasudeva, S. (2004). *The Yoga of the Mālinīvijayottaratantra: Chapters 1–4, 7, 11–17. Critical Edition, Translation & Notes.* Collection Indologie 97. Pondichéry: Institut français de Pondichéry.

Chapter 6

The Transformation of Yoga in Medieval Maharashtra

Catharina Kiehnle

Contents

1. The Songs 261

2. The God of the *Jñāndev Gāthā* 262

3. The Aim of the Devotees 264

4. The Means to Reach God 266

5. The Decline of Nāth Yoga 269

6. Bhakti Yoga 274

7. Conclusion 277

References 278

Catharina Kiehnle

Chapter 6: The Transformation of Yoga in Medieval Maharashtra

Religious Maharashtra saw many transformations during the thirteenth and fourteenth centuries. The main one was the usage of the local language for matters of religion that were formerly in the hands of Sanskrit speakers. Apart from the Mahānubhāv texts that soon were hidden from public view, the most important achievement of that age is the *Jñāneśvarī*, the Marathi *Bhagavadgītā* commentary by Jñāndev. The second transformation was the one of the local Viṭṭhala cult into the country-wide Vārkarī movement, to this day the most popular religious denomination in Maharashtra. The third one, closely connected with the other two, was the transformation of (Śaiva) Nāth Yoga into what Charlotte Vaudeville called the "nominal Vaiṣṇavism" of the Vārkarī movement.[1] Again it is Jñāndev, himself a Nāth yogi, who is supposed to be one of the main promoters of this special type of Bhāgavata religion: he included Nāth lore in his *Gītā* commentary, and many songs attributed to him contain Nāth as well as Vaiṣṇava topics. The present paper deals with the role of yoga in the Vārkarī movement.

1. The Songs

The material used here are songs (*abhaṅga*-s) from the *Jñāndev Gāthā*, a collection of texts attributed to Jñāndev. The authorship is a matter of debate. As I have shown elsewhere, the *Gāthā* may indeed contain *abhaṅga*-s composed by the author of the *Jñāneśvarī* himself, but it is extremely difficult to find out which exactly, because in the course of about 700 years many authors created songs in "Jñāndev style" and under his name.[2] In the latest *Gāthā* edition of 1995, M. Ś. Kānaḍe and R. Ś. Nagarkar separated 376 "real" ones from 730 "fake" ones. Many of the latter do indeed not look like creations of the famous poet, but even if there

1 Vaudeville 1987: 35ff.; see also Kiehnle 1989.
2 Kiehnle 1992.

may be room for discussion in several cases, it is in my opinion safest to consider the *Gāthā* as a product of what one might call the "Jñāndev school".[3] In that way it is possible to utilise it for an understanding of the history of religious ideas in Maharashtra between (roughly) the thirteenth and the sixteenth centuries. The assumption of this period seems plausible because Jñāndev is supposed to have completed his *Jñāneśvarī* in 1290, and because the *Gāthā* contains songs whose form and contents point to the age of the poet-saint Eknāth who lived from 1533–1599.[4] Close examination of all the texts will most probably also bring to light more recent ones.

For a general survey of the development of yoga as I want to give it here, I found the *Gāthā* version by P. N. Jośī (1969) very helpful. Jośī assembled most of the texts available at his time (1100 songs) and arranged them according to a larger number of subjects than his predecessors, thus facilitating a preliminary survey of the contents of the *Gāthā*. It is the basis of the present study, and the song numbers are taken from there.[5] For reasons of time, I abandoned the idea of presenting critical versions of the songs and passages quoted below; moreover, I did not include about 100 unpublished songs I found in the manuscripts. Although a flaw, I do not think that this greatly impairs the over-all impression gained from my survey. The frequency numbers mentioned in the following should also be considered as the result of work in progress. In the absence not only of a critical but also of a digital version of the *Gāthā*, the *abhaṅga*-s and terms I chose for closer inspection had to be counted "by hand", and some occurrences may have been overlooked. Still I think that the statistics are good enough to show certain proportions and to allow for the selection of representative passages.

2. The God of the *Jñāndev Gāthā*

For a better understanding of the yoga under discussion, it will be useful to examine in the beginning the ideals of the authors, that is, their idea of god. This is in most cases god Viṭṭhala of Paṇḍharpūr, represented by a black stone figure standing on a brick-like pedestal in the Paṇḍharpūr temple, hands placed on his hips, clad in a yellow garment and adorned with crocodile earrings, just as he appeared to his first Paṇḍharpūr devotee Puṇḍalīka. To this day, the Vārkarīs love

3 See also Kiehnle 1992, especially p. 135.

4 Kiehnle 1997b: 57.

5 Genuine emendations of the text in the passages quoted below are indicated by square brackets. Missing *anusvāra*-s were not added.

his shape, and it was and is their highest desire to see his statue with their own eyes, as is expressed in two famous songs:

221
1. I shall transform all existence into happiness, I shall fill the three worlds with bliss.
2. I shall go, oh mother, to that Paṇḍharpūr, I shall visit my mother's house.
3. I shall obtain the fruit of all [my] good deeds, I shall embrace Pāṇḍuraṅga.[6]

4
1. Incomparable, taking away the mind, on the waist the beautiful yellow garment, at the feet the anklets of heroic deeds – I saw the god.[7]

From a great number of passages (I stopped counting after 400 songs) it becomes obvious that for the authors the god was not only endowed with qualities (*saguṇa*), but also the highest absolute without qualities (*nirguṇa*), very often called *brahman:*

18
1. Should we call you *saguṇa* or *nirguṇa? saguṇa* and *nirguṇa* are one Govinda.
2. [He] cannot be guessed, he cannot be guessed, [what] the vedic texts call "not this, not this" is one Govinda.
3. Shall we call you gross or subtle? The gross and the subtle are one Govinda.
4. Shall we call you a form[8] or formless? The form and the formless are one Govinda.
5. Shall we call you visible or invisible? The visible and the invisible are one Govinda.[9]
6. Jñānadeva speaks through the grace of Nivṛtti – the father, the husband of goddess Rakhumā[ī], Viṭṭhala.[10]

6 *Avaghācī saṃsāra sukhācā karīna, ānandẽ bharīna tinhī loka. jāīna ge māye tayā paṃḍharpurā, bheṭena māherā āpuliyā. sarva sukṛtācẽ phaḷa mī lāhīna, kṣema mī deīna pāṃḍuraṃgī̃. pāṇḍuraṃgī̃* is either locative singular or instrumental plural (honorific), but cannot be translated literally in either way.

7 *Anupamya manohara, kā̃se śobhe pitāṃbara, caraṇī̃ brīdācā toḍara, dekhilā dev[o].* The literal meaning of *śobhe,* "looks beautiful", has been transformed into the adjective "beautiful" in the translation.

8 *Sākāru,* "with form", would be more usual in that context, but the editions are unanimous with respect to the reading *ākāru.*

9 After stanza 5, Jośī's edition contains another stanza with *vyakta* and *avyakta,* "manifest" and "unmanifest". It is absent in the Kāṇade & Nagarkar edition.

10 *Tuja saguṇa hmaṇõ kī̃ nirguṇa re, saguṇa nirguṇa eku goviṃdu re. anumāne nā anumāne nā, śruti neti neti mhaṇati goviṃdu re. tuja sthūḷa hmaṇõ kī̃ sūkṣma re, sthūḷasūkṣma eku goviṃdu re. tuja ākāru hmaṇõ kī̃ nirākāru re, ākāru nirākāru eku goviṃdu re. tuja dṛśya hmaṇõ kī̃ adṛśya re, dṛśya adṛśya eku goviṃdu re. nivṛttiprasāde jñānadeva bole, bāpa rakhumādevivaru viṭhṭhalu re.* Stanza 6 contains two "signatures" (*mudrikā*-s), *jñānadeva* and *bāpa rakhumādevivaru.* The latter is not connected syntactically with the rest of the stanza. The name Rakhumāī is usually Rakhumā in the *mudrikā-s* of the *Jñāndev Gāthā.* Viṭhṭhala should actually be written as "Viṭṭhala", but this is almost never done in Maharashtra.

The god is sometimes also described as being beyond these notions: "The husband of goddess Rakhumāī is neither endowed with form nor without form. [Although] not having become anything, he exists, oh woman!"[11] Moreover, Viṭṭhala/Kṛṣṇa was considered a special sort of *brahman* or *ātman*, one with qualities and yet all-pervading: "The father, the husband of goddess Rakhumāī, who takes away the fear from Puṇḍalīka, the highest *brahman* with form – I saw the god",[12] "Inside, outside, wholly all-pervading is Murāri."[13]

3. The Aim of the Devotees

There are hundreds of songs in which this sort of oscillation between the *saguṇa* and *nirguṇa* mode of existence is observable. One reason why god's nature was such an important issue is closely connected with the aim of the devotees. As long as it was enough for them to see and embrace the statue in Paṇḍharpūr (something which, according to R. D. Rāṇade, was actually done in the beginning of the cult),[14] the *saguṇa* form was suitable. For someone, however, who aspires to unity with the highest principle, the god's gross form is a mere garb (*veṣa*), a veil or cloak (*buṃthī*), a dramatic role (*soṃga*), a rough blanket (*ghoṃgaḍī/ghoṃghaḍẽ*), etc., as it is called in about 25 cases, e. g., "I was attracted by the dark veil, the dark form, the dark form of the self", "Cladding yourself in the veil of being a cowherd you (Kṛṣṇa) please Yaśodā's mind", "Let the idea of you and me go far away, we shall cover ourselves with one blanket alone, Hari", etc.[15] Although the Viśiṣṭādvaita term "communion" (*sāyujya*), which designates a state in which the bliss of *brahman* is experienced without loss of self-existence, is mentioned four times in the *Gāthā*,[16] the overwhelming majority of such passages shows that the authors had a complete merging with god in mind. In that sense also the Sāṃkhya term *kaivalya* occurs in 15.1 and 1008.3, which originally designated the "isolation" of spirit from matter but is here adjusted to Nāth practice and philosophy: "[The *mantra*] 'I am he' is the sweetness of *kaivalya*."[17] *Advaita*, "non-duality/

11 *Rakhumādevivaru sākāru nirākāru navhe, kãhĩ nahoni hoye toci bāīye vo* (982.3).

12 *Bāpa rakhumādevivaru, puṇḍalikā abhayakarū, parabrahma sāhākāru, dekhilā devo* (4.3).

13 *Sabāhyābhyaṃtarĩ avaghā vyāpaka murārī* (191.2).

14 Rāṇade 1961: 11–12.

15 *Sãvaḷiyẽ buṃthī sãvaḷiyā rūpẽ, sãvaḷyā svarūpẽ vedhiyelẽ* (266.1); *gõvaḷepaṇācī buṃthī gheūniyā [v]eṣa, rijhaviśī mānasa yaśodecẽ* (233.1); *mītũpaṇa jāũ de durī, ekaci ghoṃgaḍe pāṃgharũ hari* (1048.2).

16 Srinivasachari 1978: 492; 134.2, 237.2, 397.6 and 524.1, *muktī cārī* in 48.1.

17 *Sohaṃ he śirāṇī kaivalyācī* (15.1). *So 'ham* is often repeated mentally while breathing in and out during meditation. *Śirāṇī*, "sweetness, sweetmeat", is one of the rare Persian words of the *Gāthā*. Tulpule and Feldhaus (1999) translate it as "intense desire", which is, however, only the

non-diversity",[18] in contrast to *dvaita,* "duality/diversity", is a frequently chosen expression: "I saw the father, the husband of goddess Rakhumāī in the place of *brahman,* he is contained in me through his being non-dual",[19] "The feeling of duality does not have a place in us, in everything the whole deity took shape."[20] Since the highest principle is "beyond duality and non-duality",[21] and because "in the self there is neither duality nor non-duality visible",[22] the same can be said about the devotee: "The milkmaid is bereft of duality and non-duality."[23] Verbs that illustrate what happens with the individual soul in that situation are "to disappear" (*harapṇẽ, nimṇẽ, māvaḷṇẽ, lopṇẽ, virṇẽ*), "to merge" (*murṇẽ, saṃcarṇẽ, līna hoṇẽ*), "to sink, drown" (*magna/nimagna hoṇẽ, buḍṇẽ*), "to be contained" (*sāmāvṇẽ*), etc., and the authors employ metaphors like the one of waves or salt dissolving in water, the disappearance of camphor and the wick in the flame, and the mould in which the wax disappears when a figure is cast, and refer to the famous "oceanic feeling":[24]

537

1. The inner expanse bloomed in *brahman,* ah, there the mind [is] an adept as well as a seeker.
2. It made [me] different [from the world], made [me] different – I went to see [it and] was lost straight away.
3. There Ṛg-, Yajus- and Sāma[veda] were deceived, the one that is made of *brahman* blossomed in myself.
4. The husband of goddess Rakhumāī became a wave inside *brahman,* he is contained in the ocean of *brahman* and took me with him, mother.[25]

secondary meaning of the word. J. T. Molesworth (1975) notes that the original meaning is little known to the Marāṭhas.

18 Vetter (1979: 31–34) has shown that the term *advaita* refers rather to non-diversity than non-duality, but in the present context both meanings make sense.

19 *Bāpa rakhumādevivara brahmapadī̃ dekhilā, majamājī̃ sāmāvalā advaitapaṇẽ* (490.3).

20 *Dujepaṇī̃cā bhāvo āmhā̃ nāhī̃ ṭhāvo, sarvī̃ sarva devo ākāralā* (527.1).

21 *Dvaitādvaitāhūna paratẽ* (203.4).

22 *Na dise dvaitādvaita ātmā* (334.3).

23 *Dvaitādvaitavirahita gauḷaṇī* (248.1).

24 557.1, 570.3, 577.2, 694.1–3, etc.; examples for camphor: 82.1, 91.1, 392.9–10, 511.3, 536.1, 551.3, 554.1, 931.4 and 978.1.

25 *Aṃtarīcā vistāru brahmī pālhāyilā, tethe eka manu siddhasādhaku bhalā. teṇẽ kelẽ anārisẽ kelẽ anārisẽ, pāhõ gelẽ sarisẽ harapalẽ ge māye. tethe ṛgayajuḥsāma bhulale, tẽ mājhā ṭhāyī̃ phulalẽ brahmamaya. rakhumādevivara aṃtara brahmī̃ taraṃgu jālā, brahma-udadhī sāmāvalā maja gheūni māye.*

4. The Means to Reach God

According to the *Gāthā*, one of the basic requirements to reach god is a *guru*. He is not the special subject in the present chapter, but it should be understood that he ranks high in the *Jñāneśvarī* where Jñāndev praises his teacher Nivṛtti in many places. This is also the case in the *Gātha* where he is called "the king of the sant families",[26] that is, the king of the "good ones" who in this context constitute the Vārkarī community. The guru is preferably mentioned in the last stanza of an *abhaṅga:* "Jñāndev obtained knowledge accessible in secret, Nivṛtti gave it into my hands",[27] "Jñāndev asks Nivṛtti about the (innermost) desire: greater than the sky is the name."[28] One of the *mudrikā*-s in the *Gāthā,* the "signatures" of the poet in the last lines, is Nivṛttidāsa, "servant of Nivṛtti" (used about thirty times), which testifies to the reverence with which he is treated.

Apart from the name of god which will be dealt with later on, yoga was also considered an important means to reach god in the *Gāthā.* I edited and translated about 150 songs (the collections called *Lākhoṭā* and *Yogapar abhaṅgamālā*) on this topic,[29] and there are more scattered over the *Gāthā.* About 650 songs on the whole contain one or more terms from the sphere of yoga. All of them occur also in the 150 yoga songs just mentioned, which I did not include into the statistics because almost every word would have to be counted. The terms often designate states of meditation and consciousness and are also found in Pātañjala Yoga, the Nāth cult in general, and among the Buddhist and Vaiṣṇava Sahajiyās: *samādhi,* "absorption (into the object of meditation)" (37x), *sahaja,* "natural (state of mind)" (27x), *samarasa,* "union, identification" (21x, once also called *samasukha,* "happiness of union"), *unmanī,* "the state above the mind" (18x), *nirvāṇa,* "extinction" (14x), *dhāraṇā,* "binding (the mind to a place)" (9x), *śūnya,* "void" (11x), *nijadhyāsa,* "profound and repeated meditation" (Skt. *nididhyāsā,* 5x), *tur(ī)yā,* "the fourth state (of consciousness)" (2x), and *nirvikalpa,* "without conceptualisation" (2x).[30] A lesser known term used in the context of the highest state is *sattrāvī,* "the seventeenth (digit)" (15x), a phenomenon close to pure consciousness and the origin of everything according to the *Yogapar abhaṅgamālā.* In *Ṣaṭcakranirūpaṇa* 47, the commentator Kālīcaraṇa calls it *nirvāṇakalā,* "digit of extinction".[31] The four bodies (*sthūla, sūkṣma, kāraṇa, mahākāraṇa,* "gross", "subtle", "cause", "great-cause") (4x), the four stages of speech, namely *parā,* "the highest one" (14x), *paśyantī,* "the seeing one", *madhyāmā,* "the middle

26 *Saṃtakuḷīṃcā rājā* (12.1).
27 *Jñāna gūḍhagamya jñānadevā lādhalẽ, nivṛttīnẽ dilẽ mājhyā hātī̃* (64.4).
28 *Jñānadeva puse nivṛttīsī cāḍa, gaganāhunī vāḍa nāma āhe* (69.4).
29 Kiehnle 1997a.
30 This translation of *nirvikalpa* was suggested to me by K. Preisendanz.
31 Kiehnle 1997a: 139ff., Michaël 1979: 166.

one", and *vaikharī,* "the gross/solid one" (6x),[32] as well as the *tripuṭī,* "the threefold one / the three-pack" (i. e., the unity of object, subject and the relationship between the two which constitutes perception and thus the world, 33x) are listed among the elements that disappear when the highest state is reached.

By far the most popular yoga-related notion in the *Gāthā* is *dhyāna,* "meditation".[33] The term occurs, together with a few derivations of the root *dhyāṇē,* "to meditate", at least 140 times, e. g., "Jñāndev's thinking is captivated in the meditation of Kṛṣṇa"[34], "If one constantly meditates on Hari [...]",[35] etc. Except for the case of *bakadhyāna,* "the meditation of the heron" whose aim is to catch fish (a metaphor for hypocrisy),[36] *dhyāna* is practised with respect to the highest reality, which is often but not exclusively (in c 80 of about 100 cases in which the heart is mentioned) the *saguṇa* form of god in the heart, e. g., "Śrī Hari whose meditation is in the heart [...]",[37] "By the grace of the king, the wise Nivṛtti, that meditation [on Kṛṣṇa] came into [my] heart",[38] and "Jñāndev meditated [and] thus obtained the jewel that is Hari. He took it and put it into the lotus of [his] heart."[39] Although the term *dhāraṇā,* "binding (the mind to a place)" occurs only in 9 cases, derivatives of the Sanskrit root *dhṛ,* "to hold, fix", like the Marathi verbs *dharṇē,* "to hold, keep", or *sthirāvṇē,* "to become settled", occur about 25 times, often in contexts similar to those in which *dhyāna* is used: "Such a lovely form I kept in [my] heart",[40] "The husband of goddess Rakhumāī got settled in [my] heart",[41] etc. There is a special *cakra* reserved for god near the physical heart, the *hṛdayakamala,* "lotus of the heart", which occurs four times in the *Gāthā;* once it is called *hṛdayakaḷika,* "bud of the heart".[42] It corresponds to the eight-petalled lotus (mentioned twice),[43] which is different from the twelve-petalled one of the *anāhatacakra* belonging to Kuṇḍalinī Yoga.

32 According to Padoux 1975: 73, *parā vāk* is identical with the primary energy united with Śiva, *paśyantī* is the stage when differentiation starts, *madhyamā* the stage when duality solidifies, and *vaikharī* the stage of audible speech. For a discussion of the stages, see Padoux 1975: 145ff.

33 Unlike in *Tukārām Gāthā* 2.1, "beautiful is that form standing on the brick" (*suṃdara tē dhyāna ubhē viṭevarī*), it seems that the word does not appear here in the sense of "form, image".

34 *Jñānadevā citta kṛṣṇadhyānī̃ rata* (94.4).

35 *Niraṃtara dhyātā hari [...]* (115.1).

36 852.1.

37 *Śrī hari jayā dhyāna hṛdayāṃtarī̃* (151.2).

38 *Nivṛttimunirāyaprasādē̃ dhyāna tē̃ hṛdayāsī ālē̃* (22.6).

39 *Jñānadevī dhyāna kelē̃, hariratna aise sādhile, te ānuniyā ghātile hṛdayakamalik[e]* (150.3).

40 *Aisē̃ suṃdara rūpaḍē̃ hṛdayī̃ dharilē̃* (126.3).

41 *Rakhumādevivaru sthirāvalā hṛdayī̃* (497.6).

42 114.4, 189.4, 150.3, 1054.3; see also Kiehnle 1997c.

43 386.1 and 1001.18.

The *Gāthā* authors describe in at least 80 songs the role of the mind (*mana*) in their meditations, e.g., "Turning back the mind I meditated on Hari",[44] "One should fix one's meditation on a resting place, one should make the mind [think] one thought, one should remember [the name] Rāma, Rāma",[45] "Attracting the thoughts, [Kṛṣṇa] filled the eyes with pure consciousness, [and] sent the mind into meditation",[46] "In the end the mind dissolved in meditation",[47] "The mind cooled down in the state above the mind",[48] etc. In connection with the mind, descriptions of merging with the god, especially with his black form, occur about 100 times. 28 songs are exclusively dedicated to it, e.g.,

265
1. The dark highest *brahman* pleases this soul. The mind made the mind a home of dark royal glory.[49]
2. What should I do, friend, the dark one is trapping [me], the mind is hiding by itself there.
3. The father, the husband of goddess Rakhumā, [is] a dark image/reflection; in the mind the mind became one [with it] by an embrace.[50]

All this sounds to some extent similar to *Yogasūtra* 1.2, where yoga is defined as the suppression of the movements of thought, *citta-vṛtti*. In fact, these terms are also found in the songs: "My movements of thought disappeared",[51] "The movements of thought became of one form."[52] Vaiṣṇava and Advaita imagery together with Nāth yoga terminology resulted in the kind of poetry characteristic for many songs of the *Jñāndev Gāthā:*

94
1. In union the beautiful (clay-)pot dissolved [in water], and through oneness the stream disappeared together with it.
2. [In the name] "Kṛṣṇa, Kṛṣṇa" I found a straight path for the tongue together with the sense organs: the repetition [of the name].
3. In the abode of the mind, in the meditation of *samādhi,* [sitting] in the lotus seat, I meditated [on] the king of the Self.

---

44 *Mana muraḍuni hari dhyāīlā* (85.6).
45 *Visāvā to dharāve dhyāna, ekacitta karāve mana, rāma rāma smarāvẽ* (168.4).
46 *Ākarṣonī citta caitanye bharonī ṭhele locana, dhyānī̃ visarjilẽ mana* (277.6).
47 *Śekhī̃ dhyānī̃ virālẽ tẽ mana* (401.3).
48 *Unmanī̃ mana nivālẽ* (365.2).
49 A pun on the word *rāṇīva*, which can mean "darkness" as well as "royal glory".
50 *Sā̃vaḷẽ parabrahma āvaḍe yā jivā, manẽ mana rāṇivā ghara kelẽ. kāya karũ saye sā̃vaḷẽ gõvita, āpẽ āpa lapata mana tethẽ. bāpa rakhumādevivaru sā̃ṃvaḷī pratimā, man[a] manī̃ kṣ[emā] eka jhālẽ.* In stanza 3, I read *kṣemā* instead of *kṣamā* of the editions, with Tulpule & Feldhaus 1999: 806 where the passage is quoted.
51 *Harapalī mājhī cittavṛtt[ī]* (462.5).
52 *Ekākāra vṛtt[ī] jālī* (1012.5).

4. Jñāndev's thinking [was] engrossed in meditation of Kṛṣṇa, birth, old-age and death disappeared.[53]

774
1. To whom belongs this form, to whom belongs this body? Know all that [to be] the mould, the resting-place of the Self.
2. The thought of "I" and "you" should be investigated by means of discriminative knowledge. One should meditate on Govinda in this very body.
3. He arose in the thousand-petalled [lotus in the head] like the sun, different from the *tripuṭī,* [namely] the object of meditation, the meditator, [and] the process of meditation.
4. Jñānadeva says: "The form in the eye[54] – this, you should know, is called 'the place of consciousness'."[55]

5. The Decline of Nāth Yoga

Thus, all is well with yoga in the Vārkarī universe? Not entirely. The songs also reflect various degrees of devaluation of yoga. Śiva, for example, the first teacher of the Nāths, who is praised together with Śakti in the first chapter of Jñāndev's Śaiva poem *Anubhavāmṛt*[56] and who is still as important as Viṣṇu in the yoga chapter of the *Jñāneśvarī,* in the *Lākhoṭa* and in the *Yogapar abhaṅgamālā,*[57] is mentioned about sixty-three times in the songs. In a song about religious mendicants the repetition of his name is recommended,[58] and in song no. 355 the poet localises Śiva in his own body and eventually identifies him with Viṭṭhala. The equal status of the two gods is also expressed in a song in which the husband of Umā (Śiva) as well as Hari (Viṣṇu/Kṛṣṇa) appear as objects of devotion.[59] In one passage, the idea is referred to that Viṭṭhala's headgear is actually a *śivaliṅga* and that mutual respect reigns among the two gods: "Seeing the beautiful one in

53 *Samarasẽ ghaṭu virālā vinaṭu, ekarūpẽ pāṭu gelā [saṃgẽsī]. kṛṣṇa kṛṣṇa vāṭa sā̃paḍalī nīṭa, jihvesī ghaḍaghaḍāṭa iṃdriyẽsahita. manācyā bh[u]vanī̃ samādhīcyā dhyānī̃, ciṃtilā padmāsanī̃ ātmarāju. jñānadevā citta kṛṣṇadhyānī̃ rata, janmajarāmṛtyu hārapalī.*

54 The form in the eye is most probably the "blue dot" (*nīlabindu*) in the *brahmarandhra* where pure consciousness is said to reside like in a mould (Kiehnle 1997a: 119).

55 *Koṇācẽ hẽ rūpa deha hā koṇācā, ātmārāma s[ā̃]cā sarva jāṇe. mī tū̃ hā vicāra vivekẽ śodhāvā, goviṃda hā dhyāvā yāca dehī̃. dhyeya dhyātā dhyāna tripuṭīvegaḷā, sahasradaḷī̃ ugavalā sūrya jaisā. jñānadeva mhaṇe nayanā̃tīla rūpa, yā nā̃va citpada tumhī̃ jāṇā.*

56 Gokhle 1967: 3ff., Bahirat 1956: 159ff.

57 For example in *Jñāneśvarī* 6.301–324 where Śiva as well as Kṛṣṇa receive *kuṇḍalinī* in the *brahmarandhra* (Maṃgrūḷkar & Keḷkar 1994: I/330–334, Kiehnle 2004–2005: 485–489). In *Lakhoṭā* 7 (Kiehnle 1997a: 178–179), Śiva and Viṣṇu enjoy a special standing.

58 *Śivanāma śitala mukhī̃ sevī̃* (1059.2).

59 *Umecyā bhrātārā bhajāvẽ nityāni, harice kīrtanī̃ jāta jāvẽ* (986.11). *Bhrātārā* most probably stands for *bhartāra.*

the garb of a cowherd, Maheśa [is] praising the greatness of the one who glorified [him] on his head."[60] Much more frequent, however, is the "inclusivistic" method of making other gods and highest principles, whatever they may be, serve one's own (here Vaiṣṇava) cause:

139

1. Śiva teaches Bhavānī: Oh you who is dear to me like my life, meditate in your own mind [and] see the highest bliss.
2. Rāma is a friend, Rāma is a friend, Rāma is a friend, Hari Rāma is a friend.
3. [Rāma] who adorns as a spire the [hymn of] thousand names is inside, outside [and] within.[61]
4. That is one's own *dharma,* that is one's own *karma,* that is the highest *brahman,* the one secret,
5. the life of [all] creatures, the enchantment of the mind, the means to reach happiness, the collyrium of knowledge that consists in devotion:[62]
6. The father, the husband of goddess Rakhumāī, is easy to reach and [is] with form, the eternal half-mora (of the syllable *om*),[63] the bliss of (pure) consciousness [and] great happiness.[64]

Stanzas 1–3 allude to a famous verse, also put into the mouth of Śiva teaching his wife, according to which the name of Rāma is as efficient as the thousand names of the *Viṣṇusahasranāmastotra.*[65] The story is most probably also hinted at in another stanza with the words "Through the name Girijā[66] got [her] position."[67] Not only Pārvatī repeats "the name", but also Śiva himself: "The essence, the essence, the essence – Viṭṭhala, your name is the essence, therefore the one who

---

60 *Rūpa pāhatā̃ tarī ḍoḷasu, suṃdara pāhatā̃ gopaveṣu, mahimā varṇitā̃ maheśu, jeṇē mastakī̃ vaṃdilā* (208.3).

61 *Aṃtarī̃*, "inside", meaning the same as *bhītarī̃*, seems redundant here.

62 *Jñānāñjana* is the legendary "eye-salve" (Molesworth 1975 s. v.) that bestows knowledge when applied to the eyes. In the case of Rāma and his name, it seems that here devotion supersedes knowledge. Another possibility to translate *bhaktijñānācē aṃjana* is: "the collyrium of devotion and knowledge". In this case the implication would be that knowledge and devotion do not contradict each other but are acquired together through the repetition of god's name.

63 The *ardhamātṛkā* is the last part of the syllable *aum,* or an even more subtle sound after *-m* that fades into the absolute (Kiehnle 1997a: 103–104).

64 *Śiva bhavānī upadeśī prāṇapriye, nijamānasī̃ dhyāye paramānaṃdu pāhe. rāmu sakhā hari rāmu sakhā, rāmu sakhā hari rāmu sakhā. sahasra nāmāvarī kaḷasu sāje, toci to aṃtarī̃ bāhiju bhītarī̃. hāci nijadharma hēci nijakarma, hēci parabrahma varma hēci eku. jivāṃcē jīvana, manācē mohana, sukhācē sādhana bhaktijñānācē aṃjana. bāpa rakhumādevivaru sulabhu sākāru, ardhamātṛkā akṣaru cidānaṃdu sukha thora.* In stanza 3, I left *-varī* untranslated so that the general idea of the stanza will become clearer. *Cidānaṃda* in stanza 6 may also be translated as "consciousness and bliss".

65 *Rāma rāmeti rāmeti rame rāme manorame, sahasranāma tat tulyam, rāmanāma varānane.* See Bühnemann 1983: 29 and Kiehnle 1997a: 184.

66 The "Mountain-born", name of Śiva's wife Pārvatī.

67 *Nāmē pratiṣṭhā pāvalī girijā* (127.4); see also 121.1.

holds a spear in his hand (Śiva) is repeating [it] again and again",[68] "Śiva took refuge with the name, he put firm faith [in it] [...] the name is the experience of the Vedas",[69] "Tripurāri sways with love (when he hears songs about Rāma and Kṛṣṇa)",[70] etc. In one song, god and goddess (Śiva and Śakti/Pārvatī) are even made into the castanets that accompany the chanting of the Vāsudev, a Vaiṣṇava mendicant.[71] Śiva's way into insignificance ends when he is mentioned together with the soul in expressions of their unity (42x). Here, not Śiva as such is important, but the fact that god in general is identical with the soul, and especially that his name rhymes with *jīva* ("soul"). In some passages, the *-i-* in his name is even lengthened for that reason: "Where there is *jīva,* there is Śīva",[72] "*jīva* and Śīva sat down in the same row",[73] "*jīva* is Śīva",[74] etc.

Yoga (29x) and the yogis (41x) are treated in a similar way. The *Gāthā* contains, e.g., a song about the ideal yogi, the god Dattātreya:

> 424
> 1. Yonder on the peak of mount Meru, a *yogī* without form sits [practising] control of breath, applying *khecarī mudrā.*[75]
> 2. He left illusion, renounced [his] patched garment [and his] body. His mind dissolved in the bliss of *brahman.*
> 3. [By means of] the *anāhata* sound,[76] he reached the highest abode. In the pleasure of the state above the mind and the fourth state of consciousness, he sways with great joy.[77]
> 4. He bathed at Paṃcāleśvar on the shore of the Godāvarī river of knowledge.[78] Inside Jñāndev [resides] Dattātreya, the yogi.[79]

In several songs yogis are mentioned appreciatively, e.g., it is said that those are called lords among yogis who know the union of sun and moon (i.e., practise

68 *Sāra sāra sāra, viṭhobā nāma tujhẽ sāra, mhaṇoni śuḷapāṇī japatāhe vāraṃvāra* (132.1).
69 *Nāmāsi vinaṭalā śiva, teṇẽ dharilā dṛḍhabāva [...] nāma anubhava vedāṃcā* (161.3).
70 *Premẽ ḍule tripurārī* (1006.4), similarly 120.2.
71 1007.5. For the Vāsudev, see Kiehnle 2005.
72 *Jatra jīva tatra śīva* (392.5).
73 *Jīva śīva [eke] paṃktīs baisalī* (451.4), similarly *jīva śiva eke paṃktī̃* (999.11).
74 *Jīva toca śīva* (610.4).
75 *Khecarī mudrā* is achieved by bending back the tongue into the throat in order to drink the nectar (*amṛta, soma*) that is supposed to trickle down from the moon centre in the head (*Haṭhayogapradīpikā* 3.32–54).
76 The "unstruck sound" is said to be perceived by some yogis in the heart.
77 *Cha[n]da* can be translated as "intense liking, joy" as Jośī does (*man [...] ānaṃdāne ḍulat āhe*), or as "sound, reverberation", which also makes sense.
78 Pañcāleśvar is a Datta pilgrimage site not far from the Godāvarī river in the Beed District of Maharashtra.
79 *Paila merucyā śikharī̃, eka yogī nirākārī, mudrā lāvunī khẽcarī, prāṇāyāmī̃ baisalā. teṇẽ sāṃḍiyelī māyā, tyajiyelī kaṃthā kāyā, mana gelẽ vilayā, brahmānaṃdā mājhārī̃. anuhata dhvani nāda, to pāvalā paramapada, unman[ī]turyāvinodẽ chaṃdẽ chaṃdẽ ḍolatuse. jñānagodāvarīcyā tīrī̃, snāna kelẽ paṃcāḷeśvarī̃, jñānadevācyā aṃtarī̃, dattātreya yogiyā.*

Kuṇḍalinī Yoga).[80] One of the authors shows his pride of being a yogi in his *mudrikā*-s: "Jñāneśvar the royal yogi" (*jñāneśvara rājayogī*),[81] "Jñāneśvar the full yogi" (*jñāneśvara pūrṇayogī*)[82] and "Jñāneśvar the true yogi" (*jñāneśvara satyayogī*).[83] He also calls himself "knower of the truth" (*tattvajñānī*) and "himself *brahman*" (*svayaṃbrahma*),[84] so that one is tempted to consider the following stanzas as a response to these ambitious claims: "[One who] has become a 'knower of *brahman*', a 'full yogi', an adept, know him to be bound, one whose intelligence [believes in] difference. [To whom] everything appears as a form of *brahman*, he [has] understood the happiness of the Self."[85] Some of the lullabies attributed to the mythical queen Madālasā, who wanted her sons to renounce the world, bristle with yoga terminology.[86] For example, the eight limbs of yoga are enumerated among related items and are strongly recommended.[87] At the same time, the mention of Hari, Kṛṣṇa, *harināma*, "Hari's name", *rāmanāma*, "Rāma's name", *harikathā*, "stories about Hari", and *haridhyāna*, "meditation on Hari" place Madālasā's advice into a Vaiṣṇava context where yoga is less important than in the Śaiva context.[88] This can also be observed elsewhere: "The inborn life of the yogis [are the names] Rāmakṛṣṇa, Nārāyaṇa"[89] is the message of several songs containing the terms yoga or yogi. Notwithstanding the Vaiṣṇava bias, yoga is still presented in a positive manner here.

In contrast, about twenty-two passages inform in various shades of intensity about the inferiority of yoga, yogis, Aṣṭāṅga Yoga, etc., compared to devotion: "[Viṭṭhala is] the touchstone (*kasavaṭī*) of the yogis",[90] "I saw him who is difficult to reach for the yogis, oh friend",[91] "That to which the yogis direct [their] attention but never get to know, that manifested itself in Paṇḍharī",[92] "Restraint, observance, control of breath, withdrawal of the senses, all these are devices, but oh, calamities, as long as [Kṛṣṇa,] the one who is black like the *tamāḷa* tree has not

80 *Jethe caṃdra sūrya eka hotī, tethe kaici dinarātī, aisẽ je jāṇatī te yogeśvara* (478.6).

81 622.5 and 996.5. *Rājayogī* may also be translated as "the yogi who practises Rāja Yoga", derived from *rājayoga*, but the above translation fits the other *mudrikā*-s better.

82 626.5, 628.6 and 651.5.

83 654.5.

84 633.7 and 656.4.

85 *Jālā brahmajñānī pūrṇa yogī siddha, toci jāṇā baddha bheda buddhi. sarva brahmarūpa jayāsī biṃbalẽ, tayāsī kaḷalẽ nijasukha* (717.1–2).

86 999–1004, especially 1002.

87 For example, 1004.21–22. The story of Madālasā occurs in *Mārkaṇḍeyapurāṇa* 21–33 (Pargiter 1904: 113–186).

88 For example, in 999.

89 *Hẽ yogiyāṃcẽ nijajīvana rāmakṛṣṇa nārāyaṇa* (84.5).

90 *Yogiyāṃcā kasavaṭī* (4.2).

91 *Yogiyā durlabha to myā̃ dekhilā sājaṇī* (544.1).

92 *Yogī lakṣī̃ lakṣita jyātẽ, pari neṇave sarvathā [...] tẽ paṃḍhariye pragaṭalẽ* (203.4 und 6; similarly 1087.4 and 226.1).

set up his place in [one's] heart",[93] "Yoga is difficult; when one practises, it does not bring results, wherefore pure consciousness is not reached."[94] Instead, a sort of wellness programme is offered:

> 102
> 1. One should not get exhausted by the eight-limbed yoga, one should not practise restraint, observance, suppression (of the movements of the mind), king.
> 2. One should sing songs with one's voice, one should sing songs with one's voice, singing and resounding [of the name] should be heard with one's ears.
> 3. The body should be made to swing with the sound of songs,[95] one should cross the cycle of life in play and merriment.
> 4. By the name of the father, the husband of goddess Rakhumāī is obtained: this means should be applied.[96]

What sounds like a reminiscence of the beginnings of the Vārkarī movement and the first description of the cult during the thirteenth century when it was characterised as "acting and dancing" in honour of a deified folk hero,[97] exerts a stronger influence in the *Gāthā* than the few songs quoted here suggest. It is more or less the attitude manifest in the venerated *Haripāṭh*, "the recitation of Hari", a group of twenty-seven songs of the *Gāthā* in which the name of god is praised. Jośī (1969) lists a hundred more songs dedicated to that topic, and in a great number of other *abhaṅga*-s the importance of the name is mentioned in one or more stanzas. The *Haripāṭh* is recited during Vārkarī meetings throughout the year, and almost continuously for twenty-three days during the Paṇḍharpūr pilgrimage. More than 700,000 pilgrims from all over Maharashtra and Karnataka participate every year, with a large number of like-minded devotees in the background. "Say 'Hari' with your mouth, say 'Hari' with your mouth – who will count the merit" is the refrain.[98] Some of the *Haripāṭh* songs are also sung independently, such as "Keep firmly, oh mind, the one principle, the name", with the exhortation that "there is no different principle other than the name, in vain

93 *Yama niyama prāṇāyāma pratyāhāra, he sakaḷa upāya parī apāya re, jāva tamāḷanīḷa ghanasā̃vaḷā, hṛdayī̃ ṭhāṇa māṃḍūni na rāhe re* (920.7; similarly 392.8).

94 *Yoga to kaṭhīṇa sādhitā̃ sādhenā, jeṇẽ gā cidghanā na pāvije* (649.1).

95 The feminine noun *gītā* normally stands for *Bhagavadgītā*, but I am not sure whether this makes sense here.

96 *Aṣṭāṃgayogẽ na śiṇije, yama nema nirodha na kije rayā. vācā gīta gāīje vācā gīta gāīje, gātā̃ vātā̃ śravaṇī̃ aikije rayā. gītāchaṃdẽ aṃga ḍolije, līlāvinodẽ saṃsāra tarije rayā. bāpa rakhumādevivaru viṭhṭhalu nāmẽ joḍe hā upāvo kije rayā.*

97 *Naḍanācu* (*Līḷācaritra, līḷā* 508). Another version of this episode, mentioned by V. B. Kolte in his note on 508, makes Viṭṭhala a cow thief.

98 *Hari mukhẽ mhaṇā hari mukhẽ mhaṇā, puṇyācī gaṇanā koṇa karī* (48.2). I am quoting Jośī's *Haripāṭh* and not Ch. Vaudeville's edition (1969) because, although critical, the latter is not used by the Vārkarīs. In the present context, their choices are more important. Jośī's version (Jośī 1969: 40–59) agrees with the popular one published by S. V. Dāṇḍekar (1955: 63–69).

you go other paths, don't do [that]";[99] the name is "the best among all paths",[100] "among all paths the repetition of 'Hari' is easy."[101] Not only that: "Yoga, sacrifice, ritualistic rules – thereby no success [comes about], in vain [you perform] superficial things, religious acts that are hypocrisy."[102] By "the name" and its repetition practically all the aims of yoga are reached: *samādhi, samasukha, unmanī, siddhi* ("supernatural abilities"), *dhyāna* and *jīvanakalā,* the digit of life (*sattrāvī*) which is equal to the sweetness of the name:[103] "Yoga, sacrifice, action, the illusion of good and bad, they dissolved in the repetition of 'Hari'."[104]

6. Bhakti Yoga

Thus it seems that for the Vārkarīs there is no need of yoga in the classical and the Nāth sense, although the *Gāthā* contains many songs on it. Is this the triumph of one rival doctrine over the other, of the "*bhakti* movement" over yoga? I do not think so. First of all, the accomplished Nāth yogi Jñāndev himself cautions in the *Jñāneśvarī* that the fortress of yoga (*yogadurga*) is captured only by those who are *samabuddhi,* "equanimous".[105] It is much easier to do one's duty, dedicate one's actions to god and reach god by means of the path of *bhakti* (*bhaktipantha*).[106] In the *Anubhavāmṛt,* moreover, he explains that natural devotion (*akṛtrima bhakti*) leads to experiences of union with god where yoga and knowledge come to rest.[107] So the famous poet himself was aware of the different paths, although he described Kuṇḍalinī Yoga in the sixth chapter of the *Jñāneśvarī* with considerable enthusiasm.

Second, what the devotees of Viṭṭhala/Kṛṣṇa actually practise is a specialised form of yoga. They can even claim the support of *Yogasūtra* 1.23 where one learns that *samādhi* is also reached by *īśvarapraṇidhāna,* "dedication to god".[108] The

99 *Ekatattva nāma dṛḍha dharī̃ manā* (73.1), *nāmāparatē̃ tattva nāhī̃ re anyathā, vāyā̃ aṇika paṃthā jāśī jhaṇī* (73.3).
100 *Sarvamārgāṃvariṣṭha* (70.2).
101 *Sarva mārg[āṃ] sugama haripāṭha* (66.2).
102 *Yoga yāga vidhī yeṇē̃ navhe siddhī, vā̃yāci upādhī daṃbha dharma* (52.1).
103 The terms are mentioned in 55.4, 60.1, 63.2 and 50.4. See also above, p. 266f.
104 *Yoga yāga kriyā dharmādharma māyā, gele te vilayā haripāṭhī̃* (66.3).
105 *Jñāneśvarī* 12.46–57.
106 *Jñāneśvarī* 12.75–82.
107 *Anubhavāmṛt* 9.61 (Bahirat 1956: 246; Gokhle 1967: 145, stanza 760).
108 In the following, the Sanskrit quotations from the *Yogasūtra* and the "Vyāsa Commentary" are taken from Rāma Prasāda's edition (1910). The term *praṇidhāna* is rendered by O. Böhtlingk and R. Roth (1855–1875), M. Monier-Williams (1899) and V. S. Apte (1957) in several ways, such as "application, great energy, considerate behaviour, profound thinking, religious meditation, prayer", etc. In the context of the *Yogasūtra* it is often translated as "devotion", just like *bhakti* (see, e. g., Woods 1914, Hauer 1958, Satyananda Saraswati 1976,

commentary attributed to Vyāsa explains: "Through *īśvarapraṇidhāna,* a sort of devotion (*bhakti*), god, attracted [to the devotee], is merciful to him because of his (i. e., the devotee's) longing[109] alone. Alone through the longing [for god] the attainment of *samādhi* and the fruit of *samādhi* draw nearer for the yogi."[110] In *Śāṇḍilyabhaktisūtra* 1.20, *Yogasūtra* 1.23 is discussed: "*Samādhi* is reached through a subordinate (*gauṇī*)[111] [kind of devotion]",[112] and Svapneśvara comments: "There *praṇidhāna* is considered only a subordinate kind of *bhakti,* not the main one."[113] Harshananda explains: "*Parābhakti* or the highest devotion is actually the devotion that arises after the realisation of God. *Aparābhakti* or lower devotion, also known as *gauṇībhakti* is the means thereof. This latter is of the form of chanting the Lord's name, singing His glories etc. It is clear that in the *sūtras* of Patañjali it is this latter that is meant."[114] Be that as it may, this kind of *samādhi* seems to be well known also in the context of the contemplation of one's personal god. In the *Gheraṇḍasaṃhitā* it is called *bhaktiyogasamādhi,* "absorption through the yoga of devotion", and described thus:

Gheraṇḍasaṃhitā 7
14. One should meditate in one's own heart on the one whose form is one's personal deity, think [of him] by means of Bhakti Yoga, accompanied by[115] greatest delight.

Friedrich 1997, Prakash & Stoler Miller 1999, and Prabhavananda n. d. *ad loc.*); only Prasāda (1910: 40) explains *īśvarapraṇidhāna* as "feeling the omnipresence of God". In order to distinguish *praṇidhāna* from *bhakti,* I chose the rendering "dedication" for the former. This rendering fits in well with the "Vyāsa commentary" on *Yogasūtra* 2.1: "*īśvarapraṇidhāna* is the dedication of all actions to the highest teacher (god)" (*īśvarapraṇidhānaṃ sarvakriyāṇāṃ paramagurāv arpaṇam*).

109 Böhtlingk and Roth (1855–1875 s. v.) translate *abhidhyāna* as "das Richten der Gedanken auf einen Gegenstand" ("the focussing of the thoughts on an object"), adding the example *paradravyeṣv abhidhyānam,* "focussing one's thought on the possessions of others". According to Monier-Williams (1899 s. v.) and Apte (1957 s. v.), the term is used in the sense of "desiring, longing for, coveting, meditation", etc. In the context of *bhakti* "longing" makes good sense.

110 *Praṇidhānād bhaktiviśeṣād āvarjita īśvaras tam anugṛhṇāty abhidhyānamātreṇa, tadabhidhyānamātrād api yogina āsannataraḥ samādhilābhaḥ samādhiphalaṃ ca bhavatīti.*

111 *Gauṇī* is translated according to Apte (1957 s. v).

112 *Gauṇyā tu samādhisiddhiḥ.*

113 *Tatra praṇidhānaṃ gauṇabhaktir eva na pradhānam.*

114 Harshananda (1976: 63) in his English commentary on *Śāṇḍilyabhaktisūtra* 1.20.

115 The literal meaning of *pūrvaka* at the end of a compound is "preceded by", which is correct in many cases. In others it makes not much sense, and Monier-Williams (1899 s. v.) lists additional possible uses: "accompanied by, connected with, consisting in". This semantic tendency is also visible in modern Indian languages like Marathi and Hindi. Molesworth (1975 s. v.) remarks: "Its sense if explicated is still *First, preceding, antecedent*; but its service or force is that of *With, together with.* Ex. *āgrahapūrvaka With importunity [...].*" R. S. McGregor (1993 s. v.) considers *pūrvak* as a suffix forming adverbs of manner from nouns and adds as an example *ādārpūrvak* "respectfully".

15. With tears of joy and bristling of hairs, the absence of states [of mind][116] is produced. Thereby *samādhi* arises, and thereby arises the state above the mind (*unmanī*).[117]

When one compares the devotee's (*bhakta*'s) practices to the eight-limbed yoga, emphasis and details differ from the *Yogasūtra*. The followers of the *Haripāṭh* are, for example, not particularly encouraged to bother about restraint (*yama*) and observance (*niyama*). They are told that *dharmādharma*, here perhaps to be translated as "good actions and bad actions", are illusion (*māyā*) and dissolved in the recitation of "the name"[118] – and that heaps of "sins" (*pāpa*) disappear in this way.[119] However, in other songs and groups of songs like those I call *Anuṣṭhānapāṭh*,[120] selfish purpose (*svārtha*) is discouraged, and compassion with [all] beings (*bhūtadayā*), forbearance (*kṣamā*), longing [for god] (*ārta*), devotion (*bhakti*), knowledge (*jñāna*), dispassion (*vairagya*), contentment (*samādhāna*), tranquillity (*śānti*), non-injury (*ahiṃsā*)[121] and similar virtues are enjoined. In practical life, someone who has been initiated into the Vārkarī community vows to be a vegetarian.[122] Postures (*āsana*-s) in the sense of the *Haṭhayogapradīpikā* and related texts are not among the favourite occupations of the *bhakta*-s. The term occurs twice in enumerations of the eight limbs of yoga;[123] the lotus posture (*padmāsana*) is mentioned only in *Gāthā* 94.3. The two references to *āsana* in Madālasā's songs[124] may refer to a seat to sit on like in 226.1, and in 172.1 *āsana*-s are dismissed as useless (*laṭikē*). The six occurrences of the term *prāṇāyāma*,[125] though twice with a positive connotation, show the relatively low value accorded to control of breath, a practice of importance in Pātañjala and even more so in Haṭha and Kuṇḍalinī Yoga. The withdrawal of the senses (*pratyāhāra*) is mentioned only four times in enumerations of yoga practices,[126] but the numerous references to "turning back the mind" (e.g., *mana muraḍṇē, dṛṣṭi paratṇē*) and the disappearance of the constituents of perception (like *tripuṭī*) mentioned above[127] imply that the senses are withdrawn from outer and inner objects. That

116 Camanlāl Gautam (1981: 178) explains the expression *daśābhāva* as *acaitanyatā*, "state of non-consciousness".

117 *Svakīyahṛdaye dhyāyed iṣṭadevasvarūpakam, cintayed bhaktiyogena paramāhlādapūrvakam. ānandāśrupulakena daśābhāvaḥ prajāyate, samādhiḥ sambhavet tena sambhavec ca manonmanī.*

118 66.3; similarly 66.4 and 63.3.

119 For example, 20.1, 58.1, 61.2, 66.1, etc.

120 Kiehnle 1997b.

121 For example, 153.1–4, 154.1, 995.2 (see also Kiehnle 1997b: 68, 70, 71, 107).

122 Deleury 1960: 2.

123 351.3, 1004.21.

124 1002.17, 18.

125 351.3, 850.6, 920.7, 1004.21, 392.8 (*pavana abhyāsa*, "wind-practice").

126 351.3, 850.6, 920.7, 1004.21.

127 See p. 267f.

the *bhakta-s* practise the inner limbs of yoga has already been shown above: the binding of the mind to a place (*dhāraṇā*) and continued attention on a notion, contemplation (*dhyāna*), in the present context with respect to the form and name of god, occur in many songs. The ensuing *samādhi*, "[which is contemplation], appearing as the object alone, as if devoid of its nature [as a process of cognition]",[128] is not defined in the Pātañjala way in the *Gāthā*, but occurs in various descriptions and metaphors. In the following song, the transition from *dhyāna* to *samādhi* is illustrated by the lost wax technique of casting a metal image:

365
1. Watching closely I went [along, and] as I saw, I became identical [with the object of seeing].
2. [My] mind cooled down in the state above the mind, the dark highest *brahman* (Kṛṣṇa) appeared.
3. Having come, the form settled in my eyes, and as I saw, the highest *brahman* descended.[129]
4. The father, the husband of goddess Rakhumāī, Viṭṭhala, filled [himself] into the mould [of my body], discarding the wax [of my personality].[130]

7. Conclusion

One may say that the Bhakti Yoga[131] of the Vārkarīs is a shortcut version of the full-time yoga practised by "professionals" like Nāths and other monks. "For the name there is no [special] time"[132] was a motto beneficial for villagers, farmers, artisans, merchants, servants and, last but not least, women, who are among the most ardent devotees of Viṭṭhala and for whom the regular practice of postures and control of breath was no feasible option. Moreover, many of the yoga passages in the *Jñāneśvarī* and the *Gāthā* seem to be written by yogis for yogis who were well-versed in philosophy, tantric lore and terminology, and who had expert teachers to support them in theory and practice – a rare privilege. The Vārkarī cult, on the other hand, was and is a mass movement where *bhakti* with its homely

128 *Yogasūtra* 3.3: *tad evārthamātranirbhāsaṃ svarūpaśūnyam iva samādhiḥ.*

129 According to Tulpule & Feldhaus 1999, *avatarṇẽ* can also mean *aṅgāt yeṇẽ*, "to possess", as said of a ghost. If understood in a positive sense, this is what happens to the poet here.

130 *Nirakhita nirakhita gelīyẽ, pāhẽ tāva tanmaya jāliye. unmanī mana nivālẽ, sā̃vaḷẽ parabrahma bhasaḷẽ. rūpa yevoniyā̃ ḍoḷā̃ baisalẽ, pāhẽ tāva parabrahma avataralẽ. bāpa rakhumādevivarẽ viṭhṭhalẽ, mūsa otūnīyā̃ meṇa sāṃḍilẽ.* For metaphors used in the *Gāthā*, see Kiehnle 1994 and 2014.

131 The term *bhaktiyoga* is used only once, just as *bhaktipantha*, "path of devotion"; see 152.4 and 401.4.

132 *Nāmāsī nāhī kāḷaveḷa* (171.4).

images is more in demand than the yoga of the specialists. In spite of that, the *bhakta-s* transmitted the yoga songs of the *Jñāndev Gāthā*[133] and thus preserved a treasure that still waits to be recovered in its entirety.[134]

References

Anubhavāmṛt
see Bahirat 1956: 159–251.
see Gokhle 1967.

Apte, V. S. (1957). *The Practical Sanskrit-English Dictionary*. Rev. and enlarged edition. Poona: Prasad Prakashan (2nd repr. of the compact edition 1965. Delhi: Motilal Banarsidass, 2007).

Bahirat, B. P. (Trans.). (1956). Anubhavāmṛt. In *The Philosophy of Jnanadeva* (pp. 159–251). Bombay: Popular Book Depot (2nd impression 1961).

Böhtlingk, O. & Roth, R. (1855–1875). *Sanskrit-Wörterbuch. Herausgegeben von der Kaiserlichen Akademie der Wissenschaften*. St. Petersburg: Buchdruckerei der Kaiserlichen Akademie der Wissenschaften (repr. Tokyo: Neicho-Fukyū-Kai, 1976).

Bühnemann, G. (Ed., Trans.). (1983). *Budha-Kauśika's Rāmarakṣāstotra: A Contribution to the Study of Sanskrit Devotional Literature*. Publications of the De Nobili Research Library X. Vienna: Indologisches Institut der Universität Wien, Sammlung De Nobili.

Dāṇḍekar, S. V. (Ed.). (1955). *Vārkarī bhajan-saṃgrah*. Puṇe: Prācārya Dāṃḍekar dhārmik śaikṣaṇik vā sāṃskṛtik vāṅmaya prakāśan maṃḍaḷ (9th repr.).

Deleury, G. A. (1960). *The Cult of Viṭhobā*. Poona: Deccan College.

Friedrich, E. (Trans.). (1997). *Yoga, der indische Erlösungsweg: das klassische System und seine Hintergründe*. München: Diederichs.

Gautam, Camanlāl (Ed., Trans.). (1981). *Gheraṇḍa-Saṃhitā, bhāṣānuvād evaṃ vistṛt vyākhyā sahit*. Barelī: Saṃskṛti Saṃsthān.

Gheraṇḍasaṃhitā
see Gautam 1981.

Gokhle, V. D. (Ed.). (1967). *Śrījñāndevviracit Anubhavāmṛt. anek junyā poṭhyāṃce ādhāreṃ siddh kelelī navī saṃśodhit āvṛtti*. Puṇe: Nīlkaṇṭh Prakāśan.

Haripāṭh
see Dāṇḍekar 1955: 63–69.
see Jośī 1969: 40–59.
see Vaudeville 1969.

Harshananda, S. (Ed., Trans). (1976). *Śāṇḍilya Bhakti Sūtras with Svapneśvara Bhāṣya*. Mysore: Prasārāṅga, University of Mysore.

Haṭhayogapradīpikā
Haṭhayogapradīpikā of Svātmārāma, with the Commentary Jyotsnā of Brahmānanda, and English Translation by S. Iyangar. Revised by A. A. Ramanathan, and S. V. Subrahmanya Sastri. Madras: The Adyar Library and Research Centre, 1972 (repr. 1975).

133 See Kiehnle 2014.
134 For other strands of philosophy and religion in the *Gāthā*, see Kiehnle 2014.

Hauer, J. W. (Ed., Trans.). (1958). *Der Yoga, ein indischer Weg zum Selbst.* Stuttgart: Kohlhammer (3rd impression Südgellersen: Verlag Bruno Martin, 1983).

Jñāndev Gāthā
 see Jośī 1969.
 see Kānaḍe & Nagarkar 1995.

Jñāneśvarī
 see Maṃgrūḷkar & Keḷkar 1994.
 see Pradhan 1969.

Jośī, P. N. (Ed.). (1969). *Sārth śrī jñāndev abhaṅg gāthā.* Puṇe: Suvicār Prakāśan Maṇḍaḷ.

Kānaḍe, M. Ś. & Nagarkar, R. Ś. (Eds., Trans.). (1995). *Śrījñāndevāṃcā sārth cikitsak gāthā.* Puṇe: Suvidhā Prakāśan.

Kiehnle, C. (1989). Śivaismus und Viṣṇuismus in der Bhakti-Bewegung Mahārāṣṭras: Jñāndevs Saptapadi. In E. von Schuler (Ed.), *XXIII. Deutscher Orientalistentag vom 16. bis 20. September 1985 in Würzburg. Ausgewählte Vorträge* (pp. 357–363). Wiesbaden: Franz Steiner.

Kiehnle, C. (1992). Authorship and Redactorship of the Jñāndev Gāthā. In R. S. McGregor (Ed.), *Devotional Literature in South Asia: Current Research, 1985–1988. Papers of the Fourth Conference on Devotional Literature in New Indo-Aryan Languages, held at Wolfson College, Cambridge, 1-4 September 1988* (pp. 126–137). Cambridge: Cambridge University Press.

Kiehnle, C. (1994). Metaphors in the Jñāndev Gāthā. In A. W. Entwistle & F. Mallison (Eds.), *Studies in South Asian Devotional Literature: Research Papers, 1988–1991, Presented at the Fifth Conference on Devotional Literature in New Indo-Aryan Languages, held at Paris - École Française d'Extrême-Orient, 9–12 July 1991* (pp. 301–323). Paris: École Française d'Extrême-Orient.

Kiehnle, C. (1997a). *Songs on Yoga: Texts and Teachings of the Mahārāṣṭrian Nāths.* Jñāndev Studies I–II. Alt- und Neu-Indische Studien 48.1. Stuttgart: Franz Steiner.

Kiehnle, C. (1997b). *The Conservative Vaiṣṇava: Anonymous Songs of the Jñāndev Gāthā.* Jñāndev Studies III. Alt- und Neu-Indische Studien 48.2. Stuttgart: Franz Steiner.

Kiehnle, C. (1997c). The Lotus of the Heart. *Studien zur Indologie und Iranistik, 21,* 91–103.

Kiehnle, C. (Trans.). (2004–2005). The Secret of the Nāths: the Ascent of Kuṇḍalinī according to Jñāneśvarī 6.151–328. *Bulletin d'Études Indiennes, 22–23,* 447–494.

Kiehnle, C. (2005). The Vāsudev: Folk Figures and Vārkarī bhakti in the Jñāndev Gāthā. In A. Malik et al. (Eds.), *In the Company of Gods: Essays in Memory of Günther-Dietz Sontheimer* (pp. 193–210). New Delhi: Manohar.

Kiehnle, C. (2014). The Gopīs of the Jñāndev Gāthā. In Th. de Bruijn & A. Busch (Eds.), *Culture and Circulation - Literature in Motion in Early Modern India.* Brill's Indological Library 46 (pp. 160–185). Leiden: Brill.

Kolte, V. B. (Ed.). (1978). *Līḷācaritra.* Muṃbaī: Mahārāṣṭra Rājya Sāhitya Saṃskṛti Maṃḍaḷ.

Lad, P. M. (Ed.). (1973). *Śrī Tukārāmbāvāṃcyā abhaṃgāṃcī gāthā.* Muṃbaī: Government Central Press.

Līḷācaritra
 see Kolte 1978.

Maṃgrūḷkar, A. & V. M. Keḷkar (Eds., Trans.). (1994). *Upanyās, anvay, arth, ṭīpā, pariśiṣṭe va ovīsūcī yāṃsaha jñānadevī, Vi. Kā. Rājvāḍe pratītīl saṃhitā.* 3 vols. Muṃbaī: Muṃbaī Vidyāpīṭh, Marāṭhī Vibhāg.

Mārkaṇḍeyapurāṇa
see Pargiter 1904.

McGregor, R. S. (1993). *The Oxford Hindi-English Dictionary.* Oxford: Oxford University Press (36th impression, November 2009, of the first Indian impression 1994).

Michaël, T. (1979). *Corps subtil et corps causal: La description des six "Cakra" et quelques textes sanscrits sur le Kuṇḍalinī Yoga.* Paris: Le Courier du Livre.

Molesworth, J. T. (1975). *Marāṭhī-English Dictionary.* Pune: Shubhadha Sarasvat (corrected repr.).

Monier-Williams, M. (1899). *A Sanskrit-English Dictionary.* Oxford: Clarendon Press (repr. Delhi: Motilal Banarsidass, 1970).

Padoux, A. (1975). *Recherches sur la symbolique et l'Énergie de la parole dans certains textes tantriques.* Publications de l'Institut de Civilisation Indienne, Serie IN-8°, fascicule 21. Paris: Edition E. de Boccard.

Pargiter, F. E. (1904). *Mārkaṇḍeyapurāṇa. Translated with Notes.* Bibliotheca Indica New Series, Nos. 700, 706, 810, 872, 890, 947, 1058, 1076, 1104. Calcutta: The Asiatic Society (repr. Delhi: Indological Bookhouse, 1981).

Prabhavananda, Swami (Ed., Trans.). (n. d.). *Patanjali Yoga Sutras.* Chennai: Sri Ramakrishna Math, Mylapore, Chennai.

Pradhan, V. G. (1969). *Jnāneshvari (Bhāvārthadipikā): A Song-Sermon on the Bhagavadgītā. Translated from the Marāṭhī by V. G. Pradhan, edited by H. M. Lambert.* 2 vols. London: George Allen & Unwin (2nd Indian repr. Bombay: Blackie & Son Publishers, 1982).

Prakash, P. & Stoler Miller, B. (Eds., Trans.). (1999). *Yoga, der innere Weg zur Freiheit.* Frankfurt a. M.: Wolfgang Krüger Verlag.

Prasāda, R. (1910). *Patanjali's Yoga Sutras With the Commentary of Vyâsa and the Gloss of Vâchaspati Miśra. Translated by Râma Prasâda [...] With an Introduction from Rai Bahadur Śrīśa Chandra Vasu.* Sacred Books of the Hindus 4.7–9. Allahabad: Panini Office (repr. New Delhi: Munshiram Manoharlal, 1988).

Rāmarakṣāstotra
see Bühnemann 1983.

Rāṇade, R. D. (Ed.). (1961). *Jñāneśvar vacanāmṛt.* Adhyātma graṃthamālā 1. Puṇẽ: Vhīnas Prakāśan.

Śāṇḍilyabhaktisūtra
see Harshananda 1976.

Ṣaṭcakranirūpaṇa
see Michaël 1979.

Satyananda Saraswati, Swami (Ed., Trans.). (1976). *Four Chapters on Freedom: Commentary on the Yoga Sutras of Patanjali.* Munger: Bihar School of Yoga (repr. Munger: Yoga Publication Trust, 2008).

Srinivasachari, P. N. (1978). *The Philosophy of Viśiṣṭādvaita.* Madras: The Adyar Library and Research Centre.

Tukārām Gāthā
see Lad 1973.

Tulpule, S. G. & Feldhaus, A. (1999). *A Dictionary of Old Marathi.* Mumbai: Popular Prakashan.

Vaudeville, Ch. (Ed., Trans.). (1969). *L'Invocation: Le Haripāṭh de Dyāndev.* Publications de l'École Française d'Extrême-Orient LXXIII. Paris: Adrien-Maisonneuve.

Vaudeville, Ch. (1987). The Shaivite Background of Santism in Maharashtra. In M. Israel & N. K. Wagle (Eds.), *Religion and Society in Maharashtra.* South Asian Studies Papers 1 (pp. 32–50). Toronto: University of Toronto (Centre for South Asian Studies).

Vetter, T. (1979). *Studien zur Lehre und Entwicklung Śaṅkaras.* Publications of the De Nobili Research Library IV. Wien: Institut für Indologie der Universität Wien, Sammlung De Nobili.

Woods, J. H. (Trans.). (1914). *The Yoga-System of Patañjali, Or the Ancient Hindu Doctrine of Concentration of Mind, Embracing the Mnemonic Rules, Called Yoga-Sūtras, of Patañjali and the Comment, Called Yoga-Bhāshya, Attributed to Veda-Vyāsa, and the Explanation, Called Tattva-Vaiçāradī, of Vāchaspati-Miçra.* Harvard Oriental Series 17. Cambridge: Harvard University Press (repr. Delhi: Motilal Banarsidass, 1983).

Yogasūtra
- see Friedrich 1997.
- see Hauer 1958.
- see Prabhavananda n. d.
- see Prakash & Stoler Miller 1999.
- see Prasāda 1910.
- see Satyananda Saraswati 1976.
- see Woods 1914.

Chapter 7

On al-Bīrūnī's *Kitāb Pātanğal* and the *Pātañjalayogaśāstra*

Philipp A. Maas / Noémie Verdon

Contents

1. Introduction 285
1.1. The Life and Work of al-Bīrūnī 285
1.2. The *Kitāb Pātanğal* in its Socio-Historical Context 289
1.3. Al-Bīrūnī's Hermeneutic Approach to South Asian Religion and Philosophy 290
1.4. The Reception History of the *Kitāb Pātanğal* 290

2. The Search for the Sanskrit Source of the *Kitāb Pātanğal* 291
2.1. Carl Edward Sachau: A Quest in Vain 291
2.2. Surendra Nath Dasgupta: A Third Patañjali 293
2.3. Richard Garbe: The *Rājamārtaṇḍa* of King Bhoja 293
2.3.1. The Agricultural Example 294
2.3.2. The Mythological Example 297
2.4. Jean Filliozat: Al-Bīrūnī's Creativity 301
2.5. Shlomo Pines and Tuvia Gelblum: The *Yogasūtra* with an Unknown Commentary 302
2.5.1. The Medical Excursion 303
2.5.1. The Cosmographical Excursion 306
2.6. A New Hypothesis: The *Pātañjalayogaśāstra* 312

3. The *Pātañjalayogaśāstra* in Transformation 315
3.1. Explicitly Mentioned Transformations 315
3.1.1. Combining Different Layers of Text 317
3.1.2. Creating a Dialogue 317
3.1.3. Omitting Linguistic Explanations 320
3.2. Translational Strategies 321
3.2.1. Borrowing 322
3.2.2. Defining the Elements of Culture 324
3.2.3. Literal Translation 324
3.2.4. Substitution 325
3.2.5. Lexical Creation 326
3.2.6. Omission 326
3.2.7. Addition 327
3.3. Results 328

4. Conclusion 329

References 330

Philipp A. Maas / Noémie Verdon

Chapter 7: On al-Bīrūnī's *Kitāb Pātanǧal* and the *Pātañjalayogaśāstra*[*]

1. Introduction

1.1. The Life and Work of al-Bīrūnī

Abu l-Rayḥān Muḥammad bin Aḥmad al-Bīrūnī, or, more briefly, al-Bīrūnī, was a Perso-Muslim polymath who lived at the turn of the first millennium CE. Al-Bīrūnī's biography is largely unknown, because the only available source of information on the life of the scholar is the scant information scattered throughout his oeuvre.[1] Yet, it is possible to reconstruct the main events of his life. Al-Bīrūnī was born in 973 CE in today's Uzbekistan in the region known as Khwarezm, located south of the Aral Sea, which was exposed to various cultural influences from Persia, South Asia and China throughout its history.[2] Probably from 995 to 997, he left his home and stayed in Ray (a south-eastern suburb of present-day Teheran). Al-Bīrūnī also lived in ancient Gorgan, situated on the south-eastern corner of the Caspian Sea in Iran, from 1000 to 1004. He returned then to Khwarezm and lived there until 1017 when Maḥmūd, the Ghaznavid, a Muslim ruler coming from Ghazna in today's Afghanistan, subdued this region.

---

* The present chapter is partly based on Noémie Verdon's presentation at the conference "Yoga in Transformation: Historical and Contemporary Perspectives on a Global Phenomenon". There, she convincingly explained a number of characteristics of the *Kitāb Pātanǧal* as the result of al-Bīrūnī's revision of a Sanskrit source text that at this time remained to be identified. Subsequently, Noémie refined her approach to the *Kitāb Pātanǧal* by taking into account recent results of Translation Studies. When she presented a draft version of the present chapter to Philipp A. Maas, he introduced to Noémie his hypothetical identification of the *Pātañjalayogaśāstra* as a main Sanskrit source of the *Kitāb Pātanǧal*. The discussion of this hypothesis led to a joint thorough textual analysis of both the *Pātañjalayogaśāstra* and the *Kitāb Pātanǧal* as well as to a detailed discussion of previous scholarly attempts to identify the Sanskrit source of the Arabic *Kitāb Pātanǧal*. Finally, Noémie and Philipp authored the present chapter jointly by sharing their respective linguistic expertise, knowledge of South Asian and Arabic culture as well as reflections and ideas online and in two project meetings in Vienna.

1 See for instance the works of Kennedy (1970: II), Shamsi (1979), and Yano (2013).

2 Kozah 2015: 8.

From 1017 to his death, at some time between the years 1048 and 1050,[3] al-Bīrūnī remained at the Ghaznavids' court, and stayed at different places in present-day Afghanistan as, for example, Kabul and Ghazna. He also visited areas located in north-western Pakistan, such as Peshawar, and Nandana (in the Salt Range). This later period of al-Bīrūnī's life appears to be the most probable time during which the scholar participated in an exchange with South Asian intellectuals. However, the exact circumstances of this intellectual interaction remain unknown.

Al-Bīrūnī composed works on a wide range of topics, such as astronomy, mathematics, geography, history, gemmology, and pharmacology.[4] In South Asian studies, he is well known for his monograph on India, the *Taḥqīq mā li-l-Hind.* This work, which he wrote around the year 1030, is commonly referred to as the *Kitāb al-Hind* or "India".[5] In this book, al-Bīrūnī discussed a large variety of subjects related to Indian science, history, geography, culture, literature, astronomy, religion, and philosophy. He quoted abundantly from the mythological literature of the *Purāṇa*-s, from astronomical treatises, from a book that he called *Gītā,* from a work that he named *Kitāb Sānk,* and from the *Kitāb Pātanğal.*[6] The two last mentioned works are in fact Arabic translations of Sanskrit works that al-Bīrūnī prepared himself. The *Kitāb Sānk* is connected with Sāṅkhya philosophy, while the *Kitāb Pātanğal* is a rendering of a work belonging to a South Asian yoga tradition. Al-Bīrūnī rendered both works probably at some time between 1017, when he accompanied Maḥmūd in eastern Afghanistan and western Pakistan, and 1030, before he composed the *Taḥqīq mā li-l-Hind.*

Al-Bīrūnī's Arabic work on yoga is entitled "The Book by Pātanğal the Indian, on the Deliverance from the Afflictions, into Arabic, by Abū l-Rayḥān Muḥammad bin Aḥmad al-Bīrūnī".[7] In this title the word *pātanğal* is probably the Arabic transliteration of the Sanskrit word *pātañjala,* which is a *vṛddhi*-deriva-

3 Kennedy 1970: II/151; Hermelink 1977; Shamsi 1979: 273–274.

4 Boilot 1955.

5 The full title of this work is كتاب البيرونى في تحقيق ما للهند من مقولة مقبولة في العقل او مرذولة ("The Book of al-Bīrūnī on the Verification of Indian Treatises Accepted or Rejected by the Reason"). See al-Bīrūnī 1958 and trans. Sachau 1888.

6 See the lists of al-Bīrūnī's sources provided by Sachau (1888: I/xxxix–xl) and Shastri (1975).

7 كتاب باتنجل الهندى فى الخلاص من الاثقال نقل ابى الريحان محمد بن احمد البيرونى الى العربى The reading "afflictions" (lit.: "burdens", اثقال) follows the emendation for the Arabic word meaning "similarity, metaphor" (امثال) proposed by Pines and Gelblum (1966: 308f., n. 51). Al-Bīrūnī referred to the *Kitāb Pātanğal* under the title "Translation of the Book Pātanğal on the Deliverance from the Entanglements/Confusions" when he compiled a list of his own works in the year 1036 (ترجمة كتاب باتنجل فى الخلاص من الإرتباك); see Boilot 1955: 208. Moreover, in his *Taḥqīq mā li-l-Hind,* al-Bīrūnī describes his work as dealing with "the deliverance of the soul from the fetters of the body" (في تخليصِ النفسِ من رِباطِ البدنِ) (al-Bīrūnī 1958: 6, l. 2f.; for a different translation see Sachau 1888: I/8) and with "the quest for the deliverance and the union of the soul with the [object] it perceives" (فى طلب الخلاص و اتحاد النفس بمعقولها) (al-Bīrūnī 1958: 102, l. 3f.; for a different translation see Sachau 1888: I/132).

tion, i.e., a word formed by means of vowel gradation, of the proper name Patañjali. The word *pātanğal* is used to designate the authorship of a work, i.e., – as we shall argue below – the authorship of the Arabic version of the *Pātañjalayogaśāstra.* However, as was already highlighted by Hauer,[8] al-Bīrūnī used the word *pātanğal* not only to refer to the title of a book but also as a proper name of a person.[9]

Pines and Gelblum[10] suggested a different interpretation of the Arabic word *bātanğal* (باتنجل) or *pātanğal.*[11] According to them, al-Bīrūnī inserted the long *ā* in *pātanğal* "in order to ensure an approximately correct pronunciation of the foreign name" Patañjali.[12] However, in the *Taḥqīq mā li-l-Hind,* al-Bīrūnī is generally faithful in rendering the length of Sanskrit vowels into Arabic letters. Al-Bīrūnī transliterated the titles of various *Purāṇa*-s with a long *ā* at the proper positions, as for example in *bišnu-purāna* for *viṣṇu-purāṇa* (بشن پران), or in *bāğu-purāna* for *vāyu-purāṇa* (باج پران). Moreover, the orthography of the title "*Book Gītā*" (كتاب گيتا; *kitāb gītā*) corresponds to the Sanskrit title *Bhagavadgītā* in having two long vowels. Also the title of the "*Book Sānk*" (كتاب سانک; *kitāb sānk*, or سانگ; *sāng*) which is related to the classical Sāṅkhya school of thought has a long vowel. In some cases, however, a long vowel in Arabic does not represent a long vowel of a Sanskrit word, as, for example, in Arabic چتر جوك (*catur jūka*) for Sanskrit *caturyuga,* meaning "the four ages collectively". Therefore the case cannot be decided with absolute certainty.

The *Kitāb Pātanğal* consists of a dialogue between Pātanğal and "the ascetic who roamed in the deserts and jungles".[13] In this conversation, the ascetic poses questions that provide Pātanğal with the opportunity to present his exposition on yoga.

The dialogue of Pātanğal and the ascetic is structured in four chapters that al-Bīrūnī framed with his own introduction and conclusion. The title and partly the contents of the *Kitāb Pātanğal* suggest that the work is in one way or the other related to the *Pātañjalayogaśāstra,* i.e., the *Yogasūtra* of Patañjali together with

8 Hauer 1930: column 277.

9 The name Pātañjala occurs also in an Old Javanese work related to the South Asian yoga tradition, namely in the *Dharma Pātañjala.* See Acri 2011: 16.

10 Pines & Gelblum 1966: 308, n. 50.

11 The Arabic alphabet does not contain a representation of the voiceless bilabial stop *p.* Therefore, the initial letter of the word "Pātañjal" occurs in al-Bīrūnī's work either as the Arabic letter *b* (ب) or as the Persian letter *p* (پ).

12 See Verdon 2015: 133–137.

13 Trans. Pines & Gelblum 1966: 313. سأل الزاهد السايح فى الصحارى و الغياض. Instead of the word "jungle" (الغياض; *al-ġiyāḍi*), an alternative reading would be an Arabic word for desert (الفيافى; *al-fayāfī*) (Ritter 1956: 169, l. 10, and n. 4). In medieval Islam, ascetics, who roamed the deserts (سايح) of Islamic territory, were regarded as religious saints in search of Allah. See Touati 2000: 187–188.

the so-called *Yogabhāṣya*, from which, however, the *Kitāb Pātanǧal* differs considerably with regard to its form and with regard to its contents. Even so, both works are structured into four chapters. Moreover, the topics that are treated in each of these chapters as well as the titles that we find in the concluding statements of each chapter in both works roughly correspond to each other, as can be seen in Table 1 below.[14]

The chapter-concluding statements in the *Kitāb Pātanǧal*	**The chapter-concluding statements in the *Pātañjalayogaśāstra***
"Here ends the first section, (dealing with) making the heart steadfastly fixed, of Patañjali's Book." تمت القطعة الاولى من كتاب باتنجل فى اقرار القلب على مقر واحد	"In the authoritative exposition of Yoga that originates from Patañjali, in the magisterial Sāṅkhya teaching, this was the first part 'on concentration'." (*iti pātañjale yogaśāstre sāṃkhyapravacane samādhipādaḥ prathamaḥ*)
"Here ends the second section (dealing with) guidance towards the *praxis* which has been treated previously in the first section." تمت القطعة الثانية فى ارشاد الى عمل ما كان تقدم فى القطعة الاولى	"In the authoritative exposition of Yoga that originates from Patañjali, in the magisterial Sāṅkhya teaching, this was the second part called 'instruction in means'." (*iti pātañjale yogaśāstre sāṃkhyapravacane sādhananirdeśo nāma dvitīyaḥ pādaḥ*)
"Here ends the third section whose particular (subject) is recompense and the *quale* of requital." تمت القطعة الثالثة المقصورة على ذكر الجزاء وكيفية المجازاة	"In the authoritative exposition of Yoga that originates from Patañjali, in the magisterial Sāṅkhya teaching, this was the third part 'on supernatural powers'." (*iti pātañjale yogaśāstre sāṃkhyapravacane vibhūtipādas tṛtīyaḥ*)
"Here ends the fourth section, (dealing with) liberation and union, and with its ending the (whole) book has ended." تمت القطعة الرابعة فى الخلاص والاتحاد وتم بتمامها الكتاب	"In the authoritative exposition of Yoga that originates from Patañjali, in the magisterial Sāṅkhya teaching, this was the fourth part 'on separation'. And here the work ends." (*iti pātañjale yogaśāstre sāṃkhyapravacane kaivalyapādaś caturthaḥ. samāptaś cāyaṃ granthaḥ*)

Table 1: The wording of the chapter colophons of the *Kitāb Pātanǧal* and the *Pātañjalayogaśāstra* in comparison.

Although the chapter colophons of the two works differ, for example, in that the *Pātañjalayogaśāstra* designates itself as "the magisterial Sāṅkhya teaching" (*sāṅkhyapravacana*), whereas al-Bīrūnī does not refer to Sāṅkhya philosophy here at all, the degree of similarity between the two sets of colophons cannot be the result of a mere accident.

14 The text of the four chapter-concluding statements in the *Kitāb Pātanǧal* is taken from Ritter 1956: 177, l. 10, 183, l. 18, 192, l. 22 and 199, l. 1; the translations are those of Pines and Gelblum (Pines & Gelblum 1966: 325, 1977: 527, 1983: 265 and 1989: 271). The text of the concluding statements in the *Pātañjalayogaśāstra* follows Maas 2006: xxf.

1.2. The *Kitāb Pātanğal* in its Socio-Historical Context

Before we investigate the relationship of the *Kitāb Pātanğal* to possible Sanskrit sources in more detail, it may be worth recalling the socio-historical context in which al-Bīrūnī composed his work. Al-Bīrūnī composed the *Kitāb Pātanğal* during the Golden Age of the Islamic world, which lasted approximately from the middle of the eighth to the beginning of the thirteenth century CE. In this period of time, a large number of works were translated into Arabic. The most intensive phase of this important translation movement, which involved a large variety of domains, took place at the beginning of the Abbasid Caliphate (750–1258) in Bagdad. Then, Arab thinkers translated, interpreted, and commented upon many Greek philosophical works, often via intermediate Syriac translations. These works include, for instance, almost the complete oeuvre of Aristotle.[15] Indian scientific works, particularly astronomical and mathematical texts, were also studied, interpreted and rendered into Arabic.

From the ninth century onwards, Greek philosophical theories and conceptions found their way into the Arab intellectual world by means of translations of a wide range of Greek philosophical works that became subject to debates and reinterpretations. Greek philosophical conceptions were used creatively to develop new Arab philosophical and theological theories. Generally speaking, the Arab interest in ancient Greek works was to a considerable degree motivated by the desire to receive and create heuristic tools that are useful for developing and elaborating a Muslim philosophical theology.[16] Al-Bīrūnī was indebted to this intellectual milieu. Mario Kozah argues, for instance, that the exchange with his rival scholar Ibn Sīnā decisively influenced the development of al-Bīrūnī's religious and philosophical world-view as well as his methodology.[17]

For an appreciation of the scope and the meaning of al-Bīrūnī's translation work, it may be worth mentioning that the Arabic word that al-Bīrūnī used for his literary activity is *naqlu* (نقل).[18] The term actually designates in its primary meaning the activities of carrying and transporting. It is then used with a wider meaning in the sense of the transportation of ideas from a source language to a target idiom, just like the English term "transmission". Moreover, as Robert Wisnovsky et al. recall, the concept of translation implies the idea of transmission and transformation of a source text.[19] In this context, the translators of

15 Daiber 2012: 60.

16 See Daiber 2012: 43–63. On different translation projects into Arabic, see Ernst 2003: 173–174, Koetschet 2011: 11–14, and Zadeh 2011: 53–60.

17 Kozah 2015: 11f.

18 The other commonly used term is *tarjama* (ترجم) which means "to translate", but also "to interpret".

19 Wisnovsky et al. 2011: 13.

medieval Islam used different methods to transmit ideas, ranging from preparing relatively literal translations to compositing commentaries. Generally, their intention was to remain faithful to the source text, "whether that was in letter or in spirit".[20]

1.3. Al-Bīrūnī's Hermeneutic Approach to South Asian Religion and Philosophy

Al-Bīrūnī noticed, according to Wilhelm Halbfass, the similarity in difference between the ancient Greek religion and that of South Asia in so far as both religions are polytheistic and equally different from monotheistic Islam. The common difference from his own tradition provided al-Bīrūnī with a perspective that allowed for a comparison of the polytheistic Indian with the Greek religion as well as with monotheistic Islam. His view led him to a remarkably and unprecedentedly open hermeneutic approach towards the religion and philosophy of South Asia. According to Halbfass, al-Bīrūnī's hermeneutics, which is based on a "positive interest" and on a lack of missionary ambitions, may be characterised as follows:

> A clear awareness of his *own* religious horizon as a particular context of thought led him [i. e., al-Bīrūnī] to perceive the "otherness" of the Indian religious philosophical context and horizon with remarkable clarity, and he understood the difficulties of penetrating it. This clarity of hermeneutic awareness is unparalleled in the world of classical antiquity […].[21]

The intellectual background of al-Bīrūnī's literary activity already suggests that the scholar may not have intended to produce a literal translation of any Sanskrit source, but that he rather transformed his source in order to communicate the contents, as far as he understood and valued it, to his Muslim readership.

1.4. The Reception History of the *Kitāb Pātanğal*

The success of al-Bīrūnī's programme to promote knowledge of South Asian religion and philosophy in the Muslim world appears to have been rather limited. The survival of a single textual witness of the *Kitāb Pātanğal* as well as an almost complete lack of references to al-Bīrūnī's work in later Arabic or Persian liter-

20 Wisnovsky et al. 2011: 9.
21 Halbfass 1990: 26f.

ature indicate that it was received with reservation. At least one of al-Bīrūnī's Muslim readers even found his translation of the yoga work incomprehensible.[22]

Al-Bīrūnī's work did not receive much attention in medieval Islam; it became, however, the object of quite a number of modern academic studies. In these studies, the exact relationship of the *Kitāb Pātanğal* to the works of the South Asian yoga tradition, as well as possible reasons for peculiarities in al-Bīrūnī's exposition of yoga, were controversially discussed, mainly on the basis of a comparison between the *Kitāb Pātanğal* and possible Sanskrit sources. However, as we shall argue in more detail below, detecting similarities and differences between al-Bīrūnī's work and probable Sanskrit sources in order to determine the degree of faithfulness of al-Bīrūnī's literary activity cannot do justice to his oeuvre.

In the following section 2 of this chapter, we shall discuss different attempts to identify the main source of the *Kitāb Pātanğal* that scholars undertook since 1888.[23] Then, we shall present our own solution and argue that al-Bīrūnī's main source was probably the *Pātañjalayogaśāstra*.[24] In section 3, we shall initially take a fresh and thorough look at how al-Bīrūnī used his main source by taking into account what al-Bīrūnī himself related about the way he dealt with it. Following this, we shall introduce different translational strategies that al-Bīrūnī apparently used for the composition of his work. Finally, in our conclusion (section 4), we stress the fact that al-Bīrūnī composed a work that is to a considerable degree independent from its sources. Therefore, it is necessary to take al-Bīrūnī's motives and authorial intention into consideration in order to arrive at a fuller picture of his literary activity and creativity.

2. The Search for the Sanskrit Source of the *Kitāb Pātanğal*

2.1. Carl Edward Sachau: A Quest in Vain

The first western scholar to work on the *Kitāb Pātanğal* was Carl Edward Sachau. He brought the Arabic text to the attention of the academic world when he published his English translation of al-Bīrūnī's "India" in 1888 (Sachau 1888). This comprehensive survey of pre-modern South Asian culture and religion

22 See Pines & Gelblum 1966: 302, n. 1; Ernst 2003: 177.

23 The earliest history of research was already sketched by Pines and Gelblum (1966: 303–304).

24 The text version of the *Pātañjalayogaśāstra* that al-Bīrūnī knew will certainly have differed to some degree from the version of this work transmitted in modern printed editions. For a discussion of an instance of textual deviation between al-Bīrūnī's version of the *Pātañjalayogaśāstra* (as inferable from Q 46 of the *Kitāb Pātanğal*) and PYŚ 3.29, see below, p. 305f.

contains eight literal or analogous quotations from the *Kitāb Pātanǧal* as well as three references to this work.

In 1922, Louis Massignon discovered a complete text of the *Kitāb Pātanǧal,* written in the margin of a manuscript containing another work in the Köprülü Library (Köprülü 1589) in today's Istanbul. Thirty-four years later, in 1956, Hellmut Ritter published a critical edition of the *Kitāb Pātanǧal* that he based on this unique textual witness. Because this witness has come down to us in a rather bad state of preservation, Ritter conjectured a number of readings to the best of his abilities and filled some lacunae by supplementing text from parallel passages of al-Bīrūnī's "India". By providing for the first time the complete text of the *Kitāb Pātanǧal,* Ritter opened up a new chapter in the history of research. However, even before, different scholars had developed various hypotheses regarding the original Sanskrit source of al-Bīrūnī's yoga work without knowing the complete version of it.

To start with, Sachau compared the extracts from the *Kitāb Pātanǧal* in al-Bīrūnī's "India" with the *Yogasūtra* together with the *Rājamārtaṇḍa* of king Bhoja of Mālava[25] and judged the relationship between the Arabic and the Sanskrit works as follows:

> Alberuni's Patañjali is totally different from "The Yoga Aphorisms of Patañjali" (with the commentary of Bhoja Râjâ, and an English translation by Rajendralâlâ Mitra, Calcutta, 1883), and, as far as I may judge, the philosophic system of the former differs in many points essentially from that of the Sûtras. Moreover, the extracts given in the *Indica* stand in no relation with the commentary of Bhoja Râjâ, although the commentator here and there mentions ideas which in a like or similar form occur in Alberuni's work, both works being intended to explain the principles of the same school of philosophy.[26]

In his search for a possible Sanskrit source of al-Bīrūnī's work, Sachau, who was not a Sanskritist, had to rely on early translations. His choice of the *Yogasūtra* together with Bhoja's *Rājamārtaṇḍa* as a standard of comparison was more than obvious, because at Sachau's time these were the only yoga works available in English translations.[27] Sachau, however, could not find the source of the *Kitāb Pātanǧal* in Bhoja's yoga commentary. In his view, the *Kitāb Pātanǧal* is "totally different" from Patañjali's *Yogasūtra* as it appears in the English translation of Rājendralāl Mitra, obviously with regard to its form as well as with regard to its philosophical contents. The same is also true for Bhoja's commentary on the

25 Bhoja ruled in the first half of the eleventh century in Dhar, a city located in what is nowadays the western part of Madhya Pradesh. For Bhoja's date, see Pingree 1981: 336.

26 Sachau 1888: II/264.

27 See Maas 2013: 69. The first English translation of the *Pātañjalayogaśāstra* (i.e., of the *Yogasūtra* together with the so-called *Yogabhāṣya*) was only published in 1907 by Ganganatha Jha (Jha 1907).

Yogasūtra, which, according to Sachau, only shares with the *Kitāb Pātanǧal* "here and there" comparable ideas of the "same school of philosophy". In the end, Sachau's search for the Sanskrit source of the *Kitāb Pātanǧal* did not lead him to any result.

2.2. Surendra Nath Dasgupta: A Third Patañjali

Forty-two years later, Surendranath Dasgupta arrived at a similar conclusion, without, however, referring to the work of his predecessors Sachau and Richard Garbe.[28] According to him,

> [...] it is certain that this book [i.e., the *Kitāb Pātanǧal*] was not the present *Yogasūtra* of Patañjali though it had the same aim as the latter, namely, the search for liberation and for the union of the soul with the object of meditation.[29]

For Dasgupta, the *Kitāb Pātanǧal* was definitely neither an Arabic translation of the *Yogasūtra* nor, one may add, the translation of one of its commentaries. In Dasgupta's view, the two works share only their general orientation, namely liberation from the cycle of rebirths and a fusion of "the soul with the object of meditation". In his final conclusion, Dasgupta assumed that the Sanskrit source of the *Kitāb Pātanǧal* was composed by an author named Patañjali who is different from the grammatical author of the same name as well as from the author of the *Yogasūtra.*[30]

2.3. Richard Garbe: The *Rājamārtaṇḍa* of King Bhoja

As mentioned above, Dasgupta did not discuss Richard Garbe's attempt to identify the Sanskrit source of the *Kitāb Pātanǧal.* Garbe, a famous Sanskritist and at his time one of the leading specialists of Sāṅkhya and Yoga philosophy, had arrived at the conclusion

> that the Sanskrit source of the *Kitāb Pātanǧal* was probably the *Yoga Sūtras,* which in India are commonly known under the name of Pātañjala, along with the commentary of Bhojarājā (and not, as I had suspected S.Ph. 63 that of Vyāsa) [...]. I believe, however, that the use of certain similes and exemplifications shows the identity of Albērūni's exemplar with the commentary by Bhojarājā. The simile of the husked and unhusked rice grains in Albērūnī I, 55 is found in the end of Bhoja II, 13, and the two exemplifications from the legends of Nandikeśvara (Nandīśvara) and Nahuṣa at Albērūnī I, 93

28 On Garbe's attempt to identify the source of the *Kitāb Pātanǧal,* see section 2.3 below.
29 Dasgupta 1930: 60.
30 Dasgupta 1930: 64.

> occur in the same way jointly in Bhoja II, 12 (cf. IV, 2). The last mentioned agreement appears to me as especially evidentiary. If one compares the whole of Albērūni's exposition of the yoga teaching at the instances that Sachau's index contains s. v. Patañjali, the teaching appears to be blurred and occasionally wrong; one gets the impression that Albērūnī used defective information in a popular form besides the *vṛtti* of Bhoja.[31]

Garbe arrived at the opposite conclusion than Sachau, for whom, as we have stated above, the *Kitāb Pātanǧal* was neither closely related to the *Yogasūtra,* nor to Bhoja's *Rājamārtaṇḍa.* Although the German indologist acknowledged major differences between the exposition of yoga in al-Bīrūnī's work and that of probable Sanskrit sources, which he ascribed to "defective information in a popular form" (mangelhafte Information in populärer Form), he also saw striking similarities that allowed for the identification of al-Bīrūnī's source at least with a high degree of probability. In the course of his work, however, Garbe had alternated in his judgement. Initially, he was inclined to identify the *Pātañjalayogaśāstra* (i.e., the *Yogasūtra* together with its *bhāṣya)* as the most probable source of al-Bīrūnī's work. Later, however, he favoured the *Yogasūtra* together with Bhoja's *Rājamārtaṇḍa.* The reason for Garbe's change of mind was that he discovered a number of specific exemplifications, namely that of husked and unhusked rice grains as well as that of the two mythological figures Nandīśvara und Nahuṣa in al-Bīrūnī's work.

2.3.1. The Agricultural Example

All of these philosophical examples appear in Mitra's translation of the *Rājamārtaṇḍa.* However, as Garbe noticed himself in footnote 3 to the passage cited above, the part of the *Rājamārtaṇḍa* containing the example of husked and unhusked rice is missing in Mitra's edition of the Sanskrit text. The same passage

31 Garbe 1896: 41–42, translated from the original German, which reads as follows: "[...] wahrscheinlich die in Indien allgemein mit den Namen Pātañjala bezeichneten Yogasūtras nebst dem Commentare Bhojarāja's (nicht Vyāsa's wie ich S. Ph. 63 vermutet habe) gewesen [...]. Ich glaube jedoch, dass die Verwendung einiger übereinstimmender Gleichnisse und Beispiele die Identität von Albērūni's Vorlage mit dem Commentare Bhojarāja's darthut. Das Gleichnis von den unenthülsten und enthülsten Reiskörnern bei Albērūnī I, 55 findet sich bei Bhoja II, 13 Schluss, und die beiden Beispiele aus den Legenden von Nandikeśvara (Nandīśvara) und Nahuṣa bei Albērūnī I, 93 stehen ebenso neben einander bei Bhoja II, 12 (cf. IV, 2). Die letztere Übereinstimmung scheint mir besonders beweisend. Wenn man Albērūnī's ganze Darstellung der Yoga-Lehre an den in Sachau's Index s. v. Patañjali verzeichneten Stellen vergleicht, so erscheint sie freilich verschwommen und manchmal unrichtig; man hat den Eindruck, dass Albērūnī eine mangelhafte Information in populärer Form neben Bhoja's *vṛtti* benutzt habe." "S. Ph. 63" in this quotation refers to Garbe's book *Die Samkhya-Philosophie* (Garbe 1894). In the first edition of this work, Garbe assesses that the *Kitāb Pātanǧal* is to be identified with the *Pātañjalayogaśāstra,* while in the second edition he regards the *Kitāb Pātanǧal* as a rendering of the *Rājamārtaṇḍa* (Garbe 1917: 91).

is also missing in Āgāśe's edition of the *Rājamārtaṇḍa*.[32] Therefore it is at least doubtful whether this passage was an original part of Bhoja's work on yoga or whether it was added to the *Rājamārtaṇḍa* in the course of its transmission. If the latter alternative would be true, al-Bīrūnī could definitely not have silently reused Bhoja's work in his example of rice grains.

Several additional pieces of information suggest that al-Bīrūnī most probably did not use the *Rājamārtaṇḍa* as the Sanskrit source of his *Kitāb Pātanğal*. First, no evidence suggests that al-Bīrūnī ever visited Bhoja's kingdom of Mālava.[33] Second, al-Bīrūnī never mentioned a work with the title *Rājamārtaṇḍa*, and third, it is possible that al-Bīrūnī composed his work earlier than Bhoja composed his yoga work, who according to David Edwin Pingree, flourished between the years 1005–1055.[34]

For discussing the question of which work most probably was the main source of this exemplification in the *Kitāb Pātanğal* it is also relevant to notice that Bhoja was not the first author to use the exemplifications that Garbe took to be "evidentiary" (beweisend). The same illustrative examples already appear in parallel passages of a much earlier work of the philosophical yoga tradition, namely in the *bhāṣya*-passages of *Pātañjalayogaśāstra* 2.12 and 2.13, respectively.

Pātañjalayogaśāstra (PYŚ) 2.13 states that the afflictions (*kleśa*) are responsible for the maturation of karma, which cannot happen if the afflictions are removed. In order to illustrate the relation between the afflictions and the maturation of karma, Patañjali introduces the exemplification of rice grains that may or may not have husks. He says:

> As long as afflictions exist, the accumulation of karma keeps ripening. This is not the case if its root, i.e., the afflictions, is cut off. Rice grains that are covered by their husk and whose seeds are not parched can sprout; not, however, if their husk is removed or if their seeds are parched.[35]

This passage is similar to a quotation from the *Kitāb Pātanğal* appearing in al-Bīrūnī's "India",[36] which in turn corresponds to a passage from Q 29[37] of the *Kitāb Pātanğal*. The passage reads as follows:

32 Āgāśe 1904: 20.

33 However, al-Bīrūnī was well aware of the fact that Bhoja was the king of Mālava at his time (see al-Bīrūnī 1958: 152, ll. 4–6; trans. Sachau 1888: I/191).

34 Pingree 1981: 336. See section 1.4 in Verdon 2015: 187–188.

35 *Pātañjalayogaśāstra* (PYŚ) 2.13, p. 68, l. 18–69, l. 2: *satsu kleśeṣu karmāśayo vipākārambhī bhavati nocchinnakleśamūlaḥ. yathā tuṣāvanaddhāḥ śālitaṇḍulā adagdhabījabhāvāḥ prarohasamarthā bhavanti nāpanītatuṣā dagdhabījabhāvā vā* .... We take the Sanskrit word *bīja*, which we translate with "seed", to refer to the part of a rice grain that is responsible for germination, i.e., to what is called the "embryo" in modern biological terminology.

36 "The following passage is taken from the book of Patañjali: – 'The soul, being on all sides tied

> The soul *vis-à-vis* these factors [i.e., the factors that cause bondage] may be compared to a grain of rice within its husk. As long as (the grain) has the husk with it, it has the disposition (required) for sprouting and for ripening, and it alternates between its being generated and generating. When, however, the husk is removed from it, these occurrences cease. It is purified (and thus becomes fit) for permanent existence in a (changeless) state.[38]
>
> ومثال النفس فيما بينها كالارز فى ضمن القشر فانه ما دام معه كان مُعدًّا للنبات والاستحصاد ومترددا بين التولد والايلاد،
> فاذا ازيل القشر عنه انقطعت تلك الحوادث وصفا للبقاء على حال
>
> (ed. Ritter 1956: 180, ll. 1–3)

The wording of the *Kitāb Pātanǧal* can be identified as parallel to that of the *Pātañjalayogaśāstra* in as much as both passages use the example of rice grains and their husk, the presence of which determines the ability of rice to sprout. However, whereas the *Pātañjalayogaśāstra* mentions that the germination capacity of rice may be annihilated by exposing rice grains to heat, the *Kitāb Pātanǧal* does not refer to this process of sterilisation. Moreover, the two passages differ even more strikingly in that the respective examples of husked and unhusked rice grains seem to be differently contextualised. The Sanskrit work explains how future consequences of the storage of karma can be prevented, whereas the Arabic work explains that the soul is covered by ignorance like a rice grain may be covered by its husk. In the *Kitāb Pātanǧal,* the husk has to be removed in order to prevent changes of the soul, whereas, according to the *Pātañjalayogaśāstra,* removing the husk prevents the ripening of karma.

In spite of these apparent differences, it is possible to identify the passage of the *Pātañjalayogaśāstra* as a probable source of al-Bīrūnī's work if one considers the *Kitāb Pātanǧal* not as a literal translation but as an adaptation that necessarily required changes of contents. In the present case, it is quite probable that the doctrine of karma and rebirth underlying the passage of the *Pātañjalayogaśāstra,* which is foreign to Islam, called for a reformulation of the passage in al-Bīrūnī's work. Therefore, the passage of the *Pātañjalayogaśāstra* becomes recognizable as the source of the parallel passage in the *Kitāb Pātanǧal* if one considers that "ignorance" (Skt. *avidyā*), which al-Bīrūnī mentions to be the cover of the "soul" (Ar. نفس), is the most important of the afflictions (*kleśa*) in Patañjali's authoritative exposition of Yoga (see PYŚ 2.4). The conception of

---

to ignorance, which is the cause of its being fettered, is like rice in its cover. As long as it is there, it is capable of growing and ripening in the transition stages between being born and giving birth itself. But if the cover is taken off the rice, it ceases to develop in this way, and becomes stationary'" (trans. Sachau 1888: I/55; ed. al-Bīrūnī 1958: 42, ll. 7–11).

37 The abbreviation "Q" followed by a number refers to the numbering of passages in the *Kitāb Pātanǧal* in Ritter's edition that comprise the respective questions together with their answers.

38 Trans. Pines & Gelblum 1977: 524. Cf. Verdon 2015: 188f.

ignorance in the *Kitāb Pātanğal* is quite similar. There, ignorance is described as the "root" (Ar. اصل) and the "basis" (Ar. قاعدة) of the other afflictions (Ar. اثقال; lit. "burdens").[39] Viewed in this way, the removal of the "cover" of the soul in al-Bīrūnī's terminology may correspond to the removal of the afflictions from the mind (*citta*)[40] that in Patañjali's work leads to liberation from the cycle of rebirths, or, in al-Bīrūnī's words, makes the soul fit "for permanent existence in a (changeless) state".

It is possible that al-Bīrūnī's knowledge of Sanskrit was indeed "not profound" (Pingree 1983: 353) and that he had to rely on the assistance of South Asian pandits for his translation. However, the extent to which al-Bīrūnī used oral explanations is difficult to estimate. The only reference in the *Kitāb Pātanğal* to the way in which pandits assisted in the composition of the book is al-Bīrūnī's statement that the Indian books on wisdom "were read to me letter by letter" (Ar. قُرئت علىّ حرفا حرفا).[41] In the present case, however, he reused his Sanskrit source creatively in order to adapt it to his own conception of the soul and its covers.

2.3.2. The Mythological Example

The second text passage on which Garbe based his argument for identifying the *Rājamārtaṇḍa* as the Sanskrit source of the *Kitāb Pātanğal* is the exemplification referring to the two mythological characters Nandīśvara and Nahuṣa. This example occurs in al-Bīrūnī's *India*[42] as well as in Q 28 of the *Kitāb Pātanğal,* which in turn is parallel to PYŚ 2.12. The passage reads as follows:

> For instance Nandikeśvara. When he offered many sacrifices to Mahādeva, the greatest of the angels, he merited paradise and was transposed to it in his corporeal form and became an angel. (Another) instance (is) Indra, chief of the angels. When he fornicated

39 See Q 26 (trans. Pines & Gelblum 1977: 522f.; ed. Ritter 1956: 177, l. 21 – 178, l. 8), as well as the beginning of the answer to question 29 (trans. Pines & Gelblum 1977: 524; ed. Ritter 1956: 179, l. 20 – 180, l. 1).

40 The Arabic word for "soul" or "mind" (نفس) appears generally as the rendering of the Sanskrit word "mental organ" (*citta*) in the *Kitāb Pātanğal,* but in Q 26, the Arabic term "heart" (قلب) is used in order to designate the object that is afflicted by the five burdens. However, these two terms have been used as synonyms in the philosophical discussions among Perso-Muslim authors of medieval Islam. They were employed to mean "the seat of the intellectual processes" by some authors (Calverley & Netton 2012; for the concept of "heart", see Gardet & Vadet 2012). These "burdens" (Ar.اثقال) in al-Bīrūnī's work correspond to the concept of the five "afflictions" (*kleśa*) that trouble the "mental organ" (*citta*) in the *Pātañjalayogaśāstra.*

41 Ed. Ritter 1956: 167, l. 10; trans. Pines & Gelblum 1966: 309. See also Pines & Gelblum 1966: 305.

42 "The book *Patañjali* relates that Nandikeśvara offered many sacrifices to Mahâdeva, and was in consequence transferred into paradise in his human shape; that Indra, the ruler, had intercourse with the wife of Nahusha the Brahmin, and therefore was changed into a serpent by way of punishment" (al-Bīrūnī 1958: 70, ll. 13–15; trans. Sachau 1888: I/93).

with the wife of the brāhmaṇa Nahuṣa, he fell under a curse and was transformed into a snake after having been an angel.[43]

مثل نَنْدِكيشْفَرَ فانه لما اكثر القرابين لمَهاديوَ عظيم الملائكة استحق الجنة وانتقل اليها بقالبه الجسدانى وصار ملكا، ومثل
إِنْدْرَ رئيس الملائكة فانه لما زنى بامراة نَهُشْ البرهمن لُعن ومُسخ حية بعد ان كان مَلَكا
(ed. Ritter 1956: 179, ll. 13–16)

The parallel passage in Bhoja's *Rājamārtaṇḍa* has the following wording:

> In the same way as Nandīśvara's special life-form and so on became manifest in his birth here on earth, because of the power he had attained by venerating the exalted god Śiva, in this way the life-form and the duration of life of others such as Viśvamitra became manifest because of the power they attained through asceticism; and for some others only a life-form became manifest. As for example, for those who vehemently commit evil deeds, like Nahuṣa, a transformation into a different life-form and so on takes place, but Urvaśī became only a creeper in the Kārtikeya forest. In the same way, this applies for each of the three items of (1) life-form, (2) duration of life and (3) experiences in life, individually or collectively, according to circumstances.[44]

A comparison of the two passages reveals a number of differences. First, Bhoja's exemplification is more comprehensive than al-Bīrūnī's. The former does not only mention the two mythological figures of Nahuṣa and Nandikeśvara (which is a common variant of the name Nandīśvara), but also Viśvamitra, an ascetic and seer who became a Brahmin in his present life although he was born in the social class of warriors. Moreover, Bhoja cites the example of the heavenly nymph Urvaśī who was cursed to become a creeper in her present incarnation.

Furthermore, with regard to the mythological figure of Nahuṣa, the two authors refer to two different narratives. According to al-Bīrūnī, the "angel" (Ar. ملك; Skt. *deva*, "god")[45] Indra was transformed into a different life-form as a punishment for having committed adultery with the wife of the Brahmin Nahuṣa. According to Bhoja, however, it was Nahuṣa himself who was punished for a severe misdeed. In view of these differences, it appears quite unlikely that al-Bīrūnī used Bhoja's work as his main source.[46]

---

43 Trans. Pines & Gelblum 1977: 524.

44 *Rājamārtaṇḍa* 2.12, p. 19, ll. 22–26: *yathā nandīśvarasya bhagavanmaheśvarārādhanabalād ihaiva janmani jātyādayo viśiṣṭāḥ prādurbhūtāḥ, evam anyeṣāṃ viśvamitrādīnāṃ tapaḥ-prabhāvāj jātyāyuṣī, keṣāṃcij jātir eva. yathā tīvrasaṃvegena duṣṭakarmakṛtāṃ nahuṣādīnāṃ jātyantarādipariṇāmaḥ, urvaśyāś ca kārtikeyavane latārūpatayā, evaṃ vyastasamastarūpatvena yathāyogaṃ yojyam.*

45 In translating the Sanskrit term *deva* as "angel" al-Bīrūnī follows the practice of previous translators of "polytheistic Greek texts into Arabic" (Ernst 2003: 177).

46 Pines and Gelblum (1966: 303 f.) arrived at the same conclusion, without, however, discussing the pertinent text passages in detail.

This assessment is supported by the fact that the parallel passage in the *Pātañjalayogaśāstra* is closer to the *Kitāb Pātanğal* than the text of the *Rājamārtaṇḍa*. There we read:

> In the same way that the boy Nandīśvara gave up his human transformation and was transformed into a deity, so Nahuṣa gave up his own transformation as the Indra of the gods and was transformed into an animal.[47]

This passage resembles the passage from the *Kitāb Pātanğal* in that it only refers to two mythological characters, i. e., to Nandīśvara and Nahuṣa. Nevertheless, there are also considerable differences. For example, it is only al-Bīrūnī who mentions that the change of Nandikeśvara's life form was caused by his veneration of Śiva, whereas only Patañjali refers to the literary motif of Nandīśvara's turning into a god from being a boy. These differences do not, however, rule out the possibility that al-Bīrūnī used the *Pātañjalayogaśāstra* as an important source that he supplemented with other written and oral sources. The motive of Nandikeśvara's veneration of Śiva, which gained him a divine body, is narrated in *Liṅgapurāṇa* 1.43 and was probably so well-known to the audience of the *Pātañjalayogaśāstra* that Patañjali did not even need to mention it.[48] Al-Bīrūnī, however, could not expect the same background knowledge from his Muslim readership and therefore probably felt compelled to provide additional information. Moreover, al-Bīrūnī may have wanted to highlight a similarity between the Indian religion and Islam, in that the veneration of an angel leads to religious merits.

One of the differences between the Arabic and the Sanskrit work in the passage cited above in fact supports the hypothesis that al-Bīrūnī used the *Pātañjalayogaśāstra* as a main source. As we already noticed, al-Bīrūnī narrates that Nahuṣa was the husband of a woman with whom Indra had illegitimate intercourse, whereas Patañjali refers to Nahuṣa himself as the wrongdoer. This version of the myth corresponds to what we actually find in *Mahābhārata* 5.11–17 and 13.102 f. where Nahuṣa, a human, is said to have been appointed to be the king of the gods in order to replace Indra. Having reached this exalted position, Nahuṣa became arrogant, neglected his religious duties, and treated the Seers (*ṛṣi*) badly, on account of which he was cursed and transformed into a snake.[49]

---

47 PYŚ 2.12, p. 68, ll. 6–8: *yathā nandīśvaraḥ kumāro manuṣyapariṇāmaṃ hitvā devatātvena pariṇataḥ. tathā nahuṣo devānām indraḥ svakaṃ pariṇāmaṃ hitvā tiryaktvena pariṇata iti.* We read *devatātvena* ("into a deity") with manuscript Tv[Y] as against *devatvena* ("into a god") of Āgāśe's edition and manuscripts A[d] and J[d]. Furthermore, we read *nahuṣo* with manuscripts A[d], J[d], and Tv[Y] as against *nahuṣo 'pi* in Āgāśe's edition.

48 Orelskaya 1997: 240.

49 See Sörensen 1904–1925: 495a and b, s. v. Nahushopākhyāna. Al-Bīrūnī was well aware of the existence and the popularity of a book entitled *Bhāraṭa* (بهارث) (al-Bīrūnī 1958: 102, l. 13 – 104, l. 8; trans. Sachau 1888: I/132–134). He also knew that the *Kitāb Gītā* was a part of the *Kitāb*

It appears that al-Bīrūnī mistakenly combined this myth with a different one, namely with the narrative of Indra who seduced Ahalyā, the wife of the Brahmana Gautama, on account of which, according to the version of this story in the *Rāmāyaṇa*, the god lost his position of being the chief of the celestials.[50] Al-Bīrūnī's blending of the two different myths was possibly fostered by the fact that his source for the myth of Nahuṣa in connection with *Yogasūtra* (YS) 2.12 contained, just like the passage of the *Pātañjalayogaśāstra* cited above, the formulation "Indra of the gods" (*devānām indraḥ*).[51] Al-Bīrūnī may have wrongly interpreted this expression to refer as a proper name to the god Indra, instead of understanding the phrase correctly as an epithet of Nahuṣa. This apparent misunderstanding explains why, everywhere in al-Bīrūnī's work, Indra, and not Nahuṣa, figured as the wrongdoer. If this is true, the *Pātañjalayogaśāstra* is indeed a possible candidate for having been an important source of the *Kitāb Pātanǧal.*

In any case, we may notice that al-Bīrūnī's work does not provide any evidence that would justify Garbe's commitment in favour of Bhoja's work as its main source. On the contrary, as was already noticed by Pines and Gelblum, al-Bīrūnī's work in general has more in common with the *bhāṣya*-passages of the *Pātañjalayogaśāstra* than with the *Rājamārtaṇḍa.*[52]

Garbe's hypothesis on the source of the *Kitāb Pātanǧal* presumably can be explained as a result of the rather limited Indological knowledge about Sanskrit yoga works that was current at his time. The first scholar who provided an account of the literature on yoga as a South Asian system of knowledge was Henry Thomas Colebrooke. In his essay "On the Philosophy of the Hindus",[53] Colebrooke stated that the pertinent literature consisted of the *Yogasūtra* and of a commentary on the *sūtra*-s entitled "Pátánjala-bháshya" (i.e., the so-called *Yogabhāṣya*) by Vyāsa. According to Colebrooke, "both text and gloss" were commented upon by Vācaspatimiśra in his *Tattvavaiśāradī* (c 950). Moreover, Colebrooke draws attention to Vijñānabhikṣu's *Yogavārttika* (c 1550) as a fur-

---

Bhārata, although he does not frequently refer to the latter (al-Bīrūnī 1958: 21, l. 17; trans. Sachau 1888: I/29).

50 "The story has found wide favour in the epics and Purāṇas; it is alluded to twice in the *Mahābhārata,* told in detail twice in the *Rāmāyaṇa,* and then again in several Purāṇas ..." (Söhnen 1991: 73).

51 Already Pines and Gelblum noticed that "[a]l-Bīrūnī's mistake may be accounted for by his misunderstanding a Sanskrit text, especially if it used the word *indra* both as a private name and as a name of an institution or title, such as in the expression *devānām indra* which occurs in Vyāsa's version of the story here" (Pines & Gelblum 1977: 537, n. 63).

52 See Pines & Gelblum 1966: 304. For these two authors, the *bhāṣya*-passages of the *Pātañjalayogaśāstra* were, however, an independent commentary on the *Yogasūtra* that was composed by an author called Veda-vyāsa. On this authorship question, see below, p. 312.

53 Colebrooke 1827: 25.

ther commentary and to Bhoja's *Rājamārtaṇḍa* as a "third commentary". The exact nature and the relative chronology of these works were, however, unknown to Colebrooke and his immediate successors.

Therefore, academic research on the yoga works that Colebrooke listed was not, and in fact could not be, pursued chronologically and systematically. As mentioned above, the first work that appeared in a complete English translation was Bhoja's *Rājamārtaṇḍa*.[54] This work is not an independent commentary on the *Yogasūtra*, but a simplified revision of the *Pātañjalayogaśāstra*, i.e., the *Yogasūtra* together with the *bhāṣya*. The first translation of the *Pātañjalayogaśāstra* into English was published only in 1907 by Ganganatha Jha,[55] whereas the first English rendering of the *Tattvavaiśāradī* was published by Rāma Prasāda in 1910.[56]

2.4. Jean Filliozat: Al-Bīrūnī's Creativity

Although Garbe's argument in favour of the *Rājamārtaṇḍa* as the source of the *Kitāb Pātanğal* is inconclusive, it appears to have influenced Jean Filliozat in his assessment:

> It is perhaps partly in this text [i.e., the *Rājamārtaṇḍa*] that was then very recent, that al-Bīrūnī initiated himself into the Yoga of Patañjali, on which, by the way, he wrote a work in Arabic.[57]

Filliozat speculated that the *Rājamārtaṇḍa* may have partly been al-Bīrūnī's source of information about the yoga system of Patañjali. However, in contrast to Garbe, Filliozat did not regard the *Kitāb Pātanğal* as a translation of a Sanskrit work, but as an original, and to a considerable degree independent, creation by al-Bīrūnī.

54 Mitra 1883. See above, p. 292.
55 Jha 1907.
56 Prasāda 1910.
57 Renou & Filliozat 1953: 46, translated from the original French, which reads as follows: "C'est peut-être en partie dans ce texte, alors tout récent, qu'al-Bīrūnī s'est initié au Yoga de Patañjali sur lequel il a d'ailleurs écrit un ouvrage en arabe".

2.5. Shlomo Pines and Tuvia Gelblum: The *Yogasūtra* with an Unknown Commentary

Shlomo Pines and Tuvia Gelblum, who published the results of their extensive studies on the *Kitāb Pātanǧal* from 1966 onwards, were the first scholars to base their work on Ritter's critical edition of the complete text of the *Kitāb Pātanǧal*. With regard to the possible sources of al-Bīrūnī's work the two scholars remark that

> [...] most of the *Yogasūtras* themselves are traceable in the Arabic text, occurring generally in their original sequence. They have, however, been woven together with a commentary on the *Yogasūtra* [...]. The commentary used by al-Bīrūnī cannot be identified with any of the printed commentaries, despite a large number of similarities in the interpretation of the text. [...] [p. 304] It is quite possible that the source of the commentary in question is traceable to one of the numerous manuscripts of unknown commentaries housed in Indian libraries. [...] But the possibility also exists that the source in question has been lost. [...] It may be argued that the commentary in question could be related to the theistic developments evident in late commentators prior or posterior to al-Bīrūnī [...]. [p. 305] But against such argumentation one should not ignore the fact that al-Bīrūnī was a Muslim, so that in this major characteristic of his translation as well as in its minor characteristics, which likewise exhibit a good deal of 'islamization', his own interpretation, conditioned by his own cultural orientation, might have been at work. [...] [T]here is much in our text to suggest that al-Bīrūnī relied to a considerable extent on his own intelligence and autodidactic capacity in studying the sūtras and their commentary. [...] [p. 307] The Arabic translation betrays a constant effort to bring the work as near as possible to the mentality of the Muslim readers. This is evident both in the selection of the terminology and the transposition of Indian philosophical notions and problems into similar ones grounded in Aristotelian and other streams of Muslim thought. [...] Evidently, from the point of view of al-Bīrūnī and his readers, the Arabic work provides an operative or functional, though not literal, translation of the *Yogasūtra* with its commentary.[58]

For Pines and Gelblum, the *Kitāb Pātanǧal* is based on the *Yogasūtra* of Patañjali, on al-Bīrūnī's own cultural background and creativity, as well as on an unknown commentary on the *Yogasūtra*.[59] This commentary, in the view of the two authors, can neither be identified with the so-called *Yogabhāṣya*, nor with the (sub-)commentary *Tattvavaiśāradī* by Vācaspatimiśra, which provides explanations to the *sūtra*- as well as to the *bhāṣya*-passages of the *Pātañjalayoga-*

58 Trans. Pines & Gelblum 1966: 303–307.

59 In assuming that the *Kitāb Pātanǧal* is a translation of the *Yogasūtra* together with an unknown commentary, Pines and Gelblum follow Hauer (1930: columns 279–281) and Ritter (1956: 166).

śāstra, nor with Bhoja's *Rājamārtaṇḍa.*[60] Accordingly, Pines and Gelblum assume that this commentary, if it still exists, can only have survived unpublished in the form of manuscripts. Moreover, following a suggestion of Dasgupta (1930: 63 f.), they speculate on the basis of cosmographical differences between the *Kitāb Pātanğal* and the so-called *Yogabhāṣya* – which they date in accordance with Woods (1914: xxi) to a time span of 650–850 CE – that the unknown source must have been composed before the *Bhāṣya* had "attained any great sanctity or authority".[61] This assessment was accepted in scholarly literature on the history of yoga in South Asia and the *Kitāb Pātanğal,* as, for example, in Gelblum 2008 (p. 261) and in Kozah 2015 (p. 85).

2.5.1. The Medical Excursion

Pines and Gelblum (1966: 304) ruled out the possibility that their unknown commentary could be identical with the *bhāṣya*-part of the *Pātañjalayogaśāstra,* inter alia on the basis of two concrete references that al-Bīrūnī provides to the commentary he used. The first reference deals with the conceptions of the human body occurring in Q 46 of the *Kitāb Pātanğal,* which is parallel to PYŚ 3.29. There we read:

> If the complete concentration (*saṃyama*) is directed on the wheel of the navel, there arises knowledge of the arrangement of the body [YS 3.29]. By performing complete concentration on the wheel of the navel one can distinctly know the arrangement of the body. Wind, bile and phlegm are the humours. Skin, blood, flesh, sinew, bone, marrow and semen are the seven corporeal elements. This arrangement is such that each preceding element is exterior to following one.[62]

The parallel passage of the *Kitāb Pātanğal* runs as follows:

> Whoever wishes to know his own body should meditate continuously on the navel. This too belongs to the commentator's explanation. When food is digested in the belly, matter is produced from it to which (pertain) a sediment which is expurgated(?) and three residues which remain in the body. They are wind, bile and phlegm. (They) harm (?) seven things, namely the chyle, the blood, the flesh, the fat, the bones, the marrow and the semen. As for the above-mentioned matter, it is transformed into blood. Out of

60 In their footnotes, Pines and Gelblum highlighted many parallels between passages of the *Kitāb Pātanğal* and other Sanskrit works.

61 Pines & Gelblum 1966: 304. In n. 9, the two authors refer to Garbe 1894: 63 for the date of the so-called *Yogabhāṣya.* There, however, Garbe does not mention any date at all. We, therefore, inferred that the two authors actually meant the dating that Woods proposed in his famous translation. The same argument is repeated in Gelblum 2008: 262. On differences in the cosmography of the *Pātañjalayogaśāstra* and the *Kitāb Pātanğal,* see below, section 2.5.2.

62 PYŚ 3.29, p. 153, ll. 6–9: *nābhicakre kāyavyūhajñānam* [YS 3.29]. *nābhicakre saṃyamaṃ kṛtvā kāyavyūhaṃ vijānīyāt. vātapittaśleṣmāṇas trayo doṣāḥ. dhātavaḥ sapta tvag-lohita-māṃsa-snāyv-asthi-majjā-śukrāṇi. pūrvaṃ pūrvam eṣāṃ bāhyam ity eṣa vinyāsaḥ.*

the subtle (part) of the latter flesh is generated, and from its remaining gross (part) – all things that come forth from the body, such as sweat and hair and the nails. Then the fat of corpulence is generated from the flesh, the bones from fat, the marrow from bones, and the semen, which (among) these is the noblest, from the marrow. Whatever is farther from matter is more excellent. The utility of comprehending the transformations of these things and of the manner of their generation and passing away, of (the ways in which) they are useful or harmful, of the periods (in which) this (happens) and of (the relevant) measures (consists in) establishing the truth that (all) this is not good, nay that it is an evil. And this is a reason for being drawn towards the good. At this point we return to the text.[63]

ومن اراد معرفة بدنه فليدم التفكر فى السُرّة
وهذا من كلام المفسر ايضا : ان الغذاء اذا انطبخ فى الجوف حصل منه مادة لها ثقل تبرأ وفضول ثلثة تبقى فى البدن هى الريح والمرة والبلغم مضرة بسبعة اشياء هى الكيلوس والدم واللحم والشحم والعظم والمخ والمنى، فاما المادة المذكورة فتستحيل الى الدم ثم يتولد من لطيفه اللحم، ومن كثيفه الفاضل جميع ما يبرز من البدن من عرف وشعر وظفر وامثالها، ثم يتولد شحم السمن من اللحم و يتولد العظم من الشحم والمخ من العظم والمنى من المخ وهو اشرفها، و كل ما هو ابعد عن المادة فهو افضل، و منفعة الاحاطة باستحالات هذه الاشياء وكيفية كونها وفسادها ومنافعها ومضارّها واوقات ذلك ومقاديرها هى التحقق بانها ليست بشىء بل هى شر، وذلك يكون سبب الانجرار الى الخير، وقد رجعنا الى النص
(ed. Ritter 1956: 188, ll. 1–11)

This text passage of the *Kitāb Pātanğal,* which is more comprehensive than PYŚ 3.29, is clearly not a literal translation of Patañjali's work. However, in contrast to the assessment of Pines and Gelblum, the text does not show that al-Bīrūnī used a different yoga-commentary than the above-cited *bhāṣya*-passage of the *Pātañjalayogaśāstra.*

The additional information in al-Bīrūnī's text refers to different Āyurvedic theories. First, we find the conception that food is transformed into matter. Then, al-Bīrūnī mentions the three humours (*doṣa*-s) wind, bile, and phlegm, which also occur in the *Pātañjalayogaśāstra,* as products of food. Next, the Arabic author enumerates the well-known seven bodily elements and mentions the theory of food transformation from chyle to semen.[64] In view of the fact that these theories and conceptions of the human body must have been common knowledge among educated audiences of South Asia at least from the time of the composition of the *Pātañjalayogaśāstra* onwards, it was not necessary for al-Bīrūnī to take his explanation from an unknown commentary. Al-Bīrūnī probably used his own knowledge of Āyurveda in order to make his translation comprehensible to a Muslim readership. The fact that al-Bīrūnī had knowledge of

63 Trans. Pines & Gelblum 1983: 261f. The Arabic equivalent to "expurgated" in the third sentence is uncertain; Pines and Gelblum's proposition appears reasonable. By translating "harm" in "(They) harm(?) seven things", Pines and Gelblum accepted Ritter's emendation, which is probably correct.

64 Jolly 1901: 41.

Āyurveda can be concluded from al-Bīrūnī's reference to the oldest classical Sanskrit work on Āyurveda, i. e., the *Carakasaṃhitā,* in the *Taḥqīq mā li-l-Hind.*[65]

In order to assess the probability of the hypothesis that al-Bīrūnī supplemented his work with information that he drew from an unknown yoga commentary, it may be worth mentioning that none of three existing commentaries (i. e., neither the *Pātañjalayogaśāstravivaraṇa* [8th c. CE?], nor the *Tattvavaiśāradī,* nor the *Yogavārttika*) contains any explicit reference to an Āyurvedic theory of food transformation.[66]

Pines and Gelblum, however, did not base their assessment exclusively on the different contents of the two passages. For them it was even more significant that the list of bodily constituents in the *Kitāb Pātanğal* differs from that in the version of the *Pātañjalayogaśāstra* cited above in two respects: (1) Al-Bīrūnī's list starts with the item chyle instead of skin and (2) it contains the bodily element fat instead of sinew as item no. 4.[67] However, in contrast to Pines and Gelblum's view, these two deviations do not indicate that al-Bīrūnī used any other source than the *Pātañjalayogaśāstra.* The textual differences only show that the scholar had a different text version of the *Pātañjalayogaśāstra* at his disposal than the one that we find in the printed edition of Āgāśe, quoted above.[68] First, as Philipp A. Maas showed in the variants to his critical edition of the list of bodily constituents in PYŚ 3.29, quite a number of manuscripts contain the secondary reading *medas* ("fat") instead of *snāyu* ("sinew") as item no. 4.[69] This textual change was probably introduced in the course of the history of the transmission of Patañjali''s work by one or more scribes who knew that the standard list of bodily elements as it occurs in the work(s) of Vāgbhaṭa contains *medas* at the position at which Patañjali's list originally had *snāyu.*[70] Secondly, the reading *tvag* ("skin") instead of *rasa* ("chyle") that we find at the beginning of the list of bodily constituents in the printed edition is, in contrast to the view of Pines and Gelblum,[71] clearly of secondary origin. The reading *tvag* ("skin") was probably introduced by a scribe who misunderstood Patañjali's statement concerning the arrangement of bodily constituents in so far that he thought it to refer to the "physical, spatial arrangement of constituents", whereas Patañjali himself meant "the degree of their transformation from food, which is foreign to the body, to

65 Meulenbeld 1999–2002: I/116.

66 Maas 2008a: 131.

67 Pines & Gelblum 1983: 284, n. 163.

68 See note 24 on p. 291.

69 Maas 2008a: 132, n. 13.

70 Maas 2008a: 142.

71 Pines and Gelblum (1983: 284, n. 163) state that the "context shows that this variant [*rasa*] is spurious" without providing a justification for their conclusion.

semen, which is intimately related to the body, i.e., its essence".[72] It appears that al-Bīrūnī understood Patañjali correctly when he rendered his statement that "the sequence is such that each preceding is exterior to the following one" with "[w]hatever is farther from matter is more excellent". In any case, al-Bīrūnī's treatment of PYŚ 3.29 does not support the hypothesis that he used an unknown commentary as a major source for his *Kitāb Pātanğal*.

2.5.2. The Cosmographical Excursion

The second case that Pines and Gelblum take as evidence for their claim that al-Bīrūnī must have based his *Kitāb Pātanğal* on an unknown commentary of the *Yogasūtra* is the cosmographical excurse that appears in Q 46 of al-Bīrūnī's work (as well as partly in al-Bīrūnī's "India").[73] In the *Kitāb Pātanğal*, al-Bīrūnī introduced his cosmographic exposition in the following way:

> The commentator has at this point an explanatory discourse describing the world and the Earths. It seems useful to quote this discourse in an exact manner. For it is one of the sciences current among them. In the description of the existent (things) he starts with the lowest section (proceeding) towards the uppermost.[74]
>
> وللمفسر فى هذا الموضع كلام شرحى فى وصف العالم والارض وايراده على وجهه نافع فانه من المعارف الشايعة فيما بينهم، وقد ابتدأ فى وصف الموجودات من جهة السفل نحو العلو
>
> (ed. Ritter 1956: 185, ll. 16–18)

Although the following part of al-Bīrūnī's cosmography agrees with that of the *Pātañjalayogaśāstra* from a systematic point of view in so far as both descriptions start with the lowest part of the cosmos, the two expositions initially differ with regard to the listed items. Al-Bīrūnī's list consists of a sequence of entities that are recorded with their respective extent measured in *yojana*-s: "darkness", "hell", a second level of "darkness", and "earths" called "Vajra" (Ar. بَزْرَ ; *bazra*), "Garbha" (Ar. كَرْبُ ; *karbu*) and "Suvarṇa" (Ar. سوبَرْنَ ; *sūbarna*). This list of cosmographical items is odd in so far as it has, as far as we can see, no parallel in the cosmographical literatures of pre-modern Asia.[75]

72 Maas 2008a: 134.
73 "The commentator of the book of Patañjali, wishing to determine the dimension of the world, begins from below and says: […]" (trans. Sachau 1888: I/236f.; ed. al-Bīrūnī 1958: 194, ll. 6–7).
74 Trans. Pines & Gelblum 1983: 260. Ritter emended the manuscript at the end of the first sentence and inserted the name of Vyāsa (وْياص). Pines and Gelblum refute this emendation and propose the translation "the world and the earth" (العالم والارض) which fits the context well (Pines & Gelblum 1983: 275, n. 88). At the end of the second sentence, the Arabic expression (على وجهه) literally means "properly", "in the right manner", and it at least remains uncertain whether al-Bīrūnī wanted to provide a literal quotation.
75 See, also for the following part of this paper, Table 2 below.

In contradistinction to this, the *bhāṣya*-part of PYŚ 3.26 starts with a brief but quite complicated overview of the whole cosmos that apparently is intended to combine the older view of the cosmos as consisting of the three regions of the terrestrial world (*bhūrloka*), of the intermediate space (*antarikṣa*), and of the heavenly world (*svarloka*) with a more recent view, according to which the world consists of seven regions.[76] Thereafter, Patañjali lists seven hells having solid matter, water, fire, wind, space and darkness as their respective basis. This list of hells as well as the location of hells in the cosmos is quite unusual for a Brahmanical work. First of all, within the cosmos, i. e., within Brahmā's egg, hells are generally not located at the very bottom, but occupy the second position above the netherworlds (*pātāla*).[77] Moreover, the number of hells usually exceeds seven in Brahmanical works. As Willibald Kirfel showed in his authoritative survey of Indian cosmographies, the number of hells varies between twelve and 140 for the five text groups that differ according to the enumeration and arrangement of hells.[78] Early Buddhist literature, however, accepts the number of hells to be seven, although the individual names differ from those presented in the *Pātañjalayogaśāstra.*[79]

The *Kitāb Pātanğal* and the *Pātañjalayogaśāstra* agree with each other regarding the respective number of hells as well as regarding the relative position of netherworlds and hells as against the rest of the Brahmanical and Jaina literature that Kirfel surveyed. This may indicate a close historical relation between al-Bīrūnī's work and that of Patañjali, although the respective accounts do not agree exactly.

Next, al-Bīrūnī provides a list of islands or ring-continents that together with seven oceans are conceived as making up the main part of the terrestrial region of the cosmos. These islands are to be imagined as concentric circles (surrounding mount Meru) that are divided by oceans consisting of different liquids. In al-Bīrūnī's work, the sequence of islands and oceans agrees with the sequence that Kirfel found in the majority of Purāṇic sources and that he designated as the first group of texts.[80] The *Pātañjalayogaśāstra* provides a very similar list. It differs, however, with regard to the sequence of islands as well as with regard to the name of one island. Patañjali's list, which is identical with the list in Kirfel's second group of texts (consisting of passages from the *Matsya-* and the *Varāhapurāṇa*),

76 Klaus 1986: § 17.

77 See Kirfel 1920: 147. The three manuscripts A^{d}, J^{d} and Tv^{y} of the *Pātañjalayogaśāstra* that transmit in general an ancient text version whenever they share a common reading, do not at all contain the list of netherworlds that we find in the Vulgate version of the *Pātañjalayogaśāstra.*

78 Kirfel 1920: 148–173.

79 Kirfel 1920: 199–201.

80 See Kirfel 1920: 112–122.

contains the name Gomeda instead of Plakṣa.[81] The *Pātañjalayogaśāstra* and the *Kitāb Pātanǧal* agree, however, in that the island and the oceans are listed in two separate lists. This is remarkable, because from a systematic point of view a description of the terrestrial region as consisting of a sequence of island, ocean, island, etc., could be regarded as a more suitable - though less concise - choice. An additional structural parallel appears at the end of both passages where both the Arabic and the Sanskrit work refer to seven world regions and their respective inhabitants, although Patañjali does not provide the names of the first two divisions. The lists in the two works differ, however, slightly,[82] as can be seen in Table 2 below.[83] The *Pātañjalayogaśāstra* records the items (1) Earth, (2) Intermediate space, (3) Mahendra-, (4) Mahar-, (5) Jana-, (6) Tapo- and (7) Satya-loka, whereas the *Kitāb Pātanǧal* omits the third "heaven", i. e., the world region called Mahendraloka, and adds Brahmaloka as the highest region of the world. The fact that al-Bīrūnī reports his yoga source to have Brahmaloka at the highest position of the cosmos could be the result of a misunderstanding (or of a textual corruption) of the *Pātañjalayogaśāstra*. Patañjali's work indeed has a brief sentence containing the word *brahmaloka* at the end of its cosmographical passage.[84]

81 See Kirfel 1920: 122–126.

82 For Hauer (1930: column 281f.), the differences between the *Pātañjalayogaśastra* and the *Kitāb Pātanǧal* prove without doubt that al-Bīrūnī translated an unknown commentary on the *Yogasūtra.*

83 A few philological remarks are due here. In the case of the seven Pātālas, the manuscript of the *Kitāb Pātanǧal* is damaged. Ritter tried to emend this passage on the basis of the "India". In the case of the sixth island, *gomeda,* Āgāśe (1904: 150, l. 6) has *gomedha* in the main text of his edition and provides the variant *plakṣa* in parentheses without indicating his source. However, three important manuscripts of the *Pātañjalayogaśāstra,* A^d, J^d and Tv^y, read *gomeda* here.

84 See PYŚ 3.26, p. 152, l. 7: *ta ete saptalokāḥ sarva eva brahmalokāḥ.*

<table>
<tr><th>Cosmographical regions</th><th>Items listed in PYŚ 3.26 (based on Āgāśe 1904: 149f.)</th><th>Items listed in Q 46 of the Kitāb Pātanğal (based on Pines & Gelblum 1983: 260f.)</th></tr>
<tr><td rowspan="7">Seven hells (naraka)</td><td>7. Avīci, no material basis mentioned</td><td></td></tr>
<tr><td>6. Mahākāla, based on solid matter</td><td>Darkness, 18,500,000? yojana-s extent
(Ar. ظلمة; ẓulma)</td></tr>
<tr><td>5. Ambarīṣa, based on water</td><td>Naraka, 1,300,000,000 yojana-s extent
(Ar. نَرَك, naraka; جهنم, jahannam "hell")</td></tr>
<tr><td>4. Raurava, based on fire</td><td>Darkness, 100,000 yojana-s extent
(Ar. ظلمة; ẓulma)</td></tr>
<tr><td>3. Mahāraurava, based on wind</td><td>Vajra, 34,000 yojana-s extent
(Ar. بَزْرَ; bazra)</td></tr>
<tr><td>2. Kālasūtra, based on space</td><td>Garbha, 60,000 yojana-s extent
(Ar.كَرْبُ ; karbu)</td></tr>
<tr><td>1. Andhatāmisra, based on darkness</td><td>Suvarṇa, 30,000 yojana-s extent
(Ar. سوبَرْنَ; sūbarna)</td></tr>
<tr><td rowspan="7">Seven netherworlds (pātāla)</td><td>7. Mahātala</td><td></td></tr>
<tr><td>6. Rasātala</td><td></td></tr>
<tr><td>5. Atala</td><td></td></tr>
<tr><td>4. Sutala</td><td>seven Pātālas
(Ar. سَپْت پاتال; sapta pātāla)</td></tr>
<tr><td>3. Vitala</td><td></td></tr>
<tr><td>2. Talātala</td><td></td></tr>
<tr><td>1. Pātāla</td><td></td></tr>
</table>

(Continued)

Cosmographical regions	**Items listed in PYŚ 3.26 (based on Āgāśe 1904: 149f.)**	**Items listed in Q 46 of the *Kitāb Pātanğal* (based on Pines & Gelblum 1983: 260f.)**
Seven islands (*dvīpa*)	1. Jambu, 100.000 *yojana*-s extent	1. Jambu, 100,000 *yojana*-s extent (Ar. جَنْبُ دِيبَ; *janbu dība*)
	2. Śāka, double extent of the previous	6. Plakṣa, 200,000 *yojana*-s extent (Ar. پْلَكْشَ دِيبَ; *plakša dība*)
	3. Kuśa, double extent of the previous	5. Śālmala, 400,000 *yojana*-s extent (Ar. شَالْمَلِ دِيبَ; *šālmali dība*)
	4. Krauñca, double extent of the previous	3. Kuśa, double extent of the previous (Ar. كُشَ دِيبَ; *kuša dība*)
	5. Śālmala, double extent of the previous	4. Krauñca, double extent of the previous (Ar. كْرَونْجَ دِيبَ; *krawnja dība*)
	6. Gomeda (variants: Gomedha and Plakṣa), double extent of the previous	2. Śaka, double extent of the previous (Ar. شَاكَ دِيبَ; *šāka dība*)
	7. Puṣkara, double extent of the previous	7. Puṣkara, double extent of the previous (Ar. پُشْكَرَ دِيبَ; *puškara dība*)
Seven oceans	1. Lavaṇa	1. Kṣāra, 200,000 *yojana*-s extent (Ar. كْشَارَ; *kšāra*)
	2. Ikṣurasa	2. Ikṣu, double extent of the previous (Ar. إِكْشُ; *ikšu*)
	3. Surā	3. Surā, double extent of the previous (Ar. سُرَ; *sura*)
	4. Sarpis (variant: Ghṛta)	4. Sarpis, double extent of the previous (Ar. سَرْبَ; *sarba*)
	5. Dadhimaṇḍa (variant: Dadhi)	5. Dadhi, double extent of the previous (Ar. دَذِ; *daḏi*)
	6. Kṣīra	6. Kṣīra, double extent of the previous (Ar. كْشِيرَ; *kšīra*)
	7. Svādūdaka	7. Svādūdaka, double extent of the previous (Ar. سْوَاذُودَكَ; *swādūdaka*)

(Continued)

Cosmographical regions	**Items listed in PYŚ 3.26 (based on Āgāśe 1904: 149f.)**	**Items listed in Q 46 of the *Kitāb Pātanğal* (based on Pines & Gelblum 1983: 260f.)**
End of the world	Lokāloka	Lokāloka, 10,000 *yojana*-s (Ar. لوكالوك; *lūkālūka*)
		"Land of Gold", 100,000,000 *yojana*-s extent (Ar. ارض الذهب; *arḍa l-ḏahab*)
Regions above		Pitṛloka, 6,134,000 *yojana*-s extent (Ar. بِتْرِلوك; *bitrilūka*) Brahmāṇḍa (Ar. بْرَهْمانْدْ; *brahmānda*) Darkness/Tamas, 18,500,000 *yojana*-s extent (Ar. ظلمة, *ẓulma*; تَمْ, *tama*)
Seven world regions	1. Bhūrloka (Earth)	1. Bhūrloka (Ar. بْهُورْلوك; *bhūrlūka*)
	2. Antarikṣa (Intermediate Space)	2. Bhuvarloka (Ar. بْهُوبَرْلوك; *bhūbarlūka*)
	3. Mahendraloka	
	4. Maharloka	3. Maharloka (Ar. مَهَرْلوك ; *maharlūka*)
	5. Janaloka	4. Janaloka (Ar. جَنْ لوك; *jana lūka*)
	6. Tapoloka	5. Tapoloka (Ar. تَبْ لوك; *taba lūka*)
	7. Satyaloka	6. Satyaloka (Ar. ست لوك; *sat lūka*)
		7. Brahmaloka (Ar. بْرَهْمَ لوك; *brahma lūka*)

Table 2: A comparison between the cosmographies of PYŚ 3.26 and of *Kitāb Pātanğal* Q 46.

The differences in the cosmographies of the *Kitāb Pātanğal* and the *Pātañjalayogaśāstra* rule out that this particular Sanskrit work was the only source for al-Bīrūnī's knowledge of Indian cosmography.[85] It is, however, very much conceivable that al-Bīrūnī used Patañjali's exposition as an important source and adopted its content to what he knew to be the standard cosmography of his time

85 Bīrūnī's *Taḥqīq mā li-l-Hind,* ch. 21, which is entitled "Description of earth and heaven according to the religious views of the Hindus, based upon their traditional literature" (صورة الارض و السماء على الوجوه الملّية التى ترجع إلى الخبار و الرويات السمعيّة), presents indeed the cosmographical descriptions of the *Ādityapurāṇa,* the *Viṣṇupurāṇa* and the *Vāyupurāṇa,* as well as that of the commentator of the *Book Pātanğal* (Ar. مفسّر كتابِ "پاتنجل"); see al-Bīrūnī 1958: 185, l. 3–196, l. 17; trans. Sachau 1888: I/228–238.

and in the region that he visited. Therefore it is not at all obvious that the differences between the works of Patañjali and al-Bīrūnī have to be explained by the influence of an unknown commentary on the *Yogasūtra*.

Moreover, against the background of the results of recent research, the assessment of Pines and Gelblum that al-Bīrūnī composed his work before the *bhāṣya*-part of the *Pātañjalayogaśāstra* had "attained any great sanctity or authority"[86] has become difficult to maintain. As Maas argued, the *Yogasūtra* together with the so-called *Yogabhāṣya* were probably partly composed and partly compiled as a unitary work entitled *Pātañjalayogaśāstra* by a single author and redactor with the name of Patañjali. The time of the composition of the work can be dated with some confidence to c 325–425 CE.[87] At least from the middle of the eighth century onwards, the *Pātañjalayogaśāstra* was so widely known in educated circles of north-western South Asia that the famous poet Māgha reused several of its passages in his epic poem *Śiśupālavadha*.[88] The *Pātañjalayogaśāstra* was also during the following centuries widely known and referred to in Sanskrit literature. This can safely be concluded from the numerous quotations of Patañjali's work in the works of Kashmir Śaivism and other Sanskrit works.[89]

2.6. A New Hypothesis: The *Pātañjalayogaśāstra*

The *Pātañjalayogaśāstra* contains two different layers of text. The first layer, the *sūtra*-s, consists in most printed editions of 195 brief nominal phrases. Patañjali probably took these *sūtra*-s over, at least in part, from literary works of early Sāṅkhya Yoga that are now lost. The *sūtra*-s sometimes provide brief summaries of the contents of the second layer of text, the so-called *bhāṣya*, or function as headings for these contents, whereas the *bhāṣya*-part of the *Pātañjalayogaśāstra* consists of commentarial explanations of the *sūtra*-text, of polemical discussions of divergent philosophical views, of supplementary expositions, and of citations from works of pre-classical Sāṅkhya Yoga literature that are meant to support Patañjali's positions. It is this layer of text that the secondary literature from Colebrooke onwards refers to as the *Yogabhāṣya*, even though the work itself does not contain any reference to this designation.[90]

The question of how al-Bīrūnī judged the authorship the *Pātañjalayogaśāstra* and the historical relationship between its *sūtra*- and its *bhāṣya*-part is, of course,

86 Pines & Gelblum 1966: 304. The same argument is repeated in Gelblum 2008: 262.

87 Maas 2006: xii–xix and Maas 2013: 57–68.

88 Maas 2017.

89 See Maas 2006: 111f. On the status of the Sanskrit works that al-Bīrūnī chose to render into Arabic see also Verdon 2015: 100–110.

90 Maas 2006: xvf.

to some degree independent of the question of whether Patañjali actually composed his *Yogaśāstra* as a unified whole or not. In this respect, al-Bīrūnī's own testimony, which probably reflects the common view of the South Asian thinkers with whom he interacted, is more significant. As Maas showed in a recent publication, al-Bīrūnī quoted *bhāṣya*-passages of the *Pātañjalayogaśāstra* that he introduced as being part of the *Kitāb Pātanğal.*[91] This indicates that for al-Bīrūnī the book of Patañjali did not only consist of the *Yogasūtra* (as Pines and Gelblum assumed), but also of the *bhāṣya*-part of the *Pātañjalayogaśāstra.*

Nevertheless, as can be concluded from the end of the introduction to the *Kitāb Pātanğal,* al-Bīrūnī was well aware of the fact that the *Pātañjalayogaśāstra* consists of two different layers of text, i.e., of *sūtra*- and of *bhāṣya*-passages. There he stated that "[t]his is the beginning of the book of Patañjali, text interwoven with commentary".[92] If one is willing to accept that the word "text" (Ar. نصّ) refers to the *sūtra*-passages and the word "commentary" (Ar. تفسير; شرح) to the *bhāṣya*-passages of the *Pātañjalayogaśāstra,* two problems with regard to al-Bīrūnī's peculiar reference to his sources are solved. The first problem is that al-Bīrūnī neither mentioned the name of the author, nor the title of the commentary that he translated. This silence would be entirely understandable if for al-Bīrūnī the commentary was nothing but the *bhāṣya*-passages of the *Pātañjalayogaśāstra.* In this case, the author of the commentary would simply be Patañjali, and the title of the work just *Yogaśāstra,* of which *Kitāb* possibly is al-Bīrūnī's Arabic rendering.[93]

Secondly, also al-Bīrūnī's repeated references to "the commentator" in connection with Q 46 (that we have discussed above, p. 303) would cease to be problematic. Since al-Bīrūnī announced at the beginning of his work that he presents the "text interwoven with commentary", it would be not unusual for him to inform his readers of cases in which he deviates from this procedure. And exactly this is the case in Q 46, where al-Bīrūnī presented comprehensive expositions that occur not in the *sūtra*-part, but only in the *bhāṣya*-passages of the *Pātañjalayogaśāstra.*

Although it may be difficult to arrive at any definitive conclusion, the assessment at which Maas arrived on the basis of less evidence than we were able to present above appears to be a reasonable hypothesis. Most probably the *Kitāb Pātanğal* is "an Arabic version of the *PYŚ*"[94] that al-Bīrūnī supplemented with information he received from a variety of additional sources. There is no need to assume that al-Bīrūnī used an unknown commentary exclusively on the *sūtra*-s

91 Maas 2013: 59.

92 Trans. Pines & Gelblum 1966: 310; ed. Ritter 1956: 168, l. 5.

93 For possible interpretations of the word *pātanğal,* see above, p. 286f.

94 Maas 2013: 60.

of the *Pātañjalayogaśāstra* in order to account for differences between al-Bīrūnī's work and all known yoga sources. It is much more probable that al-Bīrūnī used the *Pātañjalayogaśāstra* as his main source than that he relied on a different yoga source that cannot be identified.

However, it should not go without mention that the beginning of the *Kitāb Pātanğal* contains a text passage that clearly is not a rendering of any part of the *Pātañjalayogaśāstra*. This passage, which occurs immediately after the statement "This is the beginning of the book of Patañjali", consists of two main parts: (1) a benedictory stanza, in which the anonymous speaker venerates God and "the angels and other spiritual beings" in order to secure for himself support in composing his work,[95] and (2) an introduction to the work in which the same speaker, who still refers to himself in the first person, states, among other things, the subject and the aim of the work.[96] The section ends with the statement that "my comment will have for the reader a status similar to that of sense-perception productive of conviction".[97] Apparently, Pines and Gelblum (as well as their predecessors) interpreted this section as the beginning of the unknown commentary that they regarded as the main source of the *Kitāb Pātanğal* as a whole.

We would like to argue, however, in favour of a different hypothesis. In our view, al-Bīrūnī integrated this passage into his work in order to overcome what he (or his informants) regarded as shortcomings of the *Pātañjalayogaśāstra*, namely the violation of two literary conventions for the composition of an authoritative and scholarly exposition (*śāstra*). These conventions are (1) the rule that a *śāstra* should begin with a benedictory stanza (a so-called *maṅgala* verse)[98] and (2) that a *śāstra* has to state its subject matter (*viṣaya*), its aim (*prayojana*) and the connection between the exposition and its aim (*saṃbandha*).[99] At the time when al-Bīrūnī composed his work, these literary conventions had become so widely accepted in Brahmanical circles that it was virtually impossible to compose a *śāstra* without complying with them. Al-Bīrūnī was apparently aware of these rules, and he felt the need to respond to them in his Arabic work, possibly because similar literary conventions existed also for Arabic scholarly works. It is therefore very much conceivable that either one of al-Bīrūnī informants composed a Sanskrit *maṅgala* stanza and an introduction to the *Pātañjalayogaśāstra*, which the Perso-Muslim scholar translated into Arabic in order to create a

95 Pines & Gelblum 1966: 310.

96 See Pines & Gelblum 1966: 310–313.

97 Trans. Pines & Gelblum 1966: 312.

98 On the history of the *maṅgala* verse in South Asian systems of knowledge see Minkowski 2008. On the lack of a *maṅgala* verse in the early text versions of the *Pātañjalayogaśāstra* see Maas 2008b.

99 See Funayama 1995: 181.

complete Arabic "Yogaśāstra", or that al-Bīrūnī himself composed this passage in the style of a translation.

Accordingly, Pines and Gelblum were probably not correct in assuming that the *Yogasūtra* together with an unknown commentary was the main source of al-Bīrūnī's work. However, their excellent work, which is very meticulous and offers so to say a microscopic view of the relationship between a variety of Sanskrit works that may have contributed to the composition of al-Bīrūnī's work, remains a valuable research tool. The studies of Pines and Gelblum are essential and groundbreaking for any further research into al-Bīrūnī's hermeneutic approach to yoga and other aspects of pre-modern South Asian religions and cultures.

Moreover, Pines and Gelblum were surely right in providing several explanations for the fact that the *Kitāb Pātanǧal* differs considerably from all known Sanskrit works. They suggested that al-Bīrūnī islamised and hellenised South Asian conceptions, that he used his own intelligence and creativity to communicate the ideas presented in the *Pātañjalayogaśāstra* to his audience, and that he was probably assisted in his translation by South Asian pandits.

3. The *Pātañjalayogaśāstra* in Transformation

3.1. Explicitly Mentioned Transformations

The above survey of the relationship between the *Kitāb Pātanǧal* and the *Pātañjalayogaśāstra* already provides a first assessment of the way in which al-Bīrūnī used his main source. In order to go more into detail, it may be suitable to take seriously into account what al-Bīrūnī himself related about the way he handled his main source. The following passage from the introduction to the *Kitāb Pātanǧal* is quite informative in this regard.[100]

> […] I was obliged to amalgamate in (my) translation the text with that over-lengthy commentary, to arrange the work in a way which resembles (a dialogue consisting of) questions and answers, and to omit (the parts which) are concerned with grammar and language. This is an apology which I offer because of the difference in size of the book in the two languages, if such a comparison is made. (I do this) in order that no one should think that this (difference) is due to remissness in (the rendering of) the meaning. Indeed he should be assured that it is due to a condensation of what (otherwise) would be troublesome (in its) prolixness. May God bestow His favour upon the good. This is the beginning of the book of Patañjali, text interwoven with commentary.[101]

100 The very fact that al-Bīrūnī added his own introduction and conclusion to the Arabic version of the Sanskrit work indicates that he dealt with his source freely.

101 Trans. Pines & Gelblum 1966: 310.

لذلك اضطررت فى النقل الى خلط النص بذلك التفسير المزيد، واجراء الكلام على ما يشبه السؤال والجواب والى اسقاط
ما يتعلق بالنحو واللغة، وهذا عذر قدّمته لتفاوت حجم الكتاب فى اللغتين عند المقايس بينهما حتى لا يظن ظانّ ان ذلك
لاخلالٍ بمعنىً بل يتحقق انه للتنقيح عما يعود و بالا، والله يوفق للخير بمنه
وهذا هو ابتداء كتاب باتنجل مركّباً نصه بشرحه

(ed. Ritter 1956: 168, ll. 1–5)

In this passage, al-Bīrūnī mentioned in some detail how he modified his main source when he rendered it into Arabic. This process involved the following three kinds of transformation: (1) combining the basic text with its commentary, (2) changing the structure of his source into that of a dialogue and, (3) omitting passages that are comprehensible only for readers knowing Sanskrit.

Al-Bīrūnī neither used the term "Sanskrit" nor an Arabic equivalent in order to designate the language in which his source was written. Instead, he used a number of different expressions. For example, he employed the substantive "India" as a collective term to refer to the Indians (الهند) and their language, or he chose the adjective "Indian" (الهندي) for the same purpose. In addition, he used the phrase "in the Indian language" (في الغتة الهنديّة). Moreover, in his introduction to the *Kitāb Pātanǧal*, al-Bīrūnī employed the expression "from the language of India" (من لغة الهند)[102] to refer to the source-language of his translation. The Arabic transliterations of Indian technical terms that al-Bīrūnī provided in the *Taḥqīq mā li-l-Hind* indicate, nevertheless, that the original language of these terms actually was Sanskrit. For instance, he wrote: "This is what *Patañjali* says about the knowledge which liberates the soul. In Sanskrit [i.e., in Indian] they call its liberation *Moksha* (*sic*; Ar. *mūkša*) – i.e., *the end*" (فهذا ما قال پاتنجل فى العلم المخلص للنفس ويسمّون خلاصها بلهنديّة موكش أى العاقبة).[103] In general, Arabic and Persian writers did not use the word "Sanskrit" at all.[104]

In the following (sections 3.1.1–3.1.3), we try to retrace some of al-Bīrūnī's transformations by introducing selected examples for each of the three kinds of formal transformations that al-Bīrūnī mentioned in the above quoted introduction. An understanding of how the Perso-Muslim author changed his main source, even if this source can only be hypothetically identified, contributes to an improved understanding of al-Bīrūnī's hermeneutic approach to his source and to his supplementary materials, as well as of his strategy to disseminate his knowledge of yoga.

102 Trans. Pines & Gelblum 1966: 309; ed. Ritter 1956: 167, l. 6.

103 Trans. Sachau 1888: I/70; ed. al-Bīrūnī 1958: 53, ll. 8–9. See also the lists of the Indian months, of the names of the planets, and of the zodiac signs in "The Chronology of Ancient Nations" (*Al-Āṯār al-Bāqiya*) in the tables on pp. 80, 221 and 222 of Azkaei 2001; trans. Sachau 1879: 83, 172 and 173) and tables 1–3 in Verdon 2015: 71–73.

104 See Ali 1992: 43 and Ernst 2010: 360f.

3.1.1. Combining Different Layers of Text

In the passage quoted above, al-Bīrūnī mentioned twice that he combined two different layers of text, for which he uses the Arabic words for "text" (نصّ) and "commentary" (تفسير or شرح), which we have hypothetically identified with the *sūtra-* and the *bhāṣya*-part of the *Pātañjalayogaśāstra.*[105] The *Kitāb Pātanğal* indeed presents in an integrated manner topics that are addressed in the two different layers of text of the *Pātañjalayogaśāstra.* For example, al-Bīrūnī's exposition of the five different kinds of mental activities (Ar. قوة; Skt. *vṛtti*) in Q 5, i.e., (1) grasping, understanding (ادراك), (2) imagination (تخيّل), (3) false assumption (ظن), (4) dream (رؤيا), and (5) memory (ذكر), sums up the contents of PYŚ 1.5–1.11, which deals with the mental activities of (1) valid knowledge (*pramāṇa*), (2) error (*viparyaya*), (3) conceptual thinking (*vikalpa*), (4) deep sleep (*nidrā*), and (5) memory (*smṛti*) in seven *sūtra*-s, of which six are supplemented with *bhāṣya*-passages.[106]

However, already in the *Pātañjalayogaśāstra, sūtra-* and *bhāṣya*-passages are not always separable. For example, YS 1.5 together with its introductory *bhāṣya*-passages forms a syntactical unit: "These, however, which have to be stopped although they are numerous, are the *activities* of the mind, *which are fivefold and either afflicted or unafflicted.*"[107] Accordingly, al-Bīrūnī's integration of basic text and commentary in the *Kitāb Pātanğal* is not entirely an innovation. The author rather developed further a characteristic feature that he already found in his hypothetical main source.

3.1.2. Creating a Dialogue

The second transformation that al-Bīrūnī mentioned in his introduction is the restructuration of his source into a dialogue consisting of questions and answers (I was obliged [...] to arrange the work in a way which resembles [a dialogue consisting of] questions and answers; [...] اجراء الكلام على ما يشبه السؤال والجواب اضطررت). As we already stated in the introduction,[108] in this conversation Pā-

105 Al-Bīrūnī said: "For this reason I was obliged to amalgamate in (my) translation the text with that over-lengthy commentary" (لذلك اضطررت فى النقل الى خلط النص بذلك التفسير المزيد) and "This is the beginning of the book of Patañjali, text interwoven with [its] commentary" (وهذا هو ابتداء كتاب باتنجل مركّباً نصه بشرحه).

106 Note, however, that the sequence of items no. 2 and 3 is inverted in the *Kitāb Pātanğal.* For Q 5 of the *Kitāb Pātanğal,* see ed. Ritter 1956: 171, ll. 1–13; trans. Pines & Gelblum 1966: 315–6.

107 PYŚ 1.5, p. 9, l. 3f.: *tāḥ punar niroddhavyā bahutve 'pi cittasya vṛttayaḥ pañcatayyaḥ kliṣṭākliṣṭāḥ* (YS 1.5). This passage is also discussed in Maas 2013: 63.

108 See p. 287 above.

tanğal answers the questions of an ascetic.[109] Some of these questions clearly mirror introductory questions that are already found in the *Pātañjalayogaśāstra,*[110] whereas other questions, like question no. 3 in the passage cited below, were most probably created by al-Bīrūnī himself.[111]

One of the many examples for both cases occurs in Q 2–3 of the *Kitāb Pātanğal* which run as follows:

> Q 2. What is the state of a man who has compressed within himself the faculties of his soul and hindered them from spreading out? Ans. He is not completely bound, for he has severed the bodily ties between himself and that which is other than himself, and has ceased to cling to things external to him. But on the other hand, he is not prepared for liberation, since his soul is with his body.
> Q 3. How is he (to be described) when he is in neither of the two states which have been mentioned? Ans. He then is as he really is in his essence.[112]
>
> ٢ـ قال السايل : فاذا قبض الانسان اليه قوى نفسه و منعها عن الانتشار كيف يكون حاله ؟
> قال المجيب : لا يكون على كمال الوثاق و قد قطع علايق الجسمية عما بينه و بين ما سواه وترك النشبث بالخارجات عنه ولا يكون مستأهلا للخلاص لان نفسه مع البدن
> ٣ـ قال السايل : فاذا لم يكن على احدى الحالتين المشار اليهما فكيف يكون ؟
> قال المجيب : يكون كما هو على ذاته بالحقيقة
> (ed. Ritter 1956: 170, ll. 5–11)

As Pines and Gelblum already noticed,[113] question no. 2 roughly corresponds to the introduction of PYŚ 1.3, which reads as follows:

> "When the mental organ is in this state (i.e., when its activities have ceased), then, because there is no object, the following question arises: What is the nature of the Subject whose essence it is to make the mind conscious?[114] Then, the subject of perception abides in its own form (YS 1.3). The faculty of consciousness (i.e., the Subject) is then established in its own form, like in separation (i.e., in final liberation)".[115]

At first sight, question no. 2 in al-Bīrūnī's work differs from the introductory question of PYŚ 1.3 in a number of respects. To start with, the object of enquiry differs in both works. Al-Bīrūnī's question refers to a peculiar state of a man (فاذا

109 The personal name Pātanğal only occurs in the answer to the first question. See ed. Ritter 1956: 169, l. 15; trans. Pines & Gelblum 1966: 313.
110 For example, the introductory question of PYŚ 1.24 corresponds to that of Q 12 of the *Kitāb Pātanğal,* which al-Bīrūnī quotes in his "India". See Maas 2013: 59.
111 The literary form of a dialogue was commonly used in Arabic philosophical works as well as in some Upaniṣads.
112 Trans. Pines & Gelblum 1966: 314. In the first sentence of the answer, the reading of the Arabic is uncertain. Ritter's emendation of العصمة to الجسمية ("bodily") is probably correct.
113 Pines & Gelblum 1966: 314, n. 104.
114 This translation follows the interpretation of the *Pātañjalayogaśāstravivaraṇa* p. 165, ll. 7–9.
115 PYŚ 1.3, p. 7, ll. 1–4: *tadavasthe cetasi viṣayābhāvād buddhibodhātmā puruṣaḥ kiṃsvabhāvaḥ? tadā draṣṭuḥ svarūpe 'vasthānam* (YS 1.3). *svarūpapratiṣṭhā tadānīṃ cicchaktir yathā kaivalye.*

قبض الانسان اليه قوى نفسه و منعها عن الانتشار كيف يكون حاله), whereas Patañjali enquires about the nature of the Subject (*puruṣa*). However, when the Sanskrit word *puruṣa* is not used terminologically, it frequently just means "man". Moreover, both al-Bīrūnī and Patañjali refer to a particular state. In the Sanskrit work, however, the specific state, i. e., the state of the mental organ of a yogi, is not the object of enquiry. It figures only in the conditional subclause of the main question. There, the Sanskrit compound *tadavastha* "being in this state" is a *bahuvrīhi*-compound with the anaphoric pronoun *tad* in the initial position. This pronoun refers back to the topic of the previous section of the *Pātañjalayoga-śāstra,* i. e., to the cessation of mental activities (*cittavṛttinirodha*). Al-Bīrūnī apparently understood the reference of the pronoun *tad* correctly, when he composed a simplified version of the original question, in which here, as elsewhere, he referred to the cessation of mental activities with the expression "the compressed and spread out faculties".

The Arabic and the Sanskrit work share a number of additional features that allow for an identification of the question in the *Pātañjalayogaśāstra* as the source of al-Bīrūnī's question. First, the two questions occur at identical positions in the respective work. Second, the answer to question no. 3 in al-Bīrūnī's work is a literal translation of YS 1.3. And, finally, the answer to question no. 2 in the *Kitāb Pātanğal* appears to be a translation of the *bhāṣya*-part of PYŚ 1.3, which states that the cessation of mental activities is not identical with final liberation. The Arabic translation of the original "like in separation" (*yathā kaivalye*) contains additional information that is necessary in order to communicate the full meaning of this expression to al-Bīrūnī's audience.[116] The yogi enters the state of separation only at the moment of his physical death, when the Subject (*puruṣa*) and the mental organ (*citta*) separate once and for all. Thus, al-Bīrūnī's rendering of the Sanskrit passage, in which he states that the yogi has reached an advanced state of spiritual development but "is not prepared for liberation since his soul is with his body" (و لا يكون مستأهلا للخلاص لان نفسه مع البدن), shows that his understanding of this passage corresponds to the meaning of his Sanskrit source.

Just like the previously discussed integration of *sūtra*- and *bhāṣya*-passages, al-Bīrūnī's creation of the dialogic structure of the *Kitāb Pātanğal* is a further development of a feature that already existed in the *Pātañjalayogaśāstra.*[117] Al-Bīrūnī translated some questions of his exemplar and composed new ones. In addition, he provided his work with a new narrative structure by introducing the two characters of Pātanğal and the ascetic. In this respect, his work differs clearly

116 For more details on the translational strategy of "addition", see below, section 3.2.7.

117 The quotations of al-Bīrūnī's *Kitāb Sānk* that occur in the *Taḥqīq mā li-l-Hind* show that this work, just like the *Kitāb Pātanğal,* was composed in the form of a dialogue.

from the *Pātañjalayogaśāstra,* in which questions merely introduce the topics that are discussed under the heading of the respective *sūtra*-s.[118]

3.1.3. Omitting Linguistic Explanations

In the passage quoted above from the introduction of the *Kitāb Pātanğal,* al-Bīrūnī informed his reader that he felt not only justified but obliged "to omit (the parts which) are concerned with grammar and language" (والى اسقاط ما يتعلق بالنحو واللغة),[119] in order to overcome a translational problem that is, according to his view, especially pertinent for any translator dealing with Sanskrit literature. According to al-Bīrūnī,

> a complete and accurate translation is difficult, because the commentators are concerned with grammar and etymology and other (matters) which are of use only to a (person) who is versed in their literary languages as distinct from the vernacular.[120]
>
> يعسر نقل كله وعلى ما هو عليه لاشتغال المفسرين بالنحو والاشقاق وساير ما لا ينتفع به الا المحيط بلغاتهم الفصيحة دون المبتذلة
>
> (Ritter 1956: 167, l. 21 – 168, l. 1)

Some passages of the *Pātañjalayogaśāstra* contain indeed linguistic explanations that do not correspond to any passage of the *Kitāb Pātanğal.* For example, al-Bīrūnī's work lacks any reference to the very first section of the *Pātañjalayogaśāstra,* which in its initial part discusses the exact meaning of the Sanskrit equivalent to the adverb "now" (*atha*), the meaning of the word "authoritative teaching" (*anuśāsana*) and the etymology of the word *yoga* as a derivative of the second Sanskrit root *yuj* (*yuja*) "to be aware of sth., to concentrate, to be mentally absorbed". In this way, Patañjali defines the term *yoga* as a synonym of the Sanskrit equivalent for "absorption" (*samādhi*). Then, in the second part of this passage, the author explains that *samādhi* is the common characteristic of all forms of mental awareness.[121] This explanation is rather psychological than grammatical. However, the *Kitāb Pātanğal* also does not contain any reference to this psychological excursion.

---

118 Already Pines and Gelblum assumed, although for different reasons, that the dialogic structure of the *Kitāb Pātanğal* mirrors the structure of al-Bīrūnī's main source (Pines & Gelblum 1966: 303 and 1989: 265).

119 Al-Bīrūnī's oeuvre does not contain a single reference to the grammatical work *Vyākaraṇamahābhāṣya* by another Patañjali, who lived approximately 550 years prior to the yoga author. It is therefore highly unlikely that al-Bīrūnī's just quoted statement concerning the omission of grammatical explanations from the *Kitāb Pātanğal* refers to any other work than the Sanskrit work on yoga that al-Bīrūnī translated into Arabic.

120 Trans. Pines & Gelblum 1966: 310.

121 For a discussion of the different forms of awareness and absorption see Maas 2009: 267–269.

Moreover, linguistic explanations are very rare in the *Pātañjalayogaśāstra*. Their omission in the *Kitāb Pātanǧal* therefore would hardly affect the readability of al-Bīrūnī's work. On the whole, it appears that al-Bīrūnī did not only leave out passages that would have been of interest exclusively for a readership with knowledge of the Sanskrit language, but that he omitted all passages from his *Kitāb Pātanǧal* that he thought to be of no interest to his readership. Al-Bīrūnī's work is, accordingly, the result of his conscious selection of material that his main source contained. If this assessment is correct, the mere absence of a reference to any passage of the *Pātañjalayogaśāstra* in the *Kitāb Pātanǧal* does not justify the conclusion that al-Bīrūnī's source did not contain the respective passage,[122] because it is quite probable that al-Bīrūnī's choice to communicate certain topics and to leave out other subjects is the result of the creativity involved in the composition of an Arabic work that is to a considerable degree independent of its Sanskrit source. Accordingly, it is reasonable to assume that al-Bīrūnī did not refer to this selective process when he mentioned that he omitted linguistic explanations from his work.

3.2. Translational Strategies

In section 3.1 above, we discussed the three types of transformation that al-Bīrūnī mentioned in the introduction to his work. These modifications mainly concerned the structure of his work. However, al-Bīrūnī also transformed his source in numerous other ways that result from the difficulties he was facing when he composed his work. In fact, al-Bīrūnī had set himself the difficult task to communicate Brahmanical religious and philosophical concepts that had been formulated at the time of the Guptas, i. e., probably at some time between 325 and 425 CE, to a Muslim readership of the eleventh century. This audience was not acquainted with the Brahmanical culture of the time, and it definitely lacked any awareness of the religious and philosophical milieu of classical South Asian culture. It appears therefore almost unavoidable that al-Bīrūnī took the liberty of dealing freely and selectively with his source.

The problems that al-Bīrūnī had to face when he rendered the *Pātañjalayogaśāstra* into Arabic were very much comparable with the difficulties that every translator, modern or pre-modern, in general has to cope with. The work of the linguist Vladimir Ivir helps to deal with these difficulties. Ivir identified diffi-

122 The assumption of Pines and Gelblum that the fact that some *sūtra*-s "do not appear in the Arabic version suggests the possibility that the commentary used by al-Bīrūnī had dealt with a very early version of the *Yogasūtra*, before interpolations were added" (Pines & Gelblum 1966: 304f.) has to be revised in the light of the results of the present study.

culties in the translational process as well as possible strategies to overcome them. According to Ivir, translational difficulties particularly arise when the culture in which a source was composed differs from the culture of the target language. Ivir explains that

> [...] language and culture are inextricably interwoven and [...] the integration of an element into a culture (and into the conceptual framework of its members as individuals) cannot be said to have been achieved unless and until the linguistic expression of that element has been integrated into the language of that culture.[123]

Therefore, accordingly to Ivir, "[t]ranslating means translating cultures, not languages."[124]

Ivir points out that the degree of difficulty to translate a text is conditioned by the degree of "mutual similarities" between the source culture and the target culture.[125] In the case presently under discussion, to which Ivir does not refer, the differences between the two cultures are severe. Al-Bīrūnī's Perso-Muslim culture of the eleventh century and the religious–philosophical world view of Yoga that was created some six hundred years before differ with regard to, for example, their respective theologies, the ontological status of the soul or Subject, and the qualification for religious practice of different members of the two societies. In addition, elements of the Brahmanical culture of the Gupta time do either not correspond exactly to al-Bīrūnī's cultural background, or they are entirely missing, like for example, the South Asian theories of karma and rebirth. This problematic situation may have led al-Bīrūnī to take recourse to different strategies of finding appropriate translational solutions.

According to the model developed by Ivir, there are in principle seven strategies that a translator can apply for bridging cultural gaps, each of which has inherent advantages and drawbacks: (1) borrowing, (2) definition, (3) literal translation, (4) substitution, (5) lexical creation, (6) omission, and (7) addition. In the following (sections 3.2.1–7), we briefly introduce these strategies and provide examples of how and why al-Bīrūnī applied all of them with the single exception of lexical creation.

3.2.1. Borrowing

Borrowing or importing words from the source language into the target language is a powerful but problematic strategy to overcome cultural gaps.[126] In order to introduce a loanword successfully into the target language, it is necessary to

123 Ivir 1987: 35.
124 Ibid.
125 Ivir 1987: 36.
126 Ivir 1987: 37.

ensure that the audience acquires a sufficient knowledge of the corresponding extralinguistic reality of the concept referred to by the borrowed word. An important means for this end is the definition of the loanword in the target language. However, even if a translator achieves an appropriate understanding of the reality behind a loanword for his audience, its willingness to accept the foreign term as part of its language depends on multiple socio-linguistic issues. The loanword must fit into the target language phonologically and morphologically. In addition, a general familiarity of the audience with the source language will increase its willingness to accept a new word as part of its language. Finally, the general attitude of the audience to its own language as well as to the source language may influence the success or failure of any attempt of a translator to borrow directly from a source language.

In the case of al-Bīrūnī, it appears that borrowing was a strategy that was largely at variance with his authorial intention. Al-Bīrūnī's aim was to transfer specific yogic and Brahmanical conceptions into the intellectual sphere of the Islamic culture. The importation of (technical) terms would have added a further dimension of difficulty for understanding an already complicated work. Moreover, al-Bīrūnī may also have feared that the willingness of his audience to integrate foreign Sanskrit terms into its language would have been low. Therefore, al-Bīrūnī rarely used borrowing as a translational strategy, so that not even the central term *yoga* found its way into the *Kitāb Pātanğal*. However, within the cosmographical excursion of Q 46 that we discussed above in section 2.5.2, al-Bīrūnī used Sanskrit terms that he transcribed into Arabic for the individual regions of the world even in cases where he could have easily translated the respective names into Arabic, because the names are telling, i. e., their names have a meaning, like, for example, the name Tapoloka ("The World of Heat") or Satyaloka ("The World of Truth"). An additional striking example of this procedure is al-Bīrūnī's treatment of the designations of the seven oceans that separate the seven ring continents. Each of these oceans consists of a different fluid. In the *Pātañjalayogaśāstra* and in other works dealing with cosmography, the Sanskrit names of the oceans are simply the words for these fluids, i. e., Salt [water] (*lavaṇa* or *kṣāra*), Sugar Cane Juice (*ikṣurasa*), Spirituous Liquor (*surā*), etc.[127] Although al-Bīrūnī could have easily translated these Sanskrit names into Arabic, he decided to borrow them from his source. In addition, al-Bīrūnī also provided translations of these transliterations from the Sanskrit. It appears that he used the strategy of borrowing mostly when dealing with proper names, and very rarely in the case of technical terms.[128]

127 See Table 2 on pp. 309–311 above.

128 In Q 57, however, al-Bīrūnī borrowed the Sanskrit term *rasāyana* (رسايان). See ed. Ritter 1956: 193, l. 9 and trans. Pines & Gelblum 1989: 267.

3.2.2. Defining the Elements of Culture

Defining the elements of culture makes use of knowledge shared by the members of the source and of the target culture. This translational strategy uses the common knowledge of the members of both cultures in order to reduce "the unknown to the known and the unshared to the shared".[129] What Ivir means here is that translational processes depend upon the common experiental basis of human beings, which provides the very background for communication across cultures. Even strongly culturally determined concepts can be reduced in their complexity and communicated, i. e., explained, by making reference to this common human background.

However, definitional translations are inconvenient. Because they tend to be long and complicated, they attract too much attention for themselves, which affects the immediate intelligibility of the translated text. Therefore, definitional translations should be avoided for concepts that are only part of the cultural background of the source text, and not the topic on which the discussion is focused. Otherwise, they almost certainly lead to over-translations.

Numerous instances of definitional translations occur in al-Bīrūnī's work. For example, the titles of the two first chapters of the *Kitāb Pātanğal* as transmitted in the concluding statements of the chapters contain definitions of the corresponding Sanskrit terms.[130] In his colophon to the first chapter, al-Bīrūnī defines the Sanskrit term "absorption" (*samādhi*) as "making the heart steadfastly fixed" (فى اقرار القلب على مقر واحد).[131] In the concluding statement of the second chapter, he explains the term "means" (*sādhana*) by the expression "guidance towards the *praxis* which has been treated previously in the first section" (فى ارشاد الى عمل ما كان تقدم فى القطعة الاولى).[132]

3.2.3. Literal Translation

Literal translation was probably for a long time the most prominent translational strategy in modern scholarship. It has been the ideal of academic translations that was believed to easily overcome cultural and lexical gaps, because it is faithful to its source and transparent in the target language. Ivir, however, says that

129 Ivir 1987: 38.
130 See above, p. 288.
131 Trans. Pines & Gelblum 1966: 325; ed. Ritter 1956: 177, l. 10. An alternative translation for the Arabic word *qalb*, which al-Bīrūnī used to render the Sanskrit word *citta*, could be "mind".
132 Trans. Pines & Gelblum 1977: 527; ed. Ritter 1956: 183, l. 18.

> [l]ike the other procedures discussed here, literal translation has its advantages and limitations, which need to be weighed carefully for each particular cultural element and lexical item and for each act of communication it features in.[133]

There are cases in which the extra-linguistic realities of the two cultures differ to such an extent that a literal translation does not lead to a satisfactory result. For instance, idiomatic expressions of the source language defy all attempts of literal translation. Moreover, any literal translation is inappropriate when it would result in ungrammatical or stylistically unacceptable formulations in the target language.

In general, al-Bīrūnī was not inclined to compose a literal translation for the several reasons that we already discussed above. Nevertheless, it is possible to detect some passages that consist of a literal translation of his hypothetical source. For example, the answer to question 3, "He then is as he really is in his essence" (يكون كما هو على ذاته بالحقيقة),[134] is clearly an attempt to provide a literal translation of YS 1.3: "Then, the subject of perception abides in its own form" (*tadā draṣṭuḥ svarūpe 'vasthānam*).[135]

3.2.4. Substitution

Substitution is a convenient way to bridge cultural gaps by drawing upon concepts that are "available to the translator in cases in which the two cultures display a partial overlap rather than a clear-cut presence *vs.* absence of a particular element of culture."[136] The asset of this strategy is that the substitute for the source concept is readily available for the translator and perfectly intelligible for the audience. However, the familiarity of the audience with this concept may hide certain aspects of the source concept that are not encompassed by the term used in the target language. Moreover, because the semantic overlap between the two concepts is only partial, the target concept may evoke connotations that the source concept did not justify.

Al-Bīrūnī abundantly used substitution as a translational strategy. A striking example of this is his translation of the Sanskrit term for "God" (*īśvara*) with the Arabic "Allah" (الله), for instance in Q 12, Q 13, Q 16, and Q 21 of the *Kitāb Pātanğal.*[137] Both concepts refer to the idea of a supreme being. In the case of Pātañjala Yoga, this supreme being is a special kind of Subject (*puruṣa*) that mainly serves as an object of meditation and whose role in the world is rather

133 Ivir 1987: 39.

134 Ed. Ritter 1956: 170, l. 11; trans. Pines & Gelblum 1966: 314.

135 See above, p. 318.

136 Ivir 1987: 41.

137 Ed. Ritter 1956: 173, l. 12–174, l. 5; 174, ll. 11–17; 175, l. 21–176, l. 1; trans. Pines & Gelblum 1966: 319–322.

limited.[138] In contrast, on an ontological level, Allah is unique. He is the God of judgment and retribution who determines the post-mortem fate of all human beings. In contradistinction to this, Yoga philosophy and religion takes the quasi mechanism of karmic processes to determine the welfare or otherwise of human beings in their next existences.

3.2.5. Lexical Creation

Lexical creation is the process of coining new expressions in the target language, either by creating new words or by using unusual collocations of terms. According to Ivir, it is less frequently employed than the previously discussed strategies, because it requires a large amount of creativity on the side of the translator and hermeneutical skills on the side of the audience.[139] The newly coined term is "culturally 'empty'" and thus

> ready to receive and convey the intended content [...] of the source-culture element. At the same time, such cultural neutrality has the disadvantage of masking the cultural provenance of the element in question.[140]

As far as we can see, al-Bīrūnī did not use lexical creation as a translational strategy. He did not invent new terms. Whether al-Bīrūnī used unusual collocations or not is difficult to judge. In order to detect the inventive use of expressions in al-Bīrūnī's work, it would be necessary to be almost perfectly familiar not only with his language, but also with the standard language of his time and culture.

3.2.6. Omission

According to Ivir, omission is a strategy that translators may employ not out of necessity but for pragmatic reasons. Although in principle one of the previously discussed strategies could always be used instead of an omission, a translator may decide to employ an omission when otherwise the communicative costs would be higher than the gain.[141]

In the aforementioned part of his introduction, al-Bīrūnī justified the fact that he abbreviated his source to a considerable degree with the argument that a translation of the work with all its technical contents would be difficult to understand for his readers.[142] On the whole, al-Bīrūnī's argument is based on the

138 Maas 2009: 276–280.
139 Ivir 1987: 43.
140 Ivir 1987: 44.
141 Ibid.
142 Ed. Ritter 1956: 168, ll. 3–4; trans. Pines & Gelblum 1966: 310.

same line of thought as Ivir's model of communicative costs. An example for an omission of a passage from the *Pātañjalayogaśāstra* in al-Bīrūnī's work was discussed above.[143]

It is, however, possible to differentiate several kinds of omissions in al-Bīrūnī's work. Besides omissions that are part of a translational strategy, there are also passages from the *Pātañjalayogaśāstra* that al-Bīrūnī did not incorporate into his work because he probably found them not to be of relevance for his audience. As mentioned above, these omissions are part of the creativity that he used when composing the *Kitāb Pātanğal*.[144] This type of omissions therefore appears to be the result of personally or culturally determined preferences of the author–translator.

3.2.7. Addition

Addition is a translational strategy that has to be employed whenever the author of the source expresses himself in such a way that a literal translation of his wording would leave important pieces of information unexpressed. Whereas the audience of the source culture can easily supplement these elements from their common cultural knowledge, the members of the target culture, who do not have access to this knowledge, need additional information in order to properly understand the intention of the author.

The *Pātañjalayogaśāstra* is composed in scholastic Sanskrit. In this style of literary composition, brevity of verbal expression is a characteristic feature. Accordingly, al-Bīrūnī had many opportunities to add pieces of information in his translation in order to make the work intelligible to his readership. An example for al-Bīrūnī's use of this translational strategy, already referred to above, occurs in Q 2. There, al-Bīrūnī felt the need to supplement the expression "like in separation" (*yathā kaivalye*) with two sentences:

> "He is not completely bound, for he has severed the bodily ties between himself and that which is other than himself, and has ceased to cling to things external to him. But on the other hand, he is not prepared for liberation, since his soul is with his body".[145]
>
> لا يكون على كمال الوثاق و قد قطع علايق الجسمية عما بينه و بين ما سواه وترك النشبث بالخارجات عنه ولا يكون مستأهلا للخلاص لان نفسه مع البدن
>
> (Ritter 1956: 170., ll. 7–9)

In this passage, al-Bīrūnī referred to a state that is similar to, but not identical with, final liberation. The very brief Sanskrit expression "like in separation"

143 See above, p. 320.
144 See above, p. 321.
145 Trans. Pines & Gelblum 1966: 314.

(*yathā kaivalye*), if interpreted with sufficient background knowledge of Yoga soteriology, can be understood to contain a similar content. Al-Bīrūnī's addition was an appropriate translational device, because a literal translation of this phrase would not have been comprehensible for his target audience.

Two further cases of translational additions that were motivated by al-Bīrūnī's need to provide culture specific information were discussed above in sections 2.3.2 and 2.5.1. In the first case, al-Bīrūnī informed his audience that Nandīśvara gained a divine body in consequence of venerating the god Śiva.[146] In the second case, al-Bīrūnī supplemented his work by providing Ayurvedic information that he thought necessary for understanding how and why the human body consists of the bodily elements that are listed in PYŚ 3.29.[147]

3.3. Results

The above investigation showed that in composing his work, al-Bīrūnī applied two types of transformation to his main source. The first type consists of the three transformations that he mentioned in the introduction of his work. Two of these modifications, i.e., combining different layers of text and creating a dialogue, concern the structure and the form of al-Bīrūnī's work. On the basis of a comparison of the *Kitāb Pātanğal* and the *Pātañjalayogaśāstra,* we could show that these two transformations further develop characteristic features of al-Bīrūnī's source. The third transformation, i.e., omitting linguistic explanations that would have been incomprehensible for the reader, did not lead to a structural or formal modification of the source. Because these explanations are in any case quite rare in the *Pātañjalayogaśāstra,* their omission did not have a large impact on the comprehensibility of al-Bīrūnī's work. By providing examples of these modifications, we could show that al-Bīrūnī actually put his programmatic statement into practice.

The second type of transformation results from al-Bīrūnī's more or less conscious application of different translational strategies, of which there are, according to Ivir, seven. On the basis of our comparison of selected passages from the Sanskrit and the Arabic works, it becomes evident that al-Bīrūnī used five of these strategies frequently, i.e., defining the elements of culture, literal translation, substitution, omission and addition, whereas he rarely resorted to borrowing and did not at all use lexical creations.

146 See above, p. 299.
147 See above, p. 304.

4. Conclusion

After having critically surveyed previous attempts to identify the Sanskrit source of the *Kitāb Pātanğal*, we arrived at the conclusion that at the present state of research the *Pātañjalayogaśāstra* is the most likely candidate for being the main source of al-Bīrūnī's work. Apparently, al-Bīrūnī supplemented his main source with different additional sources that were partly written and partly oral. Besides this, the cultural knowledge that he acquired naturally during his stays in South Asia will have contributed to the way in which he composed his work.

The identification of this hypothetical main source provided us with a standard of comparison that we used for further analyses of al-Bīrūnī's work. We identified two main types of transformation that al-Bīrūnī applied to his source when he rendered it into Arabic.[148] The first of these mainly consists of structural and formal transformations. The second one consists in the application of different translational strategies. Moreover, we could see throughout our study that al-Bīrūnī handled his source in a free and creative manner. He selected the topics that appeared to be most relevant and left out topics that he considered incomprehensible or irrelevant for his audience. In other cases, the scholar substituted unfamiliar South Asian concepts with ideas that he directly drew from his Islamic background. This creative process is the third and probably most important type of transformation that al-Bīrūnī applied, because it transferred a Sanskrit yoga work of approximately the fourth century into the culture of medieval Islam.

In order to estimate the creative dimension of al-Bīrūnī's work, as well as his ability (and limits) to understand his source, a comparison of the *Kitāb Pātanğal* with its hypothetical main source was therefore only a necessary first step. Understanding al-Bīrūnī's motives for deviating from his source as well as determining other reasons for differences between the *Kitāb Pātanğal* and its sources then led to a fuller picture of al-Bīrūnī's literary activity and creativity. In this way, the present chapter shows that al-Bīrūnī's aspiration was not only to provide a translation that is faithful to its source, but also to make the spiritual dimension of yoga accessible to his Muslim readership. It appears that al-Bīrūnī understood that "[t]ranslation is a way of establishing contacts between cultures",[149] or, one may add, religions and philosophies.

Future research in the hermeneutics of al-Bīrūnī requires further contextualisations of his work within the frame of the intellectual history of South

148 See also Verdon 2015 (ch. 4–6) for a more detailed discussion of why al-Bīrūnī may have used which translational strategies when he composed his *Kitāb Pātanğal* and his *Kitāb Sānk*.

149 Ivir 1987: 35.

Asia as well as with that of the Arab world. Providing a basis for such research was one of the aims of the present chapter.[150]

References

Sanskrit Manuscripts

A^d Palm leaf manuscript of the *Pātañjalayogaśāstra* in Devanagari script kept at the Lālbhaī Dalpatbhaī Bhāratīya Vidyāmandir, Ahmedabad. Ms. no. Lā. Da. Tāḍ. 34 (1).

J^d Palm leaf manuscript of the *Pātañjalayogaśāstra* in Devanagari script, ms. no. 395/2 in the *Jinabhadrasūri tāḍapatrīya graṃth bhaṃḍār-jaisalmer durg* in Jambuvijaya 2000.

Tv^y Palm leaf manuscript of the *Pātañjalayogaśāstra* in Malayalam script kept at the Oriental Research Institute, Thiruvananthapuram. Ms. no. 662. Described as no. 21 in Maas 2006: § 2.2.8.

Primary Sources

Āgāśe, K. Ś. (Ed.). (1904). *VācaspatimiśraviracitaṭīkāsaṃvalitaVyāsabhāṣyasametāni Pātañjalayogasūtrāṇi tathā BhojadevaviracitaRājamārtaṇḍābhidhavṛttisametāni Pātañjalayogasūtrāṇi.* Ānandāśramasaṃskṛtagranthāvaliḥ 47. Puṇyākhyapattana: Ānandāśramamudraṇālaya.

Al-Bīrūnī, Abū l-Rayḥān Muḥammad bin Aḥmad (1958). *Fī taḥqīq mā li-l-Hind min maqūla maqbūla fī l-ʿaql aw marḏūla.* Hyderabad: Da'irat al-Ma'arif il-Osmania Publications.

Azkaei, P. (2001). *Al-āṯār al-bāqiya ʻan al-qurūn al-ḵāliya.* Teheran: Mirāṯ-e Maktub.

Bhoja, *Rājamārtaṇḍa*
see Āgāśe 1904.

Liṅgapurāṇa
Liṅgamahāpurāṇam: With Sanskrit Commentary Śivatoṣinī of Gaṇeśa Nātu. Delhi: Nag Publishers, 1989.

Maas, Ph. A. (2006). *Samādhipāda: Das erste Kapitel des Pātañjalayogaśāstra zum ersten Mal kritisch ediert = The First Chapter of the Pātañjalayogaśāstra for the First Time Critically Edited.* Studia Indologica Universitatis Halensis. Geisteskultur Indiens. Texte und Studien 9. Aachen: Shaker.

Mahābhārata
The Mahābhārata, ed. V. S. Sukthankar et al. 20 vols. Poona: Bhandarkar Oriental Research Institute, 1933(1927)–1966.

Mitra, R. (1883). *The Yoga Aphorisms of Patanjali, With the commentary of Bhoja and an English Translation.* Bibliotheca Indica 93. Calcutta: Baptist Mission Press.

150 For a more comprehensive scholarly treatment of al-Bīrūnī's interpretation of Indian philosophies, see Verdon 2015.

Pātañjalayogaśāstravivaraṇa
Harimoto, K. (1999). *A Critical Edition of the Pātañjalayogaśāstravivaraṇa: First Pāda, Samādhipāda: With an Introduction.* Unpublished Doctoral Thesis. University of Pennsylvania.
PYŚ
Pātañjalayogaśāstra. For ch. 1 see Maas 2006, for ch. 2–4 see Āgāśe 1904.
Ritter, H. (Ed.). (1956). Al-Bīrūnī's Übersetzung des Yoga-Sūtra des Patañjali. *Oriens, 9*(2), 165–200.
YS
Yogasūtra in PYŚ.

Secondary Sources

Acri, A. (2011). *Dharma Pātañjala: A Śaiva Scripture from Ancient Java. Studied in the Light of Related Old Javanese and Sanskrit Texts.* Gonda Indological Studies 16. Groningen: Egbert Forsten.

Ali, M. A. (1992). Translations of Sanskrit Works at Akbar's Court. *Social Scientist, 20*(9), 38–45.

Boilot, J.-D. (1955). L'oeuvre d'al-Beruni: essai bibliographique. *Mideo (Mélanges de l'Institut dominicain d'études orientales du Caire), 2,* 161–256.

Calverley, E. E. & Netton, I. R. (2012). Nafs. In P. Bearman et al. (Eds.), *Encyclopaedia of Islam.* 2nd ed. http://dx.doi.org/10.1163/1573-3912_islam_COM_0833. Accessed 30 May 2017.

Colebrooke, H. Th. (1827). On the Philosophy of the Hindus. Part 1: Sánkhya. *Transactions of the Royal Asiatic Society, 1,* 19–43.

Daiber, H. (2012). *Islamic Thought in the Dialogue of Cultures: A Historical and Bibliographical Survey.* Themes in Islamic Studies 7. Leiden: Brill.

Dasgupta, S. N. (1930). *Yoga Philosophy in Relation to Other Systems of Indian Thought.* Calcutta: University of Calcutta (repr. Delhi: Motilal Banarsidass, 1974).

Ernst, C. W. (2003). Muslim Studies of Hinduism? A Reconsideration of Arabic and Persian Translations from Indian Languages. *Iranian Studies, 36*(2), 173–195.

Ernst, C. W. (2010). Fayzi's Illuminationist Interpretation of Vedanta: The Shariq al-ma'rifa. *Comparative Studies of South Asia, Africa and the Middle East, 30*(3), 356–364.

Funayama, T. (1995). Arcaṭa, Śāntarakṣita, Jinendrabuddhi, and Kamalaśīla on the Aim of a Treatise (prayojana). *Wiener Zeitschrift für die Kunde Südasiens, 39,* 181–201.

Garbe, R. (1894). *Die Sâṃkhya-Philosophie: Eine Darstellung des indischen Rationalismus.* Leipzig: Haessel.

Garbe, R. (1896). *Sāṃkhya und Yoga.* Grundriss der Indo-Arischen Philologie und Altertumskunde 3.4. Strassburg: Trübner.

Garbe, R. (1917). *Die Sâṃkhya-Philosophie: Eine Darstellung des indischen Rationalismus.* 2nd ed. Leipzig: Haessel.

Gardet, L. & Vadet, J.-C. (2012). Ḳalb. In P. Bearman et al. (Eds.), *Encyclopaedia of Islam.* 2nd ed. http://dx.doi.org/10.1163/1573-3912_islam_COM_0424. Accessed 30 May 2017.

Gelblum, T. (2008). Al-Bīrūnī, 'Book of Patañjali'. In R. S. Bhattacharya & G. J. Larson (Eds.), *Yoga: India's Philosophy of Meditation* (pp. 261–270). Encyclopedia of Indian Philosophies XII. Delhi: Motilal Banarsidass.

Halbfass, W. (1990). *India and Europe: An Essay in Philosophical Understanding.* Delhi: Motilal Banarsidass.

Hauer, J. W. (1930). Das neugefundene arabische Manuskript von al-Bīrūnīs Übersetzung des Pātañjala (Ein vorläufiger Bericht). *Orientalistische Literaturzeitung, 33*(4), 273–282.

Hermelink, H. (1977). Zur Bestimmung von Biruni's Todestag. *Sudhoffs Archiv, 61*(3), 298–300.

Ivir, V. (1987). Procedures and Strategies for the Translation of Culture. *Indian Journal of Applied Linguistics, 13*(2), 35–46.

Jambuvijaya, M. (2000). *A Catalogue of Manuscripts in the Jaisalmer Jain Bhandaras / Jaisalmer ke prācīn jain graṃthbhaṃḍāroṃ kī sūcī.* Delhi & Jaisalmer: Motilal Banarsidass & Parshvanath Jain Shwetambar Trust.

Jha, G. (1907). *The Yoga-Darśana: The Sūtras of Patañjali with the Bhāṣya of Vyāsa. Translated into English with Notes from Vâchaspati Miśras Tattvavaiśâradî, Vijnâna Bhiksu's Yogavârtika and Bhoja's Râjamârtaṇda.* Bombay: Bombay Theosophical Publication Fund.

Jolly, J. (1901). *Medicin.* Grundriss der Indo-Arischen Philologie und Altertumskunde 3.10. Strassburg: Trübner.

Kennedy, St. E. (1970). Al-Bīrūnī. In C. C. Gillispie (Ed.), *Dictionary of Scientific Biography.* Vol. 2 (pp. 147–158). New York: Charles Scribner's Sons.

Kirfel, W. (1920). *Die Kosmographie der Inder: Nach den Quellen dargestellt.* Bonn: Kurt Schröder.

Klaus, K. (1986). *Die altindische Kosmologie: Nach den Brāhmaṇas dargestellt.* Indica et Tibetica 9. Bonn: Indica et Tibetica.

Koetschet, P. (2011). *La philosophie arabe: IXe–XIVe siècle. Textes choisis et présentés.* Lonrai: Points Essais.

Kozah, M. (2015). *The Birth of Indology as an Islamic Science: Al-Biruni's Treatise on Yoga Psychology.* Islamic Philosophy, Theology, and Science: Text and Studies. Boston: Brill.

Maas, Ph. A. (2008a). The Concepts of the Human Body and Disease in Classical Yoga and Āyurveda. *Wiener Zeitschrift für die Kunde Südasiens, 51,* 125–162.

Maas, Ph. A. (2008b). "Descent With Modification": The Opening of the Pātañjalayogaśāstra. In W. Slaje (Ed.), *Śāstrārambha: Inquiries into the Preamble in Sanskrit* (pp. 97–120). Abhandlungen für die Kunde des Morgenlandes 57. Wiesbaden: Harrassowitz.

Maas, Ph. A. (2009). The So-called Yoga of Suppression in the Pātañjalayogaśāstra. In E. Franco in collaboration with D. Eigner (Eds.), *Yogic Perception, Meditation, and Altered States of Consciousness* (pp. 263–282). Österreichische Akademie der Wissenschaften, Sitzungsberichte der phil.-hist. Klasse 794 = Beiträge zur Kultur- und Geistesgeschichte Asiens 64. Wien: Verlag der Österreichischen Akademie der Wissenschaften.

Maas, Ph. A. (2013). A Concise Historiography of Classical Yoga Philosophy. In E. Franco (Ed.), *Historiography and Periodization of Indian Philosophy* (pp. 53–90). Publications of the de Nobili Research Library 37. Vienna: Verein "Sammlung de Nobili - Arbeitsgemeinschaft für Indologie und Religionsforschung".

Maas, Ph. A. (2017). From Theory to Poetry: The Reuse of Patañjali's Yogaśāstra in Māgha's Śiśupālavadha. In E. Freschi & Ph. A. Maas (Eds.), *Adaptive Reuse: Aspects of Creativity in South Asian Cultural History* (pp. 27–60). Abhandlungen für die Kunde des Morgenlandes 101. Wiesbaden: Harrassowitz.

Meulenbeld, G. J. (1999–2002). *A History of Indian Medical Literature.* 3 vols. (in 5 parts). Groningen Oriental Studies 15. Groningen: Egbert Forsten.

Minkowski, Ch. (2008). Why Should We Read the Maṅgala Verses? In W. Slaje (Ed.), *Śāstrārambha: Inquiries into the Preamble in Sanskrit* (pp. 1–24). Abhandlungen für die Kunde des Morgenlandes 62. Wiesbaden: Harrassowitz.

Orelskaya, M. V. (1997). Nandikeśvara in Hindu Mythology. *Annals of the Bhandarkar Oriental Research Institute, 78,* 233–248.

Pines, Sh. & Gelblum, T. (1966). Al-Bīrūnī's Arabic Version of Patañjali's Yogasūtra. *Bulletin of the School of Oriental and African Studies, 29*(2), 302–325.

Pines, Sh. & Gelblum, T. (1977). Al-Bīrūni's Arabic Version of Patañjali's Yogasūtra: A Translation of the Second Chapter and a Comparison with Related Texts. *Bulletin of the School of Oriental and African Studies, 40*(3), 522–549.

Pines, Sh. & Gelblum, T. (1983). Al-Bīrūnī's Arabic Version of Patañjali's Yogasūtra: A Translation of the Third Chapter and a Comparison with Related Texts. *Bulletin of the School of Oriental and African Studies, 46*(2), 258–304.

Pines, Sh. & Gelblum, T. (1989). Al-Bīrūnī's Arabic Version of Patañjali's Yogasūtra: A Translation of the Fourth Chapter and a Comparison with Related Texts. *Bulletin of the School of Oriental and African Studies, 52*(2), 265–305.

Pingree, D. E. (1981). *Census of the Exact Sciences in Sanskrit.* Series A, Vol. 4. Memoirs of the American Philosophical Society 146. Philadelphia: American Philosophical Society.

Pingree, D. E. (1983). Brahmagupta, Balabhadra, Pṛthūdaka and Al-Bīrūnī. *Journal of the American Oriental Society, 103*(2), 353–360.

Prasāda, R. (1910). *Patanjali's Yoga Sutras With the Commentary of Vyâsa and the Gloss of Vâchaspati Miśra. Translated by Râma Prasâda [...] With an Introduction from Rai Bahadur Śrīśa Chandra Vasu.* Sacred Books of the Hindus 4.7–9. Allahabad: Panini Office (2nd ed. = repr. Delhi: Oriental Books Reprint Corporation, 1978).

Renou, L. & Filliozat, J. (Eds.). (1953). *L'Inde classique: manuel des études indiennes.* Paris: Imprimerie nationale.

Sachau, C. E. (1879). *The Chronology of Ancient Nations: An English Version of the Arabic Text of the Athâr-ul-bâkiya of Albîrûnî or "Vestiges of the Past".* London: W. H. Allen.

Sachau, C. E. (1888). *Alberuni's India: An Account of the Religion, Philosophy, Literature, Geography, Chronology, Astronomy, Customs, Laws and Astrology of India about 1030. An English Edition with Notes and Indices.* 2 vols. London: Kegan Paul, Trench & Trübner (repr. Delhi: Low Price Publications, 2003).

Shamsi, F. A. (1979). Abū al-Raiḥān Muḥammad Ibn Aḥmad al-Bayrūnī. 362, 973 – CA. 443, 1051. In M. H. Said (Ed.), *Al-Bīrūnī Commemorative Volume: Proceedings of the International Congress Held in Pakistan on the Occasion of Millenary of Abū al-Rāiḥān Muḥammad Ibn Aḥmad al-Bayrūnī (973 – ca 1051 A.D.). November 26, 1973 thru December 12, 1973* (pp. 260–288). Karachi: Hamdard Academy.

Shastri, A. M. (1975). Sanskrit Literature Known to al-Bīrūnī. *Indian Journal of History of Science, 10,* 111–138.

Söhnen, R. (1991). Indra and Women. *Bulletin of the School of Oriental and African Studies, University of London, 54*(1), 68–74.

Sörensen, S. (1904–1925). *An Index to the Names in the Mahābhārata With Short Explanations and a Concordance to the Bombay and Calcutta Editions and P. C. Roy's Translation.* London: Williams & Norgate.

Touati, H. (2000). *Islam et voyage au moyen âge.* Paris: Editions du Seuil.

Vadet, J. C. (2012). Ḳalb. *Encyclopaedia of Islam.* 2nd ed. http://referenceworks.brillonline.com/entries/encyclopaedia-of-islam-2/k-alb-COM_0424. Accessed 12 September 2014.

Verdon, N. (2015). *Al-Bīrūnī's Kitāb Sānk and Kitāb Pātanğal: A Historical and Textual Study.* Unpublished Doctoral Thesis. University of Lausanne. https://serval.unil.ch/resource/serval:BIB_779D64E820E1.P001/REF. Accessed 23 February 2017.

Wisnovsky, R. et al. (2011). Introduction. Vehicles of Transmission, Translation, and Transformation in Medieval Textual Culture. In R. Wisnovsky et al. (Eds.), *Vehicles of Transmission, Translation and Transformation in Medieval Textual Culture* (pp. 1–22). Cursor Mundi: Viator Studies of the Medieval and Early Modern World 4. Turnhout: Brepols.

Woods, J. H. (Trans.). (1914). *The Yoga-System of Patañjali, Or the Ancient Hindu Doctrine of Concentration of Mind, Embracing the Mnemonic Rules, Called Yoga-Sūtras, of Patañjali and the Comment, Called Yoga-Bhāshya, Attributed to Veda-Vyāsa, and the Explanation, Called Tattva-Vaiçāradī, of Vāchaspati-Miçra.* Cambridge, Mass: Harvard University Press (repr. Delhi: Motilal Banarsidass, 1992).

Yano, M. (2013). al-Bīrūnī. *Encyclopaedia of Islam.* 3rd ed. Brill Online, 2014. http://referenceworks.brillonline.com/entries/encyclopaedia-of-islam-3/al-bi-ru-ni-COM_25350. Accessed 12 September 2014.

Zadeh, T. (2011). *Mapping Frontiers Across Medieval Islam: Geography, Translation, and the ʿAbbāsid Empire.* London: I. B. Tauris.

Chapter 8

Tibetan Yoga: Somatic Practice in Vajrayāna Buddhism and Dzogchen

Ian A. Baker

Contents

1. Vajrayāna Buddhism 337

2. Tsa Uma: The Axis of Awareness 341

3. Trulkhor: Yoga of Breath and Movement 344

4. Nyingthik: Heart Essence of Tibetan Yoga 355

5. Korde Rushen: Yoga of Spontaneous Presence 364

6. Tögal: Yoga of Active Perception 370

7. Conclusion 377

List of Figures 379

References 380

Ian A. Baker

Chapter 8: Tibetan Yoga: Somatic Practice in Vajrayāna Buddhism and Dzogchen*

1. Vajrayāna Buddhism

Tibet's Vajrayāna form of Buddhism is widely known for its monastic culture of esoteric ritual and scriptural debate. It is less well known for its Haṭha Yoga-related[1] practices that, due to their perceived potential for misapplication, are transmitted guardedly even within the tradition despite their foundational role in Vajrayāna's earliest and arguably most dynamic systems of meditation.[2] This chapter explores the developmental history of "forceful" Haṭha Yoga-related yoga and somatic practice[3] within Tibetan Buddhism as a whole while focusing

* This article is indebted to early reviews by Geoffrey Samuel, Mark Singleton, and James Mallinson. While predominantly textually based, it owes much to ethnographic research within the living traditions of Vajrayāna Buddhism and Dzogchen in India, Nepal, Tibet, and Bhutan and oral instruction by Dudjom Jigdral Yeshe Dorje, Chatral Sangye Dorje, Dilgo Khyentse Rinpoche, Dungtse Thinley Norbu, Bhakha Tulku Pema Tenzin, Yongdzin Tenzin Namdak, H. H. Sakya Trizin, H. H. the Dalai Lama, Kunzang Dorje Rinpoche, Lam Nyingku Kunzang Wangdi, Tulku Tenzin Rabgye, and Tshewang Sitar Rinpoche.

1 Haṭha Yoga is used in this essay to refer to "forceful" physically-based yogic practices that developed in medieval India within the context of Buddhist and Hindu tantra. As shown below, the term first appears in the eighth-century *Guhyasamājatantra* and in a tenth-century commentary to the *Kālacakratantra* but, in current usage, Haṭha Yoga is most often associated with "modern postural yoga", precedents for which are explored in this essay. It should be clarified, however, that the somatic techniques of Vajrayāna and Tibetan Buddhism do not necessarily reflect any direct influence from Haṭha Yoga traditions in India until the twelfth century with the dissemination in Tibet of the *Amṛtasiddhi,* Haṭha Yoga's reputed "source text" based on bodily postures (*mudrā*-s) and breathing techniques that, as revealed by James Mallinson, profoundly influenced the later development of the Haṭha Yoga tradition.

2 Yoga, in the Tibetan and Vajrayāna tradition, ultimately refers to a culminating transformation of consciousness, and not simply to the physical and breath-based practices through which liberating existential insight is achieved. Nonetheless, this essay focuses specifically on the little known Haṭha Yoga-like practices in Tibetan Buddhism that constitute a deeply embodied form of philosophical self-inquiry.

3 Derived from the Greek word *soma,* "the living organism in its wholeness", somatic practice refers to sensory–motor awareness based physical movement combined with conscious proprioception and breathing techniques that promote a unified experience of mind and body.

on its little-known applications within Dzogchen (*rdzogs chen*), Vajrayāna's coalescent "Great Perfection" cycle of practices upheld as revealing the innately liberated nature of human consciousness and the physical body. Although commonly taught today as a purely mental discipline, Dzogchen's "heart essence" (*snying thig*) transmission emphasises physically demanding preparatory exercises and prescribed postures (*stabs*, Skt. *āsana*) that push physiology - and thereby consciousness - beyond habitual limits.[4] Tibetan treatises describing the therapeutic and transformative benefits of such yogic exercises appear in the twelfth century in the "Turquoise Heart Essence"[5] and in the highly influential writings of Phagmo Drupa[6] while previously hidden wall paintings in Lhasa's Lukhang temple illustrate yogic practices linking visualisation, breath, physical *mudrā*-s, and sequential movements centuries before accounts of sequenced postural (*vinyāsa*) yoga in India.[7]

The word somatic also refers to "the body as subjectively perceived from within" which is a core aspect of tantric yoga in both its Hindu and Buddhist renditions as a means for transcending conceptuality and thereby transforming subjective experience of the mind and its perceptions.

4 See p. 365ff. for descriptions of physically demanding yogic practices in the "Continuity of Sound" (*sgra thal 'gyur*) and other foundational eleventh-century Dzogchen texts.

5 See pp. 342 and 348ff. for an account of the *Yuthok Nyingthik* (*gYu thog snying thig*), or "Turquoise Heart Essence".

6 See p. 347 for an account of the "The Path of Fruition's Thirty-two Auspicious Actions" (*Lam 'bras kyi 'phrin las sum bcu so gnyis*), "The Path of Fruition's Five-Branch Yoga" (*Lam 'bras kyi yan lag lnga sbyong*), and "Supplementary Verses on the Path of Method" (*Thabs lam tshigs bcad ma'i lhan thabs*) compiled by Phagmo Drupa Dorje Gyalpo (phag mo gru pa rdo rje rgyal po) (1110–1170).

7 See p. 358f. for the Lukhang murals and their contents. While contemporary scholarship has yet to determine the first occurrence of sequenced yoga postures specifically linking breath and movement, its fitness-oriented applications within Indian yoga are widely held to have originated in the early twentieth century as a result of transnational and colonial-era influences. However, the Lukhang murals and Pema Lingpa's "treasure text" (*gter ma*) on which they are based indicate an earlier genesis of sequenced movements, albeit within a parallel yogic tradition. Modern postural yoga differs significantly in its greater inclusion of standing postures and the substitution of extended "connected breaths" in place of "vase breaths" (*kumbhakaprāṇāyāma*) and "root lock" (*mūladharabandha*) held throughout series of dynamic movements. Internally retained breaths combined with prescribed movements are part of the purportedly ancient Kriyā Yoga, or "yoga of action" system revived by Shyama Charan Lahiri (1828–1895) in the middle of the nineteenth century and further popularised by Paramahansa Yogananda (1893–1952) from 1917 onward as well as by Swami Satyananda Saraswati from 1963 until his death in 2009. Philipp A. Maas (personal communication) points out that the term *kriyāyoga* appears several times in the *Pātañjalayogaśāstra* and is also found in the *Pañcārthabhāṣya*, Kauṇḍinya's commentary on the *Pāśupatasūtra*. It is not clear, however, in these early references whether or not Kriyā Yoga was originally practised with internally held breaths (*kumbhaka*). The full development of modern postural yoga is first associated with Tirumalai Krishnamacharya (1888–1989) and his followers. Krishnamacharya attributed his system of Aṣṭāṅga Vinyāsa Yoga to an obscure fourteenth-century text, the "Yoga Kuruntha", the transmission of which he ostensibly received from his guru, Sri Ramamohana Brahmachari, while residing for over seven years in a cave near Tibet's Mount Kailash. For a com-

Buddhist practices of physical cultivation developed within the larger context of Indian Tantrism, in particular with the emergence of the *yoginītantra* class of Buddhist Tantras between the eighth and tenth centuries. The crowning textual achievement of Buddhism's Vajrayāna, or "Adamantine Way", the Yoginī Tantras share common features with Tantric Śaivism and are based on imaginal identification with ecstatic, multi-limbed deities ornamented with human bones and signifying self-transcendent bliss and insight. The Yoginī, or "Mother" Tantras emphasise conscious realisation of the bliss–emptiness (*bde stong ye shes*) underlying all existence. They are contrasted with earlier "Father" Tantras that invoke more pacific, royally attired Buddhas such as Guhyasamāja (*gsang ba 'dus pa*) associated with "illusory body" (*sgyu lus*) practices for attaining the light body of a Buddha. Tibetans classified the "Mother" (*ma rgyud*) and "Father" (*pha rgyud*) Tantras together as "Unexcelled Yoga Tantra" (*bla ma med pa'i rgyud*, Skt. *anuttarayogatantra*), sometimes adding a third "Non-Dual Tantra" (*gnyis med rgyud*) category when both aspects are combined. As a whole, the Anuttarayoga Tantras or Yoganiruttara Tantras, as originally known in Sanskrit, involve methods for transforming sensual pleasure into enlightened awareness through techniques focused on dissolving vital winds (*prāṇavāyu*) into the body's central channel (*suṣumnā*). In Tibetan rNying ma, or "Old School" presentations of the Indian Tantras, the Anuttarayoga Tantras correspond to Mahāyoga, or "Great Yoga", to which the successive catagories of Anuyoga, "Subsequent Yoga", and Atiyoga, "Supreme Yoga" (also called Dzogchen, or "Great Perfection") were added later.[8]

Transforming early Buddhism's ascetic disposition into dynamic engagement with sensory existence, Vajrayāna expanded Buddhism's influence and applicability beyond its monastic institutions. As the eighth-century Buddhist *Hevajratantra* famously proclaims, "One must rise by that by which one falls ... By whatever binds the world, by that it must be freed."[9] Central to this endeavor was a revalorisation of the body as an essential vehicle, rather than an obstacle, to spiritual enlightenment.

The term *haṭhayoga* first appears in the eighth century in the eighteenth chapter of the "Secret Assembly Tantra" (*Guhyasamājatantra*, Tib. *gSang 'dus*

prehensive account of this subject in light of Krishnamacharya's legacy see Singleton 2010. See also Jason Birch's chapter in the present volume which demonstrates that dynamic non-seated systems of *āsana*-based Haṭha Yoga developed extensively in India from the sixteenth century onward, although previously undocumented.

8 For comprehensive accounts of the origins and development of the Hindu and Buddhist tantras and their social and institutional contexts, see Samuel 2008 and Davidson 2002 and 2005. For a clear exposition of the Yoginī Tantras' debt to Śaivite sources, see Mayer 1998 and Sanderson 2009.

9 See Farrow & Menon 1992: 173. The *Hevajratantra* further indicates that "the one who knows the nature of poison dispels the poison utilizing the poison itself."

rtsa rgyud) where it is presented as a "forceful" means for inducing noetic visions (*darśana*) as well as for "awakening" (*bodhi*) and attaining "perfection of knowing" (*jñānasiddhi*).[10] The word "forceful" recurs in the tenth-century *Kālacakratantra,* or "Wheel of Time Tantra", in the form of *haṭhena* ("forcefully") and is elaborated in Puṇḍarīka's 966 CE commentary on the *Kālacakra* entitled "[Treatise of] Stainless Light" (*Vimalaprabhā*) which defines Haṭha Yoga as a means for drawing the body's vital essences into its central channel (*madhyanāḍī*) and thereby entering unaltering present-moment (*akṣarakṣaṇa*) awareness.[11] Encyclopedic in its scope, the *Kālacakra* outlines an expedient method for attaining Nirvāṇa within the context of embodied existence (*saṃsāra*) and is the culminating expression of the Yoginī Tantras. It correlates cycles of human gestation and birth with the yogic cultivation of an "indestructible and unchanging body" (*vajrakāya,* Tib. *rdo rje'i lus*) of subtle channels, winds, and seminal essences (*nāḍī, prāṇavāyu, bindu,* Tib. *rtsa, rlung, thig le*) during recurring states of waking, dreaming, sleeping, and sexual arousal, based on a system of sixfold Vajra Yoga (*rdo rje'i rnal 'byor*).[12]

10 See Birch 2011: 535.

11 Jason Birch (ibid.) translates as follows from the *Vimalaprabhā:* "Now the haṭhayoga is explained. Here, when the unchanging moment does not take place because the vital breath is unrestrained, [in spite of] the image having been seen by means of withdrawal and so on, then [the yogin] – after having made the vital breath flow in the central channel violently through the [...] exercise of sound – can realize the unchanging moment through nonvibration by arresting the bindu of the bodhicitta in the vajra-gem placed in the lotus of the wisdom. This is the haṭhayoga." See also Mallinson (2011: 771) who describes a similar sexio-yogic technique in the circa thirteenth-century *Dattātreyayogaśāstra* that is the first Indic text to refer to Haṭha Yoga by name. The *Dattātreyayogaśāstra* describes Haṭha Yoga in the context of restraining the body's seminal essences (*bindu*) within the central channel (*madhyanāḍī*) (Mallinson 2016: 111). Mallinson also indicates that, within the later Gorakṣa tradition, Haṭha Yoga first appears by name in the *Yogabīja,* which is also the first instance of *ha* and *ṭha* referring to the body's solar and lunar currents and *yoga* as their union (Mallinson 2011: 772). As a further developed system of psychophysical purification (*ṣaṭkarma*), expansion of vital energy (*prāṇāyāma*), and physical cultivation through exercises and postures (*āsana*), Haṭha Yoga is more commonly associated with later texts such as the mid-fifteenth century *Haṭhayogapradīpikā* by Svāmi Svātmārāma and the *Śivasamhitā* as well as the more extensive seventeenth-century compilation *Gheraṇḍasaṃhitā.* All but the latter outline eight successive stages modeled on Patañjali's fourth-century CE or earlier *Pātañjalayogaśāstra,* the structure of which has been widely noted to resemble Gautama Buddha's enumeration of an Eightfold Path leading to the existential freedom of Nirvāṇa (see, for example, Larson 2012: 80). While Haṭha Yoga has been viewed by many as a pragmatic distillation of highly ritualised and exclusive forms of tantric yoga, as presented in the *Haṭhayogapradīpikā,* Birch (2011), Mallinson (2011, 2014), and Singleton (2015) have revealed a more complex development.

12 The sixfold Vajra Yoga (*rdo rje'i rnal 'byor*) is also central to the earlier *Guhyasamājatantra* and involves psychophysical techniques for attaining realisation through control of vital winds (*prāṇavāyu*), elaborating on earlier Hindu–Buddhist presentations of sixfold yoga (*ṣaḍaṅgayoga*) such as found in the *Maitrāyaṇīyopaniṣad* which is ascribed to anywhere from the third century BCE to the fourth century CE. Mallinson notes, however, that certain

2. Tsa Uma: The Axis of Awareness

As explicated in the "Stainless Light" commentary, the methods of the *Kālacakratantra* focus on concentrating vital breath (*prāṇavāyu*) in the body's central channel (*madhyanāḍī*, Tib. *rtsa dbu ma*) and cultivating seminal essence (*bindu*, Tib. *thig le*)[13] to engender the blissful adamantine body of a Buddha within an immanent metaphysical anatomy. The practice of *Kālacakra* was purportedly disseminated at the Buddhist university of Nalanda by the Kashmiri pandit and *mahāsiddha* Nāropadā (1016–1100)[14] but, in keeping with its stated purpose of

---

features of the *Maitrāyaṇīyopaniṣad* – the *suṣumnā* in particular – do not appear in any other yogic text until the seventh century CE (Mallinson 2014: 174). The *Maitrāyaṇīyopaniṣad* in all likelihood predates Patañjali's enumeration of an eight-limbed yoga (*aṣṭāṅgayoga*) in the fourth century CE and outlines a path for achieving union with *paramātman*, or "absolute being" through expansion of the breath (*prāṇāyāma*), sense withdrawal (*pratyāhāra*), contemplation (*dhyāna*), focused attention (*dhāraṇā*), concentrated inquiry (*tarka*), and unitary meditative absorption (*samādhi*). In the *Kālacakratantra*, the six stages of this "completion phase" (*saṃpannakrama*, Tib. *rdzogs rim*) consist sequentially of *pratyāhāra, dhyāna, prāṇāyāma, dhāraṇā, anusmṛti*, and *samādhi*. In the *Kālacakra* system, the "yoga of sensory withdrawal (*pratyāhara*, Tib. *so sor sdud pa*)" is practised in total darkness until the development of non-conceptualised visionary signs; the "yoga of contemplation (*dhyāna*, Tib. *bsam gtan*)" concentrates on these "empty forms" (*stong gzugs*) stilling the flow of somatic energies through the body's lateral channels; the "yoga of breath expansion (*prāṇāyāma*, Tib. *srog rtsol*)" uses vigorous methods for drawing vital energy into the body's central channel and energetic centers (*cakra*); the "yoga of focused attention (*dhāraṇā*, Tib. *'dzin pa*)" merges the previously cultivated perceptual forms with vital energies to generate indestructible seminal essences (*bindu*, Tib. *thig le*) within the *cakra*-s; the "yoga of recollection (*anusmṛti*, Tib. *rjes dran*)", during which the body's subtle essences are fused with the seminal spheres within the central channel, gives rise to four successive states of meditative bliss; while the "yoga of unitary absorption (*samādhi*, Tib. *ting nge 'dzin*)" is based upon coalescence with the supreme immutable bliss represented by the enlightened form of Kālacakra in sexual union. The "yoga of fierce heat (*caṇḍālī*, Tib. *gtum mo*)" on which the later Six Yogas of Nāropa are based reputedly forms a core component of the fifth of the six yogas in the *Kālacakra* system while, in contemporary practice, the physical movements of *'khrul 'khor* are emphasised during the initial *pratyāhāra* stage. For more detail on the sixfold yoga within *Kālacakra* see Kilty 2004.

13 *Bindu* (Tib. *thig le*) has multiple meanings depending on context. Within tantric practice it customarily refers to the energetic potency of male semen or related hormonal secretions. As the interface between consciousness and matter within the physical body, *thig le* can also be usefully compared with neuropeptides, the amino acid based molecules including endorphins that are distributed throughout the body and associated with subjective states of well-being. Candice Pert (1999) notes that information-bearing neuropeptides are concentrated on lateral sides of the spinal cord paralleling the energetic currents of the *iḍā* and *piṅgala* (Tib. *kyang ma* and *ro ma*). She also suggests that, as the physiological correlate of emotion, "peptide substrate [in the body] may provide the scientific rationale for the powerful healing effects of consciously controlled breathing patterns" (Pert 1999: 187).

14 *Bindu* (Tib. *thig le*) has multiple meanings depending on context. Within tantric practice it customarily refers to the energetic potency of male semen or related hormonal secretions. As the interface between consciousness and matter within the physical body, *thig le* may con-

being a means to enlightenment while engaged with worldly life, the *Kālacakratantra* developed a wide following outside of monastic circles and continues to this day to be transmitted among both ordained and lay practitioners.

The Kashmiri pandit Somanātha brought the *Kālacakra* teachings from India to Tibet in 1064 where they influenced the development of Buddhist practice as well as Tibet's emergent medical tradition.[15] According to lineage holder Nyida Chenagtsang, Yuthok Yönten Gönpo (gyu thog yon tan mgon po) (1126–1202) drew on the *Kālacakra*'s exposition of the subtle body and tantric physiology in his revision of the "Four Medical Tantras" (*rGyud bzhi*) and condensed its accounts of psychophysical yogas in the "Turquoise Heart Essence" (*gYu thog snying thig*),[16] his spiritual guide for Buddhist medical practitioners. Butön Rinchen Drup (bu ston rin chen grub) (1290–1364), abbot of Shalu Monastery in central Tibet, further systematised physical exercises described in the *Kālacakratantra* into practices with both therapeutic and yogic applications, including "wind meditation" (*rlung gom*) and techniques of "swift walking" (*rkang mgyogs*) that purportedly allowed adepts to cover vast distances on foot by modulating the effects of gravity.[17]

---

ceivably be related to neuropeptides, amino acid based molecules, including endorphins, associated with somatic states of well-being. Neuroscientist Candace Pert notes that information-bearing neuropeptides are concentrated on the lateral sides of the spinal cord paralleling the energetic currents of the *iḍā* and *piṅgala* (Tib. *kyang ma* and *ro ma*), and, while unproven, suggests that "peptide substrate may provide the scientific rationale for the powerful healing effects of consciously controlled breathing patterns" (Pert 1999: 187).

15 Personal communication Nyida Chenagtsang, September 2014.

16 See Chenagtsang 2013 and p. 348ff.

17 The "body exercises" called Lujong (*lus sbyong*) and "vital point exercises" called Nejong (*gnas sbyong*) that were transmitted by Butön Rinchen Drup reputedly derive from the *Kālacakratantra* and were classified as "outer" exercises to be used both by Buddhist practitioners and physicians for maintaining personal health (personal communication Nyida Chenagtsang, September 2014). Nejong, as transmitted today by Nyida Chenagtsang, consists of twenty-four sequential exercises each of which is performed with a held "vase" breath (*bum pa can*, Skt. *kumbhaka*) with the intent of balancing the body's internal energies, unblocking obstructions in the channels (*rtsa*, Skt. *nāḍī*), and pacifying diseases of mind and body (personal communication Nyida Chenagtsang, London, September 2014). Tibetan physicians prescribe specific exercises from the series to their patients in modified forms that omit the held "vase breath". Nejong is also undertaken as a preliminary practice to more demanding Trulkhor (*'khrul 'khor*) exercises that concentrate the flow of psychophysical energy within the body's central channel and lead to vibrant, coalescent states of consciousness and claimed paranormal abilities (*siddhi*). Popular accounts of "trance walkers" were reported by Lama Anagarika Govinda in *The Way of the White Clouds*, by Alexandra David-Néel in *Mystics and Magicians in Tibet*, as well as by Heinrich Harrer, the author of *Seven Years in Tibet*, in his personal diaries. The practice was reputedly maintained at Samding and Shalu Monasteries in Tibet until the depredations of Chinese occupation in 1959. Based on controlling the body's internal energy flows through specialised breathing techniques (*rlung gom*) and yogic locks (*gag*, Skt. *bandha*), "swift walking" was described by Alexandra David-Néel as follows: "The man did not run. He seemed to lift himself from the ground, proceeding by leaps. It looked as

The most direct source of Indian Haṭha Yoga practice in Vajrayāna Buddhism is a corpus of eleventh to twelfth century texts entitled *Amṛtasiddhi,* or "Perfection of the Elixir of Immortality" (Tib. *bDud rtsi grub pa*). Despite the *Amṛtasiddhi*'s explicitly Śaiva orientation, it was disseminated in Tibet from the twelfth until at least the sixteenth century[18] and was incorporated into the Tibetan canon in 1322 by the celebrated scholar Butön Rinchen Drup (bu ston rin chen grub).[19] The *Amṛtasiddhi* expounds a system of internal yoga focused on uniting the solar "female" energy (*rajas*) in the pelvic cavity with the lunar *bindu,* or seminal "ambrosia" (*amṛta*), in the cranium towards the attainment of a divinised human condition.[20] The Haṭha Yoga techniques of "great seal" (*mahāmudrā*), "great lock" (*mahābandha*), and "great piercing" (*mahāvedha*) are described for the first time in the *Amṛtasiddhi* for sequentially opening the body's inner energy channels (*nāḍī*), reversing the natural downward flow of vital energy and severing the three knots (*granthi-s*) along the body's medial axis (*madhyamā*).[21] In consequence,

> the life force flows to all places [and] mind, luminescent by nature, is instantly adorned [with the qualities] of fruition ... Such a yogin is made of everything, composed of all elements, always dwelling in omniscience ... Delighted, he liberates the world.[22]

The *Amṛtasiddhi* makes no mention of either *cakra*-s or *kuṇḍalinī,* but is clearly based on principles of tantric yoga whereby elements of a subtle anatomy are controlled through physical, pneumatic, and mental discipline leading to a divinised psychophysiological state. At the heart of this process are techniques for causing the body's vital essences to infuse its axial core (*madhyamā, suṣumnā,* Tib. *rtsa dbu ma*) and thereby induce an irrevocable self-transcending shift in awareness.[23] In its perceived transformation and optimisation of physical,

---

if he had been endowed with the elasticity of a ball and rebounded each time his feet touched the ground." See David-Néel 1937: 186.

18 Schaeffer 2002: 520.

19 Schaeffer 2002: 518.

20 Mallinson 2012: 332.

21 Ibid.

22 For a detailed introduction to the *Amṛtasiddhi* corpus and the source of this quotation, see Schaeffer 2002. For an account of the Haṭha Yoga techniques central to the *Amṛtasiddhi* see Mallinson 2012: 332. In the *Amṛtasiddhi,* the practitioner imaginatively transforms into the Hindu deity Śiva who is often presented within Vajrayāna as having been converted into a Buddha by the bodhisattva Vajrapāṇi. Within the Trika Śaivism of Kashmir, Śiva is synonymous with "pure consciousness" and non-dual awareness.

23 The body's central channel is invoked as the unconditioned self-transcendent core of human embodiment in both Hindu and Buddhist tantra. Within non-dual traditions of Śaivism, it is referred to as the "channel of consciousness" (*cittanāḍī*) and is likened to "a line without thickness", symbolizing both infinity and non-duality. Independent of its psychophysical effects, drawing vital "winds" and "essences" into the body's central channel metaphorically describes a process of psychosomatic integration in which *nāḍī* can be speculatively under-

emotional, and mental processes, the *Amṛtasiddhi* embodies the tantric ideal of *jīvanmukti* (*srog thar*), or "living liberation",[24] that lies at the heart of the Vajrayāna Buddhist understanding of yoga, a word translated into the Tibetan language as Neljor (*rnal 'byor*), or "union with the natural [unaltering] state".

3. Trulkhor: Yoga of Breath and Movement

The *Amṛtasiddhi*, or "Perfection of the Elixir of Immortality", makes the first known reference to the well-known Haṭha Yoga practices of *mahāmudrā*, *mahābandha*, and *mahāvedha*.[25] In his autobiography, the Tibetan Shangpa Kagyu master Nyenton Chökyi Sherap (gnyan ston chos kyi shes rab) (1175–1255) elaborates on these foundational yogic exercises from the *Amṛtasiddhi* after reputedly learning them from a teacher from western India who in turn attributed them to a master named Eṇadeva.[26] Described as a "Miraculous Wheel of (Yogic Movements for Realizing) Deathlessness" (*'chi med kyi 'khrul 'khor*), the physical practices of the *Amṛtasiddhi* were further codified by Nyenton Chökyi Sherap's successor, Sangye Tönpa Tsondrü Senge (sangs rgyas ston pa brtson 'grus seng ge) (1213–1285), and were subsequently transmitted within Tibet's Shangpa Kagyu suborder.[27]

Transformative exercises for amplifying innate somatic processes and expanding vitality and awareness within the body's medial core (*suṣumnā*, Tib. *rtsa dbu ma*) are referred to in Tibetan as Tsalung Trulkhor (*rtsa rlung 'khrul 'khor*), literally "miraculous wheel of channels and winds", with the Tibetan root word

---

stood as heuristic structure, *prāṇa* as primordial motility, and *bindu* as innate somatic creativity. The process culminates in a unitary awareness in which subconscious somatic intelligence aligns with conscious experience.

24 The ideal of *jīvanmukti* is referred to in a twelfth-century *Amṛtasiddhi* text compiled by Avadhūtacandra. See Schaeffer 2002: 521 for further explication of this concept. As Schaeffer further points out, Avadhūtacandra's edition of the *Amṛtasiddhi* promotes an ideal of unrestricted access markedly distinct from earlier and later tantric lineages based on secrecy and exclusivity. A similarly open ethos at the origins of Haṭha Yoga can be discerned in another early Haṭha Yoga work, the thirteenth-century *Dattātreyayogaśāstra*, which advocates its practices irrespective of ethnicity or caste. For more extensive commentary on the *Dattātreyayogaśāstra* and *Amṛtasiddhi* in the context of the historical roots of Haṭha Yoga, see Mallinson forthc. Other examples in early Vajrayāna of yogic exercises being presented openly as preliminaries to meditation include Drakpa Gyaltsen's (grags pa rgyal mtshan) twelfth-century "Miraculous Channel Wheel of the Thirty-Two Auspicious Actions" discussed on p. 350f. Drakpa Gyaltsen specifically indicates in his colophon that the movements remove obstacles to spiritual practice and "are suitable for beginners as well as advanced students" (Davidson 2005: 358).

25 Mallinson forthc.: 6.

26 Schaeffer 2002: 520.

27 Ibid.

'khor referring to a "wheel" (*'khor lo*) or "cyclical movement" and *'khrul* implying "miraculous", in the sense that all phenomena, from a Buddhist perspective, lack true existence while simultaneously "miraculously" appearing. As Trulkhor practice is integral to the Six Yogas of Nāropa, it is sometimes also translated as "illusory body movement", as "illusory body yoga" (*sgyu lus kyi rnal 'byor*) provides the context for all six yogas. Trulkhor's breath-synchronised movements are also commonly referred to as Yantra Yoga (*'khrul 'khor gyi rnal 'byor*), with the composite *rtsa rlung 'khrul 'khor* translating the Sanskrit *nāḍī-vāyuyantra,* or "instrument of channels and winds", and implying a transformative device or technology, in this case, for reconfiguring human experience.[28] The sixteenth-century Tibetan scholar–adept Tāranātha (1575–1634) described Trulkhor as "esoteric instructions for dissolving the energy-mind into the central channel and for releasing knots in the channels, primarily using one's own body as the method".[29] In his "Eighteen Physical Trainings" (*Lus sbyong bco brgyad pa*), Tāranātha consolidated yogic exercises attributed to the eleventh-century Kashmiri female *mahāsiddhā* Niguma that were disseminated in Tibet through the Shangpa Kagyu lineage originating with Khyungpo Naljor (khyung po rnal 'byor) (c 1050–1140).[30] A separate transmission of external yogic exercises in Tibet is said to have originated with Niguma's consort, Nāropadā who, in turn, ostensibly received them from his Bengali teacher Tilopadā (988–1069). Although earlier Anuttara Yoga (*bla na med pa'i rgyud*) traditions such as the *Hevajratantra* and the *Cakrasaṃvaratantra* describe internal yogic practices connected to *nāḍī, prāṇa,* and *bindu* (Tib. *rtsa, rlung, thig le*), accounts of associated physical exercises and yogic "seals" (*mudrā*) seem only to have appeared in later commentaries and redactions rather than in the original root texts. However, the *Hevajratantra* makes repeated reference to the importance of transformational dance for embodying the qualities of the deity and purifying a specified thirty-two subtle energy channels within the body. "The dance is per-

28 Following Lokesh Chandra, another Sanskritised rendering of Trulkhor is *vāyvadhisāra,* derived from the Sanskrit root *adhi-sṛ,* "to move, go, run, flow towards something" (personal communication Karin Preisendanz, January 2017) and attested in Wallace 1998: 69. Trulkhor is alternatively spelled *'phrul 'khor,* which can be interpreted as "magical wheel", with reference to the fact that the yogic exercises are to be undertaken while visualizing oneself in the non-ordinary form of a "hollow", i.e., insubstantial, tantric deity which, though appearing, is not held to be intrinsically real and can thus be considered as appearing "magically". For further elaboration of the etymology of *'phrul 'khor* and *'khrul 'khor* see Chaoul 2007a: 286 and Chaoul 2007b: 138.

29 Quoted in Harding 2010: 184.

30 Ibid. Harding's book includes translations of Niguma's foundational yogic exercises which are ascribed both medical and emancipatory effects.

formed assuming the postures of the divine Heruka [Hevajra], emanating them with an impassioned mind within a state of uninterrupted attention."[31]

References to external yogic exercises as supports for internal psychophysical processes can be found in works attributed to both Nāropa and Tilopa, but no firm dates can be assigned as to when these texts were actually produced. The "Oral Instruction on the Six Doctrines" (*Ṣaḍdharmopadeśa,* Tib. *Chos drug gi man ngag*) ascribed to Tilopa is non-extant in Sanskrit, but said to have been translated into Tibetan by Nāropa and his Tibetan disciple Marpa Chökyi Lodrö (mar pa chos kyi blo gros) (1012–1097). The text only became part of the Kagyu transmission from the fifteenth century onward. Similarly, "Vajra Verses of Oral Transmission" (*Karṇatantravajrapāda,* Tib. *sNyan brgyud rdo rje'i tshig rkang*), with a colophon attributing it to Nāropa, is also non-extant in Sanskrit, but widely held to have been translated into Tibetan by Marpa Chökyi Lodrö.[32] However, it only appears as a transmitted text from the time of Rechungpa (ras chung pa) (1083/1084–1161), a century later.[33] The verses make passing reference to six "root" Trulkhor with thirty-nine "branches", suggesting that, as with Tilopa's "Oral Instructions", the transmission of Trulkhor within the Kagyu lineage was not primarily based on texts, but on oral transmission and physical demonstrations to select initiates.

31 Farrow & Menon 1992: 209. The *Hevajratantra* further states that the dance movements "reveal the adamantine nature of the Buddhas, Yoginīs, and Mother Goddesses ... The protection of the assembly and oneself is by means of such song and dance" (p. 230). Further references to dance in the *Hevajratantra* include the following stanzas: "When joy arises if the yogin dances for the sake of liberation, then let him dance the vajra postures [of Hevajra] with fullest attention" (p. 64); "The yogin must always sing and dance" (p. 65). Although no firm dates can be established for when they first became part of the tradition, the ritual dance movements of Newar *caryānṛtya* associated with the *Cakrasaṃvaratantra* can also be considered a form of Trulkhor in their intended purpose of embodying the qualities of Vajrayāna deities. As Cakrasaṃvara's consort is the tantric meditational deity Vajravārāhī, several movements of *caryānṛtya* involve direct emulations of her visualised form, including the raising to one's lips of an imagined skull cup brimming with ambrosial nectar. In all forms of *caryānṛtya* consecrated dancers embody the qualities of specific Vajrayāna deities with the express intention of benefitting all living beings. A similar conception is central to the Tibetan ritual dances known as Cham (*'cham*) which, prior to the thirteenth century, were performed only within an assembly of consecrated initiates. Correlations can also be seen in the ritual dance movements of *tāṇḍava* as transmitted within Kashmiri Śaivism.

32 Kragh 2011: 135. See also dnz.tsadra.org for details concerning "Cakrasamvara's Oral Transmission of Miraculous Yogic Movements for Fierce Heat and the Path of Skillful Means" (*bDe mchog snyan brgyud kyi gtum mo dang thabs lam gyi 'khrul 'khor*) attributed to Marpa Chökyi Lodrö (mar pa chos kyi blo gros).

33 Kragh 2011: 138. See also the anonymously authored *gTum mo'i 'khrul 'khor bco brgyad pa* in the *gDams ngag rin po che'i mdzod,* Vol. 7 (*ja*), 537–541, fols. 19a4 to 21a2. New Delhi: Shechen Publications, 1999, listed at dnz.tsadra.org and connected with the oral transmission of Rechungpa (*ras chung snyan brgyud*).

The earliest datable descriptions of external yogic exercises in Tibetan Buddhism may be those of Phagmo Drupa Dorje Gyalpo (phag mo gru pa rdo rje rgyal po) (1110–1170) who compiled "The Path of Fruition's Thirty-two Auspicious Actions" (*Lam 'bras kyi 'phrin las sum bcu so gnyis*), using Sanskrit and pseudo-Sanskrit names to describe sequential movements.[34] Phagmo Drupa also wrote "The Path of Fruition's Five-Branch Yoga" (*Lam 'bras kyi yan lag lnga sbyong*), which consists of basic instructions for loosening the neck, head, hands and legs, as well as a manual entitled "Supplementary Verses on the Path of Method" (*Thabs lam tshigs bcad ma'i lhan thabs*) which describes six physical exercises[35] for removing obstacles and preparing the body for advanced internal yogas based on drawing psychosomatic "winds" into the body's central channel.

All traditions of Tsalung Trulkhor extol their remedial healing benefits while emphasizing their more profound transformative effects on the body and mind, including the reputed attainment of supranormal powers (*siddhi*).[36] Trulkhor is further distinguished from the medically-oriented exercises of Lujong (*lus sbyong*) and Nejong (*gnas sbyong*)[37] that Butön Rinchen Drup derived from the *Kālacakratantra* in its emphasis on sequentially performed movements with the breath held in a "vase" below the navel (*bum pa can,* Skt. *kumbhaka*) while visualizing oneself in the form of one or another non-material tantric deity, in accordance with the practice's line of transmission. As a method of self-consecration combining the Development Phase (*utpattikrama,* Tib. *skye rim*) and Completion Phase (*saṃpannakrama,* Tib. *rdzogs rim*) of Vajrayāna practice, Trulkhor is traditionally undertaken in strict secrecy with prescribed garments that symbolise interconnected psychophysical energies.[38] Vigorous and, at times, acrobatic movements combined with expanded breath and associated visual-

34 Wang-Toutain 2009: 29.

35 Ibid.

36 The attainment of supernal powers associated with yogic cultivation is rarely an admitted or admired goal within Vajrayāna Buddhism, although provisionally useful worldly *siddhi*-s such as clairvoyance, invisibility, and control of natural phenomena are claimed to this day to arise spontaneously as a result of dedicated practice. Vajrayāna's more transcendent goal, however, remains the *mahāsiddhi* of transforming egotism, greed, and aggression into empathic wisdom and unconditional compassion (*thugs rje chen po,* Skt. *mahākaruṇā*). Attaining this awakened disposition in the most expedient manner possible is viewed as the essential intent of Śākyamuni Buddha's Eightfold Path to Nirvāṇa. Dynamic, physically-based yogic practices thus infuse the expansive "path of method" (*thabs lam*) central to Vajrayāna Buddhism.

37 See n. 17. Trulkhor is further distinguished from Lujong in its tripartite purpose of clearing the body's subtle energy system, drawing seminal essence (*bindu,* Tib. *thig le*) into the central channel, and distributing it throughout the psychophysical organism to prepare it for internal tantric practices such as Fierce Heat (*caṇḍālī,* Tib. *gtum mo*).

38 Practitioners of Tsalung Trulkhor typically wear short pleated kilts called *ang rak,* the colors of which symbolise the elemental energies of space, air, fire, and water.

isations direct neurobiological energies into the body's central channel (*suṣumnā,* Tib. *rtsa dbu ma*), quelling obscuring mental activity and arousing the blissful "fierce heat" of Tumo (*gtum mo,* Skt. *caṇḍālī*) that facilitates yogic attainment during recurring cycles of wakefulness, sleep, sexual activity, and dream.[39]

Trulkhor practices in Tibet's indigenous pre-Buddhist tradition of Bön first appear in the Bön Mother Tantra (*Ma rgyud*) in a chapter entitled "Elemental Essences" (*Byung ba'i thig le*) that outlines five foundational exercises for balancing the body's fundamental constituents.[40] The practices of the Bön Mother Tantra are traditionally credited with a long line of oral transmission, but the fact that they only appeared in written form from the eleventh century makes it difficult to determine to what degree they evolved independently of Buddhist influence. Similarly, the "Great Perfection Oral Transmission of Zhang Zhung: Instructions on the Miraculous Wheel of Yogic Movements" (*rDzogs pa chen po zhang zhung snyan rgyud las 'khrul khor man ngag*) with its own tradition of Trulkhor practices also dates, in written form, to the late eleventh or early twelfth century,[41] thus making it difficult to assess Bön's possible influence on the development of Trulkhor within Tibetan Buddhism. An extensive commentary on the "Great Perfection Oral Transmission of Zhang Zhung" entitled "Profound Treasury of Space Revealing the Miraculous Wheel of Channels and Winds" (*Byang zab nam mkha' mdzod chen las snyan rgyud rtsa rlung 'phrul 'khor*) was written by a Bön scholar and meditation master named Shardza Tashi Gyaltsen (shar rdza bkra shis rgyal mtshan) (1859–1934). The text elucidates the role of Tsalung Trulkhor in Bön in supporting recognition of the mind's essential nature within the context of Dzogchen.

Within the Nyingma (*rNying ma*) tradition, the earliest transmission of Vajrayāna Buddhism to Tibet, the first textual evidence of Tsalung Trulkhor prac-

39 The unification of the body's energetic poles through the merging of *agni,* as "divine fire", and *soma,* as "cosmic nectar", through the medium of psychophysiological "winds" (*vāyu*) in a subjectively experienced "central channel" is arguably the common goal and praxis of yoga in both Vajrayāna Buddhism and Tantric Śaivism, an ideal prefigured in ancient Vedic fire rituals (*agnihotra*) and embodied in Vajrayāna rites that customarily begin with the ritual invocation of fire, wind, and water through the resonant seed-syllables (*bīja*) *ram yam kham.*

40 These practices are extensively explained in Wangyal 2011.

41 See Chaoul 2007b: 141 and Chaoul 2006: 29. Traditional accounts maintain that the *Zhang zhung snyan rgyud* first appeared in written form in the eighth century, but Chaoul points out that its later chapter on Trulkhor lists lineage holders who only lived in the last quarter of the eleventh century. Lopon Tenzin Namdak (slob dpon bstan 'dzin rnam dag), Bön's leading contemporary exponent, maintains that Trulkhor was taught in Bön prior to the eighth century as an oral teaching. Unlike Buddhism, Bön does not ascribe an Indic source for its Tsalung Trulkhor practices, but maintains that they originated in Tibet and were transmitted through the lineage of the *Zhang zhung snyan rgyud.* For the Bön presentation of Dzogchen, see Namdak & Reynolds 2006 and Namdak & Dixey 2002.

tices appears in the "Turquoise Heart Essence" (*gYu thog snying thig*), a "subtle pure vision" (*zab mo dag snang*) compiled by Sumtön Yeshe Zung (sum ston ye shes gzungs) beginning in 1157 based on original writings and teachings of Yuthok Yönten Gönpo (g.yu thog yon tan mgon po) (1126–1202), the Tibetan physician and yogic adept credited with the compilation of the earlier "Four Medical Tantras" (*rGyud bzhi*) which consolidate Tibetan medicine's approach to the prevention, diagnosis, and treatment of disease. The *Yuthok Nyingthik* was reputedly compiled after Yuthok's second of five trips to India where he presumably received direct instructions from Indian tantric masters. The "Turquoise Heart Essence" outlines the process of spiritual development to be undertaken by non-monastic practitioners, condensing the core elements of Vajrayāna Buddhism into forty root texts, the twentieth of which describes a sequence of eighteen Trulkhor exercises for refining the body's subtle energy channels in preparation for practices of Fierce Heat (*gtum mo*, Skt. *caṇḍālī*) and the yoga of sexual union (*sbyor ba, las kyi phyag rgya*, Skt. *karmamudrā*). As expounded in the *Yuthok Nyingthik,* the latter practices lead, in turn, to the realisation of Mahāmudrā and Dzogchen and the ultimate attainment of a dematerialised body of rainbow light (*'ja' lus*). The *Yuthok Nyingthik*'s concise treatise on Trulkhor entitled "The Root Text of the Miraculous Movements for Supreme Mastery which Clear the Darkness of Suffering" is supplemented with a longer commentary written by Nyi Da Dragpa (nyi zla grags pa), as requested by Drangsong Sönam (drang srong bsod nams), entitled "A Concise Synopsis of the Supreme Accomplishment of the Profound Path of the Miraculous Wheel of Yogic Movements that Clear the Darkness of Suffering" (*Bla sgrub sdug bsngal mun sel gyi zab lam 'khrul 'khor zhin bris*) and elucidates the therapeutic and yogic applications of the Trulkhor teachings of the "Turquoise Heart Essence".[42] The first two of the eighteen exercises are said to clear obscuring karmic imprints from the subtle anatomy of the body, while the following five assist in generating the transformative heat of Tumo. The subsequent eleven exercises directly prepare the body for the yoga of sexual union, held by non-monastic traditions within both Nyingma and Kagyu to be the most efficacious means for achieving the supreme realisation of Dzogchen or Mahāmudrā, as prefigured in early Vajrayāna works such as the *Guhyasamājatantra.*[43] The exposition of an eight-

42 See Chenagtsang 2013 and Naldjorpa 2014 for further details on the transmission and content of the "Turquoise Heart Essence".

43 In its later monastic contexts in Tibet, the tantric axiom "without Karmamudrā (i.e., the yoga of sexual union) there is no Mahāmudrā [supreme attainment]" – attributed varyingly to both Saraha and Tilopa – was interpreted symbolically and celibate monks and nuns practised instead with visualised "wisdom consorts" called *ye shes kyi phyag rgya* (Skt. *jñānamudrā*), in order to generate "four joys" (*dga 'ba bzhi*, Skt. *caturānanda*) of coalescent emptiness and bliss. The Four Joys are partly tantric reformulations of the Four Jhānas of Theravāda

een-set Trulkhor in the "Turquoise Heart Essence" is roughly contemporary with Phagmo Drupa's description of sets of six and thirty-two yogic exercises and, taken together, can provisionally be considered the earliest datable evidence of Haṭha Yoga-like practices within Tibetan Buddhism.[44]

Although Indian Yoganiruttara, or Yoginī Tantras such as the *Hevajra* and *Cakrasaṃvara* date to the eighth century or earlier, these systems only rose to prominence in Tibet during the second wave of Buddhist transmission from the late tenth century onward. As with the *Kālacakratantra* that was introduced in Tibet in 1064, the root texts of the *Hevajra* and *Cakrasaṃvara* do not describe sequenced yogic exercises, although the *Hevajratantra* does advocate transformational dance movements.[45] The *Hevajratantra* was translated from Sanskrit into Tibetan from 1041 until 1046 by Drokmi Sakya Yeshe ('brog mi shakya ye shes) (993–1072) in collaboration with the Indian master Gayādhara who is also said to have introduced the associated Lamdre (*lam 'bras*), or "Path of Fruition" cycle of teachings connected with the ninth-century *mahāsiddha* Virūpa. Although the *Hevajra* root tantra does not describe external yogic exercises, the Lamdre teachings associated with Virūpa do.[46] Phagmo Drupa Dorje Gyalpo's

Buddhism which are held to lead to a "state of perfect equanimity and awareness" (*upekkhāsatiparisuddhi*) without reliance on an actual or imagined consort.

44 This does not take into account the possible earlier dates of Bön Trulkhor. Furthermore, Robert Mayer has pointed out (personal communication, November 2014) that no mention can be found of Tsalung Trulkhor practices in the Nyingma and proto-Nyingma texts from the Dunhuang caves that were sealed in the early eleventh century. He notes that the only complete tantric scriptural texts to survive at Dunhuang are the *Thabs kyi zhags pa padma 'phreng* ("The Noble Lotus Garland of Methods") and the *Guhyasamājatantra* and that only passing reference is made to other important Nyingma Tantras such as the "Secret Nucleus" (*Guhyagarbhatantra*, Tib. *gSang ba snying po*) and the Śaivite derived eighth- to ninth-century "Supreme Blissful Union with All Buddhas through the Net of the Sky Dancers" (*Sarvabuddhasamāyogaḍākinījālasaṃvara*, Tib. *dPal sangs rgyas thams cad dang mnyam par sbyor ba mkha' 'gro ma sgyu ma bde ba'i mchog*). Sexual union practices are described in these pre-eleventh century works, but not in the context of *nāḍī*, *prāṇa* and *bindu* (Tib. *rtsa, rlung, thig le*) or Tsalung Trulkhor. See Mayer & Cantwell 2012: 84ff.

45 See n. 31 above.

46 See Wang-Toutain 2009: 28. There is no mention of Trulkhor practice in the *Hevajra* root tantra, only a name list of thirty-two energy channels (*nāḍī*) (see Farrow & Menon 1992: 13). The occurrence of Trulkhor within the Hevajra Lamdre (*lam 'bras*) thus seems to be a later development, either attributable to Virūpa, as Sakya tradition maintains, or possibly influenced by the propagation of the *Kālacakratantra* during roughly the same time period. However, the Lamdre cycle was introduced in Tibet twenty-three years before Somanātha brought the *Kālacakra* teachings in 1064, thus making Lamdre one of the most fertile areas for further research in regard to the development of physical yoga within Vajrayāna and Tibet. For further information on the cycles of Trulkhor within Lamdre, see the *lam 'bras slob bshad* collection edited by Jamyang Loter Wangpo ('jam dbyangs blo gter dbang po) (1847 – c 1914) and listed in the *Lam 'bras* catalogue of Lama Choedak Yuthok (available at http://www.sacred-texts.com/bud/tib/sakya-la.htm). The Trulkhor texts associated with Lamdre are also catalogued at the Tibetan Buddhist Resource Center (TBRC) as item W23649, Vol. 20, pp. 205–

early works on Lamdre Trulkhor were elaborated later on in the twelfth century by Drakpa Gyaltsen (grags pa rgyal mtshan) (1147–1216) as the "Miraculous Channel Wheel of Thirty-two Auspicious Actions" (*'Phrin las sum cu rtsa gnyis kyi 'khrul 'khor*), and he included them in his extensive "Yellow Book" (*Pod ser*) as the last of four texts for removing obstacles (*gegs sel*) on the Path of Fruition.[47] Drakpa Gyaltsen described the medical benefits of the various exercises as well as their supporting function within the Completion Phase (*saṃpannakrama,* Tib. *rdzogs rim*) of the *Hevajratanta* and the *Cakrasaṃvaratantra.*[48] Like Phagmo Drupa before him, he assigned Sanskrit-derived names to the various yogic movements[49] (see, e. g., Figure 1) and emphasised their importance in cultivating the yogic power of Fierce Heat (*gtum mo*) and other Completion Phase practices. He also advocated practising the set of thirty-two exercises once in a forward direction, once in reverse, and once in random order to make a prescribed set of ninety-six movements.[50] As Drakpa Gyaltsen assures his audience at the end of his "Yellow Book": "If one trains oneself [in the yogic exercises] as much as one can, one will achieve Buddhahood."[51]

Phagmo Drupa's initial elaboration of yogic exercises also influenced Tsongkhapa Lobzang Drakpa (tsong kha pa blo bzang grags pa) (1357–1419), the founding figure of the reformed Gelug order of Tibetan Buddhism. In his "Book of Three Certainties: A Treatise on the Phases of Training by Means of the Profound Path of Nāropa's Six Yogas" (*Zab lam nāro'i chos drug gi sgo nas 'khrid pa'i rim pa yid chos gsum ldan*) and in "A Brief Treatise for Practicing the Phases of Meditation in Nāropa's Six Yogas, Compiled from the Teachings of Jey Rinpoche by Sem Chenpo Kunzangpa" (*Nā ro'i chos drug gi dmigs rim lag tu len tshul bsdus pa rje'i gsungs bzhin sems dpa' chen po kun bzang pas bkod pa*) Tsongkhapa

267. The text, in English translation, is given as "The Profound Phases of the Path of Enlightenment of Veins, Channels, Yantra and Blazing and Blissful Heat of Caṇḍālī Yoga" (*rTsa rlung 'khrul 'khor zab lam byang chub sgrub pa'i rim pa bklags chog ma dang gtum mo'i bde drod rab 'bar ma gnyis*).

47 See Stearns 2001: 26–34. The sequence of thirty-two Trulkhor exercises in Lamdre is significant in its reference to the thirty-two subtle energy pathways listed in the Hevajra roottantra as well as to the thirty-two *nāḍī* that reputedly radiate from the eight petals of the heart *cakra.*

48 Wang-Toutain 2009: 29. The Tibetan title of Drakpa Gyaltsen's work is given as *Kyai rdo rje'i rnal 'byor las rtsa rlung.*

49 See Stearns 2001: 31 and Wang-Toutain 2009: 29. The names of Drakpa Gyaltsen's Trulkhor movements use, at times, semi-corrupted Sanskrit words to refer to animals such as lion (rendered as *singala* instead of *siṃha*), goose (*haṃsa*), peacock (*mayūra*), and tortoise (*kūrma*), but also to auspicious objects such as *vajra*-s, wheels, and immortality vases (*kumbha*), as well as to *mahāsiddha*-s such as Jālandhara and Caurāṅgī, who were also prominent Nāth adepts (Wang-Toutain 2009: 33).

50 Wang-Toutain 2009: 32.

51 Quoted ibid. Drakpa Gyaltsen further claims that practising the thirty-two exercises will result in acquiring the thirty-two major body characteristics (*lakṣaṇa*) of a Buddha (p. 46).

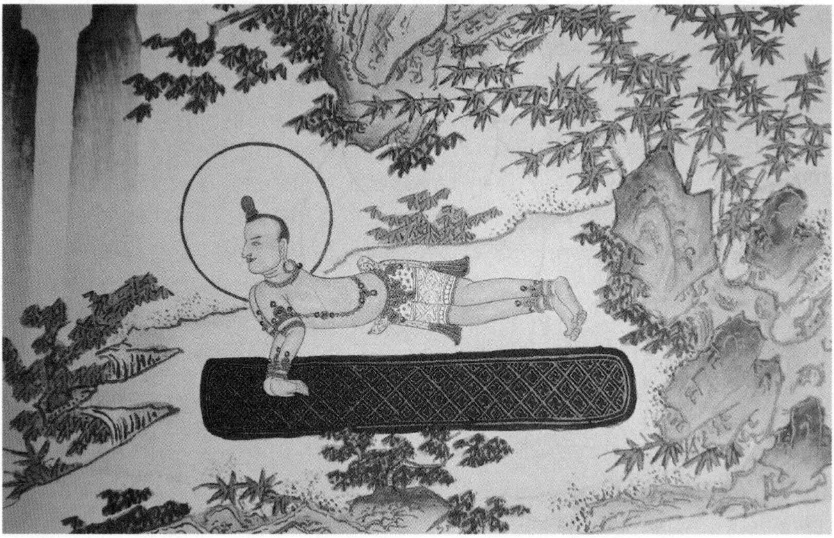

Figure 1: The Position of the Peacock described by Drakpa Gyaltsen as presented in a Qing Dynasty manuscript.

describes in detail six preliminary physical exercises based on Phagmo Drupa's twelfth-century accounts.[52] Jey Sherab Gyatso (rje shes rab rgya mtsho) (1803–1875), in his commentary to the "Book of Three Certainties", remarks that even though there are an impressive variety of exercises, "there seems to be no great advantage in doing more than the six recommended by Phagmo Drupa [as taught by Tsongkhapa] for accomplishing the inner heat [*gtum mo*] yogas."[53] Further indicating Phagmo Drupa's enduring influence, Muchen Konchok Gyaltsen (mus chen dkon mchog rgyal mtshan) (1388–1471) included a chapter entitled

52 See Mullin 1997: 58–60 and 107–109. As is customary with Trulkhor, each movement is performed while visualizing oneself as a luminously transparent tantric deity. The first exercise, "filling the body like a vase", consists of expanding the breath in the lower abdomen with a held "vase" breath. The second exercise, "circling like a wheel", involves churning the solar plexus while the third exercise, "hooking like a hook", involves stretching the arms and snapping the elbows against the rib cage to drive the lateral "winds" into the central channel. The fourth exercise, "the *mudrā* of *vajra* binding", draws vital energy down through the crown of the head while the fifth, "heaving like a dog", involves kneeling on the ground with the hands extended in front and the spine horizontal and forcibly expelling the air from the lungs. In the final exercise, the practitioner shakes the head and body, flexes the joints, pulls on the fingers to release stagnant "winds", and rubs the hands together. Textual analysis suggests that these six "proto-*yantra*-s" were a later addition to the Six Yogas of Nāropa practice and not originally taught by Tilopa, Nāropa, or even Marpa, but this does not take into account the possibility of a well-developed oral tradition outside of written texts.

53 Quoted in Mullin 1997: 58. Jey Sherab Gyatso further notes that "when stability in these practices is achieved, one will experience a sense of subtle joy that pervades the body" (p. 59).

"Thirty-two Auspicious Yogic Movements" (*rNal 'byor gyi phrin las sum cu rtsa gnyis*) in his "Little Red Volume" (*Pu sti dmar chung*), based on a prior book of oral instructions (*zhal shes*) by Lama Dampa Sönam Gyaltsen Pelsangpo (bla ma dam pa bsod nams rgyal mtshan) (1312–1375) which is almost identical to Phagmo Drupa's "The Path of Fruition's Thirty-Two Auspicious Actions" (*Lam 'bras kyi 'phrin las sum bcu so gnyis*).[54]

Over subsequent centuries Tsalung Trulkhor continued to evolve within all schools of Tibetan Buddhism, as well as within Bön. Its most celebrated exemplar, however, remains the mountain-dwelling yogi poet Jetsun Milarepa (rje btsun mi la ras pa) (1052 – c 1135) who reputedly reached enlightenment through his committed practice of Fierce Heat (*gtum mo,* Skt. *caṇḍālī*) in conjunction with Trulkhor exercises to keep his energy channels open and supple.[55] Although not named as such, the physiological "seals" and associated breathing methods used in the cultivation of Fierce Heat are an elaborated practice of the Haṭha Yoga method of *mahābandha* in which the *mūladharabandha,* or "root lock" at the perineal floor, and *uḍḍiyānabandha* in the abdominal cavity move the "illuminating fire" upward through the body's axial channel while the application of *jālandharabandha* at the throat facilitates the downward flow of "nectar" from the cranium.[56] Fierce Heat in turn, is the foundation of six psychophysical yogas (*rnal 'byor drug*) undertaken during recurring phases of waking, sleeping, dreaming, and sexual activity as well as in preparation for death.[57] These "Six

54 See Wang-Toutain 2009: 29.

55 Although there is no direct evidence of the specific yogic exercises that Milarepa practised in conjunction with his practice of Fierce Heat, the Kagyu tradition, or "orally transmitted lineage", for which he was the seminal figure, continues to transmit a set of six exercises to release blockages in the *nāḍī*-s and improve the flow of *prāṇa* during the practice of Tumo (*gtum mo*). These yogic exercises are also practised in support of the subsequent Six Doctrines of Nāropa (*nā ro'i chos drug*) in order to prevent obstructions in the channels during yogas of sexual union and more subtle practices undertaken during states of dreaming, sleeping, and dying.

56 As noted by Wang-Toutain (2009: 35), Drakpa Gyaltsen refers to *bandha*-s and *mudrā*-s in the context of his twelfth-century "Thirty-two Actions of the Miraculous Wheel of Channels" (*'Phrin las sum bcu rtsa gnyis 'khrul 'khor*).

57 Distinct from the roughly contemporary Sixfold Vajra Yoga of the *Kālacakratantra* and analogous systems within *Hevajra* Lamdre, the Six Doctrines of Nāropa (*nā ro'i chos drug*) originate with the Bengali *mahāsiddha* Tilopadā (988–1069) and distill the core Completion phase (*saṃpannakrama,* Tib. *rdzogs rim*) practices of India's principal Buddhist Tantras into an algorithm for awakening dormant capacities of mind and body and cultivating lucid awareness within normally autonomic states of consciousness. Tilopa's original introductory text on these six interconnected practices refers to them as six *dharma*-s (*ṣaḍdharmopadeśa,* Tib. *chos drug gi man ngag*), but they are commonly referred to as a system of "yoga" (*rnal 'byor*) for unifying consciousness with the total expanse of reality (*dharmadhātu,* Tib. *chos kyi dbyings*) during states of waking, dreaming, sleeping, sexual union, and death. Tilopa presents the Six Yogas as the pith essence of the most prominent Buddhist Tantras, leading to an expanded experience of reality culminating in the liberating realisation of *mahāmudrā,*

Yogas of Nāropa" (*nā ro'i chos drug*) subsequently became the basis of Tibet's Kagyu (*bKa' brgyud*), or "orally transmitted lineage".[58] Trulkhor practice within the Kagyu school subsequently diversified from the sets of six and thirty-two yogic exercises advocated by Phagmo Drupa to over one hundred and eight within the Drigung Kagyu (*'bri gung bka' brgyud*) suborder.[59] These longer and

---

interpreted to derive etymologically from *rā*, "to bestow", and *mud*, meaning "bliss". Although variant presentations exist, the series commonly begins with Illusory Body Yoga (*sgyu lus*, Skt. *māyākāya*) through which the practitioner recognises his/her body and mind as transmutable constructions of consciousness. Tilopa describes this yoga as deriving from the *Guhyasamājatantra*. The second yoga, the Yoga of Fierce Heat (*gtum mo*, Skt. *caṇḍālī*), on which all of the subsequent yogas are based, correlates with Śaivite practices for arousing the primordial energy of *kuṇḍalinī* and first appears, in Buddhist tradition, in the *Hevajra* and *Cakrasaṃvaratantra*-s. The auxiliary Yoga of Sexual Union (*las kyi phyag rgya*, Skt. *karmamudrā*) in which the practitioner engages sexually with a partner, either real or visualised, is said to derive from the *Guhyasamājatantra* while the subsequent Yoga of Radiant Light (*'od gsal*, Skt. *prabhāsvara*) is based on a synthesis of the *Guhyasamāja*- and *Cakrasaṃvaratantra*-s. The Yoga of Conscious Dreaming (*rmi lam*, Skt. *svapnadarśana*) was further said by Tilopa to derive from the *Mahāmāyātantra* while the Yoga of Liminality (*bar do*, Skt. *antarābhava*) that prepares the practitioner for a posited postmortem experience develops out of the *Guhyasamājatantra*. The Yoga of Transference (*'pho ba*, Skt. *saṃkrānti*), in which consciousness is projected beyond the *bar do* at the time of death into one or another Buddhafield, is said to originate both from the *Guhyasamājatantra* as well as from the *Catuṣpīṭhatantra*. A similar, but more condensed exposition of the Six Yogas attributed to Nāropa's consort is entitled "The Six Yogas of Niguma" (*Ni gu chos drug*) and, after its transmission to the Indian yogini Sukhasiddhi and her Tibetan disciple Khyungpo Naljor (khyung po rnal 'byor) became the basis of the Shangpa Kagyu (*shangs pa bka' brgyud*) school of Tibetan Buddhism. Within the Nyingma tradition, the Six Yogas are referred to as the "Six Yogas of the Completion Phase" (*rdzogs rim chos drug*) and are considered as revealed teachings of Padmasambhava. These and other versions of the Six Yoga doctrine, such as those found in the *Kālacakra* and *Yuthok Nyingthik*, customarily begin with cycles of physical exercises for amplifying and directing the flow of subtle energy into the body's central channel to enhance the practice of more internal yogic techniques.

58 The Shangpa Kagyu lineage originating with Khyungpo Naljor is based on an analogous system of Six Yogas associated with Nāropa's consort Niguma. The Six Yoga doctrine was also transmitted separately by Marpa Chökyi Lodrö in a condensed form known as "mixing and transference" (*'se 'pho*) in connection with the *Hevajratantra*. Marpa transmitted these practices to Ngok Chokdor and they subsequently became known as the Ngok Transmission, or *Mar rngog bka' brgyud*. According to Marpa scholar Cécile Ducher the *'se 'pho* texts make no specific mention of Trulkhor although several other texts in Marpa's collected works (*gsung 'bum*) do; see Ducher 2014. As Jamgön Kongtrul Lodrö Tayé ('jam mgon kong sprul blo gros mtha' yas) (1813–1899) points out, the "mixing and transference" instructions are based on a core verse attributed to Nāropa: "Mixing refers to awakening through meditation and transference to awakening without meditation." Kongtrul further explicates that inner heat and illusory body practices are used for awakening through meditation while transference of consciousness beyond the body (*'pho ba*) and sexual union with a consort (*las kyi phyag rgya*, Skt. *karmamudrā*) are used for awakening without meditation. See Harding 2007: 150.

59 Trulkhor practice in Drigung Kagyu is based primarily on "Cakrasaṃvara's Oral Transmission of the Miraculous Wheel of Channels and Winds" (*bDe mchog snyan rgyud kyi rtsa*

more complex systems were also periodically simplified, emphasizing five core movements combined with "vase" breaths (*kumbhaka*, Tib. *bum pa chen*), visualisation, and internal neuro-muscular "seals" (*mudrā*-s, Tib. *gag*) for harmonizing the body's five elemental winds (*rtsa ba rlung lnga*).[60]

4. Nyingthik: Heart Essence of Tibetan Yoga

Tsalung Trulkhor and versions of the six associated yogas (*sbyor drug*) developed within all schools of Tibetan Buddhism as advanced Completion Phase (*rdzogs rim*, Skt. *saṃpannakrama*) practices in monastic settings as well as among non-celibate male and female yogins (*sngags pa*). Within Tibet's Nyingma order, Tsalung Trulkhor and the "Six Yogas of the Completion Phase" (*rdzogs rim chos drug*) closely paralleled analogous practices in the Tantras and commentaries of the "new" (*gsar ma*) translation schools, but were expediently presented as revealed "treasure texts" (*gter ma*) attributed to Nyingma's iconic eighth-century patron saint Padmasambhava. The imaginal anatomy of winds and channels and the practices based on them were presented differently, however, in light of the Nyingma school's emphasis on the Dzogchen, or Atiyoga view of "self-liberation" (*rang grol*) which is held to supersede all effort-based Development and Completion Phase approaches. In Nyingma's division of the highest Vajrayāna teachings into Mahāyoga (*rnal 'byor chen po*), Anuyoga (*rjes su rnal 'byor*), and Atiyoga (*shin tu rnal 'byor*), practices connected with the psychophysical channels, winds, and vital essences (*rtsa, rlung, thig le*, Skt. *nāḍī, vāyu, bindu*) are

---

rlung 'khrul 'khor) and texts such as "The All-Illuminating Mirror: Oral Instructions on the Miraculous Wheel of Yogic Movements for Training the Body to Progress in the Practice of Fierce Heat from among the Six Yogas of Nāropa" (*Nā ro'i chos drug las gtum mo'i bogs 'don lus sbyong 'phrul 'khor gyi zhal khrid kun gsal me long*) (oral communication, Choeze Rinpoche, Lhasa, July 2010). Drigung Kagyu also includes a cycle of thirty-seven Trulkhor revealed by the Second Karmapa, Karma Pakshi (1204/1206–1283) (*karma pakshi'i so bdun*) (oral communication, Ani Rigsang, Terdrom, Tibet, August 2014). The Drigung Kagyu order was founded by Jikten Gonpo Rinchen Pel ('jig rten mgon po rin chen dpal) (1143–1217), Phagmo Drupa's principal disciple.

60 Oral communication, Tshewang Sitar Rinpoche, Bumthang, Bhutan, May 2013. Each of the body's five elemental winds (*rtsa ba rlung lnga*) supports a specific function. The "life-supporting wind" (*srog 'dzin rlung*) located in the brain regulates swallowing, inhalation, and mental attention. The "upward-moving wind" (*gyen rgyu rlung*) in the chest and thorax regulates somatic energy, speech, memory, and related functions. The "all-pervading wind" (*khyab byed rlung*) in the heart controls all motor activities of the body. The "fire-accompanying wind" (*me mnyam gnas rlung*) in the stomach and abdomen area regulates digestion and metabolism. The "downward-clearing wind" (*thur sel rlung*) located in the rectum, bowels, and perineal region regulates excretion, urine, semen, menstrual blood, and uterine contractions during labour. For further elaboration of the Five Winds, see also Wangyal 2002: 76–110.

categorised as Anuyoga, "subsequent yoga". When such techniques are used in support of the direct realisation of one's intrinsically awakened Buddha nature, the conjoined approach is often referred to with the Sanskrit-derived term "Ati Anu" (*shin tu rjes su*), or "supreme subsequent", representing a synthesis of Atiyoga and Anuyoga methods.[61]

Although no descriptions of Trulkhor can be found in original texts associated with Tibet's oldest Vajrayāna lineage, early Nyingma masters such as Rongzom Chökyi Zangpo (*rong zom chos kyi bzang po*) (1012–1088) and Nyang Ral Nyima Özer (nyang ral nyi ma 'od zer) (1124–1192) were closely associated with early "New School" proponents such as Smṛtijñānakīrti and Padampa Sangye (pha dam pa sangs rgyas) and are likely to have received transmissions from them of Tsalung Trulkhor, thus gradually introducing practices of breath and movement into the Nyingma corpus. This new material was introduced into the Nyingma tradition through the expedient means of revealed "treasure texts" (*gter ma*), "mind treasures" (*dgongs gter*), and "pure visions" (*dag snang*) that allowed Trulkhor to be recontextualised within Dzogchen's view of self-existing enlightenment. However, none of the earliest Nyingma treasure texts such as the Seventeen Dzogchen Tantras (*rDzogs chen rgyud bcu bdun*) revealed by Neten

61 Personal communication, Chatral Sangye Dorje, Yolmo, Nepal, August 1987. Vajrayāna Buddhist practice customarily consists of a Development Phase (*bskyed rim*) based on mantra recitation and visualisation followed by a Completion Phase (*rdzogs rim*) focused on the body's metaphysical anatomy of channels, winds, and essences. Dzogchen differs in its approach by "taking the goal as the path" and fusing Development and Completion Phase practices into unitary awareness (*rig pa*) of their ultimate inseparability. Dzogchen practices thus work directly with physiology and optical phenomena to reveal reality as an unfolding heuristic and creative process. Dzogchen is presented in Tibet's Nyingma school as the culmination of nine successive vehicles for transcending afflictive fluctuations of consciousness and uniting with all-encompassing awareness. The first two vehicles refer to the Hīnayāna stages of Śrāvakayāna and Pratyekabuddhayāna that lead to the solitary realisation of the *arhat,* as promoted within Theravāda Buddhism. The third vehicle, the *Bodhisattvayāna,* introduces the Mahāyāna, or greater vehicle, and cultivates enlightenment not just for oneself, but for all beings. The fourth, fifth, and sixth vehicles are the so-called Outer Tantras of Kriyātantra, Caryātantra, and Yogatantra, all of which are part of Vajrayāna, the third turning of the wheel of doctrine, but remain dualistic in their orientation. The three Inner Tantras (*nang rgyud sde gsum*) were transmitted to those deemed of higher capacity and consist of Mahāyoga (*rnal 'byor chen po*), which emphasises the Development Phase (*bskyed rim*) of imaginal perception, Anuyoga (*rjes su rnal 'byor*) which cultivates co-emergent bliss and emptiness through Completion Phase (*rdzogs rim*) practices based on a meta-anatomy of channels, winds and essences, and Atiyoga (*shin tu rnal 'byor*), the resultant non-dual dimension of Dzogchen with its liberating view of primordial, self-existing perfection. The three Inner Tantras of the Nyingma further correlate with the Unsurpassed Yogatantras (Anuttarayogatantra) of the Kagyu, Sakya, and Geluk lineages, all of which culminate in the non-dual (*advaita*) view of reality as expressed in Essence Mahāmudra (*ngo bo'i phyag rgya chen po*) which is often presented as being identical to Dzogchen in terms of view, but differing in its method.

Dangma Lhungyal (gnas brtan ldang ma lhun rgyal) in the eleventh century make any reference to prescribed sequences of transformative physical exercises.[62] In keeping with Dzogchen's non-gradualist approach to yogic practice, the Nyingma treasure texts advocate in their place spontaneous and unchoreographed physical practices that, from a Dzogchen point of view, preempt the codified regimens of Trulkhor. The fully embodied practices of Korde Rushen (*'khor 'das ru shan*) that facilitate realisation of the unbound altruistic mind of enlightenment (*byang chub kyi sems*) are described in detail in the following section of this chapter.

The clear absence of Trulkhor practices in early Nyingma "treasure teachings" (*gter chos*) is further evident from an examination of the "Heart Essence of Vimalamitra" (*Vi ma snying thig*), a three-volume compilation attributed to the eighth-century Indian master Vimalamitra, but revealed by his followers from the late tenth or early eleventh century until the middle of the twelfth century.[63] The two-volume "Heart Essence of the Sky Dancers" (*mKha' 'gro snying thig*) attributed to Padmasambhava and revealed by Tsultrim Dorje (tshul khrims rdo rje) (1291–1315/1317) in the early fourteenth century also omits any mention of Trulkhor practices. Yet, like the *Vima Nyingthik* before it, it does describe body *maṇḍala* practices of channels, winds, and vital essences (*rtsa rlung thig le*) based on yogas of sexual union.[64]

Apart from the cycle of eighteen yogic exercises described in the twelfth-century *Yuthok Nyingthik*, Trulkhor seems to have formally entered into the Nyingma corpus through the literary work of the fourteenth-century Dzogchen master Longchen Rabjampa Drimé Özer (klong chen rab 'byams pa dri med 'od zer) (1308–1364). Longchenpa synthesised earlier Nyingma treasure texts in his composite *Nyingthik Yabshi* (*sNying thig ya bzhi*) that quotes widely from the Seventeen Dzogchen Tantras, but makes no mention of Trulkhor within its multiple volumes. It is in Longchenpa's "Wishfulfilling Treasury" (*Yid bzhin mdzod*) – later catalogued as one of his "Seven Treasuries" (*mDzod bdun*) – that the first evidence occurs of Trulkhor practice in the Nyingma tradition subsequent to the "Turquoise Heart Essence".[65] The "Wishfulfilling Treasury" elucidates Buddhist cosmology and philosophical systems, but its final chapter,

62 Chögyal Namkhai Norbu (personal communication, Glass House Mountains, Australia, March 2012) maintains that the descriptions of spontaneous physical movements in the root text of the Seventeen Tantras, the *Dra thal gyur* (*sGra thal 'gyur*), represent a form of Trulkhor.

63 See Germano & Gyatso 2000: 244. The "Seventeen Dzogchen Tantras" date to the same time period and also describe body-based practices, although more synoptically than the *Vima Nyingthik*.

64 Ibid. See also the chapter by James Mallinson in the present volume.

65 Personal communication, Tshewang Sitar Rinpoche, Bumthang, Bhutan, April 2013.

"The Fruition that is the Culmination of Meditation", describes twenty Trulkhor exercises that include internal bodily massage (*sku mnye*) and sequenced stretches in support of the Dzogchen contemplative technique of Kadag Trekchö (*ka dag khregs chod*), or "cutting through [discursive mental activity] to primordial purity". Unlike the preceding forms of Trulkhor presented within Tibetan Buddhism, Longchenpa's rendition is not based on visualizing oneself as a tantric deity, but on vibrant awareness (*rig pa*, Skt. *vidyā*)[66] of one's innate Buddha Nature (*tathāgatagarbha*).[67]

Having established a clear precedent, subsequent revealed treasure texts connected to the Dzogchen Nyingthik, or "Heart Essence of Great Perfection" transmission, largely all include cycles of Trulkhor. For example, in 1366, two years after Longchenpa's death, Rigdzin Godemchen (rig 'dzin rgod ldem can) (1337–1408) revealed his highly influential "Northern Treasure" (*Byang gter*) with a Trulkhor cycle called *Phag mo'i zab rgya rtsa rlung*, based on the meditational deity Vajravārāhī. These teachings were expanded upon by the treasure revealer Tenyi Lingpa (bstan gnyis gling pa) (1480–1535) whose writings elaborated on the movement of energy through the channels during sexual union and the discipline of *vajrolī*, in which sexual fluids are circulated through the body's yogic anatomy.[68]

Longchenpa's ostensible fifteenth-century Bhutanese reincarnation, Orgyen Pema Lingpa (orgyan padma gling pa) (1450–1521), further clarified the "Ati

66 *Rig pa* is also rendered as "primordial awareness" and is experientially related to the spontaneous "recognition" (*pratyabhijñā*) of the nature of mind central to non-dual Kashmiri Śaivism.

67 In most Nyingthik, or "heart essence" systems of Trulkhor, there is no visualisation of oneself as a tantric diety because all divine forms arise from primary seed-syllables (as "vibrations") in the luminous expanse of the heart which is the ultimate deity (oral communication, Chatral Sangye Dorje Rinpoche, Pharping, Nepal, September 1992). The Trulkhor exercises described in chapter twenty-two of Longchenpa's *Yid bzhin mdzod* are less elaborate than later Nyingthik renditions for which they form the basis. The movements include interlocking the fingers against the chest and stretching them outward (no. 3), twisting the shoulders down to the hands and knees (no. 4), pushing outward from the chest with the hands held as fists (no. 5), twisting the body with the arms crossed and the hands on the shoulders (no. 6), drawing the hands along the arms as if shooting a bow (no. 8), pushing the fists outward as if against a mountain (no. 9), bending forward and backward (no. 10), joining the little fingers of the hands and forming a *mudrā* on the top of the head (no. 11), etc. For further details see the final volume of the *Yid bzhin mdzod* (p. 1579 in the edition published by Dodrupchen Rinpoche).

68 Tenyi Lingpa's elaboration of Rigdzin Godemchen's Trulkhor, as first revealed in the Gongpa Zangthal (*dGongs pa bzang thal*) – the highest Dzogchen teachings of the Northern Treasure lineage – reputedly consists of twelve preparatory exercises, thirteen principle movements, and twelve concluding movements (oral communication, Kunzang Dorje Rinpoche, Pharping, Nepal, July 1985 and correspondence with Malcolm Smith, November 2016). For an incisive, comprehensive account of the yogic technique of *vajrolī*, in which sexual fluids are drawn up the urethra, see the chapter by James Mallinson in the present volume.

Anu" practices of the "Heart Essence" tradition in his revealed treasure text "Compendium of All-Embracing Great Perfection" (*rDzogs chen kun bzang dgongs 'dus*), a chapter of which entitled "Secret Key to the Channels and Winds" (*rTsa rlung gsang ba'i lde mig*) describes a sequence of twenty-three Trulkhor exercises within the context of Dzogchen's visionary practice of "Leaping over the Skull" (*thod rgal*).[69] The practices are performed with the breath held in a "vase" (*bum pa can,* Skt. *kumbhaka*), in combination with *mūladharabandha,* and are described as "clearing hindrances" (*gegs sel*) to contemplative practice while also ensuring optimal health. The practices were eventually illustrated on the walls of the Sixth Dalai Lama's private meditation chamber in the Lukhang temple in Lhasa in the late seventeenth century (see Figure 2).[70]

Following Pema Lingpa's revelation, further cycles of Trulkhor emerged in the Nyingma tradition in "The Universal Embodiment of the Precious Ones" (*dKon mchog spyi 'dus*), a treasure text revealed by Rigdzin Jatson Nyingpo (rig 'dzin 'ja' tshon snying po) (1585–1656), as well as within the approximately contemporaneous "Accomplishing the Life-Force of the Wisdom Holders" (*Rig 'dzin srog sgrub*) revealed by Lhatsun Namkha Jigme (lha btsun nam mkha'i 'jigs med) (1597–1650/1653).[71] The trend continued with the revelation of the "Sky Teaching" (*gNam chos*) by Namchö Mingyur Dorje (gnam chos mi 'gyur rdo rje) (1645–1667) that contains a Trulkhor cycle with over sixty movements based on the Buddhist deity Vajrakīlaya (*rdo rje phur pa rtsa rlung 'khrul 'khor*).[72]

Trulkhor's place within the Nyingma "heart essence" tradition became even more firmly established with the visionary treasure revelation of Jigme Lingpa ('jigs med gling pa) (1730–1798) whose "Heart Essence of the Vast Expanse" (*Klong chen snying thig*) includes the "Miraculous Wheel of Wisdom Holders"

69 The "Compendium of All-Embracing Great Perfection" is one of three texts revealed by Pema Lingpa that elucidate the Great Perfection (*rdzogs chen*) and the only one that describes practices of Trulkhor. For a full inventory of Pema Lingpa's revealed treasures, see Harding 2003: 142–144. Pema Lingpa's system of Trulkhor expands on the simpler exercises described by Longchenpa in his "Wishfulfilling Treasury", in which there are neither forceful "drops" (*'beb*) (see n. 75) nor the "adamantine wave" (*rdo rje rba rlabs; rdo rje rlabs chu*) practice of pressing on the carotid arteries at the neck to induce intensified states of awareness (see Figure 4). For a full translation of Pema Lingpa's "Secret Key to the Channels and Winds", see Baker 2012, 2017a and 2017b.

70 For an extensive account of how Pema Lingpa's text came to be illustrated on the walls of the Sixth Dalai Lama's meditation chamber in the late seventeenth century under the direction of Tibet's political regent Desi Sangye Gyatso (sde srid sangs rgyas rgya mtsho) (1653–1705), see Baker 2017b.

71 Oral communication, Kunzang Dorje Rinpoche, Pharping, Nepal, May 1985.

72 Oral communication, Lama Tashi Tenzin, Thimphu, Bhutan, July 2014. According to Lama Tashi, this cycle concludes with *bkra shis 'beb 'khor,* or "auspicious circle of drops", in which the adept performs a clockwise series of yogic "drops" and also jumps while in lotus posture from one padded yogic seat (*'beb den*) to another. See also n. 75.

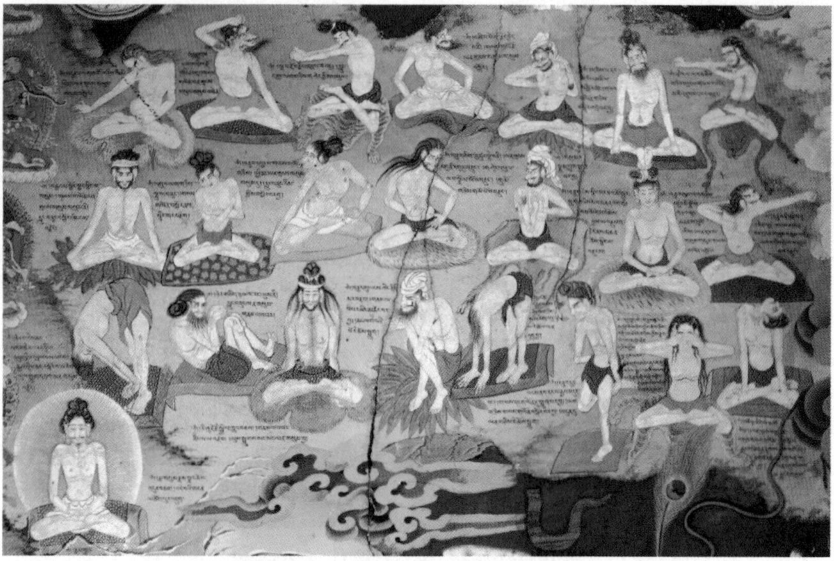

Figure 2: Mural in the Sixth Dalai Lama's private meditation chamber illustrating a sequence of twenty-three yogic movements revealed by Orgyen Pema Lingpa.

(*Rig 'dzin 'khrul 'khor*), a Trulkhor cycle of twenty-one movements elaborating on Longchenpa's yogic exercises in his "Wishfulfilling Treasury", the *Yid bzhin mdzod.* The Rigdzin Trulkhor practices consist of five initial exercises for clearing the body's elemental winds followed by eight movements that embody the qualities of eight Indian "wisdom holders" (*vidyādhara,* Tib. *rgya gar rig 'dzin brgyad*), acclaimed as enlightened contemporaries of Padmasambhava.[73] These and subsequent exercises in the series include symbolic gestures and vestiges of ritual dance together with forceful movements reminiscent of Chinese systems of *wei gong* and Yang-style *taijiquan.*[74] As in other later transmissions of Trulkhor, the series also includes intermittent controlled "drops" (*'beb*) of increasing complexity that purportedly direct the body's subtle energies into the central channel to promote expanded states of awareness (see Figures 3 and 5). The most demanding, and potentially injurious, "drops" involve leaping into the air from a standing position and landing cross-legged on the ground in the lotus posture with the breath held in a "vase" in the lower abdomen.[75] Other forceful methods

73 Personal communication, Tulku Tenzin Rabgye, Lobesa, Bhutan, October 2013. The eight Vidyadhāras are Vimalamitra, Hūṃkāra, Mañjuśrīmitra, Nāgārjuna, Prabhāhasti, Dhanasaṃskṛta, Guhyacandra, and Śāntigarbha. Sometimes Padmasambhava is added as a ninth, or as part of the eight in place of Prabhāhasti.

74 Personal observation. See also Mroz 2013.

75 *'beb,* or forceful "drops", are categorised as "small" (*'beb chung*), "medium" (*bar 'beb*), "big" (*'beb chen*), and "adamantine" (*rdor 'beb*), during which the legs are crossed in the *vajra*

for altering consciousness within the context of Tsalung Trulkhor include a technique called the "adamantine wave" (*rdo rje rba rlabs, rdo rje rlabs chu*), in reference to the pulsations of blood in the medial cranial artery when a practitioner, or spiritual preceptor, presses on the carotid arteries at the sides of the neck to induce a thought-free state of bliss and emptiness (*de stong*). The "adamantine wave" is one of twenty-one methods for pointing out the noetic state of primordial awareness (*rig pa*) described in Orgyen Pema Lingpa's "Introductory Commentary to the Pearl Garland of Introductions [to the Nature of Mind] in Six Sections" (*Ngo sprod kyi bu yig ngo sprod mu tig phreng ba le'u drug pa*) (see Figure 4).

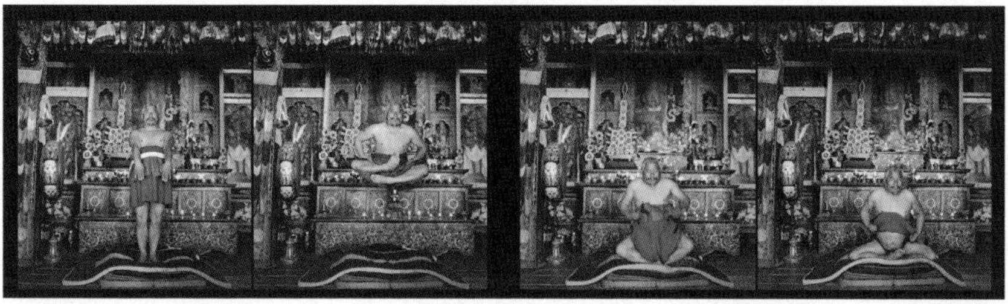

Figure 3: Tshewang Sitar Rinpoche performing an "adamantine cross-legged drop" in the Gaden Lhakhang, Ura, Bhutan.

Some subsequent "Heart Essence" treasure works such as the exclusively Dzogchen oriented *Chetsün Nyingthik* (*lCe btsun snying thig*) revealed by Jamyang Khentse Wangpo ('jam dbyangs mkhyen brtse'i dbang po) (1820–1892) make no mention of Trulkhor, whereas the roughly contemporary "All-Perfect Heart Essence" *(Kun bzang thugs thig)* revealed by Chokyur Dechen Lingpa (mchog gyur bde chen gling pa) (1829–1870) contains a Trulkhor series connected with the tantric deity Acala (mi gyo ba), the "Immovable One", that is

posture in mid air (*rdo rje dkyil dkrungs 'beb*). There are also *kyang 'beb* in which the body is extended and one drops on one's side, *chu 'beb* which are performed after first spinning in a circle, and "ornamental" *gyen 'beb* performed at the end of a Trulkhor series. It's likely that *'beb* evolved from originally gentler Haṭha Yoga practices such as *mahāvedhamudrā* which is central to Trulkhor practice in the *Amṛtasiddhi* and *Yuthog Nyingtik. Mahāvedha,* the "great piercer", is normally performed with the legs crossed in *padmāsana,* or lotus posture, the palms pressed against the ground, and the throat pulled upward in *jālandharamudrā* while holding the breath below the navel and successively dropping the backs of the thighs and buttocks on the ground to cause *prāṇavāyu* to leave the two side channels (*iḍā* and *piṅgalā*) and enter the *suṣumnā,* or central channel. James Mallinson notes, however, that *mahāvedhamudrā* as practised in the *Amṛtasiddhi* differs from the later Haṭha Yoga version and does not involve dropping onto the thighs and buttocks but sitting on the heels of the feet, which are joined and pointing downwards (personal communication, Vienna, September 2013). A similar exercise called *tāḍanakriyā,* or "beating action", is performed in Kriyā Yoga with the eyes concentrated at the point between the eyebrows in *śāmbhavīmudrā.*

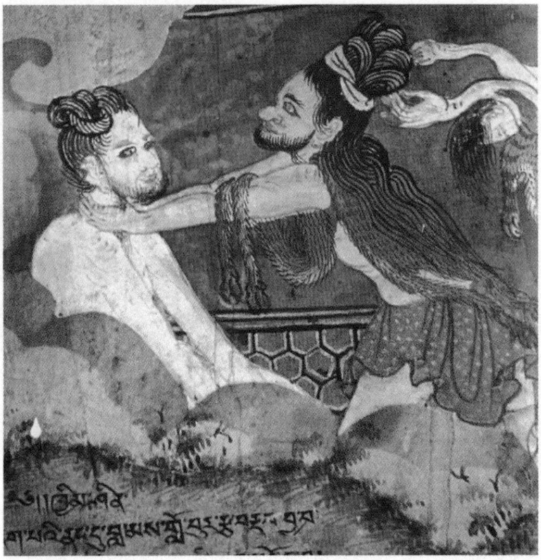

Figure 4: An illustration of the "adamantine wave" practice in the Lukhang temple, Lhasa.

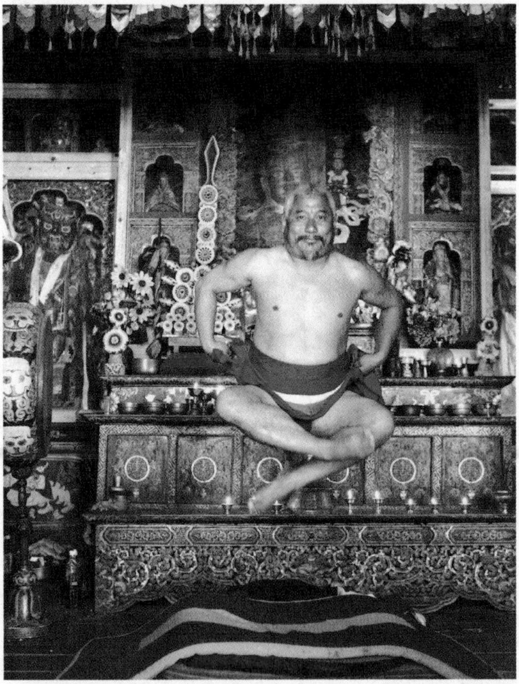

Figure 5: Tshewang Sitar Rinpoche performing an "adamantine cross-legged drop" in the Gaden Lhakhang, Ura, Bhutan.

practised within both Nyingma and Karma Kagyu traditions.[76] The later "mind treasure" (*dgongs gter*) "Heart Essence of the Sky Dancers", the *Khandro Thukthik* (*mKha' 'gro'i thugs thig*) revealed by Dudjom Jikdral Yeshe Dorje (bdud 'joms 'jigs bral ye shes rdo rje) (1904–1987) in 1928, contains a Trulkhor cycle of sixteen movements that is widely practised today both in the Himalayan world and beyond and held to have been influenced by the *Phag mo zab rgya* revelation of Rigdzin Godemchen.[77] Similarly, the "Profound Instructions of Vajravārāhī" (*Phag mo'i zab khrid*) revealed by Kunzang Dechen Lingpa (kun bzang bde chen gling pa) (1928–2006), based on prior teachings of Rigdzin Godemchen and Tenyi Lingpa, contains an extensive Trulkhor cycle with elaborate "drops".[78]

The most globally recognised contemporary form of Trulkhor is the revealed teaching of Tibetan scholar and Dzogchen master Chögyal Namkhai Norbu that he calls "Yantra Yoga", based on his 1976 commentary to a Trulkhor text entitled "Miraculous Wheel of Yogic Movements Uniting Sun and Moon" (*'Khrul 'khor nyi zla kha sbyor*) that was reputedly composed in the eighth century by the Tibetan translator Vairocana (vai ro tsa na), a contemporary of Padmasambhava. According to Namkhai Norbu, Vairocana's original text is part of a larger collection known as the "Oral Transmission of Vairo" (*Vai ro snyan brgyud*)[79] and describes seventy-five breath-sequenced yogic movements, many of which are well known within later systems of Haṭha Yoga. According to Namkhai Norbu's commentary, "A Stainless Mirror of Jewels" (*Dri med nor bu'i me long*) which was published in 2008 as *Yantra Yoga: The Tibetan Yoga of Movement*,[80] Vairocana is said to have received these yogic practices directly from Padmasambhava who, in turn, is said to have learned them from a Nepalese *mahāsiddha* named Hūṃkāra who himself reputedly learned them from Śrīsiṃha, an early Dzogchen lineage holder who lived for a considerable period at the sacred mountain Wutai Shan in western China where similar Taoist-Chan Buddhist methods of what is now called *qigong* were transmitted from before the eighth century.[81] The close parallels of the "Miraculous Wheel of Yogic Movements Uniting Sun and Moon"

76 Oral communication, Tulku Urgyen Rinpoche, Nagi Gompa, Nepal, May 1987.

77 Oral communication, Lama Nyingku Kunzang Wangdi, Bhutan, October 2011.

78 In practice, however, Kunsang Dechen Lingpa simplified the Trulkhor exercises revealed by Rigdzin Godemchen and Tenyi Lingpa as he recognised that they could be harmful if not begun at an early age (oral communication, Karma Lhatrul Rinpoche, Bangkok, January 2014).

79 The "Oral Transmission of Vairo" is part of Vairocana's collected works (*vai ro rgyud 'bum*) which were compiled in the twelfth century, thus making it speculative to date the "Miraculous Wheel Uniting Sun and Moon" to the eighth century. The text invites further independent investigation for understanding the origins and evolution of postural yoga practices in India and Tibet.

80 Clemente & Lukianowicz 2008.

81 Personal communication, Vivienne Lo, London, September 2011.

with Indian Haṭha Yoga and its potential links with Chinese systems of *dao yin* and *qigong* invite further comparative research and may eventually indicate greater transcultural origins for Tibet's Trulkhor practices than has so far been supposed. Namkhai Norbu's commentary elaborates Vairocana's system of poses and breathing practices into one hundred and eight interconnected movements adapted to a contemporary western context, giving further evidence of the heuristic nature of the Tsalung Trulkhor system which, like Haṭha Yoga, continues to evolve through its interactions and exchanges with analogous practices and increasing global knowledge and awareness of biophysical processes.[82]

5. Korde Rushen: Yoga of Spontaneous Presence

The physically embodied practices of Tsalung Trulkhor were a core component of the Vajrayāna forms of Buddhism that developed in Tibet from the eleventh century onward and, as the revealed treasure texts in the Nyingma tradition clearly indicate, Tsalung Trulkhor has been a supporting element in the transmission of Dzogchen, or Atiyoga, as well. Dzogchen is also referred to as "Supreme Yoga" (*shin tu rnal 'byor,* Skt. *atiyoga*) and, within the Nyingma tradition represents the culmination of the Development Phase (*utpattikrama,* Tib. *bskyed rim*), otherwise called *mahāyoga,* and the Completion Phase (*sampannakrama,* Tib. *rdzogs rim*), otherwise called *anuyoga,* of Vajrayāna Buddhism.[83] Dzogchen differs from Vajrayāna as a whole in its view of Buddha Nature (*tathāgatagarbha,* Tib. *de bzhin gshegs pa'i snying po*) as an innately present wakefulness rather than an indwelling potential that needs to be deliberately cultivated in order to attain freedom from Saṃsāra. Dzogchen thus characteristically "takes the end as the means" and dispenses with more gradual methods for realizing Buddhahood (*buddhatva,* Tib. *sangs rgyas nyid*). Although practices based on the body's "inner *maṇḍala*" (*nang pa'i dkyil 'khor*) of subtle energy channels are included in Dzogchen, such disciplines are traditionally viewed either as methods for removing psychophysical obstacles (*gegs sel*) or for intensifying realisation of the mind's "natural state" (*gnas lug*). Ultimately, however, the "illusory body movements" of Tsalung Trulkhor, when practised from a Dzogchen perspective, are considered to be direct expressions of enlightenment (*samyaksaṃbodhi*) rather than specific means for attaining it.[84]

---

82 Like other purely Dzogchen-oriented Trulkhor systems, Chögyal Namkhai Norbu's Yantra Yoga does not involve Anuttarayogatantra methods of deity visualisation, but envisions the body as a luminous network of energy channels. Unlike most earlier forms of Trulkhor, Yantra Yoga does not include forceful "drops".

83 See n. 59.

84 Personal communication, Tulku Tenzin Rabgye, Lobesa, Bhutan, October 2013. From another

Dzogchen is presented within Tibetan tradition as "beyond all mental concepts and free of both attachment and letting go; the essence of transcendent insight and the coalescence of meditation and non-meditation; perfected awareness free of all grasping."[85] While the unitary consciousness of Dzogchen can be directly realised without modifying the body or altering the mind in any way, its formal practice nonetheless traditionally begins with demanding physical exercises and culminates with prescribed postures and associated breathing techniques for entraining consciousness towards an incisive realisation of the primordial non-dual unity (*gnyis su med pa*) of enlightened awareness.[86] As Rigdzin Jigme Lingpa (rig 'dzin 'jigs med gling pa) (1730–1798) wrote in "Supreme Mastery of Wisdom Awareness" (*Ye shes bla ma*), one of the most revered manuals (*khrid yig*) on Dzogchen practice: "Unless the vitally important body is compliant and energy flowing freely, the pure light of consciousness will remain obscured. So take this physical practice to heart!"[87]

Initiation in Dzogchen formally entails "empowerment into the dynamic energy of awareness" (*rig pa'i rtsal dbang*). To accomplish this experientially, practitioners traditionally undertake rigorous foundational practices called Korde Rushen (*'khor 'das ru shan*) to differentiate Saṃsāra (Tib. *'khor ba*), or bounded consciousness (*sems*), from the spontaneous self-liberating awareness (*sems nyid*) of Nirvāṇa (Tib. *mya ngan 'das*). The "Continuity of Sound" (*sGra thal 'gyur*),[88] the root text of Dzogchen's esoteric "instruction cycle" (*man ngag*

---

perspective, Dzogchen considers Trulkhor exercises to be contrived means appropriate only in less direct approaches to enlightenment. As the fourteenth-century Dzogchen master Longchenpa writes in canto 31 of his "Precious Treasury of Natural Perfection" (*gNas lugs rin po che'i mdzod*): "Exhausting exercises involving struggle and strain are of short-lived benefit, like a sand castle built by a child." As he further explicates: "We strive in meditation because we desire excellence, but any striving precludes attainment ... remaining constantly at ease in uncontrived spontaneity ... non-action is revealed as supreme activity" (see Dowman 2014: 23).

85 From "Nyingthik, the Innermost Essence" (*Yang gsang bla na med pa'i snying thig*) by Rigdzin Jigme Lingpa (rig 'dzin 'jigs med gling pa), quoted in Trungpa 1972: 21.

86 The transpersonal modes of consciousness cultivated in Vajrayāna Buddhism and Dzogchen are subjects of contemporary neuroscientific research, leading to new linguistic and conceptual formulations. Some of these initiatives correlate specific meditative states with parasympathetic dominance in the brain's frontal cortex and concomitant activation of a biologically based mode of consciousness in which slow wave patterns originating in the limbic system project into the frontal parts of the brain, thereby inducing increased hemispheric synchronisation and more integral states of awareness. See, for example, Winkelman 1997: 393–394.

87 This translation and subsequent ones from the *Yeshe Lama* (*Ye shes bla ma*) are partially adapted from Chönam & Khandro 2009 and Dowman 2014, but are more indebted to Dungtse Thinley Norbu Rinpoche's oral commentary in Kathmandu in July 1987.

88 The "Continuity of Sound Tantra" is associated with the eighth-century Indian Dzogchen master Vimalamitra and is the basis of the "Seventeen Tantras of the Innermost Luminescence" (*Yang gsang 'od gsal gyi rgyud bcu bdun*) which provide the collective literary foun-

sde, Skt. *upadeśavarga*), counsels accordingly: "Perform bodily yantras [Trulkhor] while twisting and turning and alternately while prone and moving. Stretch and bend the limbs and push the body beyond its accustomed limits. Physically act out the behavior of the six kinds of elemental beings."[89] As Rigdzin Jigme Lingpa reiterates in his eighteenth-century "Supreme Mastery of Wisdom Awareness": "Then, run and jump, twist and turn, stretch and bend and, in brief, move your body in whatever way comes to mind – beyond purpose or design."[90] He further clarifies that "[f]inally you will be physically, energetically, and mentally exhausted and thus totally relaxed." Within this unbounded unitary sphere beyond the binary operations of thought, "all spontaneous actions of body, speech, and mind arise as the unity of Saṃsāra and Nirvāṇa, and thus as unobstructed Buddha-Body, Buddha-Speech, and Buddha-Mind."[91]

Customarily undertaken in solitary wilderness settings, the practices of Korde Rushen are divided into Outer, Inner, Secret, and Ultimately Secret methods for distinguishing the contents of consciousness from wakeful awareness itself until they arise indivisibly as having "one taste" (*ro gcig,* Skt. *ekarasa*). In Outer Korde Rushen, mind and body are pushed to unaccustomed extremes by acting out imaginary existences as animals, hell beings, demi-gods, or whatever the mind conceives, leading to the spontaneous recognition of the self-created, and thus mutable, nature of conditioned existence. When the capacity for physical and imaginative expression is exhausted, the practitioner enters a natural state of ease (*rnal du dbab pa*) in a posture corresponding to an open-eyed "corpse pose" (*śavāsana*) in Haṭha Yoga. The thought-free mental state is identified as the "primal purity" (*ka dag*) of the mind's essential and abiding nature rather than its transient, and potentially deceptive, expressions.[92]

---

dation for the esoteric "instruction cycle" of Dzogchen teachings known as the Dzogchen Nyingthik, or "Heart Essence of Great Perfection".

89 Dowman 2014: 11. Besides the physical body, the exercises of Outer Korde Rushen engage the voice through "chattering non-sensically or speaking in the tongues of [imagined] mythic beings", and the mind by consciously evoking positive and negative thoughts that ultimately resolve into uncontrived, non-dual awareness (see ibid.).

90 Ibid. A Dzogchen treatise entitled "Flight of the Garuḍa" by Shabkar Tsokdruk Rangdrol (zhabs dkar tshogs drug rang grol) (1781–1851) further instructs: "With the conviction that Saṃsāra and Nirvāṇa are of one taste … walk, sit, run and jump, talk and laugh, cry and sing. Alternately subdued and agitated, act like a madman … Beyond desire you are like a celestial eagle soaring through space … free from the outset like bright clouds in the sky" (quoted in Baker & Laird 2011: 115).

91 Translation based on Dowman 2014: 12. Gyatrul Rinpoche further clarifies this essential point in his commentary to "Spacious Mind of Freedom" by Karma Chagmé Rinpoche (karma chags med) (1613–1678): "If you wish to stabilize the mind, first subdue the body with the *adhisāras* [yantra yoga] … although you are ostensibly working with the body, you are indirectly subduing and stabilizing the mind" (see Wallace 1998: 69).

92 Although many Dzogchen treasure texts and commentaries elucidate the practices of Korde

The subsequent Inner Korde Rushen practices build on the cathartic dramatisations of Outer Rushen and focus inwardly on six numinous seed-syllables along the body's central channel and on the soles of the feet associated with inhibiting subconscious imprints.[93] The practitioner clears each point in turn by visualizing white, red, and blue light issuing from the antidotal seed-syllables *oṃ āḥ hūṃ* as consciousness shifts from identification with the body's materiality to direct experience of its bioluminescence (*nang gsal*).[94] As with Outer Rushen, practice sessions alternate with motionless phases of concept-free awareness in which thoughts subside within the luminous expanse of primordial awareness (*rig pa*).

Outer and Inner Korde Rushen's clearing of physical and psychosomatic obstructions prepare the bodymind for the practices of Secret Rushen, which are divided into three progressive stages of Body, Voice, and Mind. The Body phase begins with a highly strenuous isometric balancing posture – the "position of the *vajra*" (*rdo rje'i 'dug stang*). Standing with the heels together and knees bent and stretched out to the sides, the practitioner pulls his or her chin towards the larynx, lengthens the spine, and places their palms together above the crown of the head while visualizing themselves as an indestructible blazing blue *vajra* (see Figure 6). Observing the flow of energy and sensation within the body while pushing through barriers of exhaustion, pain, and perceived futility, the practitioner maintains the position until his or her legs collapse and then continues in a modified posture while sitting on the ground until capable of resuming the standing posture.[95] At the end of the session one utters the seed-syllable *phaṭ* and lies down on the ground in a state of unconditioned concept-free awareness "like a corpse in a charnel ground". When thoughts arise, one repeats the process in

---

Rushen, the summary presented here draws substantially from oral instructions given in July 1987 in Kathmandu by Dilgo Khentse Rinpoche and Dhungtse Thinley Norbu Rinpoche.

93 The precise instructions for Korde Rushen practices vary between different Dzogchen lineages. In some, the "Purification of the Six Lokas" as described here is performed prior to the Outer Rushen described above. As with all aspects of Dzogchen, the key point is never technique but the end result: integrating awareness of the mind's innermost non-dual nature within all circumstances and experience. Generally, in Inner Rushen the seed-syllables *ah su nri tri pre du* correlate with the forehead, throat, heart, navel, base of the trunk, and soles of the feet.

94 Bioluminescence within humans has been associated with photon emission resulting from metabolic processes in which highly reactive free radicals produced through cell respiration interact with free-floating lipid proteins. The thus aroused molecules can react with chemicals called fluorophores to emit "biophotons" and thus produce a subjective experience of illumination.

95 The development of increased mental and physical capacities by pushing through habitual limits recalls the biological phenomenon of hormesis whereby beneficial effects such as increased strength and resilience, growth, and longevity can result from deliberate and systematic exposure to therapeutic stress.

continuing cycles of effort and repose until the tenacious illusion of an abiding self yields to an all-pervasive, endorphin amplified awareness. As Jigme Lingpa explains in "Supreme Mastery of Wisdom Awareness", "exhausting the physical body exhausts the discursive tendencies of the mind" and leads ultimately to realisation of the mind's essential nature.[96]

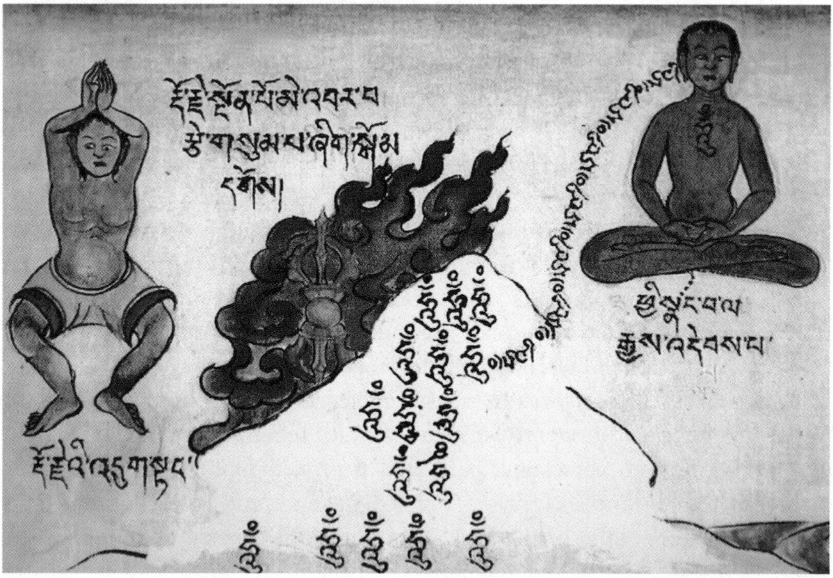

Figure 6: A Bhutanese manuscript illustrating the "secret" phase of Korde Rushen as described in the "Heart Essence of the Vast Expanse".

The intensity of the Dzogchen *vajra* position alters the flow of psychosomatic energies and encourages the emergence of adaptive mental and physical capacities as the mind progressively disengages from non-productive adventitious forms of consciousness and recovers its innate dimension of bliss, lucidity, and non-conceptual awareness. Secret Korde Rushen then continues with voice practices involving sound and vibration[97] that culminate with visualisations and intonations of the alpha seed-syllable *āḥ* to enter into direct experience of the

96 See Dowman 2014: 15.

97 In the Voice Phase of Secret Rushen the practitioner visualises and intones a blue seed-syllable *hūṃ* that multiplies until small *hūṃ*-s imaginatively fill the entire universe. The syllables and sounds of *hūṃ* then fill one's entire body propelling it imaginatively through space. The *hūṃ*-s then act like razors, dissolving all outer appearances and, turning inward, all semblance of one's physical body. At the end of the session one again lies down as in the practice of the Body Phase and remains in vivid open presence. When thoughts arise one begins the practice anew, using the primal energy represented by the seed-syllable *hūṃ* to alter habitual perceptions and attachments to consensual appearance.

pure potentiality, or "emptiness" (*stong pa nyid,* Skt. *śūnyatā*) that underlies perception and represents the ultimate Nature of Mind. Dissolving all appearances into effulgent light, the practitioner remains in a unified state of luminous cognition, or relativity, beyond conventional conceptions of time and space.

The following Ultimately Secret (*yang gsang*) Phase of Korde Rushen dynamically unifies body, voice, and mind "in order to free what has been stabilized". In a fully embodied enactment of the Deity Yoga (*lha'i rnal 'byor*) associated with Vajrayāna's Development Phase (*bskyed rim*), the practitioner manifests as a wrathful tantric deity, representing the creative volatility of sensation, thought, and emotion. As the texts prescribe, the practitioner stands with hands formed into horned *mudrā*-s while pivoting from left to right with heels rooted in the earth. With eyes rolling in the sky, loud thought-subduing laughter is emitted from the core of one's being, filling all of space with the syllables and sounds of *ha* and *hi.* As in all of the Korde Rushen practices that proceed Dzogchen's more widely known and practised contemplative techniques of "cutting through" (*khregs chod*) and "leaping over the skull" (*thod rgal*), the body is used to its fullest capacity to facilitate lucid, all-pervading awareness and freedom within all experience. As Longchenpa warns, however, no ultimate release can be obtained through deliberate, purpose driven action: "When everything is impermanent and bound to perish, how can a tight mesh of flesh, energy, and consciousness reach out to touch its indestructible core?"[98] He argues that all contrived yogas serve only to estrange us from the supreme state of being: "If we aspire to the ultimate state we should cast aside all childish games that fetter and exhaust body, speech, and mind … and realize the uncontrived unity of every experience."[99] From a Dzogchen point of view, the forceful actions of Tsalung Trulkhor are thus only useful in so far as they support the direct and ultimately effortless experience and perception of the self-effacing effulgence at the heart of every moment.[100] It is to this self-perfected and spontaneous yoga of illuminated vision that the practices of Korde Rushen and the "Miraculous Wheel of Channels and Winds" ultimately yield.

98 Translation from canto 19 of Longchenpa's "Precious Treasury of Natural Perfection" (*gNas lugs mdzod*), based on Barron 1998: 106 and Dowman 2010: 96.

99 Translation from canto 20 of Longchenpa's "Precious Treasury of Natural Perfection" (*gNas lugs mdzod*), based on Barron 1998: 107 and Dowman 2010: 98.

100 The seventeenth-century Dzogchen master Tsele Natsok Rangdröl (rtse le sna tshogs rang grol) echoes this view in his statement that for ultimate realisation of the nature of mind "you must mingle every moment of walking, sitting, eating, lying down [and thinking] with meditation. It is therefore not necessary to always maintain a specific posture or gaze." See Schmidt 1993: 92.

6. Tögal: Yoga of Active Perception

Dzogchen concurs with the larger Vajrayāna perspective that Tsalung Trulkhor practices can improve health and wellbeing and prepare the body for transformative tantric practices such as Fierce Heat (*gtum mo,* Skt. *caṇḍālī*). But the primary function within Dzogchen of all such physical practices is to harmonise the body's psychosomatic "winds" (*rlung,* Skt. *vāyu*) so that the non-dual nature of awareness becomes directly manifest through the "heart essence" (*snying thig*) contemplative technique of *lhun grub thod rgal,* literally "leaping over the skull into a spontaneous state of perfection", a method involving quiescent body postures, *mudrā*-s, subtle breathing techniques, and focused gazes (*lta ba,* Skt. *dṛṣṭi*).[101]

Lhündrup Tögal (*lhun grub thod rgal*) inverts the foundational yogic practice of sensory withdrawal (*so sor sdud pa,* Skt. *pratyāhāra*) in which sense consciousness is turned resolutely inward and instead extends perception outward, "leaping over" conventional divisions to unite experientially with a sensuous field of self-manifesting visions, based initially on entoptic phosphenes and related phenomena within the eye.[102] In "Supreme Mastery of Wisdom Awareness", Jigme Lingpa points out that the sublime visions of Tögal bear comparison with the "empty forms" (*stong gzugs,* Skt. *śūnyatābimba*) that arise as visual manifestations of consciousness during the practice of sense withdrawal in *Kālacakra.* Similarly, the *Kālacakratantra* (4.195) refers to "garlands of essences" (*thig le'i phreng ba*) that appear when gazing into the sky. The fact that the *Kālacakratantra* and the Seventeen Dzogchen Tantras seminal to Dzogchen's esoteric "instruction cycle" (*man ngag sde*) both appeared in written form in the

101 Just as Trulkhor and Korde Rushen work on the principle that intentional somatic states – from fluent postures to spontaneous movements – can influence cognition and affect not only the contents of consciousness but its primary function, the quiescent body postures and associated breathing techniques used in Tögal reconfigure visual perception, thereby altering subjective representations and experience of reality. Early Tögal texts, such as those in the eleventh-century *Vima Nyingthik,* also describe the use of a psychotropic decoction of Datura (*dha tu ra,* Skt. *dhattūra*) to accelerate the manifestation of visions, the final distillate to be introduced directly into the eyes using a hollow eagle's quill. See Baker 2004: 194. Tögal gazing techniques can also be compared with the well-known Haṭha Yoga practice of *trāṭaka* in which the practitioner stares unblinkingly at an external object.

102 From the Greek *phos,* meaning light, and *phainein,* to show, phosphenes refer to visual events that originate within the eye and brain, either spontaneously through prolonged visual deprivation or intentionally as a result of direct stimulation of the retinal ganglion cells. A perceptual phenomenon common to all cultures, phosphene patterns are believed by some researchers to correlate with the geometry of the eye and the visual cortex. Tögal visions, however, often correlate more directly with entoptic (i. e., "within the eye") phenomena such as myodesopsia, the perception of gossamer like "floaters" suspended within the eye's vitreous humor, as well as leukocytes, or white blood cells, transiting through the eye's retinal capillaries and appearing subjectively as self-existing translucent spheres.

eleventh century[103] suggests that later Dzogchen doctrines may have been directly influenced by the *Kālacakra*'s elucidation of visual forms that are neither wholly subjective nor wholly objective and, as such, illuminate the perceptual process itself. The initial visionary appearances associated with Tögal practice are vividly described by the Dzogchen master Dudjom Lingpa (bdud 'joms gling pa) (1835–1904) in his "mind treasure" (*gong gter*) "The Vajra Essence: From the Matrix of Pure Appearances and Pristine Consciousness, a Tantra on the Self-Originating Nature of Existence" (*Dag snang ye shes drva pa las gnas lugs rang byung gi rgyud rdo rje'i snying po*):

> At the beginning stage, the lights of awareness, called *vajra*-strands, no broader than a hair's width, radiant like the sheen of gold, appear to move to and fro, never at rest, like hairs moving in the breeze ... Then as you become more accustomed to the practice, they appear like strung pearls, and they slowly circle around the peripheries of the bindus of the absolute nature, like bees circling flowers. Their clear and lustrous appearance is an indication of the manifestation of awareness. Their fine, wavy shapes indicate liberation due to the channels, and their moving to and fro indicates liberation due to the vital energies.[104]

Dudjom Lingpa clarifies that, as a result of continued practice, the visions gradually stabilise and "appear in the forms of lattices and half-lattices, transparent like crystal, radiant like gold, and like necklaces of medium-sized strung crystals." Once the beginner's phase has passed, Dudjom Lingpa continues, "the visions of the absolute nature become beautiful, clear, and stable, and they take on various divine forms."[105]

The visions of Tögal gradually expand and encompass the "three bodies" (*sku gsum*, Skt. *trikāya*) of Dharmakāya, Sambhogakāya, and Nirmāṇakāya, referring, in Dzogchen, to Buddha Nature's inconceivable totality, luminous clarity, and spontaneous creativity. The visions arise through applying "key points" of posture, breath, and awareness associated with each of the three dimensions of reality. In distinction to the moving yogas of Tsalung Trulkhor, Tögal practice is performed while maintaining "three-fold motionlessness of body, eyes, and consciousness".[106] The "Garland of Pearls" (*Mu tig rin po che'i phreng ba*), one of

103 The Seventeen Dzogchen Tantras are traditionally held to have originated with the semi-legendary figure of Garab Dorje (dga' rab rdo rje) and to have been transmitted through the subsequent Dzogchen masters Mañjuśrīmitra, Śrīsiṃha, Padmasambhava, Jñānasūtra, and Vimalamitra. In the eighth century, Vimalamitra's Tibetan student, Nyangban Tingzin Zangpo (myang ban ting 'dzin bzang po) was said to have concealed these teachings for future generations and it is only after their ostensible rediscovery in the eleventh century by Neten Dangma Lhungyal (gnas brtan ldang ma lhun rgyal) that the Seventeen Tantras became the basis of Nyingma's Dzogchen Nyingthik, or "heart essence" tradition.

104 Wallace 2004: 302.

105 Ibid.

106 The earliest textual descriptions of Tögal are found in the Seventeen Dzogchen Tantras and

the principal Seventeen Dzogchen Tantras, emphasises the importance of three body positions (*bzhug stang*) described as "the postures of lion, elephant, and sage", corresponding to the Dharmakāya, Sambhogakāya, and Nirmāṇakāya, and by association with emptiness, clarity, and sensation (see Figure 7).[107] In the Dharmakāya posture of a seated lion (*chos sku bzhugs stang seng ge lta bu*) the torso is held upright (to allow the free flow of energy) with the soles of the feet placed together and the hands behind the heels in *vajra* fists (with the tips of the thumbs touching the base of the ring finger). The upper body is extended upwards with the chin tucked slightly inward (to suppress discursive thought) and the spine and back of the neck lengthened so as to allow the free flow of vital energy through the cranial arteries and associated "light channels" connecting the heart and eyes. With the breath extended outward through gently parted teeth and lips and the abdomen pulled slightly inward, the eyes are rolled inward (*ldog*) and upwards past an imagined protuberance at the crown of the head into the limitless expanse of inner and outer sky.[108] In the Sambhogakāya posture of a recumbent elephant, one's knees are drawn towards the chest (to increase metabolic heat) with the feet pointing backward and the elbows placed on the ground with the hands either positioned in front as *vajra* fists or supporting the chin (to inhibit coarse energy flow) as the spine elongates and the eyes gaze with soft-focus (*zur*) to the sides and ahead into pure visions reflecting the innate activity of conscious perception. In the Nirmāṇakāya posture of the sage (*ṛṣi*), one sits straight up (to open the channels and release the diaphragm) with the soles of the feet on the ground (to suppress the water element), one's knees and ankles together, and the arms crossed in front with elbows resting on the knees and the hands optionally tucked into the arm pits. As Jigme Lingpa clarifies in "Supreme Mastery of Wisdom Awareness",

> pulling the knees against the chest allows fire energy to blaze as luminous awareness. Slightly retracting the lower abdomen towards the spine inhibits discursive thought [presumably through the associated stimulation of the vagus nerve and the para-

their primary source, the "Continuity of Sound". All subsequent accounts of Tögal such as Jigme Lingpa's "Supreme Mastery of Wisdom Awareness" quote extensively from the original Dzogchen Tantras while offering additional commentary.

107 Personal communication, Chögyal Namkhai Norbu Rinpoche, Kathmandu, December 1993.

108 This gaze associated with the lion posture correlates with *śāmbhavīmudrā* in Haṭha Yoga, which is popularly held to synchronise the two hemispheres of the brain and lead directly to *samādhi*. In regard to the three postures as a whole, the "Continuity of Sound" specifies that "the crucial method is to apply reverted, lowered, and indirect gazes." As a result, in the lion posture "you will see with the *vajra* eye." In the posture of the recumbent elephant "you will see with the lotus eye", and in the posture of the squatting sage "you will see with the dharma eye" (personal communication Dhungtse Thinley Norbu Rinpoche, Kathmandu, July 1987).

> sympathetic nervous system] while ... placing the elbows on the knees with the hands in *vajra* fists and using them to support the throat equalizes heat and cold.[109]

In the Sage posture the gaze is directed slightly downward through half-closed eyes to control the body's vital energies and still the mind. Jigme Lingpa points out that there are many other additional postures suitable for Tögal, but that "for the innumerable heirs of tantra who prefer simplicity, the three described here are sufficient."[110]

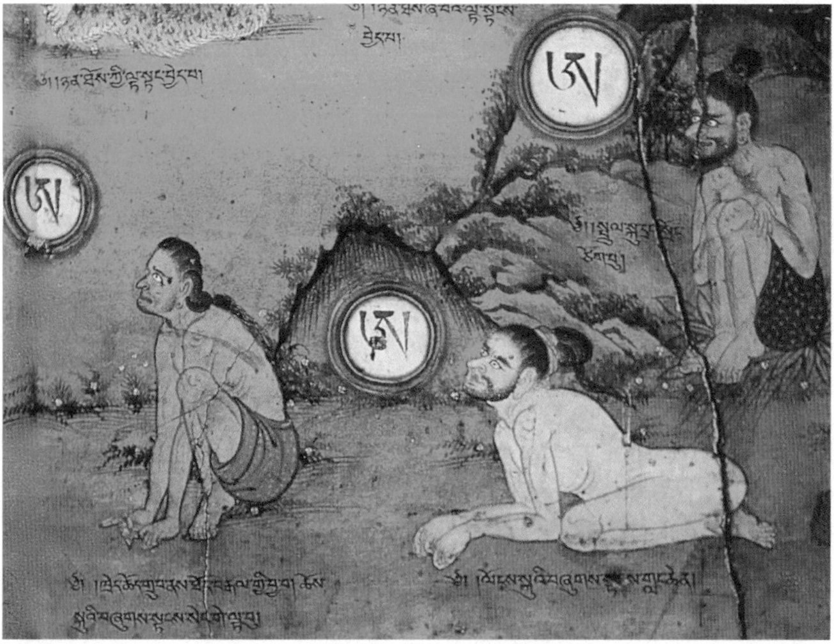

Figure 7: The primary Tögal postures of lion, elephant, and sage on a mural of the Lukhang temple.

In distinction to the nasal breathing that is predominantly used during the dynamic movements of Trulkhor, Tögal postures are combined with extended and almost imperceptible exhalations through the mouth, with the lips and teeth slightly parted and the body in absolute repose.[111] Breathing in this way diminishes the amount of oxygen circulating in the lungs and is held to free consciousness from its conditioned "karmic winds" (*las kyi rlung*) so as to more

109 See Dowman 2014: 49.

110 Ibid.

111 Exhalation and inhalation in Tögal practice are ideally naturally suspended as in the Haṭha Yoga technique of *kevala kumbhaka* in which both breathing and mental activity are spontaneous stilled.

effectively reveal the postulated "wisdom wind" (*ye shes kyi rlung*) in the heart through which consciousness ultimately transcends the corporeal body. For while Vajrayāna as a whole brings body, mind, and respiration into a renewed functional unity, Dzogchen ultimately maintains the supremacy of an integral awareness transcendent of the physical body. As such, the postures, breathing methods, and gazes associated with Tögal practice are ultimately designed to dissolve the physical constituents of the body at the time of death, transforming it into self-illuminating rainbow light. Central to this emancipating agenda are the embodied visions and progressive stages of "leaping over the skull" (*thod rgal*).

Tögal practice relies on reflexive awareness of a unitary dimension transcendent of mental experience (*khregs chod*). It is also based on sustained awareness the body's interactive "channels of light" (*'od rtsa*) through which the innate luminescence of heart-consciousness (Skt. *citta*) is perceived outwardly in progressive, self-illuminating displays (see Figures 8 and 9). As Padmasambhava declares in a chapter of the *Khandro Nyingthik* entitled "The Hidden Oral Instruction of the Ḍākinī", other teachings differentiate between channels, energy, and subtle essences; in the "heart essence" teachings these three are indivisible.[112] Padmasambhava goes on to describe the human body as a Buddha Field infused by luminescent wisdom (*'od gsal ye shes*, Skt. *prabhāsvarajñāna*) in the same way that "oil [pervades] a sesame seed". The oral instructions further clarify how, in the practice of Tögal, the body's elemental constituents manifest as five lights (*'od lnga*) and four illuminating lamps (*sgron ma bzhi*),[113] held to be purified and expanded expressions of Buddhahood (*sangs rgyas kyi go 'phang*). Through the specific postures, breathing methods, and gazing techniques of Tögal, the body's inner luminescence projects outward into the field of vision as spontaneously forming *maṇḍala*-s and optic yantras inseparable from innate enlightenment. As Padmasambhava summarises: "The nature of one's body is radiant light."[114] Rising from its center is the "great golden *kati* channel" (*ka ti gser gyi rtsa chen*)[115] which issues from the heart and through which the five lights of one's essential nature radiate (*gdangs*) outward as five-fold wisdom (*ye shes lnga*) and four successive visions (*snang ba bzhi*) leading ultimately to the body's dematerialisation at the time of death into a "rainbow body" (*'ja' lus*).

112 See Lipman 2010: 38.

113 The four lamps represent somatic sources of illumination and are most commonly listed as the "all-encompassing watery eye lamp" (*rgyang zhags chu'i sgron ma*), the "lamp of empty essences" (*thig le stong pa'i sgron ma*), the "lamp of the pristine dimension of awareness" (*dbyings rnam par dag pa'i sgron ma*), and the "lamp of naturally originated wisdom" (*shes rab rang byung gi sgron ma*).

114 Lipman 2010: 57.

115 For an elaboration of light channels in Dzogchen see Scheidegger 2007.

Figure 8: A practitioner of Tögal contemplates the "*vajra* chain" on a Lukhang mural.

The Four Visions (*snang ba bzhi*) integral to Tögal practice occur sequentially and are said to arise from the heart as visible expressions of the innate dynamism of unconditioned awareness. They also represent the manifestation of the body's channels, winds, and vital essences in their subtler reality as primordial purity, spontaneous accomplishment, and radiant compassion (*ka dag, lhun grub, thugs rje*) that correlate, in turn, with the interconnected triune Bodies of Enlightenment (*trikāya*). The visionary experiences are said to appear due to the "wind of luminosity" (*'od gsal gyi rlung*) that arises from the pristine "awareness wind" (*ye shes kyi rlung*) located in the heart. The four successive phases are described as the Direct Perception of the Ultimate Nature, the Vision of Increasing Experience, the Perfection of Intrinsic Awareness, and the Dissolution [of Phenomena] into the Ultimate Nature. Pema Lingpa points out in his fifteenth-century treasure text "Secret Key to Channels and Winds" (*Rtsa rlung gsang ba'i lde mig*) that, as the visions are physiologically based, they only arise by maintaining the key points of physical posture, "just as the limbs of a snake only become apparent when it is squeezed".[116] The first vision arises as a result of turning one's attention to naturally occurring phenomena within the "watery lamp" of the eye, as de-

116 For a translation of Terton Pema Lingpa's "Secret Key to the Channels and Winds" see Baker 2012, 2017a and 2017b. Pema Lingpa's "treasure text" illuminates the fundamental dynamics of mind and body at the heart of the Dzogchen tradition, specifically the ways in which primordial unitary awareness (*rig pa*) arises vibrantly and unconditionally in response to physiology and perception pushed beyond their accustomed limits in states of waking, sleeping, dreaming, sexuality, and near-death experiences.

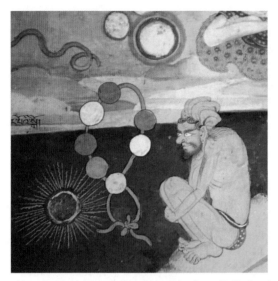

scribed above by Dudjom Lingpa. Although the garlands of pearls, gossamer threads, *vajra* chains, and transiting orbs that initially appear within one's field of vision may have naturalistic explanations as eye "floaters" and magnified red and white blood cells[117] transiting through the retinal capillaries, the entoptic events nonetheless focus awareness towards normally overlooked phenomenological processes and illuminate the ways in which a shift in perspective, or change in the way one views things, can fundamentally alter subjective experience. Central to this process is what Jigme Lingpa clarifies as "inner spaciousness shining visibly outward" within a coalescent awareness in which boundaries between inside and outside no longer obtain. The visions of the innate (*lhun gyis grub pa*) radiance of the heart develop as shape-shifting phosphenes and optical symmetries that gradually manifest anthropomorphically as male and female Buddhas within spheres of rainbow-colored light. Penultimately they resolve into four spheres – signifying the photonic essence of the four primary elemental processes within the human body – surrounding a larger central orb signifying "space", or boundless potentiality.[118] The central circle dilates through steady foveal gaze, expanding beyond circumference or periphery as the inherent luminescence of unmodified consciousness. Practised in environments of total darkness and expansive light, Tögal optimises sensory perception and leads ultimately to the posited awakening of all-encompassing luminescent and spontaneously compassionate awareness, or Buddha Mind.[119]

117 Tantric Buddhist physiology describes the body in terms of polarised red and white essences (*bindu*, Tib. *thig le*) that join at the heart at the moment of death or through tantric yogic praxis. This principle of complementary is anticipated in verse 60 of the *Yogacūḍāmaṇi Upaniṣad:* "The *bindu* is of two types, white and red. The white is *śukla* (semen) and the red is *mahārajas* (menstrual blood). … The white *bindu* is the moon; the red is the sun. It is only by the union of the two that the highest state is attained. When the red *bindu*, induced by the power of *kuṇḍalinī* together with the vital air, mixes with the white *bindu* one becomes divine. The one who realises the harmonious blending of the two *bindus* alone knows yoga" (vv. 60–64). Translation adapted from Ayyangar 1938: 288.

118 Comparisons can be made with "Haidinger's brush", an entoptic phenomenon in the visual field correlate of the macula in response to polarised light and associated with the circularly arranged geometry of foveal cones. The phenomenon appears most readily against the background of a blue sky and was first described in 1844 by the Austrian physicist Wilhelm Karl von Haidinger.

119 For further details see Baker 2012 and 2017b, and Baker & Laird 2011. As a practice of integral presence and recursive perception, Tögal can be considered a form of *sāmarasya* – the simultaneous practice of *dhāraṇā* (focused attention), *dhyāna* (contemplative meditation), and *samādhi* (coalescent unity) – leading to self-transcendent integration with the spontaneously arising visionary forms. From a Dzogchen perspective, the visionary phenomena are considered autonomous naturally unfolding perceptual processes based on the non-duality of subtle physiology and somatic awareness, resulting in a subjectively liberated experience of perception and reality.

7. Conclusion

As this chapter has hoped to emphasise, the word *haṭhayoga* first appears in Vajrayāna Buddhism's *Guhyasamājatantra* where it serves as an adjunct practice for facilitating visionary experience.[120] Although the specific method of that initial Haṭha Yoga technique remains obscure, its stated optical intention relates it with the recursive visionary practices of Tögal.[121] More characteristic Haṭha Yoga practices involving physiological *mudrā*-s were introduced to Tibet through the *Amṛtasiddhi* while the practice of Fierce Heat (*gtum mo*) central to Tibetan Buddhist lineages from the time of Milarepa is based on the intensive application of the "great seal" (*mahābandha*) which combinines *mūlabandha, uḍḍiyāṇa-bandha,* and *jālandharabandha* in conjunction with held "vase" breaths (*kumbhaka,* Tib. *bum pa chen*) and auxiliary "miraculous movements of the wheel of channels and winds" (*rtsa lung 'khrul 'khor*). Although the sequenced movements of Trulkhor predate the development of sequenced postural yoga in India and may have been directly influenced by indigenous Bön traditions, ritual dance, and yet unexplored historical connections with Chinese traditions of *dao yin,* they share a common soteriological method with Indian Haṭha Yoga and rose to prominence during roughly the same time period, as exemplified in the murals depicting Pema Lingpa's mid-fifteenth century Trulkhor cycle entitled "The Secret Key to the Channels and Winds" (*rtsa rlung gsang ba'i lde mig*).[122]

As with Indian Haṭha Yoga, the somatic practices of Vajrayāna Buddhism use dynamic means to harmonise polarised modes of consciousness through the symbolic medium of the body's central channel (*madhyamā, madhyanāḍī, suṣumnā, avadhūti*).[123] They progress, in Dzogchen, to a reorientation of somatic and attentional processes and an awakening of the heart's posited potential as an organ of recursive perception (see Figure 9). By directing attention to what is commonly overlooked the mind becomes increasingly aware of normally subconscious processes and thereby develops insight, clarity, and adaptability that

120 See Birch 2011: 535. "Visionary experience", in this context, can be associated with bringing conscious attention to subliminal perceptual events normally below the threshold of awareness. Research may ultimately suggest correspondences between interoceptive perception, i.e., supraliminal perception of autonomic physiological processes, and structural modifications of the anterior cingulate and, by extension, corresponding alterations of conscious awareness itself.

121 See also n. 11.

122 See Baker 2012 and 2017b.

123 The central channel can be partly understood in contemporary medical terms in relation to the hypothalamic–pituitary–gonadal axis that regulates the flow of mood-altering hormones within the human body. Tibetan yogic pratices such as Fierce Heat (*caṇḍālī,* Tib. *gtum mo*) cultivate proprioceptive sensation along a bioenergetic current paralleling the spine and linking the pelvic region with the interior of the brain, thus subjectively uniting experiential poles of consciousness associated with these distal regions of human anatomy.

contribute to an openness of being and expanded experience of human embodiment. Somatic practice as described in Vajrayāna and Dzogchen ultimately transcends its cultural context and points towards the awakening of collective, if unrealised, human capacities. Forceful Haṭha Yoga-like practices ultimately matter less in this process of self-transcendence than the expanded consciousness represented by "leaping over the skull" (*thod rgal*). As a deeply embodied practice, Tögal literally alters physiological processes through changing the way they are perceived, intensifying subjective experience of the bodymind as well as one's interactions with the external world.[124] The liberating reorientation of consciousness at the heart of Tögal is expressed concisely in the "All Creating King Tantra" (*Kun byed rgyal po'i rgyud,* Skt. *Kulayarājatantra*), one of Dzogchen's earliest texts: "With no need of transformation or purification, pure presence [within the body] is perfected in itself."[125] Jigme Lingpa elaborates as follows:

> The pith essence of the Great Perfection is to dwell in the natural radiance of all that occurs, at one with actions, energies, and thoughts and beyond all contrived boundaries of view and meditation; at ease in the naked clarity of the present moment.[126]

Outside the tradition of Vajrayāna, the mystically inclined poet William Blake (1757–1827) who first used the words "doors of perception" captured the essence of the self-transcendent and liberating vision of Tögal in a resonant line from his poem "The Mental Traveller": "The Eye altering alters all."[127] Applying that perceptual formula to the persistent illusion of an "I" and awakening to transpersonal dimensions of consciousness absent of cognitive and emotional strife lies at the heart of somatic practice in both Vajrayāna and Dzogchen, a process that involves altering, i. e., "making other", our embodied experience and, in so doing, promoting alternate forms of awareness that transcend perennially limiting perspectives and preoccupations. In short, seeing through the eyes of the heart into a world that is forever renewed by our perceptions and consequent interactions.

124 It echoes, for example, Gregory Bateson's concept of "creative subjectivity" in which one, in part, functions as "an artist creating a composite out of inner and outer events" (quoted in Brockman 1977: 245).

125 See Norbu & Clemente 1999: 146. The *Kun byed rgyal po* is considered the most important of the twenty-one texts of the "mind cycle" (*sems sde*) of Dzogchen, all of which emphasise the innately pure and expanded consciousness that is inseparable from enlightenment (*byang chub kyi sems*). The *Kun byed rgyal po* elaborates on more concise renditions of self-existing enlightenment such as found in the earlier six-line root text of "The Cuckoo of Awareness" (*Rig pa'i khu byug*).

126 See Dowman 2014: 36.

127 "The Mental Traveller" was never published during Blake's lifetime, but was included in a private collection of ten poems without illustrations or corrections.

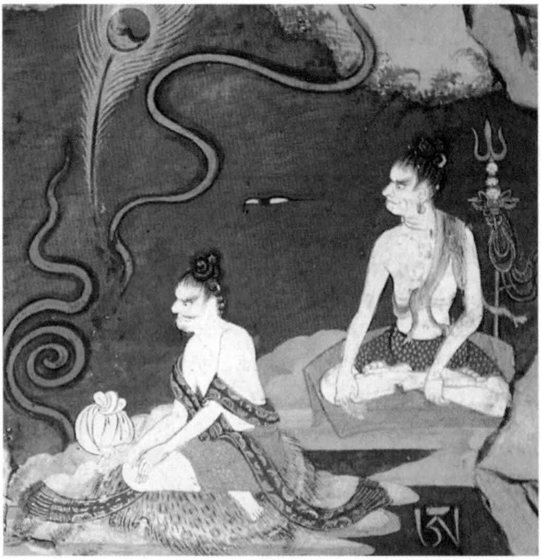

Figure 9: "Yak eye" on a Lukhang mural highlighting recursive, non-dual vision.

List of Figures

Fig. 1 "Position of the Peacock" (Skt. *mayūrāsana*) as shown in a Qing Dynasty manuscript from the Imperial Treasury illustrating the twenty-eighth of a sequence of thirty-two yogic exercises (*'khrul 'khor*) from the Hevajra Lamdre (*Lam 'bras*) as presented by Drakpa Gyaltsen (grags pa rgyal mtshan). Photograph courtesy of the Library of the Palace Museum, Beijing, China.

Fig. 2 Late seventeenth-century mural in the Sixth Dalai Lama's private meditation chamber in the Lukhang temple, Lhasa, illustrating a sequence of twenty-three yogic movements (*'khrul 'khor*) revealed two centuries earlier by Orgyen Pema Lingpa (orgyan padma gling pa) in his "Secret Key to the Channels and Winds" (*rTsa rlung gsang ba'i lde mig*). Photograph by Ian Baker.

Fig. 3 Tshewang Sitar Rinpoche performing an "adamantine cross-legged drop" (*rdo rje dkyil dkrungs 'beb*) from the twenty-one movement Rigdzin Trulkhor cycle in the "Heart Essence of the Vast Expanse" (*Klong chen snying thig*). Gaden Lhakhang, Ura, Bhutan, May 2013. Photograph by Ian Baker.

Fig. 4 A Dzogchen master presses on a disciple's carotid arteries to point out the primordial unity of emptiness and bliss (*bde stong zung 'jug*). An illustration of the "adamantine wave" (*rdo rje rba rlabs, rdo rje rlabs chu*) practice described in Orgyen Pema Lingpa's "Introductory Commentary to the Pearl Garland of Introductions [to the Nature of Mind] in Six Sections" (*Ngo sprod kyi bu yig ngo sprod mu tig phreng ba le'u drug pa*), illustrated on a corner mural in the Lukhang temple, Lhasa. Photograph by Ian Baker.

Fig. 5 Tshewang Sitar Rinpoche performing an "adamantine cross-legged drop" (*rdo rje dkyil dkrungs 'beb*) from the twenty-one movement Rigdzin Trulkhor cycle in the "Heart Essence of the Vast Expanse" (*Klong chen snying thig*). Gaden Lhakhang, Ura, Bhutan, May 2013. Photograph by Ian Baker.

Fig. 6 A Bhutanese manuscript illustrating the "secret" phase of Korde Rushen practices as described in the "Heart Essence of the Vast Expanse" (*Klong chen snying thig*). The standing "position of the *vajra*" is pictured to the left and practices of the voice, using the seed-syllable *hūṃ*, on the right. Photograph courtesy of Pelden Dorji, Bumthang, Bhutan.

Fig. 7 The primary Tögal postures of lion, elephant, and sage, as illustrated on the western mural of the Lukhang temple in Lhasa. The seed-syllable *āḥ* in the rainbow-encircled nimbus symbolises the mind's primordial "alpha" state. Photograph by Ian Baker.

Fig. 8 A practitioner of Tögal contemplates the "*vajra* chain", manifesting as a "string of pearls" backlit by the sun. Detail from the northern mural, Lukhang temple, Lhasa. Photograph by Ian Baker.

Fig. 9 The "yak eye" manifesting within pellucid space highlights the recursive vision characteristic of Tögal practice. Detail from the northern mural in the upper chamber of the Lukhang temple in Lhasa. Photograph by Ian Baker.

References

Ayyangar, T. R. S. (Ed., Trans.). (1938). *The Yoga Upanishads.* Madras: The Adyar Library.

Baker, I. (1997). *The Tibetan Art of Healing.* London: Thames & Hudson.

Baker, I. (2004). *The Heart of the World: A Journey to the Last Secret Place.* New York: Penguin Press.

Baker, I. (2012). Embodying Enlightenment: Physical Culture in Dzogchen as revealed in Tibet's Lukhang Murals. *Asian Medicine: Tradition and Modernity, 7,* 225–264.

Baker, I. (2017a). Yoga and Physical Culture in Vajrayāna Buddhism and Dzogchen, with Special Reference to Tertön Pema Lingpa's 'Secret Key to the Winds and Channels'. In *A Mandala of 21st Century Perspectives: Proceedings of the International Conference on Tradition and Innovation in Vajrayāna Buddhism* (pp. 54–101). Thimphu: The Centre for Bhutan Studies & GNH.

Baker, I. (2017b). Moving Towards Perfection: Physical Culture in Dzogchen as Revealed in Tibet's Lukhang Murals. In V. Lo and P. Barrett (Eds.), *Imagining Chinese Medicine* (pp. 403–428). Leiden: Brill.

Baker, I. & Laird, T. (2011). *The Dalai Lama's Secret Temple: Tantric Wall Paintings from Tibet.* London: Thames & Hudson.

Barron, R. (Trans.). (1998). Longchen Rabjam, *The Precious Treasury of the Way of Abiding and The Exposition of the Quintessential Meaning of the three Categories: A Commentary on the Precious Treasury of the Way of Abiding.* Berkeley: Padma Publishing.

Birch, J. (2011). The Meaning of haṭha in Early Haṭhayoga. *Journal of the American Oriental Society, 131*(4), 527–554.

Blake, W. (1863). "The Mental Traveller". In A. Gilchrist et al. (Eds.), *Life of William Blake, "Pictor Ignotus." With Selections from his Poems and other Writings* (pp. 98–102). London: MacMillan.

Brockman, J. (Ed.). (1977). *About Bateson*. New York: E. P. Duton.

Chaoul, M. A. (2006). *Magical Movements ('phrul 'khor): Ancient Yogic Practices in the Bön Religion and Contemporary Medical Perspectives*. Unpublished Dissertation. Rice University, Houston.

Chaoul, M. A. (2007a). Magical Movement ('phrul 'khor) in the Bon Tradition and Possible Applications as a CIM Therapy. In M. Schrempf (Ed.), *Soundings in Tibetan Medicine: Anthropological and Historical Perspectives* (pp. 285–304). Brill's Tibetan Studies Library 10. Leiden: Brill.

Chaoul, M. A. (2007b). Magical Movements ('Phrul 'Khor): Ancient Tibetan Yogic Practices from the Bon Religion and their Migration into Contemporary Medical Settings. *Asian Medicine, 3*(1), 130–155.

Chaoul, M. A. (2010). From Caves to the Clinic and Research: Bon Magical Movements (rtsa rlung 'phrul 'khor) Can Help People with Cancer. In *Bon: The Everlasting Religion of Tibet. Tibetan Studies in Honour of Professor David L. Snellgrove. East and West, 59*(1–4), 167–190.

Chenagtsang, N. (2013). *Path to Rainbow Body: Introduction to the Yuthog Nyingthig*. Sorig Institute Press.

Chönam, L. & Khandro, S. (Trans.). (2009). *Jigmed Lingpa, Yeshe Lama*. Ithaca, NY: Snow Lion Publications.

Clemente, A. (Trans., Ed.) & Lukianowicz, A. (Trans.). (2008). *Chögyal Namkhai Norbu, Yantra Yoga: The Tibetan Yoga of Movement*. Ithaca, NY: Snow Lion Publications.

David-Néel, A. (1937). *With Mystics and Magicians in Tibet*. London: Penguin Books.

Davidson, R. (2002). *Indian Esoteric Buddhism: A Social History of the Tantric Movement*. New York: Columbia University Press.

Davidson, R. (2005). *Tibetan Renaissance: Tantric Buddhism in the Rebirth of Tibetan Culture*. New York: Columbia University Press.

Dowman, K. (Trans.). (2010). *Natural Perfection: Longchenpa's Radical Dzogchen*. Boston: Wisdom Publications.

Dowman, K. (Trans.). (2014). *The Yeshe Lama: Jigme Lingpa's Dzogchen Ati Yoga Manual*. Charleston, NC: CreateSpace Independent Publishing Platform.

Ducher, C. (2014). *Building a Tradition: The Lives of Mar-Pa the Translator*. München: Indus Verlag.

Farrow, G. W. & Menon, I. (Eds., Trans.). (1992). *The Concealed Essence of the Hevajra-Tantra*. Delhi: Motilal Banarsidass.

Gangteng Literary Committee (2008). *The Rosary of Jewels: Biographies of the Successive Throne Holders of Gangteng*. Bhutan: Gangteng Monastery.

Germano, D. & Gyatso, J. (2000). Longchenpa and the Possession of the Ḍākinīs. In D. G. White (Ed.), *Tantra in Practice* (pp. 241–265). Princeton: Princeton University Press.

Gyatso, J. (1992). Genre, Authorship, and Transmission in Visionary Buddhism: The Literary Traditions of Thang-stong rGyal-po. In R. M. Davidson & S. D. Goodman (Eds.), *Tibetan Buddhism: Reason and Revelation* (pp. 95–106). Albany: State University of New York Press.

Gyatso, J. (1996). Drawn from the Tibetan Treasury: The gTer ma Literature. In J. Cabezón & R. Jackson (Eds.), *Tibetan Literature: Studies in Genre* (pp. 147–169). Ithaca, NY: Snow Lion Publications.

Gyatso, J. (1998). *Apparitions of the Self: The Secret Autobiographies of a Tibetan Visionary. A Translation and Study of Jigme Lingpa's Dancing Moon in the Water and Ḍākki's Grand Secret-talk.* Princeton: Princeton University Press.

Gyatso, J. (2012). Looking for Gender in the Medical Paintings of Desi Sangye Gyatso, Regent of the Tibetan Buddhist State. *Asian Medicine: Tradition and Modernity, 6*, 217–292.

Harding, S. (Trans.). (2003). *The Life and Revelations of Pema Lingpa.* Ithaca, NY: Snow Lion Publications.

Harding, S. (Trans.). (2007). *Jamgön Kongtrul, The Treasury of Knowledge: Esoteric Instructions.* Ithaca, NY: Snow Lion Publications.

Harding, S. (2010). *Niguma: Lady of Illusion.* Ithaca, NY: Snow Lion Publications.

Kilty, G. (Trans.). (2004). *K. Norsang Gyatso, Ornament of Stainless Light.* The Library of Tibetan Classics 14. Boston: Wisdom Publications.

Kragh, U. T. (2011). Prolegomenon to the Six Doctrines of Nā ro pa: Authority and Tradition. In R. Jackson & M. T. Kapstein (Eds.), *Mahāmudrā and the bKa'-brgyud Tradition. PIATS 2006: Tibetan Studies. Proceedings of the Eleventh Seminar of the International Association for Tibetan Studies, Königswinter 2006* (pp. 131–177). Beiträge zur Zentralasienforschung 25. Ambiast, Switzerland: International Institute for Tibetan and Buddhist Studies.

Larson, G. J. (2012). Pātañjala Yoga in Practice. In D. G. White (Ed.), *Yoga in Practice* (pp. 73–96). Princeton: Princeton University Press.

Lipman, K. (Trans.). (2010). *Secret Teachings of Padmasambhava: Essential Instructions on Mastering the Energies of Life.* Boston: Shambhala Publications.

Mallinson, J. (2011). Haṭha Yoga. In K. A. Jacobsen (Ed.), *Brill's Encylopedia of Hinduism.* Vol. 3 (pp. 770–781). Leiden: Brill.

Mallinson, J. (2012). Siddhi and Mahāsiddhi in Early Haṭhayoga. In K. A. Jacobsen (Ed.), *Yoga Powers: Extraordinary Capacities Attained in Meditation and Concentration* (pp. 327–344). Leiden: Brill.

Mallinson, J. (2014). The Yogīs' Latest Trick. *Journal of the Royal Asiatic Society, 24*(1), 165–180.

Mallinson, J. (forthc.). The Amṛtasiddhi, haṭhayoga's Tantric Buddhist Source Text. In D. Goodall et al. (Eds.), *Śaivism and the Tantric Traditions, a festschrift for Alexis Sanderson.* Leiden: Brill.

Mallinson, J. (2016). Śāktism and Haṭhayoga in the Śākta Traditions. In B. W. Olesen (Ed.), *Goddess Traditions in Tantric Hinduism: History, Practice and Doctrine* (pp. 109–140). London: Routledge.

Mayer, R. (1998). The Figure of Maheśvara/Rudra in the rNying ma Tantric Tradition. *Journal of the International Association of Buddhist Studies, 21*(2), 271–310.

Mayer, R. & Cantwell, C. (2012). *A Noble Noose of Methods: The Lotus Garland Synopsis. A Mahāyoga Tantra and its Commentary.* Beiträge zur Kultur- und Geistesgeschichte Asiens 73. Vienna: Verlag der Österreichischen Akademie der Wissenschaften.

Mroz, D. (2013). Towards the Motors of Tradition: A Report from the Field. Posted on Kung Fu Tea: Martial Arts History, Wing Chun, and Chinese Martial Studies, http://chinesemartialstudies.com.

Mullin, G. (Ed., Trans.). (1997). *Readings on the Six Yogas of Naropa.* Ithaca, NY: Snow Lion Publications.

Naldjorpa, K. (2014). The Traditional Methods and Practices of the Ancient Tradition of Yuthog Nyingthig. http://www.yuthok.net/node/38.

Namdak, T. (Trans.) & Dixey, R. (Ed.). (2002). *Heart Drops of Dharmakaya.* Boston: Wisdom Publications.

Namdak, T. & Reynolds, J. M. (Trans., Ed.). (2006). *Bonpo Dzogchen Teachings.* Boston: Wisdom Publications.

Norbu, N. & Clemente, A. (Trans.). (1999). *The Supreme Source: The Fundamental Tantra of the Dzogchen Semde (Kunjed Gyalpo).* Ithaca, NY: Snow Lion Publications.

Pert, C. (1999). *Molecules of Emotion: The Science behind Mind-Body Medicine.* New York: Scribner.

Samuel, G. (1993). *Civilized Shamans: Buddhism in Tibetan Societies.* Washington, DC: Smithsonian Institution Press.

Samuel, G. (2008). *Origins of Yoga and Tantra: Indic Religions to the Thirteenth Century.* Cambridge: Cambridge University Press.

Sanderson, A. (2009). The Śaiva Age: The Rise and Dominance of Śaivism during the Early Medieval Period. In S. Einoo (Ed.), *Genesis and Development of Tantrism* (pp. 41–350). Institute of Oriental Culture Special Series 23. Tokyo: University of Tokyo.

Schaeffer, K. R. (2002). The Attainment of Immortality: From Nāthas in India to Buddhists in Tibet. *Journal of Indian Philosophy, 30*(6), 515–533.

Scheidegger, D. (2007). Different Sets of Light-Channels in the Instruction Series of Rdzogs chen. *Revue d'Études Tibétaines, 12,* 40–64.

Schmidt, E. H. (Trans.). (1993). *T. N. Rangdröl, Empowerment and the Path of Liberation.* Hong Kong: Rangjung Yeshe Books.

Singleton, M. (2010). *Yoga Body: The Origins of Modern Postural Practice.* Oxford: Oxford University Press.

Singleton, M. & Mallinson, J. (2015). *The Roots of Yoga: A Sourcebook of Indic Traditions.* London: Penguin Classics.

Stearns, C. (2001). *Luminous Lives: The Story of the Early Masters of the Lam 'Bras Tradition in Tibet.* Boston: Wisdom Publications.

Stearns, C. (Ed., Trans.). (2006). *Taking the Result as the Path.* Boston: Wisdom Publications.

Trungpa, C. (1972). *Mudra: Early Songs and Poems.* Boston: Shambhala Publications.

Wallace, B. A. (Trans.). (1998). *K. Chagmé, A Spacious Path to Freedom: Practical Instructions on the Union of Mahamudra and Atiyoga.* Ithaca, NY: Snow Lion Publications.

Wallace, B. A. (Trans.). (2004). *Düdjom Lingpa, The Vajra Essence: From the Matrix of Primordial Consciousness and Pure Appearances, a Tantra on the Self-arisen Nature of Existence.* Ashland, OR: Mirror of Wisdom Publications.

Wang-Toutain, F. (2009). Introduction. In W. Luo (Ed.), *Samādhi of Completion: Secret Tibetan Yoga Illuminations from the Qing Court* (pp. 16–48). Beijing: The Forbidden City Publishing House.

Wangyal, T. (2002). *Healing with Form, Energy, and Light.* Ithaca, NY: Snow Lion Publications.

Wangyal, T. (2011). *Awakening the Sacred Body: Tibetan Yogas of Breath and Movement.* London: Hay House.

Winkelman, M. (1997). Altered States of Consciousness and Religious Behaviour. In S. Glazier (Ed.), *Anthropology of Religion: A Handbook of Method and Theory* (pp. 93–428). Westport, CT: Greenwood Press.

Part B.

Globalised Yoga

Chapter 9

Yoga within Viennese Occultism: Carl Kellner and Co.

Karl Baier

Contents

1. Occultism: A Neglected Dimension of Viennese Modernity 389

2. Kellner's Bourgeois Secular World 392

3. Theosophy, Rosicrucianism, and High-degree Freemasonry: Kellner's Bourgeois Occult World 394

4. Occult Philosophy of Nature: Hartmann, Vivekananda, and Kellner on Ether and Life Force, *Ākāśa* and *Prāṇa* 406

5. Kellner's Encounter with South Asian Yogis and His Essay on Yoga 409

6. Yoga and Ritual Sex within the Inner Occult Circle and the Early O.T.O. 421

7. A Mystical Ascension within the Pleasure Gardens: The Manuscript "Reincarnation" 427

8. Coda: Herbert Silberer's Theory of Mysticism 431

References 435

Karl Baier

Chapter 9: Yoga within Viennese Occultism: Carl Kellner and Co.

In this chapter, I will investigate the role of yoga within Viennese occultism focusing on Carl Kellner and other protagonists of this milieu who had close ties with him. In the introductory section, the term "occultism" and the state of research on Viennese occultism will be discussed. To give an idea of the background of Kellner's interest in yoga, I will be looking at his life and professional career and the fields of his occultist activities, namely his involvement in Theosophy, Rosicrucianism, and High-degree Freemasonry. The next section introduces the reader to Franz Hartmann's and Kellner's occult philosophies of nature and their striking similarities to concepts articulated some years later by Vivekananda in his famous *Raja Yoga.* After that, I will try to reconstruct core issues in Kellner's understanding of yoga. His encounter with South Asian yogis will be described, followed by an analysis of Kellner's sketch on yoga and of his manuscript "Reincarnation". Last but not least, the question of yoga and ritual sex within the so-called inner occult circle and the early Ordo Templi Orientis (O.T.O.) will be discussed. Addressing the role of yoga in his *Problems of Mysticism and its Symbolism,* the concluding part of the chapter will be an homage to Herbert Silberer, the most talented representative of second-generation Viennese occultism.

1. Occultism: A Neglected Dimension of Viennese Modernity

From the second half of the nineteenth century until the beginning of World War I, Vienna, then capital of the second-largest state in Europe, the Austro-Hungarian Empire, underwent rapid change. Many factors altered the face of this vibrant city. An increase in population (partly due to the large number of immigrants, especially Czechs and Jews from Eastern Europe) was accompanied by a strong upswing in the construction sector. Technological innovations, such as the tramway system, were introduced. A steady growth of the economy, at least from the late nineteenth century onwards, went hand in hand with rising food prices and rents. Social and economic tensions increased and cultural innovations created further frictions. Vienna became home to the cultural upper crust of the Empire. Much of the output of its cultural vanguard – from twelve-tone music to psychoanalysis – were to shape the culture of the twentieth century. The conservative authoritarian power cartel of the Habsburg dynasty, military leadership, and the Catholic Church that ruled the country was more or less hostile to the new cultural currents. Nevertheless, together with Paris, Berlin, London, and New York, Vienna became one of the centres of a cultural revolution later called "classical modernism".

It is striking that outstanding scholarly works such as the studies of Carl E. Schorske and Jacques Le Rider, as well as popular narratives of Viennese modernism, often neglect its religious innovations. Of course, city guides praise Otto Wagner's Kirche am Steinhof as a pivotal sacred building of the Viennese fin de siècle. The role of the Jews is discussed, and Herzl's Zionism is treated as part of Viennese modernity, as well as the anti-Semitic offspring of Viennese occultism represented by Guido von List and Lanz von Liebenfels – mainly because of their political relevance. Some studies interpret the mystical attitude of certain artists and writers as a symptom of the modern crisis of the individual. These exceptions aside, most of the literature at least implicitly seems to follow the rather outdated "modernisation equals secularisation" paradigm by presupposing that the Viennese modernist projects around 1900 did not comprise new forms of religion.

To compensate for this one-sidedness Robert W. Whalen goes so far as to claim that Viennese modernity was at once a basically religious phenomenon and the nucleus of classic modernism in general. "Classic modernism is the product of Viennese dreams. And these Viennese dreams were sacred dreams."[1] Although holding this (exaggerated) view, much like other explorers of fin-de-siècle Vienna, he is not interested in religious movements and writings per se, but focuses on the function of religious topics within the work of artists that belong to the codified list of proponents of Viennese modernity (Mahler, Schoenberg, Kokoschka, Klimt, Schnitzler, etc.). Whereas the religious strivings of some of the avant-garde artists are at least taken seriously, the numerous alternative religious movements of the time are only mentioned in passing as a sign of decadence.[2] Whalen is unable to see the importance of non-Christian or fringe Christian religious currents that, although excluded from the canon of Viennese modernism, were characterised by typically modern forms of religious experimentation and creativity.

1 Whalen 2007: 3.
2 Whalen 2007: 135–136.

In his seminal work *The Occult Establishment* (1976) James Webb already described the religious dimension of Viennese modernist culture in a less biased way.[3] He portrayed the circle of occultists around the fascinating polymath Friedrich Eckstein (1861–1939). The son of a Jewish paper manufacturer, a Freemason, writer, and private secretary to the composer Anton Bruckner, Eckstein was interested in Spiritism and came into contact with Theosophy through Franz Hartmann. In 1886 he met Mdm. Blavatsky in Ostende and consequently founded a theosophical lodge in Vienna. Additionally, he was involved in the neo-Rosicrucian circle of Alois Mailänder. Eckstein was a regular guest at the Café Imperial where he met his friends from the literary scene and from the occult milieu.

It was again Webb who disclosed links between Eckstein's circle and the Freudians, and for the first time described the connection of this group with occultist activities in Prague. Ten years later, Nicholas Goodrick-Clarke coined the term "modern occult revival in Vienna" for what was happening within this social stratum.[4] Very much like Webb, his article focuses on Eckstein's circle and adds some supplementary details about its history, members, and related groups. Incidentally, the term "occult revival" that Webb also uses was taken from Christopher McIntosh's famous study on Eliphas Lévi and the so-called French occult revival.[5] It is misleading insofar as it connotes the reappearance of an occultism that existed in earlier times or even since time immemorial.[6]

What emerged in Vienna and other capitals of modernity was not so much the comeback of an ancient phenomenon but the transformation and spread of relatively new forms of unchurched religiosity among the cultural and social elites of the city, and, at times, as was the case with Spiritism, within all kinds of social strata. These currents integrated elements from early-modern movements and new ideas from physics, psychology, the emerging parapsychology, and other sciences. Last but not least, due to Theosophy, there was growing interest in

3 Webb 1976: 41–47.

4 Goodrick-Clarke 1986.

5 McIntosh 1974. McIntosh triggered a kind of fashion among historians to discover "occult revivals". The "occult revival" in France was followed by a British, Russian, American, German, and – since Goodrick-Clarke – also a Viennese revival. The valuable study by Eugen Semrau on the influences of esoteric thought on Viennese modernity (Semrau 2012) takes into account the methodological improvements of recent esotericism research. Instead of postulating an occult revival he analyses "the diffusion of esoteric knowledge" around 1900 (Semrau 2012: 115–138). Semrau adds interesting information on Freemasonry to our picture of Viennese occultism. Concerning the topic of this chapter, he does not present significant new material.

6 McIntosh conceived of occultism as a kind of eternal underground of human culture. See McIntosh 1974: 11: "Occult movements and secret cults have always played a significant part in society. Like a subterranean current they have moved beneath the ground of history, occasionally bursting forth to flow for a spell in the light of day, revealing some strange and exotic fish in the process."

adding South Asian ingredients (especially yoga) to this melting pot of belief systems, symbols, and practices.

In the following, the term "occultism" is not used in an essentialist way, as by McIntosh, but as a historiographical category that designates this particular phenomenon of the nineteenth and early twentieth century. In Vienna, the most important movements within this field were Theosophy, Spiritism, psychical research, modern magic, Guido von List's Theosophy (which influenced racist Ariosophy), High-degree Freemasonry, and Rosicrucianism.

Viennese occultism was, of course, not isolated but – as Webb already saw – participated in an internationally connected middle-European network that besides Vienna had its centres in German-speaking Prague, Munich, and Budapest. Moreover, several participants in this field were affiliated to occult groups and networks of almost worldwide range. They contributed to the emergence of Vienna as a global cultural metropolis.

For the remainder of this chapter I would like to focus on one of the most interesting representatives of Viennese occultism: Carl Kellner. He was an important node in the network that constituted the relatively small but nevertheless influential and highly creative milieu of central European occultists interested in yoga.

2. Kellner's Bourgeois Secular World

Carl Kellner (1851–1905), a typical self-made-man of the Gründerzeit, was brought up in modest circumstances and eventually became an electrochemist, inventor, and industrial magnate, one of the richest industrialists of the Habsburg Monarchy.[7] His wealth was based more on his inventiveness than on his qualities as a businessman:

> Dr. Kellner [...] was undoubtedly a genius but in no sense a business man and from the business point of view a most trying and difficult man to work with. After working on a new idea a short time he would lose interest and come with something entirely new.[8]

As early as 1873, he accidentally discovered a cost-saving method for producing paper-pulp that revolutionised cellulose production and paper-manufacture. At that time he worked for Baron Eugen Hector von Ritter-Záhony at his paper mills

7 Some authors date Kellner's birth in 1850. According to *Österreichisches Biographisches Lexikon,* he was born in 1851. Sources for Kellner's biography are: *Österreichisches Biographisches Lexikon* 1815–1950 (ÖBL), vol. 3, Verlag Österreichische Akademie der Wissenschaften, Wien 1965, p. 290; Möller & Howe 1986; Weirauch 1998; Kaczynski 2012: 67–92.

8 H. W. Davis, *The Kellner-Partington Paper Pulp Company Ltd.* Salzburg: n.p., 1930, quoted in Möller & Howe 1986: 86.

in Görz (Ital. Gorizia) who supported the development of the new technique. In 1882, it was patented as the Ritter-Kellner Process.

In 1885, Carl married Marie Antoinette Delorme, the daughter of a well-known hotelier in Trieste in whose hotel Kellner lived while he was working in nearby Görz. He had four children with her, three girls and a boy. All available sources describe him as a kind and loving father who was admired by all family members. Several witnesses who participated in Kellner's private sphere affirmed that he was a charming and helpful person.

Every now and then, the Kellners displayed signs of imposture, e.g., when Carl occasionally used the doctoral degree without having finished any University study or when Marie called herself "Marion de Kellner" as if they were aristocrats.

In 1889 Kellner started one of the largest pulp manufacturing companies of the world, the Kellner-Partington Paper Pulp Company, in collaboration with the British industrial magnate and freemason Edward Partington. The headquarters of the company were in Vienna. Several factories were founded in different areas of the world, among them one in Hallein near Salzburg where the Kellner family lived in a villa.

In the early 1890s, Kellner's professional and his occultist life merged in the form of a co-operation with the Theosophist Franz Hartmann. Hartmann had developed a treatment for curing tuberculosis and other respiratory ailments using lignosulphite, a by-product of the cellulose manufacture in Kellner's factories. With the financial and technical support of Kellner, they finally opened an "inhalatorium" in Hallein in 1894 with Hartmann as director.

In the same year, Kellner patented a process that cheapened the production of alkalis and other chemical substances by using a mercury cathode cell. One year later, the Castner-Kellner Alkali Company was founded. The American co-founder Hamilton Young Castner had independently developed and patented a very similar cell. "Castner-Kellner cells were soon operating in England, Austria, Germany, France, Belgium, Italy, Sweden, and Russia."[9]

Kellner owned a large industrial laboratory in Vienna where he worked with academically trained chemists.[10] With his team he developed a large number of inventions and came up with new products like spun fibres, light bulbs, and synthetic gem-stones, many of which became registered patents. Moreover, Kellner was engaged in fundamental chemical research. In 1901, he deposited a sealed letter at the Austrian Academy of Sciences in which he advanced the

9 Kaczynski 2012: 70.
10 Weirauch 1998: 205.

argument that the chemical elements are transformable into each other. He also proposed experimental procedures to prove his theory.[11]

The work within Kellner's laboratory was apparently quite dangerous. One of his assistants died there for reasons that have remained unclear. After an accident in the laboratory in 1904, Kellner was hospitalised for a longer period of time. To complete his recovery he and his wife spent some time in Egypt. All seemed to work out well, but one month after their return to Vienna Kellner had a heart attack and died on the 7th of June 1905. He was only 54 years old. According to the medical report the cause of his death was "paralysis of the heart caused by chronic blood poisoning, due to purulence."[12] Soon after, legends arose that were structured around two myths: that of the magician who is unable to master the powers that he had evoked, and that of the magician who is cursed by another magician. Thus, commentators connected Kellner's disease and early death with his occult activities.[13]

3. Theosophy, Rosicrucianism, and High-degree Freemasonry: Kellner's Bourgeois Occult World

For the fin-de-siècle culture of Europe, North America, and South Asia, occultism was a serious religious option for the members of the upper and middle classes. With the exception of some shady characters who tried to make their fortune in the new religious market, the upstart millionaire Kellner was in good company within his wealthy occult circles.

Viennese occultism was deeply linked with the broader process of cultural transformations that encompassed innovations within the fine arts, music, literature, architecture, psychology, and other sciences. The journal *Wiener Rundschau* illustrates the close interrelatedness of these fields. The periodical for culture and arts with a focus on literature was published fortnightly between 1896 and 1901. It had a broad readership among the cultural elite of Vienna. The *Wiener Rundschau* published translations of Oscar Wilde, Walt Whitman, Leo Tolstoi, Maurice Maeterlinck, and Stéphane Mallarmé as well as the German poetry of Rainer Maria

11 See Kellner 1896b. The letter was opened by the archivists of the Austrian Academy of Science and made publicly available in the early 1980s.

12 Josef Dvorak in Weirauch 1998: 205: "Herzlähmung in Folge chronischer Eitervergiftung des Blutes."

13 Maybe his death was in a less magical way connected with his occult interests. In search for the elixir of life, Kellner very probably performed alchemical experiments in his laboratory (see below, p. 398). As mercury is of crucial importance in alchemy, he may have died from mercury poisoning. I thank Suzanne Newcombe for raising this point and for other helpful comments on an earlier draft of this chapter.

Rilke, Stefan George, and Hugo von Hofmannsthal. Very similar to French Symbolism and English Decadence, all those poets represented a new understanding of poetry and literature in opposition to the naturalistic style in literature and fine arts. Their contributions were interwoven with articles from occultists, whereas the official state religion, Catholicism, was almost totally absent.[14] Thus, the *Wiener Rundschau* became the most important public platform for the interaction between fin-de-siècle alternative religion and other areas of modernist culture in Vienna. Through their regular contributions in the *Rundschau,* the occultists positioned themselves as part of the cultural avant-garde, especially as explorers of the "cutting edge" of human knowledge where, from their point of view, ancient wisdom and the latest scientific achievements began to merge.

One of the occultist writers who regularly contributed to the journal was the physician Franz Hartmann (1838–1912), already mentioned above as collaborator of Kellner who introduced Friedrich Eckstein to Theosophy. He was a former close associate of Helena Blavatsky and had served as chairman of the Board of Control of the Theosophical Society in Adyar, Chennai. Hartmann was one of the most important theosophical writers of his time. He published many books and the monthly journals *Lotusblüthen* (1893–1900) and *Neue Lotusblüten* (1908–1913). Hartmann not only edited these journals but also wrote most of the articles himself or translated them from English. His articles on yoga were important for the popularisation of this topic within Germany and Austria.[15] In "Die Bhagavad-Gita der Indier" from 1899 he defines yoga for the readers of the *Wiener Rundschau:*

> "Yoga" is derived from Yog = to join and means the union of the human soul with God. It therefore would be an equivalent to the term "religion" if this word had not been misused like many similar ones and had not been identified with churchdom, so that it has almost lost its true meaning. Yoga is the art of self-control through the divine spirit that awakes to consciousness within us. [...] Every religious practice, insofar as it is performed selflessly and without hidden agenda, is a Yoga exercise.[16]

14 Several occultists who wrote for the *Wiener Rundschau* were members of the "Psychologische Gesellschaft" in Munich, a society concerned with psychic research, mysticism, hypnosis, etc. Its founder, the occultist philosopher and famous spiritualist Carl Du Prel, influenced the content orientation of the Viennese journal. He regularly published articles in the *Rundschau* and was in contact with poets like Rilke, Maeterlinck, and George who also wrote for the journal. Du Prel thus functioned as a kind of mentor for the emerging Viennese "occulture" that was represented by the *Rundschau.*

15 After Hartmann's death in August 1902, the 1903 issue of *Neue Lotusblüten* was published by Paul Harald Grävell von Jostenoode, who also contributed several articles to the *Wiener Rundschau.*

16 Hartmann 1899: 353: "'Yoga' kommt von Yog = verbinden, und bedeutet die Verbindung der menschlichen Seele mit Gott. Es würde dem Worte 'Religion' entsprechen, wenn dieses Wort nicht, wie so viele andere ähnliche Worte, sooft missbraucht und mit 'Kirchenthum' verwechselt worden wäre, dass es beinahe seine wahre Bedeutung verloren hat. Yoga ist die

Hartmann introduces the term as a traditional South Asian concept but at the same time uses it as a category for all kinds of religious practices that support the experience of mystical union with ultimate reality and thereby lead to the core of all religion. This view of yoga fit with the religious agenda of the *Wiener Rundschau*. Many of its writers combined a negative attitude towards the hegemonic religion ("churchdom"), on the one hand, with criticism of materialism and naturalistic art, on the other. The approval of symbolist art based on visionary experiences went hand in hand with a mystical attitude that linked the autonomy of the individual ("self-control") with the discovery of the divine spirit within oneself. As we will see, Kellner also shared the religious attitude that Hartmann associated with yoga.

Although one of the important players of Viennese upper-class occultism, Kellner did not fit into the sociological circle-structure of Viennese modernity. It is difficult to relate him to a specific group. Being a friend of Eckstein and Hartmann, Kellner was, of course, connected to Theosophy and Eckstein's circle. According to Franz Hartmann, he joined the Theosophical Society in 1887.[17]

It is unknown in which theosophical group he took part; most likely it was Eckstein's Viennese theosophical lodge. His theosophical connections are important for our topic, since the Theosophical Society was the main source of information on yoga and also provided translations of yoga scriptures.

Vienna was not Kellner's permanent residence until 1896, when the Kellner family moved from Hallein to the capital. Additionally, due to his business obligations Kellner spent a lot of time abroad. In this respect he resembled Hartmann, who also knew Eckstein and time and again would stay with him in Vienna. But as someone without permanent residence he was not fully integrated in any Viennese circle. He travelled a lot giving talks in Austria, Hungary, Germany, and Switzerland. As director of the lignosulphite inhalatorium he was based in Hallein. Time and again, Hartmann spent longer periods of time in Italy, a country that he appreciated very much and where he bought a villa in 1899.[18] Therefore, Viennese occultism consisted not only of stationary groups (with Eckstein's circle as an important upper-class institution and other, less explored groups), but also of mobile, internationally connected key players.

Kunst, durch den in uns zum Bewusstsein erwachten göttlichen Geist sich selbst zu beherrschen […]. Jede praktische Ausübung der Religion, wenn sie selbstlos und ohne Hintergedanken erfolgt, ist eine Yoga-Übung." All translations from the original German in this chapter are by the author.

17 It is very likely that Kellner and Blavatsky met. According to Karl-Erwin Lichtenecker (interview with the author, 11 February 2014), he at least possessed a photo of Blavatsky with her autograph. Blavatsky used to give autographs to visitors.

18 Lechler 2013: 150.

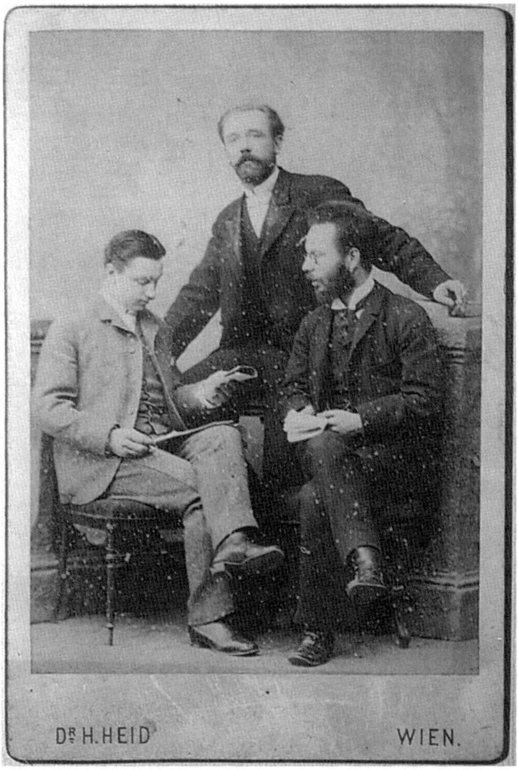

Figure 1: Carl Kellner (middle) with the Theosophists Gustav Gebhard (left) and Friedrich Eckstein (right) (photograph courtesy of Josef Dvorak).

It seems that Kellner's involvement with occultism did not start with Theosophy. Already the young Carl's decision to work in the field of chemistry most probably had occult roots. According to Paul Köthner (1902: 21) and John Yarker (1905) he inherited Rosicrucian manuscripts from his grandfather who was allegedly a Rosicrucian, manuscripts that brought him to alchemical experiments as well as to chemistry.[19] Köthner and Yarker independently claim that Kellner himself informed them about his early encounter with alchemy. Both authors had their own occult agendas and therefore one can suspect that they were interested in "occulticising" Kellner's biography.[20] Their statements have to be treated with

19 See also Kaczynski 2012: 67.

20 John Yarker (1833–1913) was an influential English high-degree freemason and theosophist who published books on Freemasonry, the mysteries of antiquity, and Modern Rosicrucianism. Paul Köthner (1870–1932) was not only a chemist who worked at the universities of Halle and Berlin, but also a freemason and occultist. After World War I, he turned away from Freemasonry and published writings in which he mixed an anti-Semitic, extreme right-wing attitude with alchemy, astrology, hermetism, etc.

caution. Nevertheless, apart from this general suspicion, in this case we do not have any reason to assume that they were spreading falsehoods.

Kellner's chemical experiments that aimed at the transmutation of chemical elements into each other can easily be understood as an attempt to use modern technology and especially high voltage electricity to pursue the old alchemical goal. Kellner himself "loved to speak of these kind of experiments as 'alchemistic'"[21] and his fellow occultists also conceived of them as such. Hartmann reports that Kellner had a special backroom for his alchemical experiments in his Viennese laboratory.[22]

In an interview with the author Karl-Erwin Lichtenecker (1929–2014), a grandchild of Carl Kellner, confirmed that according to the oral family tradition that was passed on to him by his mother Eglantine, the oldest child of the Kellners, Kellner tried to find the elixir of life, a substance (not necessarily a liquid) that would be capable of prolonging human life immensely if not produce immortality.[23]

Hartmann was the first to state that the elixir of life was the aim of Kellner's alchemical experiments. He emphasised that alchemy had been Kellner's passion:

> He was a born mystic, a 'genius' by intuition; he occupied himself with studies of occult science all his life, and his great 'hobby,' if it may be called such, was the practice of Alchemy.[24]

He connects Kellner's interest in yoga with his alchemical aspirations. Kellner would have looked for yoga practices, he says, to attain the occult powers necessary for successful alchemical work. According to Hartmann, he was first taught by Bheema Sena Pratapa and later by Sri Agamya Guru Paramahamsa (we will come back to these two men below) both staying for weeks and months in his house.[25] Kellner seemed to be very happy with the yoga he learnt from Agamya that, as Hartmann enigmatically says, was comprised of "breathing exercises and other things".[26] Hartmann quotes a passage from a letter of Kellner, stating that through Agamya's teachings, he finally found what he had been striving for all his life. One of the results would have been intensified alchemical work:

21 Dr. Carl Kellner [obituary] 1905: 2.
22 Hartmann 1923–1924: 308.
23 Lichtenecker 2014. With regard to Rosicrucian alchemy it is interesting to note that Kellner's name as a Freemason was Br. Renatus. "Renatus" means "the reborn" and may also refer to the first alchemical treatise of the Order of the Golden and Rosy Cross that was published by the founder of the Order, Samuel Richter, under the pseudonym Sincerus Renatus in 1710.
24 Hartmann 1906: 133–134.
25 Hartmann 1906: 133 and 1923–1924: 307–308.
26 Hartmann 1906: 133.

> He continued his alchemical experiments with renewed vigour, and it appears from his correspondence that his experiments in making the *Elixir of Life*, during the first stages of the process, were successful, as the material employed went through the changes described in the old books of alchemy and in the *Secret Symbols of the Rosicrucians of the 16th and 17th Century*.[27]

But, according to Hartmann, the alchemical work ultimately spun out of control. In the same article, published in 1906, he quotes two other letters from Kellner. Both deal with alchemical experiments and describe them as a fight with dark occult powers:

> (April 26, 1904): 'I am progressing favourably with my experiments. At the same time I have to contend continually with a very gruesome crowd of…. for the preparation of the Elixir. However, I begin to get accustomed to that fight, as a trainer of wild animals gets familiar with ferocious beasts. At first it seemed as if the blood would freeze in my veins; but …'
> Again he writes in answer to my objections: –
> 'I agree with you, that these arts as such are perhaps objectionable; but they are at least a new field of knowledge, and in so far they must be of some use. However, the dwellers of the threshold are to be dreaded; there are hosts of them guarding the door.'[28]

An extended version of Hartmann's article from 1906 published in German several years later again contains the two quotations from Kellner's letters, but the cited texts differ significantly.[29]

Both letters (and especially the English version) allude to a passage of Bulwer-Lytton's *Zanoni* that explains why the elixir of life is a deadly poison for all those who are not ready to face the effects it has on those who take it.[30] The elixir would sharpen the senses so that the creatures that dwell within the medium sphere between the earthly and the spiritual realm become visible and audible. Among them there would be cruel beings full of hatred called guardians or dwellers of the threshold because they prevent the unprepared from entering the spiritual realm. The dwellers are able to cause a literally killing horror within all those who have not abandoned all earthly desires by ascetic practice. It may well be that Kellner, who was familiar with Bulwer-Lytton's novel, interpreted the emotional problems that occurred along with his alchemical work by referring to *Zanoni*. But it is just as possible that Hartmann introduced the encounter with the dwellers of the threshold as a frame to interpret Kellner's early death. Obviously, he was not very interested in precise citations. He used Kellner's early death to give a theo-

27 Hartmann 1906: 134 [Hartmann's emphases].
28 Ibid.
29 Hartmann 1923–1924: 308.
30 Cf. Bulwer-Lytton 1842: 214–217.

sophical moral lesson, warning that occult experiments and yogic exercises motivated by egoistic purposes in the end would destroy the practitioner's life.

Hartmann's view that Kellner's main interest in yoga was connected to his ambition to produce the elixir of life may be exaggerated. But it is plausible that Kellner saw a strong relation between his spiritual improvements through yoga practice and his alchemical advancements, as the belief in the interconnectedness of the alchemist's state of mind and the results of alchemical laboratory work was common within his occultist milieu.

The alchemical practice that for the chemist Kellner was a valued link between his secular and occult life was in no way his individual peculiarity. Together with other German, Viennese, and Prague occultists (Gustav Gebhard and his wife, Wilhelm Hübbe-Schleiden, Hartmann, Eckstein, Graf zu Leiningen-Billigheim, and Gustav Meyrink) he participated for several years in the Rosicrucian "Bund der Verheissung" of Alois Mailänder (1844–1905).[31] Among the followers of Mailänder, alchemical thought and to a certain extent also practice was common. According to Sven Eek, Hartmann obtained from the Mailänder circle a at that time rare copy of the famous Rosicrucian work *Geheime Figuren der Rosenkreuzer aus dem 16ten und 17ten Jahrhundert* that contains several alchemical texts and illustrations.[32] As a matter of fact, he published the first English translation of this book with his theosophical commentaries in 1888 as *Secret Symbols of the Rosicrucians.*[33] A member of Mailänder's group, a carpenter and itinerant Rosicrucian and alchemist named Prestel was Mailänder's spiritual teacher. He possessed a bottle of grey salt about which he said it would be the "unfinished" elixir of life. Hartmann published an interesting explanation for Pretel's inability to reach the highest goal of alchemy. It shows that gender issues and sexuality were connected to alchemy within the Mailänder circle:

> Now, this man was not a full-fledged Alchemist, and could not make gold and the *Elixir of Life*, because, as he said, he could not find a woman sufficiently *pure*, and at the same time willing, to assist him in his labours; for, as it is known to all Alchemists, it requires the co-operation of the *male* and the *female* element to accomplish the highest process.[34]

31 The weaver Alois Mailänder lived in Kempten where he was the leader of a small Christian fringe group of factory workers and their wives. He was discovered by occult high society thanks to the leading German theosophist Wilhelm Hübbe-Schleiden at the end of 1884. From 1890 onwards he lived and taught in Dreieichenhain, a small village south of Frankfurt.

32 See Eek 1978: 609. Unfortunately, Eek does not quote any source that substantiates this claim. In his *Secret Symbols of the Rosicrucians,* Hartmann does not mention from whom he got his copy.

33 See Kaczynski 2012: 65.

34 Hartmann 1888: 235, footnote [Hartmann's emphases].

At least one other member of the group besides Prestel and Kellner, Gustav Meyrink, known for never shrinking from any form of occult practice, performed alchemical experiments.[35]

As far as I can see, from the closure of the Order of the Golden and Rosy Cross in 1787 until the end of the nineteenth century there were no larger organisations around to promote Rosicrucianism and alchemy in Central Europe. Elements of them have survived within high-degree masonic orders. Moreover, they flourished in small non-masonic groups like Mailänder's circle. Additionally, they were developed and passed on to these small groups by individuals like Prestel.[36]

Among our occultists Mailänder was famous for teaching a certain meditation technique that was considered to be of Rosicrucian origin. It can be traced back to the opera tenor, singing teacher, and Freemason Johann Baptist Krebs (1774–1851), also known by his pen name, J. B. Kerning. The occultist students of the Kerning–Mailänder tradition who were interested in South Asian wisdom, namely Kellner, Hübbe-Schleiden, Meyrink, Karl Weinfurter, and Hartmann thought it was a kind of Christian and German yoga and they appreciated it primarily because of the yoga not because of its Christian inspiration. "It is strange that Kerning already knew the yoga postures and other Indian practices," remarked Weinfurter, continuing: "At his time no translations of Indian books into European languages existed. One can only explain this through the power of clairvoyance which he acquired."[37] And Kellner writes in his sketch of yoga:

> Finally, I have to mention, that among the Christian mystics, Jakob Boehme in his discourse between the master and his disciple and J. Krebs who published on this topic in the 1850s under the pen name Kerning [...] represent the best that has ever been written in German about yoga practices, albeit in a form that might not be to everyone's taste.[38]

---

35 Binder 2009: 199–204.

36 The first important Neo-Rosicrucian organisation was the Societas Rosicruciana in Anglia founded in 1865 by English Freemasons. It spread within the English-speaking countries but was not active in the Habsburg monarchy. Some ten years later a second wave of organised Neo-Rosicrucianism emerged in the USA triggered by the occult orders founded by Paschal Beverly Randolph (1825–1875). In 1888, the Kabbalistic Order of the Rose-Croix was founded in France followed by the Order of the Martinists in 1891. In fin-de-siècle Central Europe, several interested individuals got in contact with these organisations but seemingly no successful institutionalisation took place.

37 Weinfurter 1930: 120.

38 Kellner 1896a: 6: "Erwähnen muss ich nur noch, dass unter den christlichen Mystikern Jakob Boehme in seinem Gespräch des Meisters mit dem Schüler, und der unter dem Pseudonym: Kerning in den fünfziger Jahren auf diesem Gebiete literarisch tätig gewesene J. Krebs [...] das Beste über Yogaübungen in deutscher Sprache geschrieben haben, allerdings in einer Form, die nicht nach jedermanns Geschmack ist."

The practice that reminded the occultists of yoga comprised the murmuring or silent repetition of short sentences and words with Christian background and of certain letters originally used in masonic rituals, conscious breathing, symbolic gestures, postures, and movements. The core of these exercises was concentration on different parts of the body from the feet upwards and especially on certain mystical centres. The practitioners imagined writing or saying the letters or words within these parts of the body. The meditation aimed at the awakening of the divine "inner word" to enable it to permeate and transform the human body and reconnect the human being with the universe.[39]

Like vocal coach and drama teacher François Delsarte (1811–1871), Kerning and Mailänder combined a new appreciation of the human body and physical exercises with alternative religious concepts. Thereby they laid the foundation for the occultist reception of modern physical culture and of body-centred yoga practices. The teachings of Kerning and Mailänder seemingly triggered a positive attitude towards Haṭha Yoga within Viennese and Prague occultism. As Meyrink clearly saw, the practices taught by Kerning and Mailänder contradict the theosophical concept of astral projection that aimed at separation from the physical body as the highest aim of spiritual development. The anti-ecstatic principle of "remaining in one's body" and deepening daily life consciousness enabled Meyrink to criticise astral projection as the "worst kind of schizophrenia".[40] His thanks for this insight go to Mailänder: "If the only thing I had learnt from this man was that the body must be included in the transformation of the person through yoga, he would have earned my lifelong gratitude for that insight alone."[41] Weinfurter understood the teachings of Kerning and Mailänder in the very same way:

> Master Kerning ceaselessly points to the fact that God is present *within the whole human body.* [...] Ninety-nine per cent of the occultists and Theosophists believe that human mystical development starts *within the soul. This view is one of the greatest mistakes of modern occult literature.* [...] Exactly the opposite is *true.* Mystical blossoming first happens *within the body,* taking place in the form of body sensations that nobody knows who has not experienced them and who did not enter the mystical path.[42]

39 The practices of Kerning and Mailänder and their reception within Viennese and Prague occultism are described in Binder 2009: 131–136, 195–198.

40 Meyrink 2010: 141.

41 Meyrink 2010: 138.

42 Weinfurter 1930: 222: "Meister Kerning weist unaufhörlich auf die Tatsache hin, daß Gott *im ganzen Körper* des Menschen gegenwärtig ist. [...] Neunundneunzig Prozent der Okkultisten und auch der Theosophen vermeint, dass die mystische Entwicklung beim Menschen in *der Seele* beginne! *Diese Ansicht ist einer der größten Irrtümer der modernen okkulten Literatur.* [...] Gerade das Umgekehrte ist das *Richtige.* Die mystische Entfaltung geschieht zu Anfang *im Körper*, vollzieht sich in körperlichen Empfindungen, die aber solcher Art und solchen

The Kerning-inspired exercises obviously influenced the image of yoga within Viennese occultism. Yoga was primarily understood as a practice that uses breathing exercises and postures to create certain bodily sensations that transform the whole human being and lead to a liberating experience of ultimate reality and immortality.

This concept of yoga found its way into the oeuvre of Sigmund Freud. It is Kellner's friend Eckstein whom Freud refers to when he writes in the first chapter of his *Civilization and its Discontents* (1930):[43]

> Another friend of mine, whose insatiable craving for knowledge has led him to make the most unusual experiments and has ended by giving him encyclopaedic knowledge, has assured me that through the practices of Yoga, by withdrawing from the world, by fixing the attention on bodily functions and by peculiar methods of breathing, one can in fact evolve new sensations and coenaesthesias in oneself, which he regards as regressions to primordial states of mind which have long ago been overlaid. He sees in them a physiological basis, as it were, of much of the wisdom of mysticism. It would not be hard to find connections here with a number of obscure modifications of mental life, such as trances and ecstasies.[44]

What Freud learned from Eckstein about yoga mirrors the views of the Viennese occultists. His rendering of Eckstein's understanding of yoga emphasises *prāṇāyāma,* physiological functions, and bodily sensations. But instead of references to hypnotism and somnambulism that were still common within occultism, a new and typical psychoanalytic element is added: the interpretation of yogic states as regression. Interestingly, in the quoted passage, Freud ascribes this theory to Eckstein without making mention of the psychoanalyst Franz Alexander who, as far as we know, first published it in 1922. Eckstein wrote several contributions to psychoanalysis and was able to explain yoga to Freud in a terminology that the famous psychologist could accept, although he ultimately remained sceptical about the relevance of these strange yogic states of body and mind.

Charakters sind, daß niemand sie kennt, der sie nicht erlebte, der den Weg der Mystik nicht angetreten hat." [Weinfurter's emphases].

43 According to Mulot-Déri 1988: 302, Anna Freud confirmed that Freud refers here to Eckstein. The description of his friend as a man with encyclopaedic knowledge also fits well with the reputation Eckstein had for being a polymath.

44 Freud 1962: 19–20. Cf. the original German text in Freud 1999: 430–431: "Ein anderer meiner Freunde, den ein unstillbarer Wissensdrang zu den ungewöhnlichsten Experimenten getrieben und endlich zum Allwisser gemacht hat, versicherte mir, daß man in den Yogapraktiken durch Abwendung von der Außenwelt, durch Bindung der Aufmerksamkeit an körperliche Funktionen, durch besondere Weisen der Atmung tatsächlich neue Empfindungen und Allgemeingefühle in sich erwecken kann, die er als Regressionen zu uralten, längst überlagerten Zuständen des Seelenlebens auffassen will. Er sieht in ihnen eine sozusagen physiologische Begründung vieler Weisheiten der Mystik. Beziehungen zu manchen dunklen Modifikationen des Seelenlebens, wie Trance und Ekstase, lägen hier nahe."

In an occultist context, Eckstein used a different language to describe the body experiences connected to spiritual development. In this regard, Jules Sauerwein is an important witness.[45] "Eckstein gave me certain illuminating teachings in regard to the inner life", he writes in 1929,

> which are just as precious to me now as they were twenty three years ago. It was he, who taught me, for example, that before the etheric body can be brought into a state of true equilibrium, one must reach the point, where consciousness of the various parts of the etheric body can be extended to the corresponding regions of the physical body. Under ordinary conditions we think in our head, sense our emotions and impulses in the region of the heart and sympathetic system, while in the rest of the body we are merely aware of sensory or motor stimuli. I learned from Eckstein something I had not discovered in Theosophy, namely, that before a man can be conscious of the principle higher than the physical body – the etheric body – he must learn to think in every part of his being – in other words, he must bring his visible and invisible organs into conscious spiritual activity by means of the currents circulating in the etheric body.[46]

Eckstein told Sauerwein that he had learnt this knowledge from a student of Kerning, a certain "W…" who lived in Stuttgart. This implies that he did not only practise Kerning exercises under the guidance of Mailänder, but had a second teacher. The only one to be able to fulfil this function could have been the Stuttgart-based building surveyor Weiß, the last direct student of Kerning, who died in 1916 at the age of 96. Eckstein seemingly is another representative of the blending of Kerning's occult body techniques and yoga that is so typical for Viennese and Prague fin-de-siècle occultism.

The last important element of Kellner's occultism is Freemasonry. In 1873 he was initiated at the masonic lodge Humanitas in Neudörfl and in the same year was awarded the fellow craft degree.[47] In 1875, Kellner was expelled from Humanitas because he did not fulfil his masonic duties.[48] One of the reasons for this may have been that travelling to Neudörfl was quite difficult and may have taken too much time for a busy entrepreneur and inventor.

Additionally, Blue Lodge Freemasonry (consisting of the three basic masonic degrees of entered apprentice, fellow craft, and master mason) did not fulfil Kellner's expectations. In his obituary for Kellner, Hartmann wrote about his further career within Freemasonry: "He soon turned to high-degree Freemasonry

45 Jules Sauerwein (1880–1967) was a famous French journalist who came to Vienna as a young man in 1904 and got into contact with Viennese occultism. Besides his journalistic work he translated many writings of Rudolf Steiner whom he met during his stay in Vienna. I would like to thank Rolf Speckner for providing Sauerwein's text.

46 Sauerwein 1929: 414.

47 Neudörfl was a so-called border-lodge ("Grenzloge") in Hungary close to the Austrian border. These lodges were established because at that time Freemasonry was illegal in Austria.

48 Lechler 2013: 145.

and on his long and frequent journeys he gained the highest grades and greatest honours that a mason is able to achieve."[49] In his later years, Kellner openly criticised Blue Lodge Freemasonry for having lost its secret and for only pursuing humanitarian aspirations.[50] On the other hand, he conceived of the high-degree systems as keepers of the secret of true Freemasonry. It is unknown into which systems and where Kellner was initiated between 1873 and 1895. According to Theodor Reuss, Kellner also came into contact with the Hermetic Brotherhood of Light that was founded in 1895 in Boston. In the latter year, he discussed his ambitious idea to establish an Academia Masonica, a kind of academy of High-degree Freemasonry with Reuss, a project that, if Reuss is telling the truth, was inspired by his encounter with the Brotherhood of Light. The idea of such an academy was not new:

> The Grand Orient de France operated a Grand College of Rites which had jurisdiction over all high degrees within France, and Scotland had its Supreme Council of Rites. [...] What was new was that this had not been attempted before in Germany. Many high-degree rites had not found their way to Germany, and Kellner hoped to fill this void by creating a German-language College of Rites that could administer as many of these rites as possible.[51]

It took some years until this vision became a reality. Kellner in the end collaborated with Reuss, the busy and quite dubious inventor and manager of occult organisations, and some other people from Germany's masonic milieu including Hartmann. In order to kick off this kind of organisation, it was of vital importance to collect authorisations for high-degree rites. In 1902 Kellner and his masonic collaborators managed to make a deal with Yarker who was Sovereign Grand Master of the united rites of Memphis and Misraim and of the Ancient and Accepted Scottish Rite. Yarker signed a charter for "The Sovereign Sanctuary 33°–95° etc., in and for the Empire of Germany" that authorised them to administer both rites.[52] Kellner became patron and Honorary Grand Master General of the new Sovereign Sanctuary. The "acting members" carried out the organisational work. It does not seem that Kellner as "patron" took part in it. The sanctuary was located in Berlin, where Reuss as Grand Master General ran the whole masonic order.

It also does not look as if Kellner participated in continuous masonic ritual work. Volker Lechler and Wolfgang Kistemann write about him, Reuss and Hartmann as the three leaders of the order:

49 Emanuel 1905: 2.

50 "One is just as little a true freemason if one only visits the lodges and spends money for widows as one is a true Christian if one only goes to church and gives alms" (Kellner 1903: 15).

51 Kaczynski 2012: 185.

52 Kaczynski 2012: 196.

> The three could only have sporadic contacts because they lived scattered throughout Europe. From a steady and ordered corporate work as high-degree freemasons they were literarily miles away.[53]

To become "Honorary Grand Master General" may have satisfied Kellner's ambition to occupy a leading position within the elite of occultism and to gain a kind of priestly authority. It is, however, questionable how intense his involvement really was. Nevertheless, during the last few years of Kellner's life, High-degree Freemasonry provided a kind of institutional and ritual frame for his religious practice and the social structure within which he developed and taught his worldview and occult practices, including what he and his fellow occultists conceived of as yogic exercises.

4. Occult Philosophy of Nature: Hartmann, Vivekananda, and Kellner on Ether and Life Force, *Ākāśa* and *Prāṇa*

During the first half of the 1890s, when Hartmann and Kellner collaborated to develop their lignosulphite treatment, Hartmann interpreted alchemy, Paracelsian medicine, and modern physics in light of theosophical theories that were influenced by South Asian concepts. The philosophy of nature he outlined postulates that the whole universe consists of a primary matter that modern science calls "ether" and that would be known in Indian philosophy as *ākāśa*. Ether (*ākāśa*) manifests itself in different states of vibration:

> *the difference* between *these vibrations is the foundation of all formations and expressions of power, be it in the realm of visible matter, on a higher plane that is invisible to us, or in the realm of intelligence. Above all these appearances is the cause that originates everything,* wisdom itself (self-awareness).[54]

The vibrations are caused by a living and organising force:

> This principle of life, which the Indians called "*prana*," could also be called a function of the general primary matter or "ether". It constitutes the life force of each organism.[55]

53 Lechler 2013: 150: "Die drei konnten nur sporadisch Kontakt haben, weil sie über Europa verstreut lebten. Von einer regelmäßigen und geordneten gemeinsamen Ordensarbeit als Hochgradfreimaurer waren sie, im wahrsten Sinn des Wortes, kilometerweit entfernt."

54 Hartmann 1893a: 415–416: "*[D]ie Verschiedenartigkeit dieser Schwingungen ist die Grundlage aller Formenbildungen und Kraftäusserungen [...]; über allen diesen Erscheinungen steht die Ursache, der alle Dinge ihre Entstehung ursprünglich verdanken,* die Weisheit selbst (das Selbstbewusstsein)" [Hartmann's emphases].

55 Hartmann 1893b: 27: "Dieses Lebensprinzip, von den Indiern '*Prana*' genannt, könnte auch als eine Funktion oder Eigenschaft der allgemeinen Urmaterie oder des 'Aethers' bezeichnet werden, und sie constituirt die Lebenskraft eines jeden Organismus" [Hartmann's emphasis].

For Hartmann, matter and force, *ākāśa* and *prāṇa,* are an inseparable unity. Force is matter in motion and matter is bound or incarnated energy.[56] The dual union of *ākāśa* and *prāṇa* is caused by divine will and consciousness, and constitutes a kind of *anima mundi* that enlivens the evolving cosmos as a whole and at the same time every individual being.

On the basis of these principles, Hartmann explains the possibility of the alchemical transmutation of elements into each other:

> The key to the entering of chemistry into the field of alchemy lies in a correct understanding of the qualities of "ether", or, to be more accurate, of the akâsa [sic] and its modifications, and we have good reason to believe that in this respect we are on the eve of great discoveries.[57]

Additionally, this philosophy serves him as a theoretical foundation of alternative forms of healing which he interprets as influencing the finer vibrations of ether that make up the invisible aura of the human organism. The changes within the aura cause healing effects within the gross body that conventional medicine is unable to explain.

These thoughts anticipate the emanationist cosmology developed by Swami Vivekananda in his famous *Rāja Yoga* (1896).[58] Vivekananda also conceives of the universe as "an ocean of ether, consisting of layer after layer of varying degrees of vibration under the action of Prāna."[59] Like Hartmann, he uses this concept to develop a model of health and disease that sustains the effectiveness of alternative healing methods:

> In this country there are Mindhealers, Faith-healers, Spiritualists, Christian Scientists, Hypnotists, etc., and if we analyse these different groups we shall find that the background of each is this control of the Prāna, whether they know it or not.[60]

Most likely, the convergence between Hartmann's and Vivekananda's cosmology is due to their use of the same theosophical sources as Blavatsky already speaks of *ākāśa* and *prāṇa* in the same sense although in a much less systematic way. It needs further investigation that cannot be undertaken here. The difference between Vivekananda and Hartmann or Kellner lies only in the fact that for Vivekananda *ākāśa* and *prāṇa* are correlated but basically independent principles, whereas the other two emphasise their unity.

56 Cf. Hartmann 1893a: 444.

57 Hartmann 1893a: 438: "Der Schlüssel zum Eindringen der Chemie in das Gebiet der Alchemie liegt daher einem Verständnisse der Eigenschaften des 'Äthers' und dessen Schwingungen, oder besser gesagt: des Akâsa [sic] und seinen [sic] Modifikationen und wir haben Grund anzunehmen, dass wir in dieser Beziehung am Vorabende grosser Entdeckungen stehen."

58 For Vivekananda's cosmology see De Michelis 2004: 153–168.

59 Vivekananda 1992: 158.

60 Vivekananda 1992: 149–150.

Kellner, who surely knew Hartmann's articles on alchemy and the lignosulphite treatment and may have discussed these matters with him, underlines the primacy of energy whereas Hartmann at times tends to highlight ether as the primary substance. In his manuscript "Experimenteller Beweis über die Verwandelbarkeit der sogenannten Grundstoffe", Kellner surmises that the most basic reality is energy. Matter and its different manifestations, the chemical elements and other substances, are only solidified energy.[61]

According to Köthner (1902), Kellner told him in a letter concerning his alchemical experiments that he was still not totally sure about their theoretical foundation, but that he intended to use Ostwald's theory of energy ("Energetik") to explain them. Furthermore, Köthner reports that Kellner mentioned in this letter that the alchemical writings of his grandfather gave him his first glimpses of a monistic worldview. The category "monism" was used in those days for the occultist project of a unified scientific explanation of sensory and extrasensory phenomena.[62] It was also used within mainstream science and philosophy for theories that reduce all phenomena to one single principle. The chemist and philosopher Wilhelm Ostwald was one of the most prominent monistic philosophers of his time. His philosophy aimed at overcoming the dualism of matter and mind by reducing matter to a complex of energies coordinated in space. In a further step, he applied the concept of energy to psychic phenomena and thus the notion of energy became the one and only principle underlying every phenomenon in the world.[63]

Kellner added a mystical twist to this kind of energetic monism and used it as theoretical foundation of his masonic order:

> The rite of our order is based on the insight that the general energy of the world (which we know in its lower forms as electricity, magnetism, light, warmth, etc.) manifests itself in its higher forms as love, consciousness, life, progress, etc.; that the particular part of this energy that dwells within us and constitutes our personality is as well indestructible as are all the other lower forms of energy (responsibility of all rational beings) [...]; that through the practical application of the symbols used within the rite, the forms of energy which determine our being can be further awakened and developed so that within the "higher grades" we are finally able to find our better immortal 'self' (the 'lost word') already in the present life.[64]

61 Cf. Kellner 1896b: 1.

62 For example, the German theosophical journal *Sphinx* (1886–1896) was subtitled "monthly magazine for the historical and experimental foundation of a transcendental worldview on a monistic basis".

63 Cf. Ostwald 1902.

64 Kellner 1903: 15: "Der Ritus unseres Ordens ist aufgebaut auf das Wissen: daß die allgemeine Welt=Energie (die wir in ihren niederen Formen als Elektrizität, Magnetismus, Licht, Wärme, u.s.w. kennen) sich in ihren höheren Formen als Liebe, Bewußtsein, Leben, Fortschritt u.s.w. offenbart; daß derjenige Teil dieser einen Energie, der in uns wohnt und der unsere wahre

Hartmann's attempts to connect energetic monism with South Asian concepts may have confirmed Kellner's interests in South Asian occultism as an ancient worldview that corresponds to modern science and philosophy.

5. Kellner's Encounter with South Asian Yogis and His Essay on Yoga

Being a member of the Theosophical Society and friend of Hartmann, Kellner shared the theosophical knowledge about South Asian religion, and especially yoga. He had access to theosophical articles on this topic and to translations of primary sources edited and/or translated by theosophists.

As already mentioned above, at the beginning of the twentieth century Kellner became an enthusiastic student of the Western-educated Brahmin Sri Agamya Guru Paramahamsa from Kashmir.[65] Agamya, a barrister by profession, claimed that after retiring from the High Court he stayed for several years in the Himalayas to meditate and master yoga. In public performances he demonstrated his yogic powers by stopping his pulse on command. We saw already that, according to Hartmann, Kellner learnt breathing techniques and other exercises from him and was very convinced about the results. No details about what he taught Kellner have been handed down. Several sources testify that Agamya stressed the importance of breath control to calm down the mind in his public talks in the USA and England. The descriptions of yogic exercises in his books that include, for example, the tantric concept of the rising of *kuṇḍalinī* through the *cakra*-s are too vague for a certain practice to be derived from them.

Within Kellner's occult milieu and among the general public, the guru was widely renowned as a fraudster. Hartmann was not the only one who complained that Kellner was all too trusting with regard to this dubious man. Agamya first visited Europe in 1900. It is unknown if Kellner already met him then. In 1903, during his second journey to Europe, he stayed for a while in Hallein and on this occasion, Kellner's apprenticeship ended abruptly. The "Tiger Mahatma", as was his nickname, was famous for his ferocious temper and outbursts of rage. According to oral family tradition, as passed on by Marie Kellner after the death of

Persönlichkeit ausmacht, ebenso unzerstörbar ist, wie jede andere niedrigere Energieform; daß für die höheren Energieformen ähnliche Gesetze Geltung haben wie die, welche die niederen beherrschen (Verantwortlichkeit aller vernünftigen Wesen); daß durch die *praktische* Anwendung der im Ritus gegebenen Symbole die unser Sein bedingenden Energieformen weiter erweckt und entwickelt werden können, so daß wir endlich in den 'höheren Graden' unser besseres und unsterbliches 'Selbst' (das 'verlorene Wort') schon in diesem Leben finden."

65 Cf. Kaczynski 2012: 83–86.

her husband, Agamya and Kellner had a quarrel and in the end, Agamya cursed him solemnly, probably because he had given away his secret teachings to other persons. For Kellner's widow this curse could well have been the cause of his disease and death.[66]

In 1907, Agamya visited England coming from New York. Among his students was Aleister Crowley, who attended a retreat with him that included meditation practice. Soon after, they parted in disagreement. In 1908, Agamya was finally imprisoned in England because he groped two of his female students.[67]

Several years before he met Sri Agamya Guru Paramahamsa, Kellner already became acquainted with another South Asian who visited the Western World to convince the interested public of the occult powers that yogis possess: Bheema Sena Pratapa.[68] Pratapa is said to have been a student of the University of Lahore and a member of England's Royal Asiatic Society. He led an ascetic lifestyle and at the age of twenty-nine travelled to Europe where he gave several demonstrations of what he called "yoga sleep", a state of mind in which he lost contact with the world around him, became insensitive to pain and could not be awakened unless certain movements of the hand were carried out close to his body. Pratapa claimed that during his sleep he would be in a state of bliss and union with the divine spirit. Along with Gopal Krishna, another yogi, he was an attraction for the visitors of the Millennial Exposition in Budapest in 1896, where he publicly demonstrated yoga sleep for an entire week while scientists measured his body temperature, pulse, and respiration. A scandal arose when Pratapa was accused of coming out of his yoga sleep at night in order to eat and drink, to have a smoke and to play cards with his fellow yogi. It finally turned out that most, if not all of the accusations, were baseless and that Pratapa had become the victim of a conflict between two impresarios.[69]

The public controversy about the young yogi made its way into the Austrian press and perhaps this was what made Kellner and Hartmann aware of him. In any case, they invited him to Hallein where together with the Munich theosophist Ludwig Deinhard they examined his yogic powers. For Kellner it was clear that Pratapa and his fellow yogi Gopal Krishna set themselves in the state of *nirvikalpasamādhi* during their performances.[70]

In August 1896, Kellner, Hartmann, and Deinhard accompanied Pratapa to the Third International Congress for Psychology in Munich to exhibit his yoga

66 Cf. Weirauch 1998: 201.

67 For Agamya's teaching in the USA and England, see Kaczynski 2012: 84–86.

68 For Pratapa and his encounter with Kellner, see Kaczynski 2012: 77–79.

69 Cf. the newspaper articles in *Abendblatt des Pester Lloyd*, 11 July 1896, no. 158, 1 ("Der Streit um die Fakire") and *Grazer Tagblatt*, 31 July 1896, 2 ("Eine Ehrenrettung").

70 Cf. Kellner 1896a: 19.

sleep before the scientists and to re-establish his reputation as yogi.[71] He went into yoga sleep throughout all three days of the conference from 10am to 6pm. The demonstration was not part of the official programme, but many members of the congress came to see the yogi and tried to interrupt his otherworldly state or searched for its pathological causes, both without success.

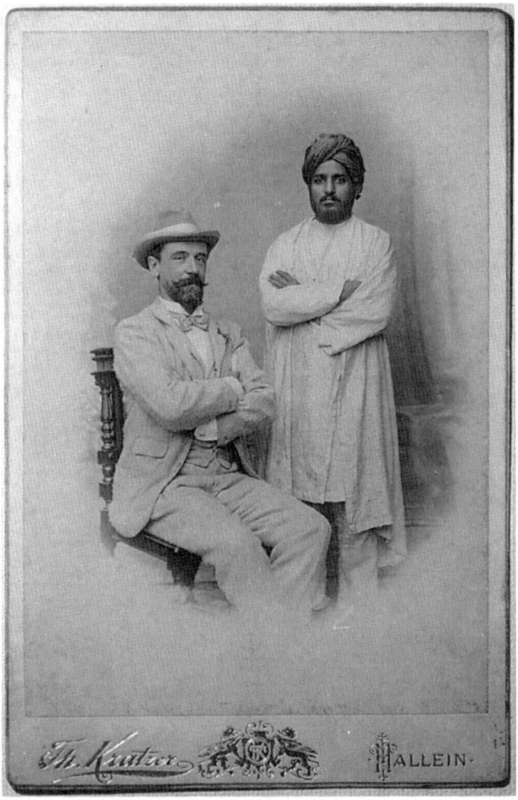

Figure 2: Carl Kellner and Bheema Sena Pratapa (photograph courtesy of Josef Dvorak).

Kellner's booklet *Yoga: Eine Skizze über den psycho-physiologischen Teil der alten indischen Yogalehre* that he dedicated to the Third International Congress for Psychology was distributed at this event. For a long time, this small 21-page treatise seemed to be lost and forgotten, but in 1989 the text was reprinted in Josef Dvorak's popular book on Satanism.[72] Another copy of Kellner's sketch is kept in

71 Kaczynski 2012: 78.

72 Dvorak 1993: 431–446. Dvorak found Kellner's sketch in the estate of the ethnologist Robert Lehmann-Nitsche that is kept in the collection of the Ibero-American Institute in Berlin (email message from Josef Dvorak to the author, 13 May 2016). He wrote seminal articles on

Oscar R. Schlag's famous esoteric library that today belongs to the Zentralbibliothek Zürich. Most of the psychologists remained sceptical about the young yogi, but Kellner's essay and also an article of Hartmann's on the yoga sleep were quoted in several newspaper articles on Pratapa's performances in Munich. The journalists now reported with much more respect about the yogi. Hartmann and Kellner definitely succeeded in restoring his reputation.

Later, Kellner's text was mentioned positively in a footnote of William James' *Varieties of Religious Experience.* James called Kellner a "European witness" who "after carefully comparing the results of Yoga with those of the hypnotic or dreamy states artificially producible by us" had come to the conclusion that yoga "makes of its disciples good, healthy, and happy men".[73] This, indeed, is one of the results of Kellner's sketch and it fits well with James' pragmatist test of religion's value by its fruits, as well as with his New-Thought inspired concept of a "religion of healthy-mindedness". James was a member of the organizing committee of the Munich congress but did not participate in it. An unidentified person who knew about James' interest in yoga must have handed Kellner's booklet to him after the congress. The essay consists of a short foreword followed by a chapter on "What is Yoga?"[74] The main part deals with "Practices to Induce and Attain Yoga".[75] The text ends with a concluding "Résumé" ("Rückblick").[76]

In the foreword Kellner writes that for several years he intended to publish the insights and experiences that he had achieved through a long and careful study of yoga. But work overload would have kept him from writing. Additionally, he hesitated to present a topic to the public that very likely would share the destiny of mesmerism (i.e., scientific and public rejection).[77] Notwithstanding these reservations, he would have decided to use the favourable moment of the presence of Bheema Sena Pratapa, and his willingness to demonstrate the scientifically testable teachings of yoga, to say what he had wanted to for a long time.

Kellner in which he, among other sources, used the stories told about Kellner in the oral tradition of the Kellner family. Cf. Weirauch 1998.

73 James 1902: 401.

74 Kellner 1896a: 5–8.

75 Kellner 1896a: 8–20.

76 Kellner 1896a: 20–21.

77 The reference to mesmerism here owes itself to the fact that Kellner's view of yoga is part of a long chain of nineteenth-century interpretations that postulated a deep similarity or even identity between yoga and mesmeric techniques and the specific states of mind they produce. He writes in his sketch: "Like hypnotism and artificial somnambulism yoga differentiates between different states, namely *dharana*, *dhiana* [sic] and *samadhi,* that correspond […] almost precisely to the stages of somnambulism known to us, whereas the state of *pratyahara* resembles the phenomena that we produce within hypnotized people by influencing their sensory perception" (7). Basu's introduction to the *Śivasaṃhitā,* Kellner's most important source, points out several convergences between yoga and mesmerism.

Kellner begins his investigation with a broad definition of yoga, very much in line with the one Hartmann gave in the *Wiener Rundschau.* Yoga, he says, comprises the practical side of each religious system. Therefore, one can find it in every holy book and also within the traditions and symbols of secret societies.[78] It consists of "certain exercises and a life style governed by certain rules that aim at dissolving the illusionary ego-consciousness (Ahankara) and reaching a union with the general world-consciousness (Atma)".[79] Insofar as this is a union with a sublime and holy object it is connected with a sense of ineffable bliss.[80] Kellner thus defines yoga as transcultural practical mysticism that represents the core of every religious system. The terms he uses for the description of mystical union are reminiscent of (neo-)vedantic thought.

Kellner states that he does not want to go further into the philosophical side of yoga because he is more interested in looking at it from a psycho-physiological perspective. For this purpose, he draws on the theory of Ambroise Liébeault, the founder of the school of Nancy, which in the 1890s had become famous as a leading school of hypnosis.[81] Liébeault's theory about the significance of the flow of attention for the generation of hypnotic states was especially innovative and Kellner applied it to yoga.

Starting from Rájendralála Mitra's translation of *Yogasūtra* 1.2, "Yoga is the suppression of the functions of the thinking principle",[82] he suggests replacing *citta,* "the thinking principle", with "attention" in the sense of Liébeault. Suppression of the changes in attention would be

> the most beautiful explanation of the induction of the state of "autosuggestion" or better "autohypnosis". [...] From a European point of view, we can say the following: Yoga is the ability to produce all phenomena of somnambulism arbitrarily through one's own free will by steady practice and a suitable way of life.[83]

78 Kellner 1896a: 6.

79 Kellner 1896a: 5. In other passages Kellner speaks of "the union of jiva and atma" (10), "the direct union of manas (literally translated 'the soul') with atma, in other words of the individual soul with the cosmic consciousness" (11) or "union of jivatma and paramatma" (19). He thereby mixes the definitions of yoga that he found in his sources, especially in the introductions of Basu and Tookaram Tatya to the *Śivasaṃhitā* and the *Haṭhapradīpikā.*

80 Kellner 1896a: 11.

81 For the theories of Liébeault, see Liébeault 1889, Gauld 1995: 319–362, and Carrer 2000.

82 Mitra 1883: 4. Kellner (1896a: 7) translates: "Yoga ist die Unterdrückung der Veränderungen des Denkprinzipes."

83 Kellner 1896a: 7–8: "Entkleiden wir daher diesen Fundamentalsatz Patanjali's seines indischen Charakters und setzen wir statt seinem '*Chitta*' (Denkprinzip) das Wort; [sic] '*Aufmerksamkeit*' im Sinne der Libeaultschen [sic] Anschauung, so haben wir die schönste Erklärung zur Herbeiführung des Zustandes der 'Autosuggestion' oder besser gesagt der 'Autohypnose' [...]. Wir können daher auf 'abendländisch' sagen: Yoga ist die durch andauernde Übung und geeignete Lebensweise erlangte Befähigung zur willkürlichen Selbsthervorrufung aller Erscheinungen des Somnambulismus" [Kellner's emphases]. Kellner's

The practitioner creates a state of steady flow of attention towards a suggested object that leads to a somnambulic state in which identification with the object can take place.

Kellner's opting for this approach is not surprising insofar as theories of hypnosis and autosuggestion were among the most promising scientific approaches that offered explanations for yogic experiences and powers at the end of the nineteenth century. As we saw, Kellner knew about the criticism of mesmerism and that it could threaten the reputation of yoga. He obviously did not want to fall into this trap, but tried to connect to a more recent, less academically controversial theory, even though among occultists mesmeric theories were still highly regarded. Liébeault's place within the history of psychology is somewhere halfway between mesmerism and the new psychologies of hypnotism and suggestion.

Kellner's definition of yoga fit well with the programme of the congress. Many papers on psycho-physiological topics as well as on hypnotism, somnambulism and suggestion were presented. Ambroise Liébeault himself spoke on "Communication des pensées par suggestion mentale".[84] One entire section dealt with the "Psychology of sleep, dream, hypnotic and related phenomena".[85] As no speaker at the conference addressed phenomena and concepts from outside the Euro-American world, Kellner's sketch and Pratapa's performance were very avant-garde.

More surprising than his recourse to Liébeault is the fact that Kellner's view of yoga includes a clear plea for Haṭha Yoga. At the end of the nineteenth century the four hegemonic schools concerning the interpretation of yoga, namely Theosophy, Neo-hinduism, academic orientalism, and psychology, were still clinging to a predominantly negative image of Haṭha Yoga, whereas already in the early years of Theosophy, certain elements of it were evaluated positively and popularised. From the second half of the 1880s onwards, South Asian theosophists and Sanskrit scholars started to translate, edit, and comment select major works of this form of yoga. They developed less prejudiced views and sometimes even recommended certain Haṭha practices. Kellner adopted this new trend. Haṭha Yoga, he writes, is the most interesting type of yoga "from a pure physiological point of view".[86] And not only that, according to him, the psycho-physiological dimension ensures its superiority among the different yogas. Haṭha Yoga practices "possess the most formidable hypnogenetic means" and therefore

study of the *Yogasūtra* is also documented by a manuscript that contains his translation of the first sixteen *sūtra*-s of the third *pāda*.

84 Cf. *Dritter Internationaler Congress für Psychologie in München* 1897: 427.

85 *Dritter Internationaler Congress für Psychologie in München* 1897: 348–382.

86 Kellner 1896a: 12.

they are able to create the yogic state in the simplest possible matter and faster than other yoga techniques.[87]

The yoga texts he refers to in his essay are Rájendralála Mitra's translation of the *Yogasūtra* and three translations of Haṭha Yoga texts: Srischandra Basu's translation of the *Śivasaṃhitā* from 1887 and translations of the *Haṭhapradīpikā* and the *Gheraṇḍasaṃhitā*. He does not correctly quote the last two, but in all likelihood he used the translations of T. R. Srinivasa Iyangar (1893) and again Srischandra Basu (this time called Vasu, 1895). All three translations were published by theosophical publishing houses and represent the positive attitude of the elite of Indian theosophists towards Tantrism and Haṭha Yoga.

Basu's introduction to his translation of the *Śivasaṃhitā* is the source that Kellner explicitly and implicitly quotes or paraphrases most often. Basu repeats the negative attitude of Theosophy towards Haṭha yogis while, at the same time, affirming the value of their breathing techniques. *Prāṇāyāma*, he says,

> facilitates the liberation of the spirit. There are different modes of bringing about this result but the one proposed by the Yogi through the regulation of the breath, is the easiest, and safest, and what is its greatest recommendation, requires no external accessories. Fumigation, dancing, music &c., have been employed by various mystics to bring about trance, but all these mean the help of external adjuncts.[88]

In the same vein, the theosophist Tookaram Tatya who wrote the introduction to Srinivasa Iyangar's English translation of the *Haṭhapradīpikā* identified breath-control with Haṭha Yoga:

> The regulation of breath for the purpose of checking the fluctuations of the thinking principle is called Hatha-yoga [...]. Raja-yoga begins where Hatha-yoga, properly followed, ends. It would therefore be unwise to consider the Hatha-yoga as nothing more than a dangerous gymnastic feat, for a moderate practice of it has been found by experience to be both conducive to health and longevity.[89]

Basu's and Tatya's views of Haṭha Yoga and the experiences that he had with body-centred meditation à la Kerning-Mailänder may have inspired Kellner to become one of the earliest (if not the first) proponents of Haṭha Yoga in Europe. Following the two South Asian commentators, for Kellner the core discipline of this yoga is a "systematized regulation of breath".[90] Thanks to the use of the psychological and physiological effects of controlled breath, "the Haṭha Yoga practices have the best hypnogenetic means. Therefore they are the easiest practices leading to the yogic state and the fastest reaching that goal".[91]

87 Kellner 1896a: 9.
88 Basu 1887: 17.
89 Tatya 1893: xii.
90 Kellner 1896a: 8.
91 Kellner 1896a: 9.

Kellner exemplifies the polysemy of yoga terms and instructions by explaining the different layers of meaning of the term Haṭha Yoga.[92] He first mentions the interpretation that *ha* means moon and *ṭha* the sun. He adds that the union of sun and moon could be related to a certain breathing technique that unites the breathing through the left and the right nostril in the area in-between the eyebrows in order to attain salvation. *Haṭha,* the union of sun and moon could also refer to the union of *prāṇa* and *apāna,* the downward and upward moving breath (*vāyu*) within the navel region. On a philosophical level, it would mean the union of *jīva* (moon) with the *ātman* (sun).

It is worth mentioning that a symbolism of heavenly opposites and their union was well known to Kellner from his occult background. The rooftop of Kellner's villa in Vienna was decorated with a large figure holding in one hand the sun and in the other one the earth. Josef Dvorak interpreted this figure as a representation of Baphomet (a popular symbol of the union of polarities in occultism). But it actually depicts the title vignette of the first volume of Carl von Eckartshausen's *Aufschlüsse zur Magie* from 1788. The vignette shows the eternal oneness as divine creator of the cosmos holding in his hands the primordial duality of sun and earth from which the manifold phenomena of the created world emerge. Two chains connect sun and earth with a four-stringed lyre that represents the tetrachord as symbol of cosmic harmony.

In alchemy the union of sun (sulphur) and moon (mercury) has a prominent place within the production of the philosopher's stone and the elixir of life. It was often depicted as a hierogamy between a king and a queen.

Within the context of his argument in favour of Haṭha Yoga, Kellner mentions other forms of yoga (Mantra Yoga, Bhakti Yoga, and Laja [sic] Yoga, etc.) in passing without detailed description. Only Rāja Yoga stands out being characterised as "crown of yoga".[93] Following Tookaram Tatya, he does not identify it with the *Yogasūtra* but with the highest, redeeming state of mind that is the general aim of yoga.

He then uses Patañjali's eightfold path as a system of subdivisions that he believed to be accepted in all forms of yoga. He interprets *yama* as religious regulations which do not only have a moral purpose but also a psychological one, because they create the state of inner calm that is necessary for yoga. *Niyama* is defined as a purification of the outer and inner man. More attention is given to *āsana.* Kellner proposes explaining the yogic poses as mimetic enactment of states of the mind:

92 Ahead of the Indology of his time, today Kellner's understanding of Haṭha Yoga is anchronistic. Cf. Birch 2011.

93 Kellner 1896a: 11.

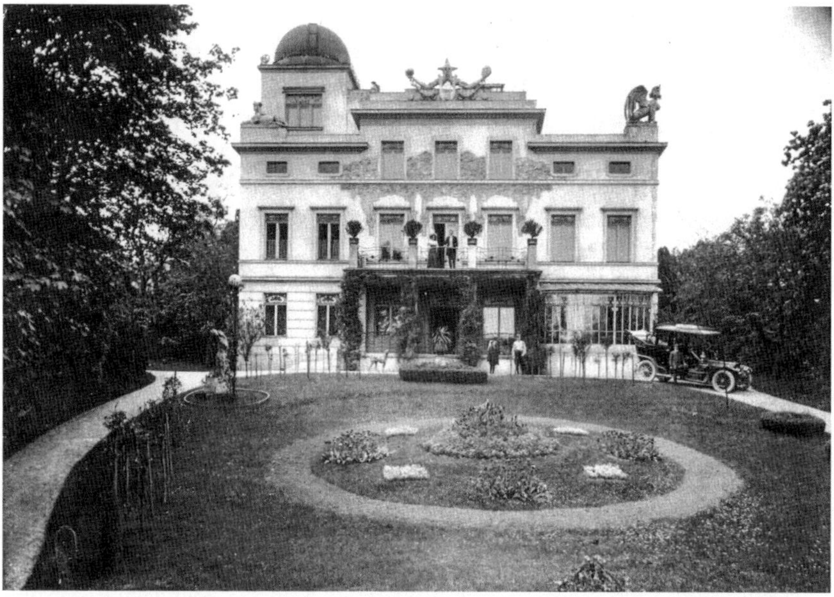

Figure 3: The villa Hochwart of the Kellner family in Vienna (photograph courtesy of Josef Dvorak).

> It is clear that if we want to develop inner concentration we have to adopt a pose that harmonises with the inner processes. The actor who has to represent a hero will walk in a different way than when he has to perform a bon vivant. It is also well known that we change our body posture as soon as our emotions change. Well, the yogi attempts to influence the inner through the outer by adopting a pose from the start that fits to the state of mind he wishes to put himself in.[94]

During the 1880s, a significant cultural change concerning attitudes towards the human body took place. Modern physical culture had come to Vienna from England and the USA. In keeping with the times, Kellner became a passionate sportsman. His trainer Georg Jagendorfer, then "the strongest man in town", was the owner of a gymnasium in the centre of Vienna where he taught his speciality,

94 Kellner 1896a: 13: "Es ist klar, dass wir eine Stellung einnehmen müssen, die mit unseren inneren Vorgängen in Einklang steht, wenn wir eine innere Konzentration vornehmen wollen. Der Schauspieler, der einen Helden vorzustellen hat, wird auch anders einherschreiten als wenn er einen leichtsinnigen Lebemann gibt. Ebenso ist ja der Wechsel der Körperstellungen bei Gemütsbewegungen bekannt. Der Yogi sucht nun von aussen nach innen zu wirken und passt gleich seine Stellung demjenigen Zustand im Vorhinein an, in den er sein Gemüte versetzen will."

Indian club swinging, as well as rhythmic gymnastics, wrestling, and boxing. Jagendorfer also worked as private trainer of Kellner's children in Hallein.[95]

In line with modern physical culture, Kellner highlights that a yogi should live according to the principle of *mens sana in corpore sano*: "The Yogi needs a strong and in all of its parts totally healthy body. He has to possess perfect body control."[96] Nevertheless, he did not recommend the *āsana*-s described in the Haṭha Yoga scriptures for the purpose of physical training, because he thought they would be too difficult for Westerners. Referring to the thirty-two *āsana*-s of the *Gheraṇḍasaṃhitā* he refuses to publish them in his sketch "because they can only be performed by the so-called contortionists of our circuses and vaudevilles".[97] In this context he quotes *Yogasūtra* 2.46 to underline that the yogic postures should be firm and comfortable.[98] Their main purpose should be to support inner concentration and in the West, e.g., one should not use *padmāsana,* etc., but easier sitting poses to promote attention and inner calm.

Kellner is therefore a good example of the type of modern man whose interest in self-cultivation is at the same time open to the latest techniques in Western physical culture as well as yoga exercises from South Asia. Not least because of his knowledge about the practices of Kerning–Mailänder, he appreciates the importance of the body for meditation. If the modern forms of *āsana* practice had existed in his time, he surely would have integrated them into his practice.

The fourth constituent of the eightfold path, *prāṇāyāma,* is treated in the most detailed fashion. Here is the point where Kellner brings in the Haṭha Yoga practices that interested him most. He mentions several of the breathing exercises from the Haṭha Yoga scriptures. Furthermore he introduces the system of the ten *vāyu*-s, lists fourteen *nāḍī*-s, and outlines the role of both within yogic practice:

> The yogi shifts his consciousness, condenses his attention on one of the vayus and on a nadi and connects this imagination in a certain asana with the breath. This kind of combination is called mudra. Altogether there are 25 mudras (among them some very strange ones)![99]

The practice of *mudrā,* then, would bring about the higher limbs of yoga. Through the practice of *mudrā*-s and the other yogic disciplines, the yogi de-

95 For Kellner's relation to Viennese fin-de-siècle physical culture, see the remarks of Josef Dvorak in Weirauch 1998: 193.

96 Kellner 1896a: 12–13.

97 Kellner 1896a: 14.

98 On *Yogasūtra* 2.46, see the chapter by Philipp Maas in the present volume.

99 Kellner 1896a: 17–18: "Der Yogi versetzt sein Bewusstsein, verdichtet seine Aufmerksamkeit auf einen der genannten Vayus und auf ein [sic] Nadi, und verbindet diese Vorstellung in einer [sic] gewissen Asana mit dem Atem. Eine solche Kombination nennt man ein Mudra und so gibt es 25 Mudras (worunter einige sehr sonderbare)!"

velops *pratyāhāra*, the ability to suppress his sensory perceptions and to deliberately replace them with arbitrary imaginations. Kellner compares this state of mind with the state of a hypnotised person. He briefly describes the practice of *saṃyama* as fixation of the *citta* to one spot (*dhāraṇā*), followed by a steady stream of attention towards this spot (*dhyāna*) culminating in a union of the seer with the seen (*samādhi*). This process leads to the development of *siddhi*-s, paranormal powers, and finally to redemption through union of *jīvātmā* and *paramātmā*. Kellner connects a defence of Pratapa and his fellow yogi to the introduction of the topic of the *siddhi*-s.

In the "Résumé" of his article, Kellner once again addresses the psychologists that attended the Munich conference. He tries to convince them that the ancient yoga teachings are deserving of careful study. The practice of yoga is summed up as "a kind of pursued autosuggestion and autohypnosis" that could be used to produce positive physiological and psychological changes.[100]

It is worth mentioning that throughout his whole sketch, Kellner does not deny what he calls the philosophical aspects of yoga. Nevertheless, he develops a secularised psychosomatic model of yoga and, in the end, opts for the use of yoga as a therapeutic tool without any religious or philosophical frame. This is a new strategy within the occultist advocacy of yoga. He does not want to confront mainstream science as Blavatsky did, but tries to defend yoga with arguments that were able to draw scientific approval.

As several researchers have observed, Kellner's sketch contains spelling mistakes and errors. He was evidently in a hurry while writing the piece. One of his mistakes has an important history of reception. In his list of the ten *vāyu*-s Kellner mentions a "Nâpa" and correlates it with the "function of insemination".[101] This *vāyu* is not mentioned in Kellner's primary source concerning the *vāyu*-s, which is the *Gheraṇḍasaṃhitā*. It was probably only a spelling error: he wrote "Nâpa" instead of the correct *nāga*.[102] But this does not explain Kellner's view about the function of this *vāyu*. *Nāga* is traditionally associated with burping and vomiting and not with insemination.

Years later, in the legendary jubilee edition of the *Oriflamme* published in September 1912, Kellner's dubious "Nâpa" *vāyu* was used by Reuss to substantiate a tradition of ritual sex in the O.T.O. dating back to Kellner whom he called "the spiritual father of the O.T.O."[103] I will return to this matter in the next section.

100 Kellner 1896a: 20.

101 Kellner 1896a: 17.

102 Cf. Möller & Howe 1986: 139–140; Weirauch 1998: 194–196.

103 Reuss 1912: 3.

There is no allusion to sacred sexual intercourse in Kellner's yoga booklet. Except for the "Nâpa" *vāyu,* only one passage in his sketch refers to sexuality. "Asanas", Kellner writes, "are supposed to influence the circulation within the lower extremities and the sexual drive and to be training for willpower".[104] The only practice that he describes in more detail is a *prāṇāyāma* called *sahita* and a Sufi breathing technique without any sexual connotations, both taken from Basu's introduction.

Although sexual practices are not directly mentioned, it is not difficult to derive a yoga technique of dealing with "the function of insemination" from Kellner's description of *mudrā* and from the "Nâpa" *vāyu* he introduced. The yogi takes a convenient position that facilitates the influence on the sexual drive. Then he focuses his attention on "Nâpa" *vāyu* and a *nāḍī* using a certain breathing technique to calm the mind and create a steady flow (of blood according to Basu, quoted by Kellner) towards the brain and thus sublimates the sexual drive. Maybe Kellner's acquaintance with a practice like this made him erroneously project the function of insemination into the system of the *vāyu*-s.

With regard to ritual sex, it is important to note that Kellner's general concept of yoga is based on a kind of asceticism. For him *vairāgya,* renunciation, is one of the master keys to yoga. Only somebody who refrains from earthly wishes and desires can attain the inner peace that is necessary to attain the higher stages of yoga: "Through the mastering of his thoughts and his body, the yogi becomes a virtuous man. As he subjugates his drives and inclinations to his original will and because he focuses this will towards the good, he becomes an 'authentic personality'."[105]

Again, Kellner's interpretation of yogic renunciation probably integrated a concept from Basu's commented translation of the *Śivasaṃhitā.* In keeping with his Sanskrit source, Basu emphasises that celibacy is not necessary for success in yoga. Furthermore, referring to the Sikh guru Arjun he prefers the state of the householder yogi who lives a married life and moderates his sexual desires to that of the completely abstinent ascetic.[106] Kellner could read in Basu's translation of the *Śivasaṃhitā* and the other Haṭha yoga texts that through the preservation of semen during sexual intercourse (or by drawing it up again through the penis after ejaculation together with the woman's generative fluid) the householder can become a fully liberated yogi.[107] The following section deals with a closer ex-

104 Kellner 1896a: 14.

105 Kellner 1896a: 21: "Durch die erlangte Herrschaft über seinen [sic] Gedanken und seinen Körper, wird der Yogi ein 'Charaktermensch'; und dadurch, dass er seine Triebe und Neigungen seinem eigentlichen Wollen unterwirft und letzteres auf das Gute gerichtet sein lässt, eine 'Persönlichkeit' […]."

106 Basu 1887: xx; see also pp. iv and xxx.

107 Basu 1887: 33–35. Cf. James Mallinson's chapter on *vajrolīmudrā* in the present volume. The

amination of the question whether Kellner – motivated by what he found in yoga scriptures or other sources – experimented with sexual practices.

6. Yoga and Ritual Sex within the Inner Occult Circle and the Early O.T.O.

Kellner considered his Sovereign Sanctuary to be a superior alternative to the Christian churches because of its methods to achieve union with the eternal, divine source of the universe:

> Naturally, churchdom is occupied with solving the question of "the lost word", i.e., "the lost eternal life", but it always refers the searcher to the path of grace and always sets it up as a gift, not as something that one can attain or has attained by oneself. Our order gives every searcher the opportunity to unite with the cosmic consciousness, the primordial creativity already within this life in a conscious and deliberate way through practical means.[108]

The "practical application of the symbols" of high-degree masonic rituals was meant to trigger the awakening and development of the energies from which all human life emerges – a process intended to culminate in the discovery of the practitioner's immortal self.[109] The Sovereign Sanctuary promised verbal instructions concerning these practices to all members who have reached the necessary stage of spiritual development. The available texts about the order that were published while Kellner was still alive do not explain what kinds of "practical means" were offered and what the "practical application of the symbols" in this context would mean. But it is clear that the masonic rituals and initiations were supplemented by special teachings dealing with practical occultism.

In fact, it seems that there existed a small "Inner Occult Circle" within the order that focused on occult practices. The "Inner Triangle" that is sometimes

---

positive attitude towards sexuality presented in Basu's edition of the *Śivasaṃhitā* according to Ida Craddock even inspired Vivekananda. See Schmidt 2010: 126: "While Vivekananda had consistently proclaimed celibacy as a spiritual ideal to his American audiences, Craddock heard that he had offered a select few a glimpse of 'the higher truth'. 'I have been shown a book,' she noted in 1900, 'which he was said to have circulated among his more advanced disciples in Chicago. […] It is called *The Esoteric Science and Philosophy of the Tantras. Shiva Samhita.*'"

108 Kellner & Reuss 1903: 50: "Das Kirchentum beschäftigt sich naturgemäß auch mit der Frage 'vom verlorenen Wort', i. e. 'dem verlorenen ewigen Leben', sie verweist den Suchenden aber immer auf den Weg der Gnade und stellt es stets als ein Geschenk und nicht als etwas Selbstzuerwerbendes oder Erworbenes hin. Unser Orden stellt es jedoch in die Möglichkeit eines jeden einzelnen Suchenden, mittelst praktischer Mittel sich mit dem Weltbewußtsein, der Ur-Schöpferkraft, bewußt und selbst gewollt schon in diesem Leben zu vereinen."

109 Kellner 1903: 15.

mentioned in connection with this circle points to a leadership team (Kellner, Reuss, and Hartmann, if I were to hazard a guess) with Kellner as the leading authority because of his experience in occult practice. The aim of this circle was to offer a training course based exclusively on oral instructions for the higher grades of the order. The whole project is reminiscent of the "Esoteric Section of the Theosophical Society" (later called the "Eastern" or "Esoteric School of Theosophy") and its "Inner Group", both working independently from the Theosophical Society except for the fact that only (high-ranking) theosophists were admitted into it.

There is not much known about the practices that were taught in this group. Its philosophical and religious concepts as well as its occult practices were still in the making when Kellner died. One year after his death, Max Dotzler provided some indications – and referred to yoga:

> The inner occult circle of the order was established within the frame of the order, because the practices of the occult circle were introduced and transmitted absolutely independently from the ritual and the doctrines of the order. The first stages of the practices are of Templar (Rosicrucian-gnostic) origin, the higher practices or stages with breathing exercises and yogi [sic] from which I have received a sample, are yogism, pure yoga exercises [...].[110]

This looks like a mixture of exercises from the Kerning–Mailänder tradition and practices that were considered to be yogic *stricto sensu*, i. e., exercises originating in South Asia. Within these techniques obviously breathing played a prominent role.

A letter of Reuss to Franz Held in 1903 indicates that Kellner was the authority for meditation within the Sovereign Sanctuary. Held, who may have been a candidate for the Inner Occult Circle, complained about headaches caused by the exercise of sitting. Reuss answered: "I cannot help you. But you are free to report this result to Br. Kellner himself and seek his advice. If one does not tolerate water, one cannot learn to swim."[111] The announcement of Carl Kellner's serious illness, published by The Inner Triangle in the *Oriflamme* in 1904, affirms the regular practice of meditation within the Inner Occult Circle. The brothers of the circle were asked to unite themselves with the Inner Triangle "in their daily

110 Dotzler 1906: 62: "Der innere okkulte Kreis des Ordens wurde im äußeren Rahmen des Ordens gebildet, denn die Übungen des okkulten Kreises wurden absolut unabhängig von dem Ritual und der Ordenslehre eingeführt und gegeben. Die ersten Stufen der Übungen sind templerischen (rosenkreuzerisch-gnostischen) Ursprungs, die höheren Übungen bezw. Stufen mit Atemübungen und Yogi [sic], von denen ich eine Probe bekam, sind Yogismus, reine Yogaübungen [...]."

111 Reuss 1906: 109.

meditations" by including the wish that "our leader" should remain on the earthly plane.[112]

The practice of meditation was one thing, but the real hot spot of the Inner Occult Circle was the integration of sexual magic into High-degree Freemasonry in theory and practice.

1. Theoretically it was integrated through the interpretation of the masonic symbols and rituals from the perspective of phallicism or what Reuss more precisely called the Lingam–Yoni cult: the worship of the male and female sexual organs and sexual intercourse as primary symbols of Divine creativity and the insight that this worship is the source of all religion.[113] As Dotzler asserted in 1906, neither the Scottish, nor the Memphis or the Misraim rite per se comprised an interpretation of their rites in the sense of the Lingam–Yoni cult. But what the Sovereign Sanctuary claimed was "that all masonic rites from the purest Blue Lodge Masonry to the Memphis rite with its 95° possess the symbols, mystical signs and words of sexual magic, the Lingam–Yoni cult, etc.! The members of the rites have *lost* the interpretation of the symbols, signs and words!"[114] The secret instructions within the Inner Occult Circle aimed at restoring this lost knowledge.

2. The Lingam–Yoni cult implied the concept of sexual intercourse as something holy. Reuss wrote in 1906:

> Finally, the act of communion in love has to become a religious act again as it has been in ancient times and as it still is, unknown to the crowd, within certain ceremonies and feasts of the Catholic church. The act of procreation was at all times a divine act of creation, a divine action and formed the hidden foundation of every higher religious cult.[115]

Moreover, Dotzler equates the exercises that were based on this insight with certain yogic exercises of the Haṭha Yoga scriptures quoted by Kellner in his sketch on yoga, practices in which the organs of reproduction play a role "for the attainment of certain yogic states".[116] Seemingly, exercises were taught that used

---

112 Das innere Dreieck 1904.

113 Cf. Pendragon 1906.

114 Dotzler 1906: 60: "Wohl aber besitzen alle freimauerischen Riten von der reinsten Johannismaurerei der ersten drei symbolischen Grade bis zum Memphisritus mit 95° die Symbole und die mystischen Zeichen und Worte der Sexualmagie, des Lingam-Yoni Kultes etc.! Die Mitglieder der Riten haben die Deutung der Symbole, Zeichen und Worte *verloren!*" [Dotzler's emphasis].

115 Nothung 1906: 18–19: "Endlich muss aber der Vereinigungsakt der Liebe wieder eine Religionshandlung werden, wie er es in alten Zeiten war und wie er es, der Menge unbewusst, in der katholischen Kirche gewesen ist und in gewissen Zeremonien und Festen derselben gefeiert wird. Der Zeugungsakt war zu allen Zeiten ein göttlicher Schöpfungsakt, eine göttliche Handlung und bildete die verborgene Basis jedes höheren Religionskultus."

116 Dotzler 1906: 63.

sexual excitement and/or sexual intercourse within a ritual frame to attain certain occult goals and altered states of consciousness. Reuss and Dotzler called this kind of practice "sexual magic", a common term within occultist circles.

If one follows the oral tradition of the Kellner family, then at least Kellner practised ritual sex. Karl-Erwin Lichtenecker narrated that his mother Eglantine told him about a room in the Villa Hochwart which Carl and Marie Kellner retired to time and again. No other family member was allowed to enter it.[117] According to Lichtenecker, Eglantine became curious and asked her parents what they were doing within this room. She finally got the answer that they were performing a ritual that aimed at "intimacy pushed to the utmost limit" (*auf's Äußerste gesteigerte Innigkeit*) in order to break through to things that usually are unknown. The talks that he had with his mother about this issue left no doubt for Lichtenecker that both performed a sex ritual that aimed at an experience of transcendence.

If we accept this as true, open questions still remain. Lichtenecker did not receive any detailed information about the ritual and so we do not know from this source what they were actually doing. At this point of our investigation, two things have to be considered.

Reuss asserts that the Hermetic Brotherhood of Light (HB of Light) was the source of the Rosicrucian esoteric teachings taught within the Inner Occult Circle.[118] This small brotherhood was an offshoot of the Hermetic Brotherhood of Luxor (HBL). John Patrick Deveney explored the HB of Light and was able to identify some of its members. According to him, they departed from the HBL because of differing views about ritual sex. The practice within the HB of Light was to arouse, preserve, and control the sexual energy without ejaculation, whereas the sex magic of the HBL in the tradition of Paschal Beverly Randolph advocated focusing on these goals at the moment of the simultaneous orgasm of both partners.[119] If Kellner was instructed how to perform sex magic within the HB of Light, he learnt the non-orgasmic version of it.

Several statements of Reuss and Dotzler support the assertion that the Sovereign Sanctuary followed the save-the-semen school (Deveney's term) of ritual sex. Dotzler admitted in 1906 that the secret practices of the order had already been

117 Lichtenecker 2014. A similar "occult room" existed in the villa of the rich German theosophist Gustav Gebhard in Elberfeld. In this case the room was reserved for the meeting of the closest friends from Gebhart's theosophical circle. The existence of this room was known within Viennese occultist circles. Cf. Hevesi 1901: 49–50. Perhaps it inspired Kellner to create this kind of space within his Viennese villa for his special purposes. He could have also read in Basu that householders and family men should create special rooms for yoga practice in their homes (Basu 1887: xvi–xvii).

118 Reuss 1912: 15–16.

119 Email message from John Patrick Deveney to the author, 28 April 2016.

popularised in the writings of Harry W. Bondegger, Ramacharaka, and other authors.[120] He claims originality only with regard to the date, not with regard to the content of the occult teachings of the Inner Circle: "All these popular writings have been published after Kellner and Reuss decided to pass on certain practices."[121] Bondegger and William Walker Atkinson, who used the pseudonym Yogi Ramacharaka for his writings on yoga, were New Thought authors. Both supported methods to preserve the semen and to sublimate sexual arousal into higher energies that were widespread within the New Thought movement.

In his *The Hindu Yogi Science of Breath* (1904) Ramacharaka (i. e., Atkinson) described a practice called "the transmutation of the reproductive energy".[122] While breathing rhythmically one should imagine drawing "etheric pranic energy" upwards from the sexual organs to the solar plexus or to the brain with each inhalation. The transmuted sexual energy would be stored in the solar plexus or the brain and could be used for different purposes. Ramacharaka emphasises that this yoga exercise "is specially recommended when one feels the instinct most strongly, at which time the reproductive energy is manifesting and may be most easily transmuted".[123] At the beginning of the twentieth century more and more translations of New Thought texts that recommended this kind of sexual practice became available on the German book market. The first German edition of *The Hindu Yogi Science of Breath* was published in 1909 with the title *Die Kunst des Atmens der Hindu-Yogi.*

In 1901 Bondegger translated Hiram E. Butler's *Practical Methods to Insure Success* into German.[124] Butler's ideas about a chaste association of the sexes are one of the topics of this book that influenced, according to Deveney, the sexual practices of the HB of Light. Among the books Bondegger edited for the German New Thought book series "Talisman-Bücherei" is also one on "Love and Marriage" written by a Mahatma Arkaja Brahma (most probably a pseudonym of Bondegger). Referring to Butler, the Mahatma praises the advantages of total sexual abstinence, especially for those who aspire full adepthood in yoga. Married people should practice moderation and the transmutation of sexual energies by concentrating on the finer vibrations that permeate the body.[125]

Furthermore, the save-the-semen practice fits very well with Kellner's understanding of yoga as an ascetic practice based on self-control and restraint of

120 Dotzler 1906: 63.

121 Ibid.

122 Ramacharaka 1904: 78–80.

123 Ramacharaka 1904: 79.

124 Cf. Butler 1901. (*Praktische Methoden den Erfolg zu sichern. Die Geheimnisse des Geschlechtslebens*). There were eight editions between 1901 and 1930, also in the Talisman-Bücherei (no. 43) published by the Rudolph'sche Verlagsbuchhandung in Dresden.

125 Mahatma Arkaja Brahma c 1911: 45–48.

earthly desires. The sexual reform that Reuss propagated connects the rediscovery of the holiness of sexual union with the ethical duty of men to take the responsibility for the results of the act of reproduction. The combination of these two points also becomes very reasonable in light of the practice of restrained ejaculation within ritual sex.

In the legendary jubilee edition of the *Oriflamme* published in September 1912 Reuss exposes sexual magic as the secret of the O.T.O. and of all religion.[126] He does this mostly by repeating what Kellner, Dotzler, and he published already between 1896 and 1906 about the practice of the Inner Occult Circle and the Lingam-Yoni cult. Additionally, he reveals "a certain yoga practice" called "the transmutation of the energy of reproduction" to inform the "true seekers" about the kind of sexual exercises they can expect when they join the order.[127] He starts the description of this practice with a reference to Kellner's sketch of yoga. Reuss quotes Kellner's list of *vāyu*-s and points out that sexual magic deals with the sixth *vāyu* called "Nâpa" located in the organs of reproduction. What follows is an accurate paraphrasing of the exercise of the transmutation of sexual energy from Ramacharaka's *The Hindu Science of Breath.*

Thus it seems that the early O.T.O. practised the same New Thought techniques of controlling and directing sexual arousal without orgasm that were already known within Kellner's Inner Occult Circle. Reuss was only innovative in that he integrated sexual magic into the higher grades instead of restricting its practice to a circle that worked independently of the rites of the order although recruiting its members from there.

The above argument tried to show on the basis of the material available that the occult practices of the Inner Occult Circle of the Sovereign Sanctuary and the early O.T.O. were very probably predominantly body-centred practices from the Kerning-Mailänder tradition and New Thought save-the-semen exercises that were partly identified with ideas found in translations of Haṭha Yoga scriptures. Some elements from South Asian teachers might have also played a role (e.g., certain *prāṇāyāma*-s or teachings about the *cakra*-s, *vāyu*-s, *mudrā-s* and the ascent of the *kuṇḍalinī).* At the current stage of research this is purely hypothetical, as we do not have any valid information about the yoga teachings Kellner and others might have received from there. Within the early O.T.O. the Kerning-Mailänder exercises may have lost their importance or vanished completely, whereas sexual rituals and the sexual interpretation of religious symbolisms gained priority. Later, new sexual practices that Kellner and Reuss would never have thought of were introduced by Aleister Crowley.

126 Reuss 1912: 21–23.
127 Reuss 1912: 22.

7. A Mystical Ascension within the Pleasure Gardens: The Manuscript "Reincarnation"

The only original testimony of Kellner's own yoga practice is a small note, undated and handwritten, with the title "Reincarnation". I conclude this chapter by taking a look at this document that was provided to the author by Kellner's great-granddaughter Erika Plutzar. It seems that Kellner, at a later point, changed the manuscript by altering its title to "3 Reincarnationen" and adding very short notes at the left bottom edge about two other reincarnations. Here, only the elaborate text is given, translated, and commented on.

Reincarnation [sic]

Asana ist stetig, die Athem des Lebens sind unter den
Zügeln des Geistes – die azurne Flamme erscheint –
das Ich begiebt sich in die Flamme – und schaut
zurück – weit zurück – halt – – da seh ich uns
Beide – eine Stadt – glatte Häuser – Thürme –
viereckig – ich trage eine nach vorne gebogene Mütze
einen gelben Mantel – Du – oh wie schön! –
weiche glitzernde Seidenstoffe verhüllen nur
wenig die schlanken und üppigen Formen Deines
Körpers – ja das bist Du – aus diesem Auge
leuchtet die gleiche liebe Seele – – Nacht –
– die Sterne glitzern und funkeln – – es ist
eine der grossartigen Sternen Nächte auf den
Ebenen Chaldäas – –
– und das ist das alte grosse Babylon –
und ich bin ein Priester – ein Diener der – Schamaja –
und ich steige auf den Feuerthurm und opfere
Opfere der Gottheit – das Feuer, denn das Feuer
ist das Licht, und das Licht glänzt aus
den Sternen, und aus der Sonne – –
Die Sonne aber ist das grosse Licht und
alles Leben kommt von diesem Licht – .
Alles Licht aber ist ein Licht – denn man
kann nicht sagen, es sei dieses oder jenes!
Licht ist Licht – . Und darum ist das
Licht meines Opferfeuers – dasselbe Licht, wie
das der Sterne, wie das der Sonne – und
mein Leben dasselbe Leben wie das
meiner Menschen Brüder und Schwestern –
Und mein Feuer brennt und ich spreche den
alten Segen in aramäischer Sprache –
Der Opferthurm steht aber in den Lustgärten des

Fürsten – und die Brunnen plätschern der Spring-
quell steigt – die Blumen duften – die Vögel aber
schweigen – denn sie warten auf das Licht des Tages
– und während des Wartens – – schlafen sie. –

Asana is steady, the breaths of life are under the
reigns of the mind – the azure flame appears –
the ego puts itself into the flame – and looks
back – far back – stop – – there I see both of
us – a town – smooth buildings – towers –
rectangular – I wear a cap folded forward
a yellow robe – You – oh how beautiful! –
soft glittering silk fabrics barely veil
the slim and opulent forms of your
body – yes this is you – out of these eyes
shines the same dear soul – – night –
the stars glitter and sparkle – it's one
of these amazing starry nights on the
Chaldean plains – –
– and this is the grand old Babylon –
and I am a priest – a servant of – Schamaja –
and I climb the fire-tower and I am sacrificing
Sacrificing the deity – the fire, because the fire
is the light, and the light shines out
of the stars and out of the sun – –
The sun, however, is the great light, and
all life comes from this light – .
Every light is but one light – because one
cannot say that it is this or that!
Light is Light –. And therefore the
light of my sacrificial fire is – the same light as
that of the stars, as that of the sun – and
my life the same life as that
of my human brothers and sisters –
And my fire burns and I pronounce the
old blessing in Aramaic language –
The sacrificial tower stands within in the pleasure gardens of
the ruler – and the fountains ripple the gusher
rises – the fragrance of flowers is in the air – but the birds
keep silent – because they are awaiting the light of day
– and while they are waiting – – they sleep. –

The beginning of the text refers to yoga practice. The yoga term *āsana* is mentioned and also the mastering of the *vāyu*-s (the "breaths of life" in Kellner's diction). The result of this practice is a visionary state of mind in which the practitioner develops one of the *siddhi*-s, the power to recall previous lives.

To come into contact with his past lives Kellner uses a certain technique. After an azure flame appeared before his inner eye, he immerses himself into the flame and looks back. The motive of the blue light may be influenced by a passage of Basu's introduction to the *Śivasaṃhitā* in which he comments on the removal of obscuration of the light as result of *prāṇāyāma* (*Yogasūtra* 2.52):

> The light here alluded to is the pure *sattavic* light which the Yogi sees in his heart when in deep contemplation. It is the same light which the mesmerised subjects of Baron Reichenbach saw issuing from the poles of magnet, &c. When mesmerising, we have invariably found that the first thing that the mesmerised person sees, is utter darkness, as black as night. Slowly in this darkness, as soon as his eyes are closed, there are seen flashes of blue light which growing stronger, the subject begins to see a blue atmosphere surrounding him. This is the chidakas of the Vedantins, the region of imagination. This light gives way to a pure white electric light, very brilliant, and described as more pleasant, clear and luminous than that of the sun.[128]

The transition from the realm of imagination symbolised by the blue light to a region of formless pure white light is also part of Kellner's vision. The imaginary journey into the past ends when two persons appear before Kellner's inner eye, which he identifies as "us". The sequence that follows describes an ascent from individual earthly appearances to the universal heavenly Divine light, followed by a renewed attention to and blessing of the multitude of individual things.

The images that appear in this part of Kellner's vision are not directly referring to yoga or Hindu symbols (except the widespread symbolisms of the sun and light that one can also find in South Asia). Rather, they reflect the high esteem of Chaldea, the home of the famous Chaldean oracles and their theurgy within Rosicrucianism and Theosophy. As already Josef Dvorak has pointed out, Kellner's notion of being a priest and servant of the Schamaja most probably refers to Bulwer-Lytton's *Zanoni,* where "the starry truths which shone on the great Shemaia of the Chaldean Lore" are mentioned.[129] In the first chapter of the first volume of *Isis Unveiled,* Blavatsky quotes this passage and uses "Shemaia" as a synonym for the old Oriental or universal Kabbala, the highest possible wisdom on this earth whose few adepts live "on the shores of the sacred Ganges", as well as in Thebes or Luxor.[130] In Kellner's Theosophical ambience the truths of the Chaldean lore were identical with the wisdom religion that has been almost forgotten in the West but is still alive in South Asian traditions like yoga.

Kellner finds himself and a woman, most probably his wife, in a town that turns out to be antique Babylon. He is wearing a robe and a ceremonial cap and recognises himself as a priest of the Schamaja. His female companion is almost

128 Basu 1887: xlxii [Basu's emphasis].
129 See Bulwer-Lytton 1842: 123.
130 See Blavatsky 1877: I/17.

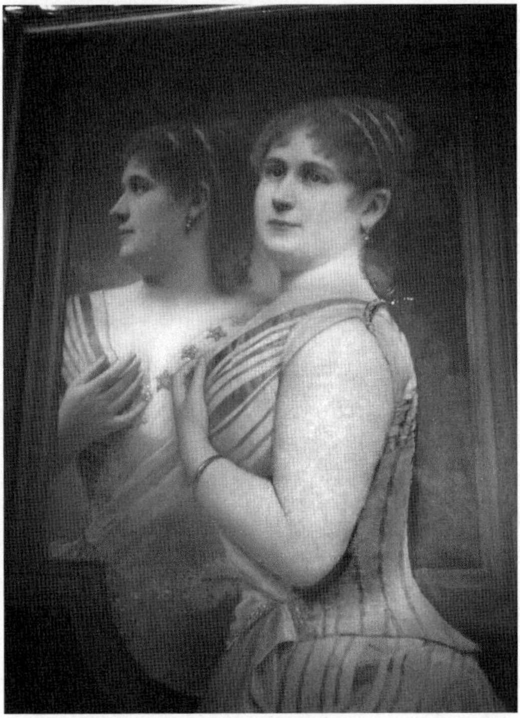

Figure 4: Carl Kellner's wife Marie Antoinette. Painting in possession of the family of Karl-Erwin Lichtenecker (photograph: Karl Baier).

naked and he praises the beauty of her body and her shining eyes within the starry night. This erotic episode of the vision is followed by a scene in which Kellner as priest is climbing up a fire tower to perform a fire sacrifice. The erotic atmosphere and love for his companion is the beginning of a mystical ascent. Kellner climbs up the tower to sacrifice the fire. The one Divine light and life is evoked as present in everything, thereby connecting and unifying everything including Kellner and his human brothers and sisters. What started as sexual attraction and love for his wife ends in a universal communion with the cosmos and especially all human beings. Kellner's monistic cosmology of the one energy emanating from divine consciousness and leading cosmic evolution to higher forms of love is presented in a poetic and visionary way. In his "Introduction into the Esotericism of our Order"[131] Kellner derived an ethic of responsibility from this monism. His vision articulates the emotional and energetic side of this responsibility: the union of all human brothers and sisters. Kellner's description of his yoga experience contains no explicit sexual rite, but nevertheless follows

131 See Kellner 1903.

the same logic as the above-mentioned New Thought techniques of transmutation of sexual energy – and may also be influenced by a New Thought inspired reading of Haṭha Yoga sources.

After the climax of the whole vision, the experience of mystical union, Kellner returns to the individual realities. He sees the sacrificial fire and himself pronouncing a blessing in Aramaic. The surroundings of the fire tower become present, picturesque pleasure gardens with fountains, flowers and sleeping birds that still await morning, whereas Kellner has already touched eternal light.

8. Coda: Herbert Silberer's Theory of Mysticism

Herbert Silberer (1882–1923) was the flashiest second-generation representative of Viennese fin-de-siècle occultism. His outstanding oeuvre and his tragic suicide aptly mark the end of this period and the emergence of a new level of occultist theory.

Silberer's father Victor was a self-made man very much in the style of Kellner – successful in business, Austrian politics, and sports. Kellner and Victor Silberer were friends and Kellner's daughter Eglantine was engaged to Herbert Silberer for a while.[132] Herbert, a passionate balloonist like Victor, worked as journalist, psychoanalyst, and private scholar but never succeeded in becoming financially independent from his father.[133]

In 1909 he applied for a charter at the Martinist order in Paris. His in-depth study of Rosicrucianism and alchemy is probably connected with his affiliation to Martinism.[134] For members of his generation interested in these topics it was an obvious step to join one of the new Rosicrucian organisations.

In 1910 he became a member of the Viennese Psychoanalytic Society, the most important psychoanalytic association of the time that met on Wednesdays at Freud's flat. He irregularly participated in it until the end of his life. Silberer remained an outsider within this group but nonetheless presented his ideas during lectures at the Wednesday meetings and also published ground-breaking psychoanalytical contributions to the interpretation of dreams and symbols and to the comparative psychology of mysticism.[135] He was the first scholar who investigated the connections between alchemy and the psychology of the un-

132 Cf. Weirauch 1998: 193. The relationship between his mother and Silberer was affirmed by Karl-Erwin Lichtenecker in his interview with the author.

133 Nitzschke (1997: 11–15) points out the problematic relationship between Herbert Silberer and his father.

134 Kodek 2009: 326.

135 For Silberer's role within psychoanalysis, see Nitzschke 1988: 10–18.

conscious, as C. G. Jung, the champion of this field, thankfully acknowledged.[136] His distinction between the psychoanalytical and anagogical sense of symbols, dreams, and imaginations that was also adopted by Jung, aimed at reconciling the psychoanalytical approach with a hermetic-theosophical (in the premodern sense of the term "theosophical") interpretation. An English version of his opus magnum *Probleme der Mystik und ihrer Symbolik* (1914) was published in New York in 1917 and had considerable success in the United States.[137]

Rather late in his short life, in 1919, Silberer was initiated into the masonic lodge Sokrates in Vienna.[138] In two talks at the Grand Lodge of Vienna he applied his theory of symbolic thinking to masonic work.

Many essential matters of Viennese fin-de-siècle occultism including yoga are present in his writings. The psychoanalyst Wilhelm Stekel, with whom Silberer collaborated (although Stekel had fallen out with Freud), sums up his occult interests and practices:

> He scrutinized astrology, tried to check the long-distance effects of the stars on individuals and conducted profound studies in alchemy. [...] He experimented a lot with sexual magic and finally also engaged himself with the practices of Raja-Joga [sic]. Through them he successfully immersed himself into deep meditation that at its climax looked like a state of apparent death.[139]

The starting point and centre of *Problems of Mysticism and its Symbolism* is an analysis of the different layers of meaning of "Parabola", a text from *Geheime Figuren der Rosenkreuzer aus dem 16ten und 17ten Jahrhundert.* Silberer maintains a deep affinity between Freemasonry, Rosicrucianism and alchemy based on a common language of signs and symbols that dates back to the ancient European World.[140] He derives the basic structure of the mystical path from this system of symbols and illustrates its universality by pointing to parallels within Christian mysticism, Sufism, and above all yoga.

Silberer defines mysticism as "that religious state which struggles by the shortest way towards the accomplishment of the end of religion, the union with the divinity; or as an intensive cultivation of oneself in order to experience this union".[141] Whereas this definition is very close to Hartmann's definition of yoga in the *Wiener Rundschau,* his description of the different steps on the mystical

136 Jung 1971: 336.
137 Silberer 1917.
138 Kodek 2009: 327.
139 Stekel 1924: 412: "Er studierte Astrologie, versuchte die Fernwirkung der Gestirne auf das Einzelindividuum nachzuprüfen, machte tiefgründige Studien über Alchemie. [...] Er machte viele sexual-magische Experimente und kam auch zu den Raja-Joga-Übungen [sic], bei denen ihm eine innere Versenkung bis zum Bilde des Scheintodes gelang."
140 In this regard he follows the historian of Freemasonry Ludwig Keller (1849–1918).
141 Silberer 1917: 254–255.

path includes many elements from psychoanalysis.[142] For Silberer, mysticism is a process of introversion (a psychological terminus technicus coined by Jung) that starts by entering into the underworld of the unconscious and then leads to a fight with demons and dragons, the infantile and crude desires and drives. This confrontation can fail and one can lose oneself by becoming a sorcerer who tries to satisfy his egocentric desires through magical means, or by becoming a schizophrenic, desperate, or suicidal person. If it ends well, one is reborn through the control of the unconscious impulses and is capable of experiencing union with the divine. The key to this transformation of the human being is sublimation:

> This Freudian term and concept is found in an exactly similar significance in the Hermetic writers. In the receptacle where the mystical work of education is performed, i. e., in man, substances are sublimated; in psychological terms this means that impulses are to be refined and brought from their baseness to a higher level. Freud makes it clear that the libido, particularly the unsocial sexual libido, is in favourable circumstances sublimated, i. e., changed into a socially available impelling power.[143]

According to Silberer, the mutability of sexual desire is known in the mystical traditions as well as in Freud's psychology:

> I observe that the mystical manuals show that the most active power for spiritual education is the sexual libido, which for that reason is partially or entirely withdrawn from its original use. (Rules of chastity.) "Vigor is obtained on the confirmation of continence." (Patañjali, Yoga-Sutra, II, 38.) These instruction books have recognized the great transmutability of the sexual libido. (Cf. ability of sublimation in the alchemistic, as well as in the Freudian terminology.)[144]

Another important dimension of the mystical ascension is the unification of dualities. Like Kellner before him, Silberer mentions the union of sun and moon as the symbolic meaning of Haṭha Yoga and he addresses the similarity to European alchemy that Kellner also must have recognised but did not refer to in his sketch on yoga (maybe out of respect for his audience at the Psychological Congress in Munich):

> It is probably worthy of notice that the Yoga-Mystics, like the alchemists, are acquainted with the idea of the union of the sun and the moon. Two breath- or life currents are to be united, one of which corresponds to the sun, the other to the moon. The expression Hathayoga (where hatha = mighty effort. Cf. Garbe, Samkhya and Yoga, p. 43) will also be interpreted so that Ha = sun, tha = moon, their union = the yoga leading to salvation. (Cf. Hatha-Yoga-Prad., p. I.).[145]

142 Freud, Jung, Stekel, and others.
143 Silberer 1917: 256.
144 Silberer 1917: 303.
145 Silberer 1917: 360.

In line with the alchemical symbolism that uses the sexual union of king and queen as an equivalent to the union of sun and moon, Silberer stresses that not only the union of the two stars, but also the mystic marriage (*hieros gamos*) between man and woman is a widespread symbol for the mystical transcending of dualities, be it the duality of the seer and the seen in general or of the soul and God at the peak of mystical experience. He is convinced that the sexual symbolism is dangerous because it easily could be taken literally. The use of the unconcealed sexual act as a symbol would lead to a degeneration of religion.[146] If Stekel is right and Silberer experimented with sex magic, and if his practice was coherent with the ideas developed in his major work, it is hard to imagine that his ritual sex was not based on the principle of sublimation of the sexual drive.

Several signs in Silberer's work announce a new era. His writings are more systematic and academic than those of the older generation of Viennese occultists. Hartmann's and Kellner's writings on yoga are not mentioned at all. He prefers to quote academic works like Richard Garbe's *Sāṃkhya und Yoga* (1896), the writings of Paul Deussen, or Leopold von Schroeder's translation of the *Bhagavadgītā*. Only if no other translation of a yoga text was available did he use theosophical editions. Silberer evaluates Hartmann's English edition of *Geheime Figuren der Rosenkreuzer aus dem 16ten und 17ten Jahrhundert* as a "poor translation of the German original".[147]

Silberer was very negative about Theosophy in general. In *Durch Tod zum Leben* ("Through Death towards New Life"), an extended study from 1915 written under the sway of the beginning of World War I, he radically dissociates from the theosophical movement using the name "Theosophisticism" to distinguish Blavatsky's modern Theosophy from the old Theosophy that in his view is the only one worthy of this name. He recommends an unbiased study of ethnology and psychoanalysis to the "Theosophisticists". Following Hans Freimark, he also attacks the tendency of Theosophy and Rudolf Steiner to reify the human mind.[148]

In a friendlier, but nonetheless critical way, he connects his own project to Kerning's Freemasonry.

> To-day, too, there is a royal art. Freemasonry bears this name. Not only the name, but its ethical ideal connects it with the spirit of the old alchemy. This statement will probably be contradicted and meet the same denial as did once the ideas of Kernning [sic] (J. Krebs), although I think I am on different ground from that of this poetic but, in my eyes, all too uncritical author.[149]

146 Cf. Silberer 1917: 204–205.
147 Silberer 1917: 436.
148 Cf. Silberer 1997: 310.
149 Silberer 1917: 378.

The fin-de-siècle occultists of the Habsburgian Empire used a pseudo-scientific language that had no chance of being taken seriously by mainstream science, or they articulated themselves in two quite different languages depending on whether they addressed an occult or a scientific audience. Silberer succeeded in connecting his occult thought with psychoanalytical theory in a way that enriched both. Psychoanalysis was a disputed discipline but it was, at least, accepted as a problematic but nonetheless interesting scientific alternative with a certain lobby inside academia. The way in which the Viennese psychoanalytical occultist interprets yoga and other religious practices and topics already breathes the spirit of the Eranos conferences. Historically, Silberer's work functions as a link between the religionist form of academic research represented by the Eranos circle and fin-de-siècle occultism.

References

Basu, S. (Trans.). (1887). *The Esoteric Philosophy of the Tantras: Shiva Sanhita.* Calcutta: Heeralal Dhole (repr. New Delhi: Cosmo Publications, 2004).

Binder, H. (2009). *Gustav Meyrink: Ein Leben im Bann der Magie.* Prag: Vitalis-Verlag.

Birch, J. (2011). The Meaning of haṭha in Early Haṭhayoga. *Journal of the American Oriental Society, 131*(4), 527–554.

Blavatsky, H. (1877). *Isis Unveiled: A Master Key to the Mysteries of Ancient and Modern Science.* 2 vols. New York: J. W. Bouton.

Bulwer-Lytton, Sir E. (1842). *Zanoni.* Leipzig: Bernhard Tauchnitz Jun.

Butler, H. E. (1901). *Praktische Methoden den Erfolg zu sichern: Die Geheimnisse des Geschlechtslebens.* Carl Georgi's Bücherei 4. Berlin: Carl Georgi's Bücherei.

Carrer, L. (Ed., Trans.). (2002). *Ambroise-August Liébeault: The Hypnological Legacy of a Secular Saint.* College Station, TX: Virtual.bookworm.com.

Das innere Dreieck (1904). An alle Schüler des okkulten Kreises. *Oriflamme, 3,* 8.

De Michelis (2004). *A History of Modern Yoga: Patañjali and Western Esotericism.* London: Continuum.

Dotzler, M. (1906). Schreiben des Br. Max Dotzler an die Herren Held in Hamburg und Adriány in Nürnberg. *Oriflamme, 5*(2), Neue Serie, 58–64.

Dritter Internationaler Congress für Psychologie in München (1897). München: Lehmann.

Dr. Karl Kellner [obituary] (1905). *Volksfreund Hallein, XV. Jahrgang, Nr. 39,* 30 September 1905, 1–2.

Dvorak, J. (1993). *Satanismus: Schwarze Rituale, Teufelswahn und Exorzismus. Geschichte und Gegenwart.* 2nd ed. München: Heyne.

Eek, S. (Ed.). (1978). *Damodar and the Pioneers of the Theosophical Movement.* Adyar: Theosophical Publishing House.

Emanuel (pseud. Franz Hartmann). (1905). Obituary Br. Dr. Carl Kellner. *Oriflamme, 3*(6), 1–2.

Freud, S. (1962). *Civilization and its Discontents. Newly Translated from the German and Edited by James Strachey.* New York: W. W. Norton.

Freud, S. (1999). *Gesammelte Werke.* Vol. XIV: *Werke aus den Jahren 1925–1931.* Frankfurt am Main: Fischer Taschenbuch Verlag.

Gauld, N. (1995). *A History of Hypnotism.* Cambridge: Cambridge University Press.

Goodrick-Clarke, N. (1986). The Modern Occult Revival in Vienna 1880–1910. *Theosophical History, I*(5), 97–111.

Hartmann, F. (1888). *Magic: White and Black, or: The Science of Finite and Infinite Life Containing Practical Hints for Students of Occultism.* 3rd rev. and enlarged edition. London: George Redway.

Hartmann, F. (1893a). Das Wesen der Alchemie. *Lotusblüten, I. Semester (Heft IV–IX)*, 411–447.

Hartmann, F. (1893b). *Ueber eine neue Heilmethode zur Heilung von Lungentuberkulose, Katarrh, Influenza, und anderen Krankheiten der Athmungsorgane vermittelst der Einathmung gewisser Gase und Dämpfe aus der bei der Cellulosefabrikation gebrauchten Kochflüssigkeit. Nebst einem Anhange, bezugnehmend auf verschiedene noch wenig erforschte, aber im Alterthum wohlbekannte Entstehungsursachen von Krankheitserscheinungen.* Leipzig: Verlag von Wilhelm Friedrich.

Hartmann, F. (1899). Die Bhagavad-Gita der Indier. *Wiener Rundschau, 15,* 15 June 1899, 250–259.

Hartmann, F. (1906). The Danger of "Experimenting in Occultism". *The Occult Review, III,* 133–135.

Hartmann, F. (1923–1924). Dr. Karl Kellner, ein Opfer des Okkultismus. *Theosophie, XII,* 306–309.

Hevesi, L. (1901). *Mac Eck's sonderbare Reisen zwischen Konstantinopel und San Francisco.* Stuttgart: A. Bonz' Erben (repr. Norderstedt: Vero Verlag, 2013).

James, W. (1902). *The Varieties of Religious Experience: A Study in Human Nature.* Being the Gifford Lectures on Natural Religion Delivered at Edinburgh in 1901–1902. New York: Longmans, Green, and Co.

Jung, C. G. (1971). *Mysterium Coniunctionis.* Gesammelte Werke 14.2. Freiburg i. Br.: Olten.

Kaczynski, R. (2012). *Forgotten Templars: The Untold Origins of Ordo Templi Orientis.* n.p.: R. Kaczynski.

Kellner, C. (1896a). *Yoga: Eine Skizze über den psycho-physiologischen Teil der alten indischen Yogalehre. Dem III. Internationalen Congress für Psychologie gewidmet.* München: Kastner & Lossen.

Kellner, C. (1896b). "Experimenteller Beweis über die Verwandelbarkeit der sogenannten Grundstoffe". Manuscript. Wien: Austrian Academy of Sciences. Archive Registration Number VS 319.

Kellner, C. (1903). Einführung in den Esoterismus unseres Ordens der A. und A. Freimaurer. *Oriflamme, 2,* 15–16.

Kellner, C. & Reuss, Th. (1903). Das Geheimnis der Hochgrade unseres Ordens. Ein Manifesto des Großorients. *Oriflamme, 11*(6), 48–50.

Kodek, G. K. (2009). *Unsere Bausteine sind die Menschen: Die Mitglieder der Wiener Freimaurer-Logen 1869–1938.* Wien: Löcker.

Köthner, P. (1902). Die Goldmacherkunst im Mittelalter und in der Gegenwart. *Zeitschrift für Naturwissenschaften, 75,* 1–24.

Lechler, V. (2013). *Heinrich Tränker als Theosoph, Rosenkreuzer und Pansoph. Unter Mitarbeit von Wolfgang Kistemann.* Stuttgart: Selbstverlag Volker Lechler.

Lichtenecker, K.-E. (2014). Interview with the author, 11 February 2014.

Liébeault, A.-A. (1889). *Le sommeil provoqué et les états analogues.* Paris: Octave Dion.

Mahatma Arkaja Brahma (c 1911). *Liebe und Ehe.* Dresden: Rudolph'sche Verlagsbuchhandlung.

McIntosh, Ch. (1974). *Eliphas Lévi and the French Occult Revival.* New York: Samuel Weiser.

Meyrink, G. (2010). The Transformation of the Blood. In M. Mitchell (Ed.), *The Dedalus Meyrink Reader* (pp. 120–185). Swatry: Dedalus.

Mitra, Rájendralála (1883). *The Yoga Aphorisms of Patanjali With the Commentary of Bhoja Rájá and an English Translation.* Calcutta: J. W. Thomas.

Möller, H. & Howe, E. (1986). *Merlin Peregrinus: Vom Untergrund des Abendlandes.* Würzburg: Königshausen und Neumann.

Mulot-Déri, S. (1988). Alte Ungenannte Tage. Zu einer Biographie Ecksteins. In F. Eckstein, *'Alte Unnennbare Tage!': Erinnerungen aus siebzig Lehr- und Wanderjahren* (pp. 295–328). Wien: Wiener Journal Zeitschriftenverlag.

Nitzschke, B. (1988). Die Gefahr, sich selbst ausgeliefert zu sein: Herbert Silberer, zum Beispiel. In B. Nitzschke (Ed.), *Zu Fuss durch den Kopf: Wanderungen im Gedankengebirge. Ausgewählte Schriften Herbert Silberers. Miszellen zu seinem Leben und Werk* (pp. 7–79). Tübingen: edition discord.

Nitzschke, B. (1997). Vorwort: Herbert Silberer – Skizzen zu seinem Leben und Werk. In H. Silberer, *Probleme der Mystik: Durch Leben zum Tod. Der Seelenspiegel* (pp. 9–19). Sinzheim: Archiv für Altes und Geheimes Wissen.

Nothung, das neidliche [sic] Schwert (pseud. Theodor Reuss). (1906). Ehefrage, Sexualreform und Frauenlogen. *Oriflamme, 5*(1), Neue Serie, 12–21.

Ostwald, W. (1902). *Vorlesungen über Naturphilosophie.* Leipzig: Veit & Comp.

Pendragon (pseud. Theodor Reuss). (1906). *Lingam–Yoni oder die Mysterien des Geschlechts-Kultus als die Basis der Religion aller Kulturvölker des Altertums und des Marienkultus in der christlichen Kirche sowie Ursprung des Kreuzes und des Crux Ansata.* Gross-Lichterfelde, Berlin: Verlag Willsson.

Ramacharaka, Yogi (pseud. William Walker Atkinson). (1904). *Science of Breath: A Complete Manual of The Oriental Breathing Philosophy of Physical, Mental, Psychic and Spiritual Development.* Chicago: Yogi Publication Society.

Reuss, Th. (1906). Brief Reuss an Franz Held vom 19. August 1903. *Oriflamme, 5*(2), Neue Serie, 108–111.

Reuss, Th. (1912). Mysteria Mystica Maxima. *Oriflamme, 7 (Jubiläums-Ausgabe)*, 21–23.

Sauerwein, J. (1929). A Glimpse of the Beyond. *Anthroposophy, 4*, 413–419.

Schmidt, L. E. (2010). *Heaven's Bride: The Unprintable Life of Ida C. Craddock, American Mystic, Scholar, Sexologist, Martyr and Madwoman.* New York: Basic Books.

Semrau, E. (2012). *Erleuchtung und Verblendung: Einflüsse esoterischen Gedankenguts auf die Entwicklung der Wiener Moderne.* Innsbruck: Studienverlag.

Silberer, H. (1997). *Durch Tod zum Leben: Eine kurze Untersuchung über die entwicklungsgeschichtliche Bedeutung des Symbols der Wiedergeburt in seinen Urformen, mit besonderer Berücksichtigung der modernen Theosophie.* In H. Silberer, *Probleme der Mystik und ihrer Symbolik. Durch Tod zum Leben. Der Seelenspiegel* (pp. 298–354). Sinzheim: Frietsch-Verlag (repr. of *Durch Tod zum Leben.* Beiträge zur Geschichte der neueren Mystik und Magie 4. Leipzig: Heims, 1915).

Silberer, H. (1917). *Problems of Mysticism and Its Symbolism.* New York: Moffat, Yard and Co.

Stekel, W. (1924). In memoriam Herbert Silberer. *Fortschritte der Sexualwissenschaft und Psychoanalyse*, Vol. 1. Leipzig: Franz Deuticke, pp. 408–420.

Tatya, T. (Ed.). (1893). *The Haṭha-yogapradipika of Svātmārām Swāmi. Translated by T. R. Shrinivās Iyāngār.* Bombay: Theosophical Publication Fund (repr. Adyar: The Theosophical Society, 1972).

Timms, E. (2013). *Dynamik der Kreise, Resonanz der Räume: Die schöpferischen Impulse der Wiener Moderne.* Weitra: Bibliothek der Provinz.

Vivekananda, S. (1992). *Rāja Yoga.* In *The Complete Works of Swami Vivekananda.* Vol. 1 (pp. 119–314). Mayavati Memorial Edition. 14th repr. Calcutta: Advaita Ashrama.

Webb, J. (1976). *The Occult Establishment.* La Salle, IL: Open Court Publishing Company (repr. Glasgow: Richard Drew Publishing, 1981).

Weinfurter, K. (1930). *Der brennende Busch: Der entschleierte Weg zur Mystik.* Lorch (Württemberg): Renatus-Verlag (7th ed. Bietigheim: Karl Rohm, c 1965).

Weirauch, W. (1998). Eine Reise nach Wien. Bei den Quellen des OTO. Interview mit Josef Dvorak. *Flensburger Hefte, 63*/I, 171–220.

Whalen, R. W. (2007). *Sacred Spring: God and the Birth of Modernism in Fin de Siècle Vienna.* Grand Rapids, USA: Eerdmans Publishing Company.

Yarker, J. (1905). Obituary of Dr. Karl Kellner. *Ars Quatuor Coronatorum, 18*, 150.

Chapter 10

Yoga, Nature Cure and "Perfect" Health: The Purity of the Fluid Body in an Impure World

Joseph S. Alter

Contents

1. Introduction 441

2. Yoga: The Problem of Consciousness and Perfection 444

3. Nature Cure: Purification and the Perfectibility of Health 447

4. Healing and Consciousness in Rishikesh: From the Unity of Disease to the Yoga of Synthesis 450

References 457

Joseph S. Alter

Chapter 10: Yoga, Nature Cure and "Perfect" Health: The Purity of the Fluid Body in an Impure World

1. Introduction

This chapter seeks to provide an answer to the question of why *āsana* and *prāṇāyāma* came to be understood within the framework of Nature Cure in modern India, as institutionalised in the Central Council for Research on Yoga and Naturopathy. The focus is on the correlation between purification and embodied perfection, and the way in which impurity is understood to be problematic for health as well as for the development of transcendent consciousness. Swami Sivananda's early publications on healing and medicine are used to show how a biomedical doctor who renounced the world and established the Divine Life Society – what became one of the most influential centers for the development of modern yoga – integrated elements from yoga and Nature Cure into his understanding of the body, embodied impurity and the perfection of health.

The opposition of purity and pollution has structured arguments about the nature of many aspects of social life in South Asia, encompassing ritual, social hierarchy, auspiciousness, and diet among many other features of culture. The dynamics of exchange based on principles of caste identity has in particular stimulated considerable debate, ranging from Dumont's dualistic thesis[1] to Marriott's three-dimensional, cubic model of transaction based on Hindu categories.[2] The literature generated by this and related arguments has produced phenomenal insight into the nature of the body and embodied practices that show how health is linked to problems of philosophy and metaphysics.[3] Two interrelated aspects of the body in this regard – and the nature of bodily substances specifically – will be examined here in order to help explain the popularity of yoga in contemporary India – a popularity that does not simply reflect its ancient philosophical heritage, whatever that can be made to be in terms of

1 Dumont 1970.
2 Marriott 1990.
3 See Daniel & Pugh 1984: Leslie 1976; Leslie & Young 1992.

ideology. The argument presented here, about what is often mistakenly said to be a pure expression of profound philosophical idealism, is based on a materialist conception of the history of the body in modern practice: yoga's popularity is a function of hybridity on a number of different levels involving the meaning and experience of both the structural opposition of purity and pollution as a binary pair, and the fluid nature of the body. Yoga takes shape as practice in historically contextualised environments where the meaning and significance of fluidity, purity and pollution changes over time.

Yoga in contemporary India takes on as many forms as it does elsewhere around the world, ranging from upscale urban studios to institutionalised routines and individualised practice.[4] What may distinguish India as a context for understanding yoga is the fact that high end studio forms of practice – as can be found at Ananda Spa in the Himalayan town of Rishikesh – are found cheek by jowl, so to speak, with forms of practice that seek to lay claim to ancient heritage and authenticity, precisely because they are Indian,[5] and then more "traditionally Indian" than anywhere else precisely because they are in specific places like Rishikesh, the so-called birthplace of classical yoga.[6] In other words, the question of authenticity and heritage is heavily marked in India, not because the heritage is necessarily there in India – the "that art thou" of *tat tvam asi* being, quite literally, neither here (in the West) *nor* there (in India) – but because its location in space and time is rendered highly problematic by the multiplicity of forms at play in the reality of the contemporary moment.

In relation to modern history, yoga in contemporary India has been institutionalised and professionalised in a way that is somewhat unique and distinctive. Although intimately linked to discourses of Orientalism that highlight ineffable, arcane and esoteric attributes,[7] it has taken shape under rubrics of science, medicine, athletics and religion, as these discursive rubrics, and the practices therein, have themselves been shaped by the conflicted ideals of colonial and postcolonial nationalism.[8] More specifically, yoga in modern India has been shaped by a long history of institutionalisation and professionalisation in relation to medicine. Although the history of this development has defined many aspects of global practice, in India there is considerable continuity between early twentieth century experiments with health and healing and the structured regimentation of *āsana* and *prāṇāyāma* in most forms of public performance, including schools, hospitals, jails, ashrams and neighbourhood parks as well as in popular television programmes.

4 Singleton 2010.
5 Alter 1997, 2004.
6 Strauss 2005, 2008.
7 See Urban 2010.
8 Alter 2004, 2006, 2008a, 2008b, 2014.

While there are large, private organisations that highlight specific features of modern yoga's concern with health, healing and athleticism,[9] and well established social movements that have played an important role in popularisation[10] – as well as numerous charismatic figures who have defined specific techniques such as the Raja of Aundh's *sūrya namaskār,* Dr. Shanti Prakash Atreya's yogic wrestling,[11] and Raojibhai Patel's auto-urine therapy[12] – one of the interesting and important features of yoga in modern India is the professionalisation of practice within the structure of government administration as this relates to ideas about public health in middle-class Indian consciousness.[13]

In many ways the Central Council for Research on Yoga and Naturopathy (CCRYN), established in the 1990s and then incorporated under the Ministry of Ayurveda, Yoga and Naturopathy, Unani, Siddha and Homoeopathy (AYUSH) in 2014, can be seen as a state institution that establishes the legitimacy of yoga – and the legal status of licensed, commercial practitioners – in terms of healing and health care within a framework of medical pluralism. Beyond legitimacy, the structure of CCRYN support and control, which has taken various forms over the past thirty years, has played a major role in postural yoga's popularisation where, in many contexts, practice is mechanical, mundane and mass-produced to a degree that is at the opposite extreme from what might be imagined in the shadow light of Orientalism's mystical and magical take on the subject.

There are many organisations that offer teacher training programmes with certification of various kinds, but the overarching structure of national level certified training under the authority of the CCRYN reflects a history of professionalisation that is intimately linked to histories of science, medicine and public health, both in colonial India and elsewhere. Significantly, it also reflects a particular kind of institutionalised spirituality that blends health, governmentality and consciousness. Although by no means linear, an influential and well-marked trajectory in this development connects early innovators such as Swami Kuvalayananda and Shri Yogendra directly to the CCRYN. Almost all forms of contemporary practice in India have been influenced, either directly or indirectly, by this discursive trajectory; a discourse of health and healing that defines the applied significance of *āsana* and *prāṇāyāma* in practice.[14]

As the AYUSH designation for the central research council suggests, yoga and naturopathy are thought to be two parts of a single system of health care, the other systems within the administrative structure being Āyurveda, Unani, Siddha

9 Alter 2004: 73–108; 2011: 149–178.
10 Alter 1997.
11 Alter 2013b.
12 Alter 2000: 146–154; 2004: 181–210.
13 Alter 2000: 55–82.
14 Alter 2004: 109–141.

and homeopathy. Both the structure of AYUSH itself as well as the conjunction of yoga and naturopathy within this framework of pluralism reflects a number of interesting historical patterns and developments, some of which will be touched on below. But the most basic question is clear and unambiguous: how do we make sense of the structural conjuncture of yoga and naturopathy in the context of India? It must have more to do with feeling, in some ineffable sense, than with logic, pure and simple, since the range of medical options available in South Asia includes Āyurveda, as well as a spectrum of home remedies very similar to Nature Cure treatment, as this form of treatment was formalised in nineteenth century Europe. As will be argued here, one aspect of this "feeling" is the correlation of purity and self-purification with a particular kind of perfectibility in embodied experience and the development of a set of practices – including the publication of books – that articulate the significance of this experience.

2. Yoga: The Problem of Consciousness and Perfection

A great deal has been written about yoga from a number of perspectives. Many key philosophical, metaphysical and historical questions are coloured by a complex intellectual history that has suffered under the burden of colonialism, nationalism and post-colonialism's various disciplinary manifestations.[15] The arguments within this intellectual history are important, but no attempt is made here to sort out particular questions on specific points of scholarship. Rather an effort is made to distill out from this body of literature basic themes that transcend different interpretations. The risk is obvious: over-generalisation and the interest-driven selection of themes to make "disinterested", objective claims. Nevertheless, and other problems – of terminology, classification and categorisation – notwithstanding, the distillation of generalisations is a useful exercise since, following the logic of parsimony, the most persuasive arguments are based on making the fewest abstract assumptions.

One aspect of yoga is especially helpful in this respect – it is an embodied form of practice, regardless of the extent to which there are questions about the distinction between mind and body. Yoga is something you do, and therefore practice is anchored in experience rather than imaginative speculation, where anything is possible. While this is true for yoga in general, it obviously has particular significance for the practice of yoga in the experience of people whose lives can be understood in the grounded context of history and culture; that is, in a context that includes more than just the idealised experience of yoga in the imagination. The further back in time one goes the less is known about "context"

15 De Michelis 2003 and 2008; Singleton & Goldberg 2014; White 2014.

although terminology is often revealing – "gymnosophist" being a case in point in relation to the classical world.[16] In any case, philology almost always provides a critical perspective on the obscured nature of the body at specific points in time.[17]

Much has been made – and maligned – about Orientalist misperceptions of this and that in the characterisation of arguments that relate to the pervasive problem of consciousness in South Asian schools of philosophical thought. It is easy to see how intellectual attempts to understand the problem lead to pejorative generalisations about nihilism, negativism, self-mortification and detachment from the world at large, especially from perspectives of incipient colonial ethnocentrism.[18] It is also easy to see how a critical intellectual history of these kinds of generalisations produces various forms of reactionary revisionism, including derivatively discursive generalisations with both overtones and pervasive undertones of nationalism.

Notwithstanding the problematic ways in which Orientalism provokes nationalist responses, it is necessary to take the compromised contingency of consciousness seriously as an ontological problem in the context of South Asian philosophical speculation in order to understand what makes yoga possible as a form of modern practice. On one level – as is manifest clearly in the gross body – the problem is characterised as obstruction, impurity and pollution on the one hand, and, on the other, by impermanence. In essence, change reflects the contingency of reality in consciousness. The body manifests this in all of its aspects, gross and subtle alike.[19] Although our sense of self is permanent, hair, tears, feces, urine, saliva, breath, blood, semen, ear wax, finger and toe nails, sweat, light in the eyes, and consciousness all reflect the impermanence of material reality as the body changes through time, until death.[20] And, needless to say, death defines a particular kind of problem heavily marked by the impermanence of material existence and the derivative consequences of this for the living, pollution, impurity and the "accretions" of karma being paramount. In conjunction with this it is important to keep in mind the process of decomposition and decay which follows death, as bodily substances continue to flow and mix into the environment.[21] On this point fire plays a significant role, both in terms of ritual purification and with respect to the "physics" of transubstantiation.

One can imagine two possible solutions to the problem of time in relation to consciousness – flow with it or stop the flow. However, these are not at all the

16 Alter 2013a; see also Alter 2009 for the term "yoga" in the modern context of pre-modern East Asian history.
17 See Maas 2008; Mallinson 2012; Wujastyk 2009; White 2012; Zysk 2007.
18 See Urban 2010.
19 See Samuel 2013.
20 See Keyes & Daniel 1983.
21 Bloch & Parry 1982; Parry 1994.

same kind of solution; they are not on the same plane of reality. To flow with time is to simply embody consciousness of change rather than to transcend consciousness which is itself a material manifestation of contingency. The idea of rebirth is perhaps the best example of this, turning what appears to be linear into the idea of an endless cycle.[22] There are also other examples of how ritual performances play with the fluidity of time and substance in order to engage the problem of contingency. In keeping with health and medical issues, Āyurveda provides some striking examples that are especially apropos.

In many ways Ayurvedic medicine is structured around the epistemological problem of growing old.[23] Rasāyana therapy causes the body of a person who is aging "gracefully" to first radically decompose into a fluid mass of decay and then reconstitute itself into an adamantine form of its previously organic self. Rasāyana enables an immortal king to take advantage of Vājīkaraṇa therapy without suffering the consequences of semen loss; although, even in the logical contrivance of this scenario, "real" immortality is vested not in endless priapic potency, but in the health and strength of progeny and lineage.[24] It is difficult to escape the flow of time while living in the material body.

Ayurvedic references allude to a key point that will be examined in more detail with reference to yogic practice, namely the correlation of purity, health and immortality. In a way that directly reflects the problem of contingency in creation – and in procreation as a reproduction of the action of creation – perfect health is an impossible ideal. Instability is endemic to the most elemental aspect of life. More refined degrees of purity approximate perfection. And this, I think, is a key point. Purity in the context of Ayurvedic practice – and also, as we will see, in yoga – is not defined in opposition to categorical impurity, but rather in terms of refinement, as in the image of a diamond-like body. However, the term's polysemy encourages a degree of connotational blurring, such that purity is to perfection as cleanliness is to godliness. Somewhat surprisingly, however, degrees of "perfection" can be manifest in substances that are, in other contexts, regarded as rather impure, such as in the case of urine.[25] It is polluted and polluting in the context of ritual practices of various kinds, and yet with regard to auto-urine therapy it is conceptualised as a "perfect" articulation of re-cycling, and all that this can be made to mean within a framework involving the embodied flow of substances and time. In a somewhat different but comparable way, blood – and the gendered dynamics of containment[26] – suggests the subtle complexity of purity, perfection, and pollution in the flow of bodily substances.[27]

22 Keyes & Daniel 1983.
23 Alter 1999.
24 Alter 2011: 179–212.
25 Alter 2004: 181–210.
26 Selby 2005.

If Āyurveda struggles with the imperfectability of time that flows through bodies and bodies flowing through time, yoga is about stopping the flow and embodying the end of time, so to speak.[28] The literature on yoga makes this very clear, although it also makes it very clear that to understand what this means, and to put that understanding into practice, is anything but clear and obvious. And this is the critical point. Up until the end of the nineteenth century, yoga was inherently arcane, esoteric and secretive, but also perfectly clear about what could be achieved – the power of perfection and the perfection of embodied power.[29] The seductive potential of embodied perfection rubbed off onto the notion of "purity" as a realist construct in the rapidly globalizing cultural context of late colonial India. Refined techniques for self-purification invoked the power of yogic perfection in terms of a practical means by which to discover its hidden secrets.[30] Combined with Nature Cure, Yoga provided a practical, applied solution to the problem of contingency in the care of health – albeit with intimations of immortality – without getting caught up in the cyclical flow of time, as did the once and future patients of Caraka and Vāgbhaṭa.

3. Nature Cure: Purification and the Perfectibility of Health

At almost exactly the same time that individuals were experimenting with the practice of yoga in different parts of the world at the fin de siècle, Nature Cure started to become popular in the cultural crucible of urban India. To understand how and why a reactionary form of radically alternative nineteenth century European medicine sparked the early twentieth century imagination, it is important to keep at least five historical developments in mind.

First, what goes around comes around, to put it colloquially: Orientalism – and with it elements of Sāṃkhyan philosophy[31] – helped to shape articulations of nature and naturalism within the context of eighteenth century German romanticism, as romanticism provided the ideological – and aesthetic – backdrop for the practice of Nature Cure in the nineteenth century. There are intriguing hints that the embodied practice of yoga itself may have filtered into early European consciousness.[32] And it is interesting to note how the *Yogasūtra* played into arguments about broad themes in philosophy,[33] including debates about the

27 Copeman 2009.
28 Sarbacker 2005; White 1989 and 1996.
29 De Michelis 2003; Samuel 2008; White 2009.
30 Sarbacker 2008.
31 Larson 1969; Larson & Bhattacharya 1987.
32 Marchignoli 2002.
33 See White 2014.

methods of dialectical reasoning as against holistic relativism.[34] To be sure, the transmigration of Nature Cure to India at the turn of the last century owes a small debt to the fact that German Romanticism survived Hegel's early nineteenth century critique of its Indian sources of inspiration, as outlined by the brothers Schlegel, Humboldt and Schopenhauer. However, not too much should be made of all this, since the connection between Indology, romanticism and Nature Cure is oblique at best; a more linear history connects Nature Cure to Hippocrates, but even then without much more than the four elements being the *arche.* There is hardly a hint of Galenic humoralism in the "industrial strength" Nature Cure of the late nineteenth century!

Second, the end of the nineteenth century was characterised by dramatic medical innovations such as germ theory and vaccination, but also by an epidemiological transition manifest as a crisis of public health involving wide spread infectious diseases and broad based antipathy toward institutionalised medicine – and fear of iatrogenesis – especially in late industrial Europe. This extended to many parts of the world, including urban India.[35] Concerns about health and the problems of health care were compounded by the time and space compression of the epidemiological transition in places such as India.

Third, the structure of colonial medicine in the practice of public health involved broad based regulations to control the movement and behavior of populations, and these regulations often involved doing things to people, and to their bodies and environments, that did not allow for a great deal of choice and freedom, to put it mildly.[36] This provoked considerable interest in alternative forms of medicine – and the indigenisation of biomedicine[37] – as a kind of self-preservation based on self-treatment that sometimes had political implications.

Fourth, science came to define an epistemology of modernity in a way that was profoundly imperial by the turn of the century, as well as increasingly reductive, deterministic, and hegemonic.[38] Perhaps on account of this, the discursive field of science also became increasingly global at this time in ways that might be characterised as "trans-colonial" rather than nationalistic, given the flow of creative ideas about science and alternative "science" among activists in India, Europe, the United States and elsewhere. Although space does not permit a full discussion here, the work of J. S. Haldane and his son J. B. S. Haldane reflects a remarkable articulation of scientific holism – albeit from within the bracket of Cartesian empiricism – that blends into fiction, philosophy and a politics of

34 See Baier 1998 and 2009, and Halbfass 1988 for a discussion of Indology, German philosophy and Orientalism.
35 Berger 2013; Bashford 2004.
36 Arnold 1993; Pati & Harrison 2009.
37 Mukharji 2009.
38 Habib & Raina 2007.

inspired socialism.[39] Trans-colonial critiques of modernity – and experiments with the embodiment of alternative life-styles – further animated the thinking of charismatic figures as diverse as Mohandas Gandhi, Bernarr McFadden, Sylvester Graham, John Ruskin and Leo Tolstoy.

Fifth, the politics of nationalism produced profound ambivalence about the relationship between cultural heritage and modernity as reflected in arguments about the purity and power of language and languages, the reification and consolidation of beliefs and practices into "religious systems", and the practice, delineation and theorisation of traditional medicine. Ambivalence about the nature of Ayurvedic modernity[40] – how to reconcile humours with germ theory, for example[41] – created a space for new forms of medical practice that were at once unambiguously modern and unambiguously alternative as well as detached from the burden of a community's imagination concerning problems of traditional authenticity and the preservation of the purity of received wisdom. On this point, yoga's counter-cultural mystique and insistence on the obscure secrecy of true knowledge allowed for creative, uninhibited interpretations in the experimental domain of applied "clinical" practice.[42] Since yoga was *not* medical, its application *as* naturopathic medicine was less problematic with respect to the relationship between heritage and modernity.

While various cultural factors stimulated the development of Nature Cure, especially ritualised forms of bathing in early modern Europe, its invention is closely associated with technology – albeit simple technology, at least at first – as a means by which to use "nature" in order to solve problems of highly invasive and dangerous forms of institutionalised biomedicine.[43] This involved a reconceptualisation of nature and health, manifest clearly in Vincenz Priessnitz's account of his early nineteenth century "invention" of water therapy using wet cloth wraps after watching a deer heal itself of a wound by bathing in a stream. More than likely this was an invention in the sense that Priessnitz – who by no stretch of the imagination could have been the first person to cover a wound with a wet cloth – contextualised the provincialism of what he was doing in terms of the big-picture of Europe, professionalised medicine and European modernity around him. By the late 1830s he had established a spa near the town of Gräfenberg. During the course of his long career this Czech "peasant" treated artists, intellectuals and wealthy industrialists throughout Europe including a large number of the Austrian aristocracy.

39 Adams 2000; Sarkar 1992.
40 Berger 2013; Langford 2002.
41 Leslie 1976; Leslie & Young 1992.
42 Alter 2004.
43 Kirchfeld & Boyle 2005. See Singh 1980 for Europe and India, and Whorton 1982, 2000 and 2002 for the United States.

4. Healing and Consciousness in Rishikesh: From the Unity of Disease to the Yoga of Synthesis

While the history of Nature Cure's development is interesting on many levels and important as a general framework for understanding what follows, for our purposes here it is only necessary to focus on Louis Kuhne's theory of the Unity of Disease. This was explained in his book *The New Science of Healing,*[44] which had a significant impact on the practice of self-care in India.[45] Kuhne developed his theory based on dietary and hydrotherapeutic techniques he used to heal himself. He then established a large sanatorium in Leipzig in the 1880s where he experimented with various technologies to administer treatment using only air, water, earth and sunlight.

Kuhne's theory of the Unity of Disease is critical for understanding how yoga *āsana* and *prāṇāyāma* were incorporated into the techno-holism of Nature Cure, alongside bathtubs, showers and solariums of various sizes and shapes. Three features of the theory are particularly important. First, bodies heal themselves, and any attempt to use drugs or perform surgery is harmful and counterproductive. Second, diseases, no matter how different from one another, are, in fact, just symptoms of a more basic, singular problem: toxicity. Toxicity is a chronic condition of life lived in an unnatural mode. Of course this begs a key question, with intimations of Sāṃkhyan dialectics: what is the nature of nature, and how is it integrated into "natural" existence? Third and perhaps most controversial, symptoms of distress, no matter how traumatic, are positive signs of the body working to purge toxins and restore health.

On a fundamental level, therefore, Kuhne's theory of the Unity of Disease defines human existence as an existential problem that begs the question of the absolute purity of nature in human experience, as experience is predicated on culture and cultural perception. The contrivance of purity in the elements earth, water, sunlight, and air provides a logical – and ultimately materialised – mechanism to work toward a resolution of this problem. But, quite obviously, consciousness as a reflection of culture prohibits a resolution that is quite that simple. Can you completely purge culture from the body? Priessnitz's account of the "bathing" deer is simply a particular example of the way in which culture distorts our perception of the reality of the environment as a cultural construction of nature. Significantly, however, practitioners of Nature Cure from Priessnitz through Kneipp to Kuhne – and on through a range of practitioners of yoga in India – located the possibility of perfection in the configuration of natural

44 Kuhne 1892.
45 Singh 1980.

elements involving the body, ecology and the environment in the context of modernity.

Kuhne's book *The New Science of Healing* was translated into Telugu, Urdu and Hindi around the turn of the century, followed shortly thereafter by Adolf Just's manifesto "Return to Nature!".[46] These books inspired a large number of individuals to experiment on themselves, some of whom advocated Kuhne's approach using just tubs, douches and showers and others who experimented with related techniques, including *āsana, kriyā* and *prāṇāyāma.*[47]

Having examined many of the earliest cases in which scientific experimentation was used to understand the medical application of *āsana* and *prāṇāyāma,* my goal here is to more thoroughly work out the correlation between philosophy, yoga and Nature Cure by examining the work of Swami Sivananda, a biomedical doctor who renounced the world in the early 1920s, established the Divine Life Society Trust in Rishikesh in 1936, and wrote extensively about the health benefits of yoga from a unique vantage point. A number of scholars have interpreted Sivananda's teaching from the standpoint of religion and philosophy and have examined aspects of yoga philosophy and practice within the framework of the Divine Life Society,[48] but few have focused directly on his understanding of medicine and health.

Obviously Swami Sivananda's philosophy of yoga and health cannot be reduced down to the principles of Nature Cure, and, as a medical doctor who had worked in Malaysia for many years he was not a purist. He recognised the value of drugs in the treatment of disease. However, in light of the structural conjuncture of yoga and Nature Cure in modern India, extending from Vivekananda to the CCRYN, Sivananda's work can shed light on some important general questions concerning how existential and metaphysical problems came to be linked to the problems of the body and health.

Although it is Sivananda's teachings about the practice of yoga and healing that are of primary concern, it is his understanding of *brahmacārya* – what he called the foundation or cornerstone of *sādhana* – that provides particular insight on his conceptualisation of health, purity and the relationship among the body, transcendence and the world. First published in 1934, ten years after he took *sannyās dīkṣā* on the banks of the Ganga at Rishikesh, Sivananda's *Practice of Brahmacharya*[49] is a remarkable book in many ways. Drawing on an eclectic range of sources from many different parts of the world, including the homegrown literature on yoga and sexuality,[50] it is, with the ambiguities of tantra in

46 Just 1903.
47 Alter 2000 and 2014.
48 See Strauss 2008.
49 Sivananda 1934.
50 See Alter 2008a; Burley 2008.

yoga notwithstanding,[51] an unambiguous critique of sex and sexual desire in human experience, but also a broad ranging critique of modernity at large.

> "Wake up, friends, from this mire of illusory Samsara now. Passion has wrought great havoc in you as you are drowned in Avidya. How many millions of fathers, mothers, wives and sons you have had in previous births! The body is full of impurities. What a shame it is to embrace this filthy body! It is mere foolishness only."[52]

Sivananda makes his argument for celibacy by showing how sex and sensuality have corrupted society and weakened the body. Although very critical of a culture of modernity that encourages sensuality and the gratification of desire, what is important about Sivananda's argument is that he locates the root of the problem in consciousness itself, rather than simply in the affected trappings of colonialism's "debased" culture. It is the scale and scope of the problem in the context of colonial modernity that turns what is fundamentally a pervasive problem of contingent consciousness into a particular problem of immoral materialism manifest in the embodied impurity of thoughts, words and deeds.

Like many others writing about the practice of yoga, Sivananda not only emphasised the importance of self-purification, but often referred to the body as "filthy" and "dirty". On one level this is fairly straight forward, and fits into the distinction between the subtle and the gross body in many formulations. However, what is significant is the way in which the filth of the body is characterised both in terms of tangible, somewhat obvious things, as well as by a range of things that cross the spectrum from gross to subtle, but remain, nevertheless, associated with tangible, material substances.

Semen provides the clearest case in point, since it signifies a substance that is metonymical of sex, lust, attachment, desire and many other things. It is the material essence of a basic problem of sensory consciousness that extends through desire to reproduction, rebirth and the whole structure of illusion in the nature of material reality. An important feature here is that the syntagmatic chain of these correlations establishes a connection between this substance that flows out of the body and a range of mental processes and states that are themselves aspects of the gross body and also reflect – especially in the mind of a medical doctor – the material nature of the painful, fluid and illusory world at large.

> Poets describe in their fanciful, passionate moods that honey flows from the lips of a young, beautiful lady. Is this really true? What do you actually see? The stinking pus from the sockets of the teeth that are affected with dreadful pyorrhea, the nasty and abominable sputum from the throat, and foul saliva dribbling on the lips at night – do you call all this as honey and nectar? And yet, the passionate, lustful and sex intoxicated

51 White 2003.
52 Sivananda 1934: 8–9.

> man swallows these filthy excretions when he is under the sway of excitement! Is there anything more revolting than this![53]

Sivananda's identification of sex as especially "dirty" and "filthy" is important also in that it shows that the problem of purity and purification is not simply skin deep, so to speak. The body is "filthy" in a way that includes but extends beyond the fact that, for example, food and water enter it and then exit as feces, urine, sweat and other "dirty" things. Although very much on the pure end of the spectrum when contained within the body, once it flows out semen signifies impurity on a number of correlated registers, including profligate waste, pollution and a lack of self-control. Moreover, there is the critical problem of semen's key role in reproduction, which opens the door to time … that goes on and on or around and around and around. It is the driving force behind rebirth and the accumulated impurity of "millions of fathers, mothers, wives and sons", as described above.

Air, in many ways, presents a related but slightly different logical problem. It flows in and out through different orifices in various gross ways, but also transubstantiates into subtle *prāṇa* (*prāṇ*) and animates the body. However pure the agency of *prāṇ*, breathing is a gross act, just as sex is a gross act in relation to the flow of semen and the subtle vitality of pure *ojas* otherwise contained within the body. First published in 1935, and in sixteen subsequent editions through 1997, Sivananda's *The Science of Pranayama*[54] is an extended discussion of the therapeutic use of *prāṇ* by means of breathing techniques and exercises. Although not unique, since Kuvalayananda[55] and Yogendra[56], among others, published very similar books, it is a dramatic example of how the logic of material purification works to effect healing through the agency of breathing as a "gross" bodily function. On the one hand, breathing purges toxins from the body, preventing the development of asthma, consumption and other respiratory diseases by purifying the blood and lungs and improving the function of the heart.[57] But at the same time

> [b]y the practice of Pranayama, the purification of the Nadis, the brightening of the gastric fire, hearing distinctly of spiritual sounds and good health result. When the nervous centers have become purified through the regular practice of Pranayama, the air easily forces its way up through the mouth of the Sushumna, which is in the middle […] After such entry it is that the Yogi becomes dead to the world, being in that state called Samadhi. Drawing up the Apana and forcing down the Prana from the throat, the Yogi free from old age, becomes a youth of sixteen. Through the practice of Pranayama

53 Sivananda 1934: 30–31.
54 Sivananda 1997.
55 Kuvalayananda 1933, 1935.
56 Yogendra 1931, 1935.
57 Sivananda 1997: 66–67.

> chronic diseases, that defy Allopathic, Homeopathic, Ayurvedic and Unani doctors will be rooted out.[58]

Sivananda's teaching about the practice of yoga – with strong but somewhat sanitised tantric undertones – fits into his understanding of health as a problem that has both subtle and gross manifestations. On one level it could be argued that "health" is an inappropriately mundane term to use in relation to refined forms of advanced yogic practice. While it may well be true that the gross nature of healing puts a drag on the subtle insight of transcendence, what is apparent in Sivananda's teaching – given his orientation toward enlightenment and a divine life – is the logical power of conflation manifest in the discourse and practice of *āsana* and *prāṇāyāma* in the context of modernity. The potentiality and subtle purity of *ojas* and *prāṇ* are residual in the material manipulation of semen, breath and the body as a whole. In light of Sivananda's writing on the subjects of semen and breath specifically one is better able to appreciate his general perspective on health, as articulated in *Health and Happiness*[59] and *Yogic Home Exercises.*[60]

In *Health and Happiness* – which contains a number of chapters on Nature Cure and a poem in which *prakṛti* as Mother Nature is meta-anthropomorphised into the supreme Naturopath – he starts by identifying the causes of disease:

> Failure to answer the calls of nature in time poisons the system and exerts as bad an effect on the health of man as an obstructed drain or a sewer and retention of solid refuse of a town have on the health of the community at large.[61]

In *Yogic Home Exercises* – which contains chapters on biomedical physiology; bathing, fasting, sleeping and "yogic diet"; the importance of *brahmacārya;* a full course of yogic exercises; *prāṇāyāma* and relaxation – Sivananda writes:

> By drinking pure water, by eating pure and wholesome food, by observing carefully the laws of health and hygiene, by taking regular exercise and cold baths in the morning, by practicing Japa and meditation, by right living, right thinking, right action, right conduct, by observing Brahmacharya, by living in the open air and sunshine for some time daily, you can have wonderful health, vigor and vitality.[62]

Nature Cure provides a logic of healing in the elemental structure of *prakṛti* that involves self-purification, and it is the power of this conflation – which works for Sivananda and others in the opposite direction of the logic they felt manifest in the practice yoga – that provides a cultural framework for the material manip-

58 Sivananda 1997: 19.
59 Sivananda 1984.
60 Sivananda 1939.
61 Sivananda 1984: ix.
62 Sivananda 1939: xv.

ulation of the body through the practice of *āsana* and *prāṇāyāma* in a corrupt and contaminated world.

One thing that makes Sivananda a fascinating figure is his cosmopolitan perspective on the world.[63] Born into an upper-middle class, upper-caste Tamil family in 1887, Kuppuswamy Iyer – as he was then known – attended S. P. G. College in Trichinopoly when Rev. H. Packenham Walsh was principal during the first decade of the nineteenth century. There he performed Shakespeare and became interested in medicine, later publishing a popular journal on health called *Ambrosia.* After training at the Tanjore Medical Institute and working in a pharmacy clinic in Madras he migrated to Malaysia to pursue a professional career, returning "home" to India in 1923, only to work tirelessly to try and remake it through an endless process of reflection on what it could or should be in the context of global modernity.

While in Malaysia Kuppuswamy Iyer became a member of the Royal Institute of Public Health, the Royal Asiatic Society and an Associate of the Royal Sanitary Institute. He also published several books on health, a number of which, such as *Home Remedies, Fruit and Health,* and *The Practice of Nature Cure* were inclined towards the principle of the Unity of Diseases. In this way – and notwithstanding his professional training in Osler's Medicine under Dr. Tirumudiswami – Iyer was very much like Gandhi, the London-trained South African Gujarati lawyer who returned to India in 1914. Although different with respect to many specific beliefs and practices, in its genesis the Divine Life Society reflects a structural position in the cultural history of nation building that is comparable to that of Sabarmati Ashram and Sevagram, albeit with the focus on *sādhana* and self-purification rather than *satyāgraha* and politics.

Following the establishment of Sivanandashram in 1932 and the founding of the Divine Life Society Trust in 1936, Sivananda published a large number of books on yoga, health and spirituality. Where Gandhi's writing from the same period is largely concerned with the embodiment of Nature Cure as *svarāj* – albeit with a spiritual and moral orientation drawn in part from the *Gītā* – and Shri Yogendra and Swami Kuvalayananda's books focus primarily on yogic physical culture, physical education, and medicine, Sivananda's publications incorporate many of these features, but do so within the framework of a philosophy of yoga, sanitised Tantra and neo-Vedānta. Apart from insight into the history of the structural conjuncture of yoga and Nature Cure provided by the similarities and subtle contrasts between the views of all of these authors, it is also important to keep in mind that Nature Cure unto itself, without any particular investment in yoga philosophy, flourished in the first half of the century based on purely techno-medical applications, as exemplified by Krishna Swaroop Shro-

63 See his "Autobiography" (Sivananda 1989).

triya, Dr. Lakshmi Narayan Choudhri, Dr. Kulranjan Mukherjee and Dr. Baleshwar Prasad Singh[64].

Several of Sivananda's early books provide critical insight on the way in which the philosophy of Nature Cure shapes the practice of yoga and how the embodied philosophy of yoga, in turn, provides powerful justification not just for the purifying practices of hydrotherapy, solar therapy, fasting, and enemas, but for contemplation and meditation as well. Thus, Nature Cure provides a broad framework within which very different aspects of yoga, articulated in aphorisms and *āsana*-s, enemas and enlightenment, celibacy and *samādhi,* are integrated into developmental practice based on the rubric of *aṣṭāṅga,* as the neological connotations of this formulation mistakenly suggest a linear connection between the abstractions of the *Yogasūtra* and the magical alchemy of the *Haṭhayogapradīpikā.*[65]

The need for purity in practice permeates Sivananda's writing about the subtle importance of the "messy" interface between physiology and metaphysical insight. The idea of purification allows him to articulate a perfectly realist synthesis.

The *Handbook of Instructions on Yogic Exercise*[66] was among Sivananda's early publications under the auspices of the Divine Life Society, although it was preceded by *Memory Culture,*[67] *Happiness is Within,*[68] *Control of Evil Habits,*[69] *Select Spiritual Gems,*[70] and *Yoga for Health,*[71] along with several others. Among numerous books on practical methods of healing and staying healthy, including the *Practice of Nature Cure* (1952), Sivananda's *Health and Happiness: A Comprehensive Presentation of the Fundamental Laws of Health and Hygiene*[72] is a broadly philosophical discussion of natural healing and self-purification, as is *Yogic Home Exercises* (1939), an expanded and updated version of the *Handbook.* In any case, the sheer range of Sivananda's writing under the banner of the Trust shows how various different kinds of daily practice - mundane and mystical - were regarded by him as important and fundamentally congruent within the framework of a pure, divine life.

Especially in the early years, Sivananda was writing - mostly in English, but sometimes in Tamil - for a middle-class Indian audience, albeit in a cosmopolitan mode. This is important to keep in mind since the globalisation of yoga

64 Singh 1980.
65 See White 2014.
66 Sivananda 1939.
67 Sivananda 1936.
68 Sivananda 1937b.
69 Sivananda 1937c.
70 Sivananda 1937d.
71 Sivananda 1937a.
72 Sivananda 1984.

tends to be interpreted from a vantage point colored by colonial Orientalism and the post-colonial export of *āsana* and *prāṇāyāma* to Europe and the United States. The arrival in Rishikesh of four lads from Liverpool in 1968 – five years after Sivananda's death – helped define the trajectory of this history, anticipated by Eliade's academic visit in the late 1920s, and the subsequent publication of *Yoga: Immortality and Freedom.*[73] But from 1930 through 1960 Sivananda helped to clearly define how the practice of yoga worked in relation to the philosophy of Nature Cure, and how Nature Cure allowed for the "ideals" of yoga to transubstantiate into an alternative conception of embodied health in colonial and early post-colonial society.

With the body clearly in mind, Gandhi was ambivalent on the question of the logical place of *āsana* and *prāṇāyāma* in trying to reconcile the *Gītā,* Karma Yoga and Kuhne's theory of the Unity of Disease.[74] Swami Kuvalayananda commented on the *Yogasūtra,* but was somewhat preoccupied with laboratory experiments at the institute he founded for the scientific study of yoga,[75] and Yogendra and others focused on exercise routines and physical education, even though the *Yogasūtra* was used – and abused – to make sense of this.[76]

Intent on the construction of a divine life following seven years in Malaysia working to heal Tamil plantation workers, Sivananda had the mind more clearly in body, and understood how the power of self-purification through the practice of *prāṇāyāma* and other techniques might resolve, for technocrats and bureaucrats, some of the residual problems of embodied consciousness in the binary opposition of colonialism and nationalism, as well as in the synthesis of this dialectic in modernity. In any event, the Central Council for Research on Yoga and Naturopathy – which is indebted to the likes of Sivananda, Gandhi, Kuvalayananda and Yogendra, as well as a host of lesser souls – is a perfectly Nehruvian institution in the sense that it is a discovery of an idealised Indian modernity deeply felt in the grounded context of a hybrid middle-class consciousness that cannot escape the vagaries of time.

References

Adams, M. B. (2000). Last Judgment: The Visionary Biology of J. B. S. Haldane. *Journal of the History of Biology, 33*(3), 457–491.

Alter, J. S. (1997). A Therapy to Live by: Public Health, the Self, and Nationalism in the Practice of a North Indian Yoga Society. *Medical Anthropology, 17,* 309–335.

73 Eliade 2009.
74 Alter 2000.
75 Alter 2004.
76 Alter 2014.

Alter, J. S. (1999). Heaps of Health, Metaphysical Fitness – Ayurveda and the Ontology of Good Health in Medical Anthropology. *Current Anthropology, 40,* S43–S66.

Alter, J. S. (2000). *Gandhi's Body: Sex, Diet, and the Politics of Nationalism.* Critical Histories. Philadelphia: University of Pennsylvania Press.

Alter, J. S. (2004). *Yoga in Modern India: The Body Between Science and Philosophy.* Princeton, NJ: Princeton University Press.

Alter, J. S. (2006). Yoga at the Fin de Siècle: Muscular Christianity with a "Hindu" Twist. *International Journal of the History of Sport, 23*(5), 759–776.

Alter, J. S. (2008a). Ayurveda and Sexuality: Sex, Sex Therapy, and the 'Paradox of Virility'. In D. Wujastyk & F. M. Smith (Eds.), *Modern and Global Ayurveda: Pluralism and Paradigms* (pp. 177–200). Albany: SUNY Press.

Alter, J. S. (2008b). Yog Shivir. In M. Singleton & J. Byrne (Eds.), *Yoga in Modern India: Contemporary Perspectives* (pp. 36–48). New York: Routledge.

Alter, J. S. (2009). Yoga in Asia – Mimetic History: Problems in the Location of Secret Knowledge. *Comparative Studies of South Asia, Africa and the Middle East, 29*(2), 213–229.

Alter, J. S. (2011). *Moral Materialism: Sex and Masculinity in Modern India.* New Delhi: Penguin Books.

Alter, J. S. (2013a). Sex, Askesis and the Athletic Perfection of the Soul: Physical Philosophy in the Ancient Mediterranean and South Asia. In G. Samuel & J. Johnston (Eds.), *Subtle Bodies* (pp. 120–148). London: Routledge.

Alter, J. S. (2013b). Yoga, Body-building and Wrestling: Metaphysical Fitness. In D. Diamond (Ed.), *Yoga: The Art of Transformation* (pp. 87–95). Washington, DC: Smithsonian Institution Press.

Alter, J. S. (2014). Shri Yogendra: Magic, Modernity, and the Burden of the Middle-class Yogi. In M. Singleton & E. Goldberg (Eds.), *Gurus of Modern Yoga* (pp. 60–81). New York: Oxford University Press.

Arnold, D. (1993). *Colonizing the Body: State Medicine and Epidemic Disease in Nineteenth-century India.* Berkeley: University of California Press.

Baier, K. (1998). *Yoga auf dem Weg nach Westen: Beiträge zur Rezeptionsgeschichte.* Würzburg: Königshausen & Neumann.

Baier, K. (2009). *Meditation und Moderne: Zur Genese eines Kernbereichs moderner Spiritualität in der Wechselwirkung zwischen Westeuropa, Nordamerika und Asien.* 2 vols. Würzburg: Königshausen & Neumann.

Bashford, A. (2004). *Imperial Hygiene: A Critical History of Colonialism, Nationalism and Public Health.* Houndmills: Palgrave Macmillan.

Berger, R. (2013). *Ayurveda Made Modern: Political Histories of Indigenous Medicine in North India, 1900–1955.* Basingstoke: Palgrave Macmillan.

Bloch, M. & Parry, J. (1982). *Death and the Regeneration of Life.* Cambridge: Cambridge University Press.

Burley, M. (2008). From Fusion to Confusion: A Consideration of Sex and Sexuality in Traditional and Contemporary Yoga. In M. Singleton & J. Byrne (Eds.), *Yoga in the Modern World: Contemporary Perspectives* (pp. 184–203). London: Routledge.

Copeman, J. (2009). *Veins of Devotion: Blood Donation and Religious Experience in North India.* Studies in Medical Anthropology. New Brunswick, NJ: Rutgers University Press.

Daniel, E. V. & Pugh, J. F. (Eds.). (1984). *South Asian Systems of Healing.* Contributions to Asian Studies 18. Leiden: E. J. Brill.

De Michelis, E. (2003). *A History of Modern Yoga: Patañjali and Western Esotericism.* New York: Continuum.

De Michelis, E. (2008). Modern Yoga: History and Forms. In J. Byrne & M. Singleton (Eds.), *Yoga in the Modern World: Uses, Adaptations, Appropriations* (pp. 17–35). London: Routledge.

Dumont, L. (1970). *Homo Hierarchicus: An Essay on the Caste System.* Chicago: University of Chicago Press.

Eliade, M. (2009). *Yoga: Immortality and Freedom.* Mythos: The Princeton/Bollingen Series in World Mythology 56. Princeton, NJ: Princeton University Press.

Habib, S. I. & Raina, Dh. (Eds.). (2007). *Social History of Science in Colonial India.* Oxford in Indian Readings - Themes in Indian History. New Delhi: Oxford University Press.

Halbfass, W. (1988). *India and Europe: An Essay in Understanding.* Albany, NY: State University of New York Press.

Just, A. (1903). *Return to Nature! The True Natural Method of Healing and Living and the True Salvation of the Soul.* Vol. 1: *Paradise Regained.* New York: Lust Publications.

Keyes, Ch. F. & Daniel, E. V. (Eds.). (1983). *Karma: An Anthropological Inquiry.* Berkeley: University of California Press.

Kirchfeld, F. & Boyle, W. (2005). *Nature Doctors: Pioneers in Naturopathic Medicine.* 2nd ed. Portland, OR: NCNM Press.

Kuhne, L. (1892). *The New Science of Healing; or, the Doctrine of the Oneness of all Diseases Forming the Basis of a Uniform Method of Cure, without Medicines and without Operations: An Instructor and Adviser for the Healthy and the Sick.* Leipzig: Louis Kuhne (trans. by Th. Baker of *Die neue Heilwissenschaft oder die Lehre von der Einheit aller Krankheiten und deren darauf begründete einheitliche, arzneilose und operationslose Heilung: ein Lehrbuch und Ratgeber für Gesunde und Kranke.* 3rd greatly augmented ed. 1891).

Kuvalayananda, S. (1933). *Asanas.* Bombay: Popular Prakashan.

Kuvalayananda, S. (1935). *Pranayama.* Lonavla: Kaivalyadhama S. M. Y. M. Samiti.

Langford, J. (2002). *Fluent Bodies: Ayurvedic Remedies for Postcolonial Imbalance.* Durham: Duke University Press.

Larson, G. J. (1969). *Classical Sāṃkhya: An Interpretation of its History and Meaning.* Delhi: Motilal Banarsidass.

Larson, G. J. & Bhattacharya, R. Sh. (Eds.). (1987). *Sāṃkhya: A Dualist Tradition in Indian Philosophy.* Encyclopedia of Indian Philosophies 4. Princeton, NJ: Princeton University Press.

Leslie, Ch. (Ed.). (1976). *Asian Medical Systems: A Comparative Study.* Berkeley: University of California Press.

Leslie, Ch. M. & Young, A. (Eds.). (1992). *Paths to Asian Medical Knowledge.* Comparative Studies of Health Systems and Medical Care. Berkeley: University of California Press.

Maas, Ph. A. (2008). The Concept of the Human Body and Disease in Classical Yoga and Āyurveda. *Wiener Zeitschrift für die Kunde Südasiens / Vienna Journal of South Asian Studies, 51,* 125–162.

Mallinson, J. (2012). The Original Gorakṣaśataka. In D. G. White (Ed.), *Yoga in Practice* (pp. 257–272). Princeton: Princeton University Press.

Marchignoli, S. (2002). Che cos'è lo yoga? Traduzione ed egemonia alle origini dell'Indologia tedesca. In F. Squarcini (Ed.), *Verso l'India, Oltre l'India: Scritti e ricerche sulle tradizioni Intellettuali Sudasiatiche* (pp. 87–102). Milano: Mimesis.

Marriott, M. (Ed.). (1990). *India through Hindu Categories.* Contributions to Indian Sociology, Occasional Studies 5. New Delhi: Sage Publications.

Mukharji, P. (2009). *Nationalizing the Body: The Medical Market, Print and Daktari Medicine.* London: Anthem Press.

Parry, J. (1994). *Death in Banaras.* Cambridge: Cambridge University Press.

Pati, B. & Harrison, M. (Eds.). (2009). *The Social History of Health and Medicine in Colonial India.* Routledge Studies in South Asian History. London: Routledge.

Samuel, G. (2008). *The Origins of Yoga and Tantra: Indic Religions to the Thirteenth Century.* Cambridge: Cambridge University Press.

Samuel, G. (2013). The Subtle Body in India and Beyond. In G. Samuel and J. Johnston (Eds.), *Religion and the Subtle Body in Asia and the West: Between Mind and Body* (pp. 249–266). New York: Routledge.

Sarbacker, S. R. (2005). *Samādhi: The Numinous and Cessative in Indo-Tibetan Yoga.* SUNY Series in Religious Studies. Albany: State University of New York Press.

Sarbacker, S. R. (2008). The Numinous and Cessative in Modern Yoga. In M. Singleton & J. Byrne (Eds.), *Yoga in the Modern World: Contemporary Perspectives* (pp. 161–183). London: Routledge.

Sarkar, S. (1992). Science, Philosophy, and Politics in the Works of J. B. S. Haldane, 1922–1937. *Biology & Philosophy, 7*(4), 385–409.

Selby, M. A. (2005). Narratives of Conception, Gestation and Labour in Sanskrit Ayurvedic Texts. *Asian Medicine: Tradition and Modernity, 1*(2), 254–275.

Singh, S. J. (1980). *History and Philosophy of Naturopathy.* New Nature Cure Research Series. Lucknow: Nature Cure Council of Medical Research.

Singleton, M. (2010). *Yoga Body: The Origins of Modern Posture Yoga.* Oxford: Oxford University Press.

Singleton, M. & Goldberg, E. (Eds.). (2014). *Gurus of Modern Yoga.* New York, NY: Oxford University Press.

Sivananda, S. (1934). *Practice of Brahmacharya.* Rishikesh: The Divine Life Society (repr. 1993).

Sivananda, S. (1936). *Memory Culture.* Rishikesh: Sivananda Ashram.

Sivananda, S. (1937a). *Yoga for Health.* Rishikesh: Sivananda Ashram.

Sivananda, S. (1937b). *Happiness is Within.* Rishikesh: Sivananda Ashram.

Sivananda, S. (1937c). *Control of Evil Habits.* Rishikesh: Sivananda Ashram.

Sivananda, S. (1937d). *Select Spiritual Gems.* Rishikesh: Sivananda Ashram.

Sivananda, S. (1939). *Yogic Home Exercises: Easy Course of Physical Culture for Modern Men and Women.* Bombay: D. B. Taraporevala Sons (repr. 1977).

Sivananda, S. (1952). *Practice of Nature Cure.* Rishikesh: Sivananda Publication League.

Sivananda, S. (1984). *Health and Happiness: A Comprehensive Presentation of the Fundamental Laws of Health and Hygiene.* 3rd ed. Rishikesh: The Divine Life Society.

Sivananda, S. (1989). Autobiography of Swami Sivananda. Rishikesh: The Divine Life Society.

Sivananda, S. (1997). *Science of Pranayama.* 16th ed. Rishikesh: The Divine Life Society.

Strauss, S. (2005). *Positioning Yoga: Balancing Acts across Cultures.* Oxford: Berg.

Strauss, S. (2008). "Adapt, Adjust, Accommodate": The Production of Yoga in a Transnational World. In M. Singleton & J. Byrne (Eds.), *Yoga in the Modern World: Contemporary Perspectives* (pp. 49–73). London: Routledge.

Urban, H. B. (2010). *The Power of Tantra: Religion, Sexuality, and the Politics of South Asian Studies.* London: Palgrave Macmillan.

White, D. G. (1989). Why Gurus are Heavy. *Numen, XXXI,* 40–73.

White, D. G. (1996). *The Alchemical Body: Siddha Traditions in Medieval India.* Chicago: University of Chicago Press.

White, D. G. (2003). *Kiss of the Yoginī: "Tantric Sex" in its South Asian Contexts.* Chicago: University of Chicago Press.

White, D. G. (2009). *Sinister Yogis.* Chicago: The University of Chicago Press.

White, D. G. (2012). Introduction. In D. G. White (Ed.), *Yoga in Practice* (pp. 1–23). Princeton: Princeton University Press.

White, D. G. (2014). *The Yoga Sutra of Patanjali: A Biography.* Lives of Great Religious Books. Princeton: Princeton University Press.

Whorton, J. C. (1982). *Crusaders for Fitness: The History of American Health Reformers.* Princeton, NJ: Princeton University Press.

Whorton, J. C. (2000). *Inner Hygiene: Constipation and the Pursuit of Health in Modern Society.* Oxford: Oxford University Press.

Whorton, J. C. (2002). *Nature Cures: The History of Alternative Medicine in America.* Oxford: Oxford University Press.

Wujastyk, D. (2009). Interpreting the Image of the Human Body in Pre-modern India. *International Journal of Hindu Studies, 13*(2), 189–228.

Yogendra, Sh. (1931). *Yoga Personal Hygiene.* Bombay: The Yoga Institute.

Yogendra, Sh. (1935). *Simple Meditative Postures.* Bombay: The Yoga Institute.

Zysk, K. G. (2007). The Bodily Winds in Ancient India Revisited. *Journal of the Royal Anthropological Institute, 13,* S105–S115.

Chapter 11

Sāṃkhya in Transcultural Interpretation: Shri Anirvan (Śrī Anirvāṇa) and Lizelle Reymond

Maya Burger

Contents

1. Introduction 465

2. Two Biographies or Where Two Worldviews Meet 468

3. Shri Anirvan's Sāṃkhya Interpretation 473

4. *Prakṛti, Puruṣa* and the Void 475
4.1. *Prakṛti* 475
4.2. *Puruṣa* 477
4.3. The Void 477

5. Conclusion 480

References 481

Maya Burger

Chapter 11: Sāṃkhya in Transcultural Interpretation: Shri Anirvan (Śrī Anirvāṇa) and Lizelle Reymond

1. Introduction

Sāṃkhya,[1] one of the ancient philosophical systems of India, is often believed to have completed its productive phase several centuries ago. However, in the persons of Shri Anirvan[2] and Lizelle Reymond it provides the conceptual frame for a philosophical encounter and dialogue. By studying the intellectual biography and thinking of the two protagonists, we learn about their individual life stories and just as much about their respective roots, histories and contexts. This framework implies that the focus of the present chapter is not the history of Sāṃkhya, but a microhistorical study of its impact on Lizelle Reymond who received and translated Shri Anirvan's Sāṃkhya first for a Western and then for an Indian readership. She brought a modern and "translated" Sāṃkhya to the West, thereby documenting its plasticity and adaptability proper to the Indian context and subsequently manifest on a transnational level.

As a contribution to the history of Indian yoga and the issue of its transformation over time, the study of the encounter between Shri Anirvan and Lizelle Reymond provides a modern example of how yoga is conceptualised within the frame of a Sāṃkhya revived in a transnational setup.

Lizelle Reymond,[3] a Swiss Orientalist, travelled in 1948 to Almora where she spent a year in a Brahmin family,[4] before sharing four years with Shri Anirvan, a Bengali scholar and yogi. Together they opened a residence near Almora they

1 Indian terms are transliterated according to the international standard of transliteration. In quotes from Anirvan and Reymond, they appear as used by the authors.

2 Proper names are written without diacritics.

3 The Library of Lausanne University has inherited the bequest of Reymond consisting in the original type-written letters of correspondence with Anirvan and photographs.

4 Reymond put down her experiences during that year in writing: *Ma vie chez les brahmanes* (translated into English under the title *My Life with a Brahmin Family*). This book is a relatively rare testimony of a Western woman in an Indian family, with quite stereotyped perspectives on Brahmanical worldviews.

called Haimavati, which was supposed to have become a centre of learning for scholars interested in the study of traditional knowledge systems and spirituality,[5] but failed to fulfil their shared hopes. However, the encounter of these two personalities left us with the legacy of a modern interpretation of Sāṃkhya and Yoga: Shri Anirvan, the master who refuses to be one, and Lizelle Reymond, the disciple who will in turn become a teacher in Switzerland. Their significance for this history does not seem to have been studied or acknowledged, and this chapter is a step towards filling this desideratum.

Modern history of yoga is best studied from the perspective of a connected history, in our case between India and Europe.[6] Attention to the circulation of ideas, stories, texts, persons and material objects helps to avoid essentialised constructs, to accentuate processes and to make use of dynamic approaches.[7] Microhistories, as postulated by Carlo Ginzburg (1980), invite us to pay careful attention to peculiar stories in specific settings and, in our case, to approach yoga in a detailed exemplary manner. Case studies may yield enough information to contribute to a better understanding of wider contexts within which these microstories unfold and are part of, and thus reflect them.

Lizelle Reymond and Shri Anirvan belong to the period after the Second World War, after the Independence of India; in this pre-Saidian period, the East–West polarity still meant something quite concrete for them. While Europe was at that time located at the top of the globe, and was, so to speak only on a cultural level, the centre of intellectual and modern innovations and possibilities,[8] for Lizelle Reymond (in a very post-theosophical move[9]) the East had something she

5 Anirvan and Reymond had indeed planned to build an international cultural centre for philosophical and spiritual exchanges.

6 Wilhelm Halbfass, with his *India and Europe,* remains for me a solid example how we may understand, from the perspective of a hermeneutics of encounter, the processes of exchange between India and Europe. Romain Bertrand is yet another example, with S. Subrahmanyam, who tries to construct a recent history in a symmetric way, capable of studying the two poles of the relation in a balanced way: *L'histoire à parts égales* (Bertrand 2007 and 2011; Subrahmanyam 2007).

7 Anirvan and his Sāṃkhya interpretation can be studied in many ways. In this paper he is studied from the angle of his relation to Reymond and the angle of cultural translation. Hence his elaborate commentaries and exegesis are not part of this chapter that emphasises the transnational aspect of Anirvan in relation to the topic of the conference "Yoga in Transformation: Historical and Contemporary Perspectives on a Global Phenomenon" (Vienna, 19–21 September 2013). Another angle would be provided by the comparison of Anirvan and Shri Aurobindo – an intellectual, not a personal encounter, yet one that exemplifies the reception and transformation of Western ideas by Shri Aurobindo, their reinterpretation and reception by Reymond, via Anirvan. Both Anirvan and Aurobindo share a thinking combined with spiritual practice or that is the outcome of such practice and experience.

8 On the general debates and issues, see Ashcroft et al. 1995.

9 Be it in certain writings of the Romantic Movement, or in the theosophy of H. P. Blavatsky, the Orient could also be seen as the origin of wisdom, or the wisdom-religion. Blavatsky was quite

thought the West had lost. She shared with Jean Herbert[10] the conviction that modern Indian thinkers and especially spiritual masters were not known and had to find their place among Western thinkers. She met Ramanamaharshi, Swami Ramdas, Shri Aurobindo and Ma Anandamoyi and wrote the biography of Sister Nivedita (*The Dedicated*). In this sense, Lizelle Reymond may be qualified as a cultural translator, inhabiting two spaces at the time or incorporating what Homi Bhabha calls the "space in-between".[11] Anirvan, no less than Lizelle Reymond, is a "translated" person,[12] though he never left India, but through his knowledge of European languages had access to key ideas in various fields.

Cultural translation is much more than going from East to West or vice versa, or between tradition and modernity, woman or man, past or present. Translation is actually the key term of the type of intellectual occurrences this chapter wishes to elaborate, and it addresses the many layers of the intricate processes of going back and forth between different social and cultural realities, and, in our case, psychological and philosophical reflexions related to the meaning of Sāṃkhya-yoga.

To study the Sāṃkhya of Shri Anirvan does not mean, however, to study an interpretation of a pure, old Indian Sāṃkhya in modern times, but rather an additional version of something that has been a historical and cultural construct since we have known about it.[13] It is the assertion of something composed, enshrined by the term *sāṃkhya*. Shri Anirvan does use the word *sāṃkhya* and Lizelle Reymond calls *his* teaching Sāṃkhya. Combining textual analysis with a historical perspective allows us to acknowledge the necessity to view Shri Anir-

---

instrumental in promoting the idea that the Orient, especially India, had something to teach which the West had lost. This idea would have a lasting impact on certain perspectives of India (theosophy, anthroposophy, new-age). See, for instance, the first issue of the Indian edited journal *The Theosophist* (1879–1880) in which Blavatsky recognised India as still harbouring some of the ancient wisdom and inviting Indian authors to be proud of their heritage and knowledge.

10 Jean Herbert was married at that time to Reymond and together the couple published many books on modern Indian authors and introduced their thinking to the West, which was an innovative step with long-lasting consequences.

11 See Bhabha 1994: 10: "The border line work of culture demands an encounter with 'newness' that is not part of the continuum of past and present. It creates a sense of the new as an insurgent act of cultural translation. Such art does not merely recall the past as social cause or aesthetic precedent; it renews the past, re-figuring it as a contingent 'in-between' space, that innovates and interrupts the performance of the presence."

12 To take up Salman Rushdie's term of "having been born across the world, we are translated men" (Rushdie 1992).

13 This specification may seem superfluous, but it is important to distance the present study from any perspective that would contrast pure and "degenerated" versions of Sāṃkhya. The idea is more precisely to accept any version of Sāṃkhya studied in its precise setting. There is no idea of a true or authentic version, whereas to stipulate an earlier or a more complex version may make sense for certain type of research.

van's thinking and interpretation against the backdrop of his encounter with Lizelle Reymond (and with us reflecting about their encounter), and his effort to translate his knowledge into a language capable of explaining his view to himself and to her, as much as to a wider audience, one that is mainly European and Indian.

Clearly Lizelle Reymond and Shri Anirvan created a collaborative project, where Indian and European, more specifically, Bengali and Swiss parties came together and fostered new philosophical interpretations of the world.[14] They proposed answers to the problems of contemporary societies in the quest for meaning and fulfilment. Lizelle Reymond wished to present a new luminary, Shri Anirvan, as a formidable thinker, philosopher and yogi. Shri Anirvan, in accordance with his experience, applied Sāṃkhya to the needs of a modern world. He saw Sāṃkhya as a philosophical system capable of answering the psychological challenge of modernity, or at least he saw it as providing the structural framework to explain the modern world.

2. Two Biographies or Where Two Worldviews Meet

The biographies of the two authors explain and describe the intertwining of two lives, but also of their ideas, expectations, appropriations and what was actually possible in the precise life-span of their encounter after the Second World War.

Lizelle Reymond (see Figure 1 below) was born in Switzerland in 1899 and joined the United Nations in 1920 in New York as a librarian, before travelling to and writing about India. During the first half of the twentieth century, she was known for the books she published with Jean Herbert on living spiritualties of India.[15]

She was later known in France and Switzerland for having, on the one hand, contributed to opening a Gurdjieff group in 1956 in Switzerland, based on the teachings of Georges Gurdjieff (1866–1949), an esotericist of the first half of the twentieth century of Armenian origin who lived and was active in Paris from 1924 until his death. On the other hand, she brought Tai chi chuan, a Chinese martial art, to Paris and Geneva in the early 1960s. She is the bridge between Shri Anirvan and the West and she is the first person to have written extensively about Shri Anirvan in the West, where he had apparently not entered the history of yoga as a

14 Irschick (1994) emphasised a similar pattern of interconnectedness in the context of South India, but focused more on the socio-political realm, without always accounting for all power-related asymmetries.

15 "Spiritualités vivantes" is the series founded by Herbert and herself in 1946 with the publisher Albin Michel in Paris. They had actually started their publications with a Swiss editor in Neuchâtel, Delachaux et Niestlé, before switching to Albin Michel.

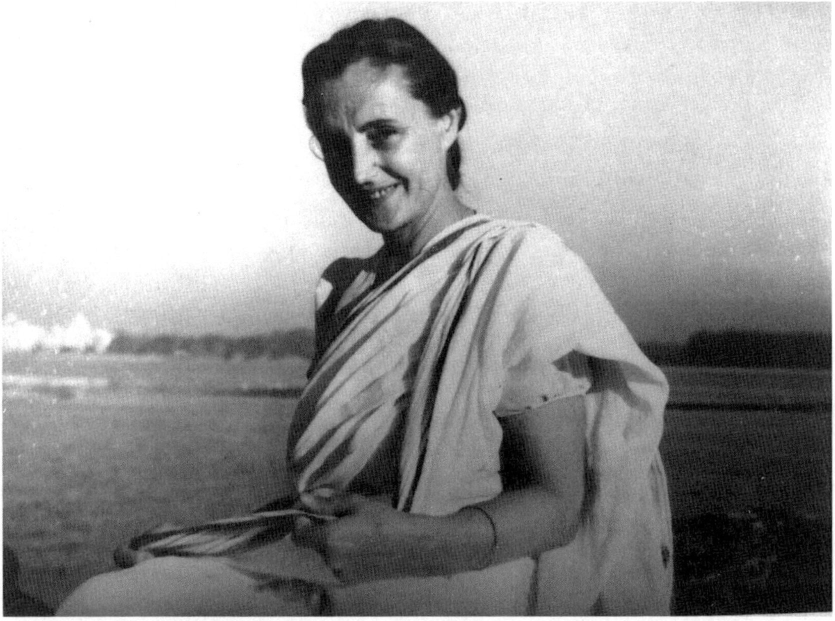

Figure 1: Lizelle Reymond

genuine and important participant.[16] Shri Anirvan himself had advised Lizelle Reymond to study Gurdjieff on her return from India in 1953.[17] From a transnational perspective, with the association to this movement, not only was *she* connected to it, Sāṃkhya also turned out to be a means of communication with the Gurdjieffian system of thought.

Lizelle Reymond wrote about her life with Shri Anirvan twelve years after leaving India in 1953. This was the interval that he had requested in order to make sure that her knowledge and understanding had deepened and matured. She continued to travel back and forth between India and Europe, had an intensive epistolary exchange with Shri Anirvan and had her writings corrected by him, until his death in 1978. The very fact that most of the information we get from Lizelle Reymond stems from a correspondence is important, as this is a type of reading that is close to a dialogue and reveals or contains an element of the in-between-ness of cultures in its very shape.

16 There are biographies by Dilip Roy (1982) and Ram Swarup (1983) in English; Reymond's writings on Anirvan are among their sources.

17 Anirvan learnt about Gurdjieff through a book he received from a bookshop in Allahabad, which was Ouspensky's *In Search of the Miraculous* (more explicit in its French title, *Fragments d'un enseignement inconnu*, which is actually the subtitle of the English version) (Ouspensky 1949a and 1949b). It is the narration of the eight years of work Ouspensky spent with Gurdjieff. The latter had agreed to this publication.

Her first book on (or by) Shri Anirvan is *La vie dans la vie,*[18] published in 1969. From our perspective of a connected history and in terms of book history, it is particularly interesting to note that she translated the English correspondence into French for this publication. The book is and was often used to determine the life story of Shri Anirvan, since he had told it to her. In 1983, after his death, an English translation of the book was published in Calcutta and many changes can be noticed. The proclaimed author is now only Shri Anirvan, and Lizelle Reymond is named as the compiler, with the parts concerning her missing. The correspondence is now (re-)published in the original English, no longer the translated version. The book is called *Letters from a Baul.* Gurdjieff, regularly named by Lizelle Reymond in her French version, is absent from the English edition (replaced by a more generic term such as "any adept of samkhya"). The book is for many a reference book on Shri Anirvan. The subtitle in French is *Pratique de la philosophie du sâmkhya d'après l'enseignement de Shrî Anirvân,* whereas in the English version it is *Letters from a Baul: Life within Life.*[19] These changes were made by Lizelle Reymond after Shri Anirvan's death and thus reflect events in her life and her active role in the history of yoga (nationally and transnationally). She died in 1994 at the age of 95.

Our second protagonist, Shri Anirvan (see Figure 2 below) was from a Kayastha family and was born in 1896, three years before Lizelle Reymond, as Narendra Candra Dhar in Mymensingh, which is in modern-day Bangladesh. He studied Sanskrit at the University of Calcutta and took *saṃnyāsa* from Nigamananda who had his *āśrama* in Jorhat in Assam.[20] He stayed at this *āśrama* up until 1930 and was forced to work very hard during the day to build the *āśrama.* Lizelle Reymond quotes Shri Anirvan as saying:

> For a space of fourteen years, my guru laid upon me the burden of working in silence, without news of the outside world, without letters. I helped to cut down trees, dig canals, make bricks, and build houses; such was my daily task. In the evening I taught Philosophy and Sanskrit, and learned to live an inward life meticulously controlled, and thus gradually to possess my True Being by accepting automatic obedience to another. When the soil has been well prepared the tree will thrive. At night, when we meditated,

18 The second book is *Le pèlerinage vers la vie et vers la mort.*

19 Sāṃkhya was evidently important to Reymond, but less so to the community of Aurobindo who was responsible for this Indian edition.

20 It is Shanti Ashrama known as Saraswata Matha or Assam Bongiya Saraswata Matha founded in Jorhat in 1919 by Swami Nigamananda (1880–1935). The latter was a yoga and spiritual master better known in the Eastern part of India. Although he was initiated in the lineage of Shankara, he is known as a master of yoga and tantra and for his life of deep experiences. There can be no doubt that Anirvan learnt much from him; however, what is important for us is the fact that *he left* the Ashrama and, at the same time, any institutional affiliation, in order to promote an independent way of thinking in accordance with his *own* worldview and what *he* expected to be necessary for his time.

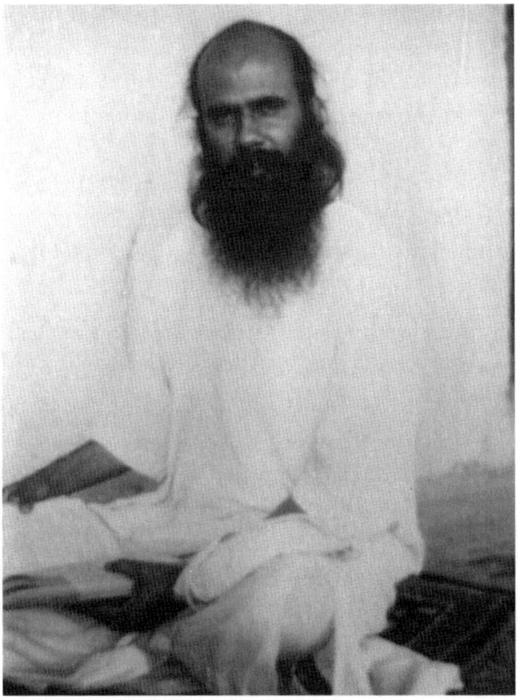

Figure 2: Shri Anirvan

> the smoke of surrounding braziers reminded us of all those who were living on the by-products of the trees which we had felled.[21]

Shri Anirvan developed a technique to live the outer life independently from his inner life and experiences. There are no other independent sources on his training in yoga (*āsana*-s, *prāṇāyāma,* meditation), but the text contains information open to interpretation: "obedience to another" likely means to his Guru Swami Nigamananda; "to live an inner life meticulously controlled", describes exactly what he later called "Antaryoga" and Sāṃkhya, and "meditated at night" confirms that Shri Anirvan himself could have had the spiritual experiences about which he taught authoritatively and which he recognised in the ancient scriptures.

In 1930 he left the *āśrama* to become an independent teacher, tutoring and travelling across North India. He identified his attitude and lifestyle with that of the Bauls and it is likely that he knew some representatives of this group personally. By qualifying himself as a Baul, he asserted his freedom from institutions and religions, and his need to proceed only by way of self-discovery (a key-motif

21 *My Life with a Brahmin Family* pp. 163–165.

in all of his documented life). This is one of the reasons why he did not feature as a guru nor called himself a guru, but viewed himself as a catalyser. The profound inner reorientation manifests outwardly in the change of the name Nirvanananda Saraswati, the name given to Shri Anirvan on the occasion of his initiation as a sadhu.[22]

He agreed to present his views in French (which he knew fluently) through Lizelle Reymond; hence we may conclude that he intended to reach a Western or universal readership. He himself stated that he used the language of psychology, which to him is a universal language:

> I know how difficult it is to explain deep spiritual values. That is why I think the best link between the things of the beyond with the things of this world is that of practical psychology. Psychology speaks a universally known language.[23]

We have almost no information regarding the eighteen years preceding Shri Anivan's meeting Lizelle Reymond. She extracted from him information about his life, though he did not care in the least about the events of the outer world.[24] In 1942, he met a group of Aurobindo adherents and was motivated to translate Aurobindo's work *Life Divine* into Bengali, which was applauded as a masterpiece by the Bengali recipients.[25]

The same year, in 1953, Haimavati in Almora was closed and Shri Anirvan travelled again, finally settling during his last years in Calcutta where he died in 1978, sixteen years before Lizelle Reymond.

He owned an impressive library in Almora and worked incessantly, besides leading a meditative life. Lizelle Reymond recounts that he would not speak for days, and rarely at all unless asked a question. He led a very simple and secret life, helped by friends who appreciated his exegesis on the various texts he would disclose during rare but long nights of discussion.

Shri Anirvan wrote extensively in Bengali and was accepted and reputed as a Vedic scholar. There can be no doubt that he had spiritual experiences, though he would never speak directly about them. However, he delved into the ancient texts

---

22 Even though the exact meaning of this name for Anirvan remains unknown, the literal meaning of the name Nirvanananda, "he who rejoices in *nirvāṇa*", sharply contrasts with that of Anirvan, "he who does not have (i.e., has not reached) *nirvāṇa*".

23 *Letters from a Baul* p. 12. He interprets metaphysical concepts as "spiritual values". "Psychology" is used in a Western sense.

24 The most complete bibliography can be found at http://anirvan-memories.blogspot.ch/p/english-translations-of-some-bengali.html (accessed 6 June 2014).

25 Anirvan invested several years of his life in this translation which was first published in 1953. It is considered the best exposition of Aurobindo's words and thoughts in the Bengali language. In the context of this chapter, it is not possible to further expand on this work. However, it is likely that even though he maintained his own philosophy, Anirvan felt an affinity to Aurobindo's thinking.

to find words and structures to give name and form to his experiences. This attitude or quest appears as a *sādhana* in its own right. The language he used to render and expose his spiritual, historical and philosophical options is accessible and designed for readers in a contemporary world, most notably in *Antaryoga* and in *Letters of a Baul,* which has been translated in various languages. He is therefore a protagonist of the intellectual history of Sāṃkhya in India, as well as an exponent of a universal art of living, based on his vision of Indian traditions.

3. Shri Anirvan's Sāṃkhya Interpretation

What are the particularities of Shri Anirvan's Sāṃkhya? Most of the information presented here is taken from *La vie dans la vie, Letters from a Baul: Life within Life* and *Antarayoga,*[26] which is a systematizing practice-oriented instruction on yoga following the eight limbs as set forth in the *Yogasūtra* but including extensive passages with tantric elements. This is complemented with references taken from his book entitled *Buddhiyoga* and his commentaries on Upaniṣads.

Sāṃkhya for Shri Anirvan serves as a means for having a rational exposure to inner living, to inwardly-turned experiences. It is for him a scientific language and in accordance or "matchable" with his claim that psychology is the common "spiritual" language for speaking about it.

In the general introduction to his commentaries on the *Īśopaniṣad,* he writes about two ways, and one can easily recognise his preference:

> The Samkhya propounded by Kapila is one of the oldest Indian philosophies. It is 'Munidhara' – the Muni Tradition or 'Tarka Prasthan,' which is Reason, the way of the Rationalist. Vedanta, on the other hand, is 'Rishi dhara' – The Rishi Tradition or "Mimansa Prasthan," the way of the critical analysts. The one looks within himself, whereas the other looks without. The Muni closing his eyes goes within and sees himself or the Atman, and the Rishi with eyes wide open sees gods or Brahman everywhere.[27]

For Shri Anirvan Sāṃkhya is a way to explain yoga, especially his experience of yoga. Yoga is the practical side of Sāṃkhya and he states, in *Antarayoga,* that its goal is not only a means to stop the chaotic activity of the mental, but also to develop the personality and to lead life to its perfection. "Yoga is the only scientific means to make appear the person who is in you."[28]

---

26 The French version writes "Antarayoga", whereas the English version has "Antaryoga".

27 *Ishopanishad,* General introduction, p. 1. http://anirvan-memories.blogspot.ch/p/english-translations-of-some-bengali.html (accessed 6 June 2014).

28 "En vérité, le yoga est la seule manière scientifique de faire apparaître la personne qui est en vous" (*Antarayoga* p. 116).

> He who practices a spiritual discipline (*sādhanā*) will use Samkhya to learn how to look at the movements of the Great Nature in all its manifestations without interfering with its movements, to recognize its imprint on everything and to observe the ability of prakriti to pass imperceptibly from one plane of consciousness to another. [...]
>
> Long and meticulous work is indispensable in order to discover that emotion of any kind creates a passionate movement, which takes man out of himself. In this case *yoga* teaches how to check any impetuous movement by emptying the mind of all images. The superabundant energy is thus brought back to the self. But *the purpose of Samkhya is that this energy, having returned to the self, should also be directed consciously towards the outer life, that it should become openly active without disturbing the inner or outer prakriti.* In this way life-energy is purified. It becomes creative. Of course, this state can only last for a few minutes, and the ordinary man immediately reappears with his train of habitual reactions within the play of manifestation.
>
> This moment of illumination (*sattva*) and this word is right even if the moment be brief, is a look into oneself and at the same time a look outside oneself (*śivadṛṣṭi*). Symbolically, it can be compared to the piercing look of Purusha into himself and upon the active Prakriti around him. To accept Prakriti in its totality is pure sahaja. In a subtle manner, beyond "I like and I don't like," it brings a possibility of modification in the densities of the intrinsic qualities (*guṇas*) of the lower prakriti and shows the path by which a higher Prakriti can be reached.[29]

This long quotation may stand as one example out of many others. It shows how the technicality of Sāṃkhya terminology almost disappears in English (replaced by expressions such as "movement of Great Nature"). Certain Sāṃkhya terms are retained (*puruṣa, prakṛti*) or added to the translation (*sattva*). Readers with some knowledge of what is called "classical Sāṃkhya" may be at an advantage. Certain indicative statements imply an authority, which is likely to stem from Shri Anirvan's own experience, such as "[i]n a subtle manner", "beyond 'I like and I don't like,' it brings a possibility".

Shri Anirvan speaks of two types of Sāṃkhya: the first is philosophical and was formulated by Ishvara Krishna, recognised by Shri Anirvan as meant for the yogi and the anchorite, and is regarded by him as a profoundly negative philosophy. It represents what is known about Sāṃkhya in the West. The second Sāṃkhya is a mystical path enshrined in the Vedas and the Upaniṣads, which in the course of centuries has found a clear expression in the Purāṇas and the Tantras, especially in the later scriptures. Here, the world is not denied, which is one of the main features of his view. The second Sāṃkhya, to which he also refers as Kapila

29 *Letters from a Baul* pp. 5–7 [my emphasis].

Samkhya, is more important to him, and it encompasses the entire Indian tradition from the Vedas to the Tantras and Purāṇas.[30]

Further, Shri Anirvan sees Sāṃkhya as a conscious effort to understand "what is there". It means, plainly, to make use of all that is available to enlarge the plane of consciousness, revealing the relation between the known and the unknown universe.

Shri Anirvan's spirituality is qualified by Lizelle Reymond as Sāṃkhya and it is the way he is presented to the West, but it is also the way he wished to be seen. Sāṃkhya is a way for him to structure and to explain the world, and as a frame it can even be used to explain other religions.[31] Sāṃkhya had become for him, and for Lizelle Reymond, a way to understand and to explain life, and yoga is the means of living it:

> As soon as one withdraws consciously from prakriti, if only for an instant, its movement ceases. One emerges from it having touched the point of creation. This point gives extremely pure sensation. It is often reached through "spiritual death," which is beyond all energy, beyond cogitations [...].[32]

Three key terms are selected to exemplify Shri Anirvan's reinterpretation of yoga as it is rendered in his collaboration with Lizelle Reymond.

4. *Prakṛti, Puruṣa* and the Void

4.1. *Prakṛti*

The two types of Sāṃkhya are projected onto the concept of *prakṛti* which has a lower and a higher aspect. Shri Anirvan also speaks of an individual *prakṛti* and a great one. The latter is called "Mother" or "Nature" with a capital N.

> The philosophical Samkhya takes into consideration only the lower prakriti, which is merely a complex of the qualities of *sattva, rajas,* and *tamas,* permanently intermingled, although one of them must necessarily predominate. But a pure quality (*śuddha sattva*) can also exist, which is neither touched nor soiled by *rajas* and *tamas.* This, then, would be the highest Prakriti that is many times mentioned in Puranic and Tantric literature. This idea of pure sattva reigns over all the practical philosophies of the Hindu mystics.[33]

30 His notion of "Kapila Samkhya" was likely derived from the *Bhāgavatapurāṇa*, in which (3.25–33) Sāṃkhya is exposed in the dialogue between Kapila and Devahūti.

31 See, for instance, in *Letters from a Baul* in the chapter on Sāṃkhya, how he reads Christianity with the help of his view of Sāṃkhya (p. 21).

32 *Letters from a Baul* p. 24.

33 *Letters from a Baul* p. 19.

For Shri Anirvan, *prakṛti* contains everything that exists. It is the divine womb of all manifestation and reveals three different degrees:

1. Everything which we are made of: soul, intelligence, ego, life, mind, and the animal matter of our body. If it is possible to recognise the terms (*puruṣa, buddhi, ahaṃkāra, manas*) here, there is no equivalent for *life,* which is a personal and very important term for Shri Anirvan and Lizelle Reymond (and Reymond introduced the terminology in *La vie dans la vie,* which she decided was central to his thinking as the capacity to live a "detached, or spiritual" life within the ordinary life).
2. The very principle of our possible evolution on all planes of our psychic and physical being.
3. The divine energy (*śakti*) in its most subtle elements. "In one sense all is materiality [...] there is no difference between spirit and matter; it is only a question of different densities."[34]

Prakṛti and *puruṣa* are also seen as psychological and physical entities, which give a gendered perspective to Shri Airvan's teaching of Sāṃkhya. This can be seen for instance in his differentiation between men and women, and their ways of practising yoga, as shown in *Antarayoga* (pp. 25–26). Sāṃkhya is a graduated series of experiences, consciously lived (p. 41), but the experience is not the same for woman (renewed by nature) and man (who has to practise asceticism).

This gendered philosophy formulated in *Antarayoga* was addressed to a probably mixed audience in Calcutta. When he writes to the female Lizelle Reymond, Shri Anirvan uses plain imperatives on how to deal with *prakṛti:*

> Hold back your prakriti in all the spontaneous movements that may arise in you, so that it does not flow out or become diverted toward the prakriti of others. This calls for no withdrawal on your part; but it allows you to prevent heavy matters from becoming agglutinated with other disordered heavy matters. Then you will be able to observe the movements and erratic nature of others and this will help you to catch sight of your own movements. At that point, some control can be exercised, but only of yourself. This state of transparency has a relation to what one can also call "self-remembering," if one clearly understands that prakriti includes the entire being in the multitude of its conscious and unconscious manifestations."[35]

Shri Anirvan has several ways to speak about his convictions, either in a descriptive way or in an imperative way (as in this example), or in a personal way, quoting his "I" experience, which is far less frequent than the first two ways.

34 *Letters from a Baul* p. 21.
35 *Letters from a Baul* pp. 83–84.

4.2. *Puruṣa*[36]

Shri Anirvan speaks far less about *puruṣa* than *prakṛti*, but of course the interplay of the two is indispensable. *Puruṣa* is "Spirit" in his words, it is what watches *prakṛti* from afar. *Puruṣa* is, whereas *prakṛti* is and also does:

> Purusha can do nothing for us, since we are the slaves of prakriti. Purusha is outside of time and beyond our understanding, whereas prakriti exists in time. It is at once the aggregate of the qualities (*guṇas*) that we can evaluate and the aggregate of the movements and impressions (*saṁskāras*) of all those qualities that make up our life. Purusha is a flash of perception, while prakriti operates in an integral mechanism.[37]

The important relation of *puruṣa* to *prakṛti* is further explained:

> It is essential to build one's life around two principles: that of letting go and that of contraction. *The moment of complete, conscious "letting go" is when Purusha is in dissociation from Prakriti.*[38] Such a moment lasts only as long as several very calm respirations; this creates the naked universe, stripped of the "I".[39]

Expansion is the creative movement corresponding to introspection. The one inevitably leads to the other, that is, expansion in itself leads to letting go when one finds the inner point of balance.

The third selected term designates the aim of Sāṃkhya and yoga.

4.3. The Void[40]

When Shri Anirvan talks about the end or the goal he generally speaks about the Void: "In any case, one must turn to the Void, which is the beginning as well as the end of all things."[41] Every creation is generated in the Void:

> Every master of Samkhya speaks about the plurality of "I"s. He will say, in different ways, that at the start, the "I" towards which all the "I's" converge is only theoretically the Void. Through a meticulous discipline you draw close to an "I" from which you can calmly observe yourself. From there the world is seen with all its mechanical movements; from there, for brief moments, you may have a glimpse of that "I" which is the Void.[42]

---

36 *Puruṣa* is hardly ever translated by Anirvan, which is not the case with *prakṛti*.

37 *Letters from a Baul* p. 20.

38 My emphasis.

39 *Letters from a Baul* p. 27.

40 Anirvan rarely uses the term *kaivalya*. Most of the time, the term used for the goal of his Sāṃkhya-yoga is "Void", written with an initial capital letter.

41 *Letters from a Baul* p. 23.

42 *Letters from a Baul* p. 73.

From an editorial point of view, we note that in the French version "every master of samkhya" was Gurdjieff: "Gurdjieff parle beaucoup de la pluralité des 'moi'."[43] Thus, the passage documents how Shri Anirvan's Sāṃkhya is re-imported to India after having been appropriated or at least confirmed by its analogy with ideas of a Western teacher and movement; Sāṃkhya is Gurdjieff in the spiritual path of Lizelle Reymond, and may stand here as a good example of the circulation of ideas and discourses.[44]

The reference to the aim invites us to read once more what Shri Anirvan and Lizelle Reymond have to say about the spiritual path they envisage (Life in the life!). In the *Letters from a Baul,* Shri Anirvan expounds on ways to proceed to experience the Void:

> There are two ways to escape from the chain of prakriti, since everything on every plane exists in such a way that experiences are endlessly repeated. Both of them are very exacting. One of the ways is upward and consists in the initiation into *sannyāsa* of the monks who roam about India wearing the ochre or the white robe, or of the layman who resolutely enters, at a particular time in his life, upon the hermit's "cave life" in order to live a spiritual experience. The other way tends downward. For man and woman alike, it is like the degradation of prostitution: the abandoning of castes and of the social framework. By this movement they deliberately cease to submit to the true Law and put themselves under a lower set of laws. It is not giving that counts, for giving remains a proof that one has something to give. What counts is to experience the most complete dissatisfaction with oneself and to see it with open eyes until one gets down the bedrock. This is the movement that causes prakriti, uncovered and unmasked to react. At this moment something as yet unperceived can begin to break through. It is the energy (*śakti*) that becomes the matrix or the Void. There only can something take shape and be born when the time comes. Bedrock represents the eternal Prakriti busy with ceaseless creation, for such is her function, indifferent to everything taking place around her. This is one of her movements. She has another movement, opposite to it, which must also be discovered. According to one of her Laws, she gradually pushes her children into Purusha's field of vision. Meeting the piercing look of Purusha, whose function it is to "see," is an instant of total understanding, a giving up of oneself. How can one describe that look? What one knows of it cannot be communicated. And besides, it would be useless to try. All what one can do is to wait with much love and be ready to meet it. Is it possible to guess when Prakriti will make the gesture for you? Is it possible to know why she does so?[45]

In this passage, the perspective identified with Sāṃkhya reveals many combined perspectives, tantric and psychological, which are also able to explain the expe-

43 *La vie dans la vie* p. 166.

44 It may also be seen as an attempt of Reymond to recast Anirvan in a fully Indian context and as belonging to a traditional knowledge system – the way she wanted him to be seen.

45 *Letters from a Baul* pp. 25–26.

riences of Shri Anirvan.[46] The psychological tone of his explanations recalls how he was interested in psychoanalysis and psychology as a language that could be used to explain spiritual experiences.

The following is a statement introducing an identification of Sāṃkhya with psychology that speaks not only a universal language, but even a scientific one, which could be equated with "modern" and "competitive":

> Samkhya is the only religious philosophy that speaks a psychological language, hence a scientific language. Everything can be explained from the point of view of Samkhya. It is the basis of the Buddhist *piṭakas,* as well as of the Sufi precepts. It is no more concerned with rites or with dogmas than are the *Upanishads.*[47]

Again it is relevant for the present purpose to notice that the French version has one paragraph more:

> Ceux qui font pénétrer ces idées très larges dans le courant de la pensée accomplissent une chose importante. En cela, Georges Ivanovitch Gurdjieff, qui a suivi cette méthode dénuée de tout artifice, est un pionnier en Occident. Il est très en avance sur son temps, de là les attaques virulentes dont il est l'objet.[48]

This way of presenting Shri Anirvan's Sāṃkhya from the perspective of Lizelle Reymond's biography must not leave the impression that it was a one-way road. Gurdjieff may not have found his way back to Indian uses of Sāṃkhya thought, but other influences in this chapter of modern Sāṃkhya philosophy are explicitly acknowledged; hence in *Buddhiyoga* we read under the title "New Hopes":

> We may take Russell's view as representative of the Western mind's conception of the aim of existence and call his ideal world the neo-Rationalist's Utopia, reflecting the dominating trend of Rational Realism in modern philosophy. Kapila, who is at the head of the Indian Rationalists had suggested no Utopia and modern Realism might look upon him as an escapist. But he has also offered to humanity a way of thinking and a pattern of living which might be named Spiritual Realism to mark it from the Rational Realism of the West. Whether this brand of Realism is rational or irrational remains to be seen. We may concede that both Kapila and Russell are Realists in two spheres of philosophical living which might not after all contradict each other, although modern Realism is naturally suspicious of anything that smacks of the spiritual.[49]

It is interesting that Shri Anirvan uses the term "New Hopes" as a title, which could also indicate that he hopes for something in spite of his inclination towards renunciation, and shares the ideal of Lizelle Reymond to teach something to the world.

46 The quote shows, structurally speaking, how the polarity of *prakṛti* and *puruṣa* has become more easily accessible to the West with tantric descriptions.

47 *Letters from a Baul* p. 12.

48 *La vie dans la vie* p. 97.

49 *Buddhiyoga* p. 239.

5. Conclusion

Shri Anirvan combines an on-going yoga tradition and a psychological approach of self-discovery based on a rethinking of the tradition. To separate these two spheres or dimensions, at least from a heuristic perspective, helps to situate him both in the Indian scene and the international one. However, his Sāṃkhya is simultaneously present in both and is an example of the impossibility of separating these spheres any longer. The conjuncture of various contributions, Indian and Western, creates a powerful movement of interpretation and regeneration. The result does not belong to either sphere, neither the Indian nor the Western, but constitutes an epistemic force through interpretations and translations, which are meaningful to those who elaborate and transmit them.

If Shri Anirvan invited Lizelle Reymond to seek out the company of Gurdjieff's followers, he may not have really understood what this could mean or imply. For him, nothing is esoteric; he uses the most rational system to structure his thoughts and experiences, whereas Gurdjieff's writings are hermetic and difficult to access.[50] However, there are points of convergence, at least in certain content elements, such as the fourth way of Gurdjieff that is a way outside any institution and based on self-discovery.[51]

It is of course illusory to measure or even account for the direct or indirect influences Shri Anirvan and Lizelle Reymond had on the Gurdjieff movement (Gurdjieff himself was inspired by his travels in Asia and interest in Buddhist and Indian thinking), and the most we can do is speak of a network of influences and exchanges. However, in the larger history of yoga and transformation, it is interesting to note that Lizelle Reymond's contribution to the "West" was not in the realm of postural, meditative or "well-being" yoga, but on a more esoteric level if we take her connection to the Gurdjieff group, and on a more philosophical and psychological level if we see her contribution more as being her connection with Shri Anirvan. Shri Anirvan used psychology as an introspective means to reflect on the world. It is through introspection and meditation that he developed a conscious and reflective mind, which quite aligns him with thinkers such as Aurobindo or even Gurdjieff.

---

50 See Moore 2006; Needleman 2006.

51 "On y accède par quatre étapes. Les Fragments d'un Enseignement inconnu parlent abondamment des deux premières. Ensuite Ouspensky s'est tu car il avait quitté Gurdjieff. Tout son enseignement personnel ultérieur, qui est très important, développe ces deux dernières étapes dont il relate les développements et les expériences vécues avec son maître. Par contre, les livres de Gurdjieff ouvrent les frontières des deux dernières étapes. Celles-ci sont habilement dissimulées dans le récit mythique. Ces étapes sont: la pluralité des 'moi'; un seul 'moi'; point de 'moi'; le Vide" (*La vie dans la vie* p. 67). It should be noted that this quote is absent from the English version.

What occurred in history as the biographies of Shri Anirvan and Lizelle Reymond turns out to be a microhistory that opens up a view on much larger movements. The biographies of Shri Anirvan and Lizelle Reymond turn into microhistories which are part of much larger contexts (macrohistories), such as, for example, the history of Sāṃkhya, the propagation of "Inner" Yoga as an alternative of yoga practice less visible than Āsana Yoga, the growing acceptance of psychological and spiritual insights and experiences – which may have multiple, independent or simultaneous causes – integrating different traditions, and research into the mechanics of encounter and translation of cultures, the prerequisites of such encounters.

Shri Anirvan's interpretation of Sāṃkhya is psychological and follows the way Lizelle Reymond understood it and wanted to present it to the world. It first reached a French audience before it also joined the ranks of Indian contemporary interpretations and exegesis by a spiritual master who is recognised in India as a scholar as well as a yogi. His interpretation in certain publications can however never be separated from Lizelle Reymond who gave it a shape that has been certainly adapted in the English version, but also remains largely similar to the original French one.

The Sāṃkhya that is presented here is not only a philosophical system with yoga as its practical side, it also appears in its "translated" form, suitable for a modern world, as a skilful, rational, attentive, consciousness-oriented, positive way of life that includes its renunciation.

References

Works by Shri Anirvan

Antarayoga
Shrî Anirvan (2009). *Antara Yoga: Le Yoga intérieur.* Collection Le Maître et le disciple. Gollion: Infolio.

Buddhiyoga
Anirvan (1983). *Buddhiyoga of the Gītā and Other Essays.* New Delhi: Biblia Impex.

Gitanuvachan
Trans. by Smt Kalyani Bose. http://anirvan-memories.blogspot.ch/p/english-translations-of-some-bengali.html. Accessed 6 June 2014.

Ishopanishad. Sri Anirvan's Commentary on Ishopanishad
Trans. by Sri Gautam Dharmapal. http://anirvan-memories.blogspot.ch/p/english-translations-of-some-bengali.html. Accessed 6 June 2014.

Letters from a Baul
Reymond, L. (Comp.). (1983). *Letters from a Baul: Life within the Life.* Calcutta: Sri Aurobindo Pathamandir.

Letters written by Sri Anirvan
Trans. by various authors. http://anirvan-memories.blogspot.ch/p/english-translations-of-some-bengali.html. Accessed 6 June 2014.
Mandukya Upanishad (based on talks by Sri Anirvan)
Trans. by Sri Gautam Dharmapal. http://anirvan-memories.blogspot.ch/p/english-translations-of-some-bengali.html. Accessed 6 June 2014.
'Pather Sathi', The Eternal Companion in Divine Quest
Part I. *A Translation of 'Pather Sathi', a Collection of Letters to one of his Followers, dated from December 10, 1964 to May 7, 1978.* Trans. from the original Bengali by Kalyani Bose. http://anirvan-memories.blogspot.ch/p/english-translations-of-some-bengali.html. Accessed 6 June 2014.

Works by Lizelle Reymond

The Dedicated
Reymond, L. (1953). The Dedicated: A Biography of Nivedita. Madras: Samata Books.
Ma vie chez les brahmanes
Reymond, L. (1957). *Ma vie chez les brahmanes.* Paris: Flammarion.
My Life with a Brahmin Family
Reymond, L. (1958). *My Life with a Brahmin Family*, trans. L. Norton. London: Rider (French original: *Ma vie chez les brahmanes*).
Le pèlerinage vers la vie et vers la mort
Reymond, L. & Shrî Anirvân (2009). *Le pèlerinage vers la vie et vers la mort.* Gollion: Infolio.
La vie dans la vie
Reymond, L. & Shri Anirvan (1969). La vie dans la vie: Pratique de la philosophie du sâmkhya d'après l'enseignement de Shrî Anirvân. Genève: Mont-Blanc.

Secondary Sources

Ashcroft, B. et al. (Eds.). (1995). *The Post-Colonial Studies Reader.* London: Routledge.
Bertrand, R. (2007). Rencontres impériales. L'histoire connectée et les relations euro-asiatiques. *Revue d'Histoire Moderne et Contemporaine, 54*(4bis), 69–89.
Bertrand, R. (2011). *L'Histoire à parts égales: Récits d'une rencontre, Orient-Occident (XVIe–XVIIe siècle).* Paris: Seuil.
Bhabha, H. (1994). *The Location of Culture.* London: Routledge.
Blavatsky, H. P. (Ed.). (1879–1880). *The Theosophist: Monthly Journal Devoted to Oriental Philosophy, Art, Literature and Occultism,* 1.
Ginzburg, C. (1980). *Le fromage et les vers: L'univers d'un meunier du XVIe siècle,* trans. M. Aymard. Paris: Flammarion (Italian original: C. Ginzburg, *Il formaggio e I vermi è un saggio storico.* Torino: Einaudi, 1976).
Halbfass, W. (1988). *India and Europe: An Essay in Understanding.* Albany: State University of New York Press.

Irschick, E. (1994). *Dialogue and History: Constructing South India 1795–1895*. Berkeley: University of California Press.

Moore, J. (2006). Gurdjieff, Georges Ivanovitch. In W. J. Hanegraaff (Ed.), *Dictionary of Gnosis and Western Esotericism* (pp. 445–450). Leiden: Brill.

Needleman, J. (2006). Gurdjieff Tradition. In W. J. Hanegraaff (Ed.), *Dictionary of Gnosis and Western Esotericism* (pp. 450–454). Leiden: Brill.

Ouspensky, P. D. (1949a). *Fragments d'un enseignement inconnu: La voie de la connaissance*, trans. Ph. Lavastine. Paris: Stock (English original: *In Search of the Miraculous: Fragments of an Unknown Teaching*).

Ouspensky, P. D. (1949b). *In Search of the Miraculous: Fragments of an Unknown Teaching*. New York: Harcourt, Brace.

Roy, D. (1982). *Six Illuminates of Modern India*. Bombay: Bharatiya Vidya Bhavan.

Rushdie, S. (1992). *Imaginary Homelands: Essays and Criticism 1981–1991*. London & New York: Granta Books & Penguin.

Subrahmanyam, S. (2007). Par-delà l'incommensurabilité: pour une histoire connectée des empires aux temps modernes. *Revue d'Histoire Moderne et Contemporaine, 54*(4bis), 34–53.

Swarup, R. (1983). Introduction. In Anirvan, *Buddhiyoga of the Gītā and Other Essays* (pp. vi–xvi). New Delhi: Biblia Impex.

Chapter 12

Christian Responses to Yoga in the Second Half of the Twentieth Century

Anand Amaladass

Contents

1. Introduction 487

2. Diversity of Views on the Relationship Between Yoga and Christianity 488
2.1. Reservations about the Western Reception of Yoga in General 489
2.2. Reservations Based on Theological Arguments 492

3. Positive Responses to Yoga 493

4. The Impact of Yoga on the Christian World 496

5. Can Yoga Enrich Non-Asian Religious Practices? 498

6. Conclusion 500

References 501

Anand Amaladass

Chapter 12: Christian Responses to Yoga in the Second Half of the Twentieth Century

1. Introduction

During the second half of the previous century a yoga boom swept the globe. The Christian response to yoga during that period was very ambivalent. There is no such thing as *the* Christian response. It has its own history of mixed views ranging from an enthusiastic or cautious approach to hostile reactions. Not only did some modern Protestant evangelicals oppose it, also the Roman Catholic Church officially issued a warning against Eastern methods of meditation in a letter to the Catholic Bishops in 1989.[1] The modern Hindu response is also very vehement, yoga being "a victim of overt intellectual property theft", etc.[2]

This chapter presents the diversity of Christian response to yoga, first the reservation about Asian methods in general and then the reservation about adapting yoga from a Christian theological point of view; secondly, it highlights the positive response to yoga and the *de facto* impact of yoga in the Christian world and concludes with an open mind that yoga can enrich non-Asian, in particular the Christian religious practices.

1 "The expression 'eastern methods' is used to refer to methods which are inspired by Hinduism and Buddhism, such as 'Zen,' 'Transcendental Meditation' or 'Yoga.' Thus it indicates methods of meditation of the non-Christian Far East which today are not infrequently adopted by some Christians also in their meditation. The orientation of the principles and methods contained in this present document is intended to serve as a reference point not just for this problem, but also, in a more general way, for the different forms of prayer practiced nowadays in ecclesial organizations, particularly in associations, movements and groups." This is the endnote no. 1 of the "Letter to the Bishops of the Catholic Church on Some Aspects of Christian Meditation" issued on 15 October 1989; http://www.vatican.va/roman_curia/congregations/cfaith/documents/rc_con_cfaith_doc_19891015_meditazione-cristiana_en.html. Accessed 7 June 2016.

2 See Jain 2012.

2. Diversity of Views on the Relationship Between Yoga and Christianity

During the period in question a wide diversity of opinions on this subject emerged. Five main attitudes are identified by David Burnett in his book on Hinduism (Burnett 1992). First, there is the view that all religions naturally include yoga. Adherents of this view would argue that all faiths, by the very fact that they are spiritual, are fundamentally devotional yoga. Yoga is not a discipline restricted to Hinduism, it is also found in Buddhism, in some forms of Sufism, as advocated, for example, by Idries Shah, and of course in Christianity.

Second, there are those who regard yoga as the lost secret of Christianity. Burnett cites Maharishi Mahesh Yogi who initially claimed that the world religions had failed because they lost the techniques of yoga. As there is no historical evidence for such an argument, Burnett refutes him.

Third, some Christians have regarded yoga not as part of a religious system but as a scientifically confirmed applied philosophy as it has been presented by Transcendental Meditation (TM) and other neo-Hindu movements. In this model, yoga and religion are considered as different entities that complement one another, as do science and literature. Barnett points out that the US courts however, after careful consideration of TM, could not see how yoga could be severed from its roots as a spiritual discipline of Hinduism.[3]

Fourth, some hold the view that yoga is demonic. This has been the typical response of many evangelicals to the subject. This is an extreme reaction. Certain types of yoga, such as tantric yoga, do involve paranormal and occult phenomena. This, however, cannot be said about Haṭha Yoga, which was essentially developed to facilitate other more advanced forms of yoga, according to Burnett.

Finally, yoga has been considered a spiritual discipline that may be used by a Christian for his/her own spiritual development. The writings of Jean-Marie Dechanet, a French Benedictine monk, have been influential in promoting this view. Dechanet considers Christian yoga as a preparation for communion with God, an emptying of oneself to appreciate more fully the grace of God. Dechanet is very clear in his position with regard to yoga:

> The essential point is to understand thoroughly and to admit *that it is not a question of turning a given form of yoga into something Christian*, but of bringing into the service of

---

3 Maharishi Mahesh Yogi, founder of TM, claimed his movement to be an educational technique rather than a religion and received both federal and state funding. At some stage, due to financial dealings, the matter went to the court. On 19 October 1977, US District Judge H. Curtis Meanor declared: "No inference was possible except that the teaching of the SCI/TM and the *puja* are religious in nature." That led to an eighteen-month long legal battle with the court finally affirming the earlier ruling (Burnett 1992: 199).

> Christianity and of the Christian life (especially when this is given up to contemplation) the undoubted benefits arising from yogic disciplines. Everything in yoga, therefore, that promotes dialogue, the basic Christian dialogue, may be boldly considered as fit for adaptation. On the other hand, whatever makes for involution and isolation must be banished.[4]

Many Christians had sympathy for Dechanet's view, but also had reservations. For example, some argued that if yoga is so important for spiritual development, why did Jesus not teach this, or some similar practice? Dechanet recognises the dangers of Rāja Yoga as well as other forms.[5] Can yoga be neutral? David Burnett raises this question and answers it himself as follows:

> Almost all Christians would answer negatively, arguing that any benefits that may be gained from Hatha Yoga can be achieved equally well through prayers and contemplation upon the Holy Bible.[6]

Burnett concludes this section in his book by pointing out the Christian position. In the biblical vision there is no question of separation from the world nor of absorption (*samādhi*) into the ultimate reality, but a continuous relationship between God and his people.

2.1. Reservations about the Western Reception of Yoga in General

Obviously, among the Christians in the West there was much scepticism towards taking over Hindu practices and elements from Asian religions in general. Even a quite unorthodox protestant like Carl Jung observed in his *Yoga and the West* that the European is so constituted that he "inevitably" makes the worst possible use of yoga. Nevertheless he recognises that some sort of yoga, some form of yogic discipline, is needed in the West. "Western civilization", he says,

> must first of all be liberated from its narrow barbarism. If we are to succeed in doing this we shall have to penetrate more deeply into what is properly human in man. This knowledge cannot be acquired by copying, 'aping' other people's methods, which came to birth in very different psychological conditions. The West will have to create its own Yoga, Yoga built on Christian foundations – and in time it will do so.[7]

This attitude is found also among other great minds who wrote on Indian themes. For example Hermann Hesse (1877–1962), the celebrated author of the novel "Siddhartha", says that the Europeans should search for their spiritual renewal

4 Dechanet 1984: 17–18.

5 Dechanet 1984: 15–17.

6 Burnett 1992: 203.

7 C. G. Jung, Le yoga et l'occident. In *Approches de l'Inde: Textes et études*, ed. J. Masui. Paris: Cahiers du Sud, 1949, pp. 324–329, quoted in Dechanet 1965: 9.

not in some foreign past, through superficial taking over of the Asian wisdom tradition, but find the source within themselves:

> We are different, but we have become outsiders here without the right of citizenship. We have lost our paradise long ago. The new one that we want to build lies in us and in our own northern future, not in the warm oceans of the East.[8]

But this awareness dawned on Hesse after his exposure to the Eastern shores. He must have been deeply immersed in the world of Hinduism, Buddhism, Daoism, and Confucianism, before he could discover for himself anew his own Christian tradition.[9]

Some yoga teachers were exacting radical transformations in their students requiring extended periods of serious *sādhanā* and study. Some other Indian gurus in the West modernised their teachings and tolerated behaviour that would not be found in India. This trend has been noticed by social scientists and theologians. Two studies devoted to this phenomenon could be mentioned here: *Turning East* by Harvey Cox (1977) and *The Light at the Centre: Context and Pretext of Modern Mysticism* by Agehananda Bharati (1976). Cox wrote it as a Christian theologian and Bharati was an Austrian-born Hindu monk and professor of anthropology. Both Cox and Bharati do not go into the deeper analysis of the problem. Cox's book is more of a travelogue than an in-depth investigation. Bharati insists that his work is social science.

Cox investigated a number of Eastern meditation techniques. He talked with members of the International Society for Krishna Consciousness (ISKCON) and sat with a Zen Buddhist meditation group. Finally he found peace in the company of Benedictine monks and pointed out that the West has its own systems of worship and pathways for meditation. However, he failed to recognise that the background of most young Americans was not that of his generation:

> Religious education does not play a prominent role in the upbringing of the "television" generation whose imagination is captured more by superheroes (or super-villains) than by Biblical tales. For those who do attempt to make a connection with their mythic origins, quite often the exotic is the most appealing.[10]

Bharati, on the other hand, lived the life of the sixties a generation earlier. His training in Indian languages and cultures opened avenues to the exotic for him long before affordable travel facilities made India accessible to the masses. He seems reluctant to accept the legitimacy of the new Americanised meditation movements, preferring to lend credibility to the more Hinduised groups such as ISKCON:

8 Hesse 1970: 283.
9 Cf. Gellner 2001.
10 Chapple 1985: 102.

> However towards the end of his analysis he sees that America is ripe for the freedom which successful meditation produces, and predicts that yoga will wane in India, just as Buddhism and Christianity disappeared from the places of their origin.[11]

Bharati believes in the possibility of a true rapprochement between the East and the West. But he is critical of people who are advocating pseudo-esoteric eclecticism, because they lack intuition for the genuine and the spurious. It is because their knowledge of Indian traditions stems from translations and from talks with English-speaking Hindus, most of whom themselves represent a mixed tradition. Bharati is convinced that without a thorough knowledge of Sanskrit, and at least one more modern Indian language, in both speech and writing, one can never be a competent writer on India.[12]

In a similar way, Louis Renou pointed out that tradition is not something one learns by intuition or after some breathing exercises. It is the thought-process of old masters commented on by successive masters – yoga or Vedānta – captured in their origins, their historical development, etc., and not in the syncretism contaminated by Christianity, psychoanalysis and Theosophy, in search of primordial wisdom dispersed in humanity, the *philosophia perennis.*[13]

Renou is very strong in his language about the several varieties of neo-Hinduism amalgamated with Western data in a Hindu guise, claiming to interpret Hinduism. Most often they draw from a false terminology, arbitrary interpretations, and randomly selected texts of some sects. And he adds, "let us not forget, India is a land of charlatans."[14]

One could summarise the historical situation within which the Christian reception of yoga took place as follows:

1. The orientalistic dispute based on typologies of "the West" and "the East" was still very important.
2. Three groups were involved within the encounter with South Asia: the Indologists, the theologians, the non-church individualistic spiritual seekers and interested lay Christians from different churches and denominations.
3. Christian as well as non-Christian people in the USA and Europe were primarily interested in South Asian religions because of their mystical dimensions and their practices of meditation including meditative body exercises. Little informed about the traditional reality of the Hindu world of

11 Ibid.

12 Cf. Bharati 1980: 17.

13 Cf. L. Renou, *Sanskrit et culture: L'apport de l'Inde à la civilisation humaine.* Paris: Payot, 1950, pp. 61–62, quoted in Maupilier 1974: 292.

14 L. Renou, *L'Hindouisme.* Collection que sais-je. Paris: Presses Universitaires de France, 1951, pp. 34 and 123–124: "L'Inde, ne l'oublions pas, est la terre bénie des charlatans"; quoted in Maupilier 1974: 292.

yoga, they used formulae and postures in a spirit immediately practical to regain religious experiences or to revive the tired Christian emotions.
4. Some Indologists like Bharati or Renou claimed to have privileged access to the "real Indian tradition". They criticised the eclecticism and superficiality of the popular approaches.
5. Several Christian theologians studied yoga on a practical level as well as on the basis of a philological study of the old Sanskrit texts. They also often took a critical stance towards popular forms of yoga.
6. The positive approach to yoga by Dechanet aims at facilitating contemplative prayer when everything seems to be making this more difficult. "The Christian in praying does not have to search for his own self nor to forget himself in the manner of Orientals, but to open himself to the word of God, for it is solely in this and by this that he can find himself and exist."[15]

2.2. Reservations Based on Theological Arguments

In the first half of the twentieth century, the distinction between revealed and natural religion was predominant and the influence of this distinction was still to be felt in later decades. This theological position does not allow accepting non-Christian religions as "revealed". In 1950, Alan Watts, at that time still speaking as an Episcopalian theologian, complains that Western man remains unconscious of his inner being, of the truly subjective realm. That would be the reason why he is unable to distinguish the subjective character of oriental metaphysics from extremely introverted ego-centricity.[16] This he illustrates by quoting Maritain's essay "The Natural Mystical Experience and the Void". The title itself can be said to really beg the question. As Watts further argues, there are no solid grounds at all for calling Hindu realisation a *natural* experience as distinct from the *supernatural* experience of the Christian mystics.

Watts further states that

> apparently Maritain thinks it natural because it is possible to produce this mystic experience by the personal effort of yoga, whereas the Christian experience is solely the gift of God, for which the soul can only prepare. This is to introduce a distinction between yoga and Christian mystical theology which simply does not exist.[17]

Vedānta theology would involve no such idea as producing realisation by one's own effort or action. Śaṅkara, the Vedāntin, points out that

15 Dechanet 1984: 27.
16 Watts 1972: 190.
17 Watts 1972: 190, n. 1.

> realization is by knowledge and not by action. For Brahman constitutes a person's Self and it is not something to be attained by that person. And even if Brahman were altogether different from a person's Self, still it would not be something to be obtained; for as it is omnipresent it is part of its nature that it is ever present to everyone.[18]

Śaṅkara explicitly states in his *Vivekacūḍāmaṇi* (v. 3) that there are three things difficult to obtain by human effort alone, these being attainable only by divine favour or God's grace (*devānugraha*): to be born as a human being (*manuṣyatva*), the desire for ultimate liberation (*mumūkṣutva*) and the protecting care of a perfected sage (*mahāpuruṣasamśrayaḥ*).

> Maritain goes on to suggest that what is experienced in oriental mysticism is the *esse* of the soul rather than God, presupposing an absolute discontinuity between the *esse* or being of man and the being of God – which is natural enough in Thomism where God is always the object of love and knowledge. Furthermore, Maritain seems to be familiar only with the mono-ideistic type of *yoga* which excludes everything from consciousness other than the point of concentration. But mono-ideism is as much a Christian as a Hindu practice, and furthermore is never anything but a preparative means.[19]

Watts thus was one of the pioneers who paved the way to a theological understanding of South Asian yoga practices that conceives them as a means for a truly revelatory experience of the ultimate reality that Christians call God.

3. Positive Responses to Yoga

Many Christian thinkers who came to India were busy with Indian spirituality, which includes the study and practice of yoga. Pierre Johanns,[20] Olivier Lacombe,[21] Abbé Jules Monchanin[22] (1895–1991), Henri le Saux (Abhishiktananda) (1910–1973)[23], and Bede Griffiths are prominent Catholic examples.

18 Commentary on *Vedāntasūtra* 1.1.4, trans. G. Thibaut, *The Vedânta-Sûtras*. Sacred Books of the East 34. Oxford: The Clarendon Press, 1904, pp. 32–33, quoted in Watts 1972: 169.

19 Watts 1972: 190, n. 1. Watts furthermore states: "*Moksha* itself, the supreme spiritual state of *yoga*, is an inclusive and not at all an exclusive state of consciousness and is in no sense, as Maritain suggests, a purely negative experience which, because of the identity of negatives, cannot be properly distinguished from a negatively described God. One wonders how a philosophy can know anything about the *esse* of the soul, when it is so heavily committed to the principle *nihil est in intellectu quod non prius fuerit in sensu*" (Watts 1972: 169).

20 Johanns 1996.

21 Lacombe 1986.

22 Cf. Monchanin 1956 and 1962.

23 Abhishiktananda, who was fully immersed in the Indian spiritual traditions, still seems to have doubts and scruples at times about the possibility of adapting yoga for Christians, as he writes in his diary about yoga as follows: "Can it still be Christianized? For a long time I thought so. More and more I have come to doubt it. For this 'personal' or transpersonal attainment of the absolute, and even the decisive and committed search for it, conflicts with

Additionally, several popular self-help books introduced yoga to a Christian audience (e.g., Hayden 1966).

The Benedictine monk Bede Griffiths, to focus on one important figure of Catholic intermonastic spiritual dialogue, has several publications to his credit. His first book, *The Golden String* (1954), and a sequel to this book, *The Marriage of East and West* (1982), highlight his position as a Christian mystic towards the Eastern wisdom traditions. Pertinent to our theme is his book *Return to the Centre*[24] the last chapter of which is devoted to yoga. Griffiths points out that the underlying philosophy of Patañjali is the separation of body and spirit, and the goal of yoga is to free consciousness from any taint of mortality. But he is in agreement with Aurobindo's integral yoga, where matter and life and consciousness in man are seen to be evolving towards divine life and divine consciousness in which they are not annihilated but fulfilled. According to Griffiths,

> This is the goal of a Christian yoga. Body and soul are to be transfigured by the divine life and to participate in the divine consciousness. There is a descent of the spirit into matter and a corresponding ascent, by which matter is transformed by the indwelling power of the Spirit and the body is transfigured [...] For a Christian this has already taken place in the resurrection of Christ. In his body, matter has already been transformed, so as to become a spiritual body which is the medium of the divine life.[25]

Several individuals bear witness positively to their experience of yoga, how they benefited from this practice. Anthony Grey, for example, was a British correspondent who was arrested for political reasons. With all this experience he wrote three books, one of which is on yoga, and there he writes that this book is the one he cherished most and that he spent two hours daily on yoga practice.[26] So also Périclès Korovessis, a Greek political prisoner, after he was freed writes how he was supported by yoga.[27]

In India, especially after the Second Vatican Council, Catholic Christian groups tried to adapt yoga techniques to their Christian spirituality. Even if they did not take the whole of yoga as their life-style, they brought in some form of yoga or Zen as part of their spiritual praxis. Dechanet's book on yoga was a source of inspiration for many educated Christians in India. Based on this, some of the Christian writers prepared text books to meet the needs of these groups. Swami Amaldas was a student of Griffiths who recommends yoga as a method of prayer

---

Christian dogma and the Church, which being grafted onto history, is obliged to attribute an absolute value to time in order to preserve its own value as absolute. What is beyond the 'mind' is opposed to all absoluteness at the level of the 'mind'" (Abhishiktananda 1998: 135).

24 Griffiths 1976.

25 Griffiths 1976: 137–138.

26 Déclaration de l'Agence France-Presse, October 1969; quoted in Maupilier 1974: 289.

27 *La filière : Témoignages sur les tortures en Grèce.* Collection Combats. Paris: Éditions du Seuil, 1969, p. 25, quoted in Maupilier 1974: 289.

by a Christian. Amaldas recommends yoga as a means for higher life and as a method for the integration of human nature as a whole. The author sees universal man in all five elements such as earth, fire, water, etc. filled with biblical echoes. He also describes a meditation on the trinity.[28] The word "yoga" is used here as a general term for spirituality in the process of inculturation.[29]

Another development among the Christians in India was to combine the Spiritual Exercises of St. Ignatius with yoga practice.[30] In the tradition of St. Ignatius there is a practice among Catholics to go on an annual retreat for eight days (some continue it for thirty days) – a time of prayer and meditation. The spiritual directors started to include some sessions of yoga practice with selected exercises. The *Bhagavadgītā* (*Gītā*) allowed them to offer this combination.

First of all, the *Gītā* (2.48) defines yoga as attaining a *samatva* attitude (*samatvaṃ yoga ucyate*), equanimity between the polarities (*dvandva*-s) like heat and cold, praise and blame, gold and mud, etc. St. Ignatius gives the same type of examples in his Spiritual Exercises and calls it "indifference" – whether it is honour or dishonour, riches or poverty, health or sickness. So *samatva* could be translated as "indifference" in the Ignatian sense. R. C. Zaehner in his translation of the *Bhagavadgītā* renders yoga as "spiritual exercise" and refers to Ignatius of Loyola in his commentary (on *Gītā* 2.48) in order to acknowledge his indebtedness.[31]

The second point of similarity is what the *Gītā* (6.10–19) describes as the physical conditions for the practice of yoga, giving hints on the conducive place, the suitable posture, etc., which St. Ignatius calls *Annotations* in the Spiritual Exercise. The third striking similarity is the goal of yoga. In the Ignatian view, the goal is "seeing God in all things and all things in God" and in the *Gītā*'s language it is "seeing the self in all things and all things in the self". Thus yoga entered into Christian spiritual practice on the basis of the *Bhagavadgītā*, if not through Pātañjala Yoga.

28 Amaldas 1974.

29 Matus 1992; Vineeth 1995; Ravindra 2005.

30 For example, Amaladass 1987.

31 Zaehner 1973: 146. There was also strong criticism by Hindu thinkers like Krishna Warrier from Kerala that this translation was "catholic" and did not reflect the real *Gītā*, etc. However, on this point Zaehner is right.

4. The Impact of Yoga on the Christian World

Yoga has in fact challenged the Christian world, where every non-Christian religion was declared as anonymous Christianity, while the other side has responded in kind. Christianity was perceived as an incomplete or "unfulfilled" Buddhism and John's Gospel as "anonymous Vedānta" etc.

The author of *Christian Yoga,* Jean-Marie Dechanet, wrote this book in French in 1955 (*La Voie du Silence).* It was translated into many languages and offered an occasion to rediscover the early Christian sources of prayer techniques and meditations. Reference is made to *The Way of a Pilgrim* revealed to the West in about 1925, in which a pilgrim in search of salvation discovers with astonishment the secret of uninterrupted prayer at the school of a *starets* (master or guru) and from the *Philokalia.* The *Philokalia* is a collection of writings by the Fathers of the Eastern Church (some thirty of them) from the third to the fifteenth century and exists in three versions: Greek (1792), Slavonic (1793) and Russian. It is a storehouse of the secrets of prayer or rather of a form of prayer that can with certainty be traced back to about 1250 CE and that has marked the whole development of Greco-Russian spirituality from then on.[32]

A very important part of the "inner asceticism" propagated by the *Philokalia* is played by the "Jesus Prayer", uttered in a particular bodily position with a special way of breathing. The aim of the Jesus Prayer was to produce *hesychia* ("quiet") in the sense of inner stillness and silence of the heart and those who practise it are known as Hesychasts.[33] The standard form of the Jesus Prayer is found first in the "Life of Abba Philemon", a sixth-century Egyptian monk. The first significant reference to a physical technique linking the recitation of the Jesus Prayer with the rhythm of breathing is to be found in the writings of Nicephorus the Hesychast, a thirteenth-century monk of Mont Athos. Nicephorus recommends that the one praying sit with the chin resting on the chest and the gaze focusing on the navel. Next, the rhythm of respiration is to be slowed down. While thus engaged the one praying should focus inwardly upon the place of the heart.

The question was raised whether there was a direct influence of yoga on the practice of the "prayer of the heart". Western scholars dismiss this question saying that one cannot historically prove such an influence, though from the time of Alexander the Great (356–242 BCE) there was certainly a cultural exchange between the Hellenic world and India, and the Buddha legend was known from the writings of Clement of Alexandria.[34] The teacher of Plotinus (203–269) was said to have been a Buddhist monk Ammonius Sakka (175–242) and Plotinus

32 Cf. Dechanet 1974: 173–174; Jungclaussen 1974.

33 Zawilla 1993.

34 Cf. Bergh van Eysinga 1904; Benz 1951.

became the focus of attention in the history of philosophy as an intellectual bridge to India.[35] But the question still remains unanswered where this aspect comes from – namely, this practice of prayer accompanied by breathing exercises and a specific posture of the body. Some Catholic spiritual writers do acknowledge the fact that there is close resemblance to yoga, but do not go further.[36]

The challenge of yoga led to several discussions among Christian thinkers who showed the differences between the Christian approach to prayer and meditation and that of yoga. Emmanuel Jungclaussen, a German Benedictine monk and teacher of the Jesus Prayer, for example, pointed out the commonalities and differences. Yoga stems from the concept of death and rebirth, Hesychasm has dying and being born-again, the resurrection with Christ in the mystery of baptism as an obvious presupposition. Hesychasm is only the most external consequence of the mystery of baptism. Both yoga and Hesychasm demand moral preparation (*yama* and *niyama* – Christian virtues) and both demand a spiritual master (guru or *starets*). Both require certain withdrawal into oneself, silence and regulated breathing practice. The recitation of the name of Jesus and Om is said to have a healing effect. The goal in both is calming the inner world and thus reaching the ultimate reality. This leads to the question about the unity of religious consciousness of mankind. In both forms Jungclaussen recognised the same religious genius that searches for the Absolute.[37]

Another example for a positive reception would be the study of Psalms under the inspiration of yoga. Eulogia Wurz analysed the yoga techniques and granted that yoga is certainly an *instrumentum salutis,* although it is different from the Christian approach. What is striking is his use of the term yoga in the Christian context. He talks of the "Yoga-way of Christ" and states that "our yoga is Jesus Christ" and "the whole life is Christ-Yoga", reminding us of Aurobindo's phrase "the whole life is yoga":

> The whole life must be *yoga,* if one wants to master the art and to speak of the effective *mantra.* The whole life must be oriented towards God, if one wants to obtain grace, to pray the psalm perfectly.[38]

Exposure to yoga prompted the Christian world to enter into a serious discussion, to show how the Christian belief system differs from the world of yoga. Walter Schmidt, in his book on yoga in Germany, responded to Dechanet's

35 Cf. Jungclaussen 1971.

36 See P. B. T. Bilaniuk, in his article on "Eastern Christian Spirituality" (1993: 329): "Hesychasm has long been known as an aesthetico-mystical teaching together with psychosomatic practice which in many respects calls to mind the practice of yoga"; see also Ware 1987: 566.

37 Cf. Jungclaussen 1971: 62–66; see also Monchanin 1956: 1–10.

38 Wurz 1971: 101.

book.[39] Dechanet understands yoga as a method which can be used by Christians. Schmidt thinks that this is secularizing yoga. The external procedure of traditional yoga techniques is not to be separated from their inner content of Hindu philosophy. Yoga methods are thus not simply neutralisable. Yoga is not as objective as mathematics.

As a result of this discussion, dialogue-oriented theologians asserted that Schmidt is right in the sense of pointing out the differences between Hindu and Christian worldviews. But it also became clear that one cannot not stop there and remain isolated from the religious other by absolutising one's own perspective. One should not attempt to neutralise one another. The uniqueness of each perspective is to be acknowledged – Christian or Hindu. One speaks in terms of a personal God and the other refers to an impersonal Absolute; one attains salvation and the other ultimate liberation, one is self-centred and the other oriented towards God's grace. Such language of demarcation and the related concepts come from their respective worldviews – anthropocentric or cosmo-centric, i. e., an anthropocentric or karmic understanding of history. However, they need not exclude one another; they could be seen as complementary. They are at the crossroads perhaps and new ways of thinking could emerge in the process of encounter.

Some others pointed out the differences but did not rush to the conclusion that both could mutually enrich both spiritualities – Hindu and Christian. Albert Cuttat says:

> In the world of the spirit it is the clear differentiation which really unites without mixing up, while a uniform type of blurring the borders in reality only separates, because genuine values could never be exchangeable, never actually be equivalent.[40]

The implication of this approach is that yoga and Christian spiritual practice cannot be juxtaposed against one another, but that there must be a way of viewing them hierarchically. That is to say, yoga is not in a position to fulfil the sanctification of the monotheistic Christian religion, but the other way around is possible, according to Cuttat.

5. Can Yoga Enrich Non-Asian Religious Practices?

Other theologians referred to the *Pātañjalayogaśāstra* as helping to bridge many of the chasms that became apparent in the discussion of yogic meditation practices and their transmittal to the West. Patañjali's Yoga would deal explicitly

39 Schmidt 1967.
40 Cuttat 1965: 22.

with states of affective experience (*samādhi*), listing several varieties and diverse means to achieve them

> For cross-cultural purposes its emphasis on practice is extremely useful, as it discusses process, not doctrine or belief. Fundamentally, yoga explains how and why we hold beliefs and feelings, it does not dogmatically dictate *what* to believe, feel or do.[41]

From this point of view, yoga is essentially a technique. It is a phenomenological investigation of suffering and its transcendence, its sole presupposition being that humankind is plagued with discomfort and suffering (*duḥkha*) and that this suffering can be overcome by reaching a state of liberation. The *Yogasūtra* states: "Suffering that has yet to manifest is to be avoided" (YS 2.16).[42] If Patañjali's analysis of suffering and of the means to avoid it is true, then yoga can be applied by any individual seeking self-fulfilment of a spiritual kind.

Part of the appeal of yoga lies in the many diverse means it prescribes. The student of yoga is told that liberation is achieved through well-cultivated practice and detachment (YS 1.12–14). One who has applied faith (*śraddhā*), vigour (*vīrya*), mindfulness (*smṛti*), absorption (non-dual awareness) (*samādhi*) and discernment (*prajñā*) is said to gain success (YS 1.20). Another way is to devote one's meditation to the primal teacher (*īśvara*), who remains untainted by the ravages of change inflicted by association with material things (*prakṛti*).

Appropriate behaviour in interpersonal relationships is seen to be another tool for self-development: "One should cultivate friendship with the joyful, compassion for the sorrowful, gladness toward those who are virtuous, and equanimity in regard to the non-virtuous; through this, lucidity arises in the mind" (YS 1.33). The emphasis is here on flexibility, being able to recognise a situation and act as called for. Breathing is seen as a means to achieve the stability of mind (YS 1.34). By recognizing the most fundamental of life's processes, closeness to the self is achieved. Other practices prescribed in the *Yogasūtra* include directing one's consciousness to one who has conquered attachment (*vītarāga*), or meditating on an auspicious dream experience, centring the mind in activity or cultivating thoughts which are sorrow-less and illuminating, or by any other means as desired (YS 1.35–39).

The purpose of these various practices is to diminish the influence of past actions which were guided by selfish or impure motives (*kleśa*-s) and generate suffering; *kleśa* is described further as "seeing the atman which is eternal, pure, and joyful, in that which is non-atman, non-eternal, impure and painful" (YS 2.5).

41 Chapple 1985: 103.

42 *Heyaṃ duḥkham anāgatam*. See Bryant 2009: 212.

The yogic practices of transformation begin at the ethical level. For the yogi, freedom is found through disciplined action. By restraint from violence, stealing, hoarding and wantonness and through the application of truthfulness the influences of the self-centred past are lessened. Cultivation of purity, contentment, forbearance, study and devotion to a chosen symbol (*īśvarapraṇidhāna*) establishes a new way of life, constructing a new body of free and responsible action (Chapple 1985: 107).

Much of the debate seems to be based on some generalised presuppositions and misinterpretation of the key terms concerning the *Yogasūtra*. The spirit – matter (*puruṣa* – *prakṛti*) dichotomy is an example. It is true that there are different schools of Hindu thought with different understanding of this duality. But the *Yogasūtra* does not mean to say that matter is annihilated at the end, but rather that a rightful relationship between them should be restored and that they interact reciprocally. Different meditative paths are suggested as means to reach this level. In the same way the state of *samādhi* is not simply absorption into the ultimate reality, but a transformed state of consciousness. Secondly, some disciplinary practices or ethical prescriptions are part of any spiritual growth and they need not be taken as a claim that one can achieve salvation by one's own effort or denying the role of grace in this process. Hence a right understanding of yoga without prejudice need not be seen as opposed to the Christian vision of reality and salvation. Moreover, the Christian apprehension seems to be based on contradictory interpretations by some Hindu yoga masters.

6. Conclusion

With regard to the discussions concerning the relationship of yoga and Christianity within the second half of the twentieth century the opposing parties expressed certain legitimate concerns. On the one hand, one has to respect the pastoral concerns of the authorities of the Christian traditions, i. e., to train their followers, warn them against possible dangers and thus protect them from aberrations, while preserving their identity. On the other hand, those who talk about a subject like yoga must take time to understand what the yoga traditions themselves are saying about their beliefs and convictions, which presupposes the knowledge of the source language and a certain openness to perceive the differences in others rather than only their own. Unreliable secondary sources and a biased approach could jeopardise the mutual relation and make them isolated, and as a result even cause them to harm themselves.

It is undisputed that Yoga has had an impact on the whole world. There are many who practise yoga in the West to escape their stressful life-situation, to gain mental health, etc., without going into the theological implications of the yoga systems with their Hindu religious–philosophical background.

The predominant Christian theological position towards yoga or Eastern meditation techniques in general has been to adapt them within the framework of faith. This has been summed up in a German guidebook to meditation following the tradition of Karlfried Graf Dürckheim as follows:

> Meditation is not the privilege of the Far-East, but it is the innermost mainspring of all wisdom traditions. The East has made us aware of this truth, which was forgotten in the West. Eastern wisdom can enrich us very much on the way to contemplation, only if we open ourselves to it with caution and prudence, just like the Fathers of the Church who have understood in their time to take and baptize all the riches that Greek culture offered them. They were convinced that every truth, wherever it appears, is already an expression of God's Word [...][43]

References

Abhishiktananda (1998). *Ascent to the Depth of the Heart: The Spiritual Diary (1948–1973) of Swami Abhishiktananda (Dom Henri Le Saux). A Selection, edited with Introduction by R. Panikkar. English Translation by D. Fleming and J. Stuart.* Delhi: ISPCK.

Amaladass, A. (1987). The Bhagavadgita as Basis for a Retreat. *Ignis, 16*, 13–18.

Amaldas, B. (1974). *Yoga and Contemplation.* Tiruchirappalli: Shantivanam Ashram.

Baier, K. (1998). *Yoga auf dem Weg nach Westen: Beiträge zur Rezeptionsgeschichte.* Würzburg: Königshausen & Neumann.

Benz, E. (1951). *Indische Einflüsse auf die frühchristliche Theologie.* Wiesbaden: Verlag der Akademie der Wissenschaften und der Literatur.

Bergh van Eysinga, G. A. van den (1904). *Indische Einflüsse auf evangelische Erzählungen.* Göttingen: Vandenhoeck & Ruprecht.

Bharati, A. (1976). *The Light at the Centre: Context and Pretext of Modern Mysticism.* Santa Barbara: Ross-Erikson.

Bharati, A. (1980). *The Ochre Robe.* Santa Barbara: Ross-Erikson.

Bilaniuk, P. B. T. (1993). Eastern Christian Spirituality. In M. Downey (Ed.), *The New Dictionary of Catholic Spirituality* (p. 329). Collegeville, MN: Liturgical Press.

Bryant, E. F. (2009). *The Yoga Sūtras of Patañjali: A New Edition, Translation and Commentary with Insights from the Traditional Commentators.* New York: North Point Press.

Burnett, D. G. (1992). *The Spirit of Hinduism: A Christian Perspective on Hindu Thought.* Tunbridge Wells: Monarch Publications.

Chapple, Ch. (1985). Yoga and Cross-Cultural Religious Understanding. In Z. P. Thundy et al. (Eds.), *Religions in Dialogue: East and West Meet* (pp. 101–126). Lanham: University Press of America.

43 Goettmann & Goettmann 1989: 18.

Cox, H. (1977). *Turning East: Why Americans Look to the Orient for Spirituality and what that Search can Mean to the West.* New York: Simon & Schuster.

Cuttat, J. A. (1965). *Asiatische Gottheit – christlicher Gott: Die Spiritualität der beiden Hemisphären.* Einsiedeln: Johannes Verlag.

Dechanet, J.-M. (1965). *Yoga in Ten Lessons*, trans. S. F. L. Tye. London: Burns and Oates (Engl. trans. of J.-M. Dechanet, *Yoga chrétien en dix leçons.* [Paris]: Desclée de Brouwer, 1964).

Dechanet, J.-M. (1974). *Yoga and God*, trans. S. Fawcett. London: Search Press (Engl. trans. of J.-M. Dechanet, *Journal d'un yogi.* 2 vols. Paris: Courrier du Livre, 1967–1969).

Dechanet, J.-M. (1984). *Christian Yoga.* Tunbridge Wells: Search Press.

Eliade, M. (1970). *Yoga, Immortality and Freedom.* Princeton, NJ: Princeton University Press.

Frei, G. (1958). Christliches Mantram-Yoga: Das Herzensgebet. In W. Bitter (Ed.), *Meditation in Religion und Psychotherapie* (pp. 19–28). Stuttgart: Ernst Klett Verlag.

Gellner, Ch. (2001). Literatur und Weltreligionen: Östlich-Westliches bei Hesse, Brecht, Grass und Muschg. In P. Tschuggnall (Ed.), *Religion – Literatur – Künste.* Vol. 3 (pp. 344–356). Anif: Verlag Mueller-Speiser.

Goettmann, A. & Goettmann, R. (1989). *Meditieren im Atem Gottes: Ein Übungsweg für Christen.* Freiburg i. Br.: Herder.

Griffiths, B. (1954). *The Golden String.* London: Havel Press.

Griffiths, B. (1976). *Return to the Centre.* London: Collins.

Griffiths, B. (1982). *The Marriage of East and West: A Sequel to The Golden String.* London: Collins.

Hayden, E. W. (1966). *Everyday Yoga for Christians: Seven Simple Steps to Victorious Living.* London: Arthur James.

Hesse, H. (1970). *Gesammelte Werke.* Vol. 4. Frankfurt am Main: Suhrkamp Verlag.

Jain, A. R. (2012). The Malleability of Yoga: A Response to Christian and Hindu Opponents of the Popularization of Yoga. *Journal of Hindu-Christian Studies, 25,* 3–10.

Johanns, P. (1996). *To Christ Through the Vedanta: The Writings of Reverend P. Johanns S. J.*, comp. Th. de Greeff. 2 vols. Bangalore: United Theological College.

Jungclaussen, E. (1971). Yoga und Herzensgebet. In U. v. Mangoldt (Ed.), *Yoga Heute* (pp. 29–67). Weilheim: Otto Wilhelm Barth Verlag.

Jungclaussen, E. (Ed.). (1974). *Aufrichtige Erzählungen eines russischen Pilgers.* Freiburg: Herder.

Lacombe, O. (1986). *L'Élan spirituel de l'hinduisme.* Paris: O. E. I. L.

Maritain, J. (1941). The Natural Mystical Experience and the Void. In J. Maritain (Ed.), *Ransoming the Time* (pp. 255–289). New York: Charles Scribner's Sons.

Matus, Th. (1992). *Yoga and the Jesus Prayer Tradition: An Experiment in Faith.* Bangalore: Asian Trading Corporation.

Maupilier, M. (1974). *Le Yoga et l'homme d'Occident.* Paris: Éditions du Seuil.

Monchanin, J. (1956). Yoga et Hesychasme. In J. Monchanin et al. (Eds.), *Entretiens 1955* (pp. 1–10). Pondichéry: Institute Français d'Indologie.

Monchanin, J. (1962). *Die Eremiten von Saccidananda: Ein Versuch zur christlichen Integration der monastischen Überlieferung Indiens*, trans. M. Mayer & M. Vereno. Salzburg: Otto Müller Verlag.

Ravindra, R. (2005). *The Yoga of the Christ: The Way to the Centre.* Adyar, Chennai: The Theosophical Publishing House.

Renou, L. & Filliozat, J. (1947, 1953). *L'Inde classique: Manuel des études indiennes.* 2 vols. Paris: Payot.

Schmidt, W. (1967). *Yoga in Deutschland: Verbreitung - Motive - Hintergründe.* Stuttgart: Kreuz Verlag.

Vineeth, Fr. (1995). *Yoga of Spirituality: Christian Initiation into Indian Spiritual Traditions.* Bangalore: Vidya Vanam Publications.

Ware, K. (1987). The Eastern Christianity. In M. Eliade (Ed.), *The Encyclopedia of Religion.* Vol. 4 (pp. 566–567).

Watts, A. (1972). *The Supreme Identity: An Essay on Oriental Metaphysic and the Christian Religion.* New York: Vintage Books.

Wurz, E. (1971). Der Yoga des Psalters. In U. v. Mangoldt (Ed.), *Yoga Heute* (pp. 69–108). Weilheim: Otto Wilhelm Barth Verlag.

YS. *Yogasūtra*
see Bryant 2009.

Zaehner, R. C. (Trans.). (1973). *The Bhagavad-Gītā with a Commentary Based on the Original Sources.* London: Oxford University Press.

Zawilla, R. J. (1993). Hesychasm. In M. Downey (Ed.), *The New Dictionary of Catholic Spirituality* (pp. 471–473). Minnesota: The Liturgical Press.

Chapter 13

Following the Transcultural Circulation of Bodily Practices: Modern Yoga and the Corporeality of Mantras

Beatrix Hauser

Contents

1. Introduction 507

2. Models of Dissemination 509

3. Fragments of the Anthropology of Globalisation 513

4. The Contingency of the Body 515

5. Mantras and *Vokalatmung* 518

6. Conclusion 523

References 525

Beatrix Hauser

Chapter 13: Following the Transcultural Circulation of Bodily Practices: Modern Yoga and the Corporeality of Mantras*

1. Introduction

As a social anthropologist my interest in the current popularity of yoga practice around the globe is twofold: (1) Having become part of everyday culture at several places, the yoga boom provides a promising social field to explore how notions of the self and the body, of health, spirituality and wellbeing are negotiated in present-day societies. This requires intimate and detailed "thick" descriptions of what seems normal or natural at a particular research site vis-à-vis its wider social, religious and cultural environment. In this way ethnography may contribute to our understanding in what ways yoga is important for the life of various kinds of people. (2) Furthermore, yoga can be seen as an example of translocal cultural flows within a process commonly labelled as globalisation, shaped by increasing personal mobility, new forms of transnational interdependencies and advances in communication technology. There is indeed a coincidence in time between the accelerated global circulation of ideas, routines and commodities on the one hand and the recent popularity of yoga on the other. Research objectives in this field require data not only from one location and point in time, but a multi-sited and/or an ethnohistorical approach.[1]

In the following I will take up the second interest and focus on some of the premises that come with the conceptualisation of postural yoga as a global practice and on the explanatory force of related models of thinking. No doubt, notions on the global spread and usefulness of yoga have come to dominate popular discourse, replacing previous views on yoga as an exotic and fairly inaccessible skill that required adaption to the abilities and needs of "modern

* I am grateful to the organisers and participants of "Yoga in Transformation: Historical and Contemporary Perspectives on a Global Phenomenon" for their helpful comments and questions on my contribution. In particular, I would like to thank Anne Koch and Karl Baier for their stimulating critique on a draft version of this paper.

1 See Hauser 2013.

Western people"[2]. Today it seems as if yoga exercises are accessible to all kinds of people who will benefit in similar ways. From an anthropological standpoint I have doubts as to what extent yoga is a universal method irrespective of sociocultural context. There certainly are collective patterns of assessing postural yoga and these vary along social lines. Moreover, yoga differs in its experiential possibilities. The range of experiences can't be explained solely by contrasting schools of (Neo) Hatha Yoga, such as Iyengar Yoga versus Kundalini Yoga.[3] My intuition is that the effectiveness of yoga as a bodily practice to increase mental and physical health correlates with a distinct cultural *imaginaire* of the self in the world, the attentiveness to the body and of the conditions for wellbeing. Similar to an anthropology of biomedicine[4] it is now time to adopt a self-reflexive stance and to critically (re-)consider the sociocultural dimension in various settings of teaching, learning and practising yoga. A focus on moral concepts, everyday rituals and modes of representation that come with yoga, for instance, promises insights on changing patterns of self-care or on para-religious concepts of human transformation.

The aim of this chapter is much more modest. It focuses on the epistemic conditions underlying how we approach changes in postural yoga within the globalised world. I wish to evaluate some of the recent studies on the transnational dissemination of yoga practice and explore how the process of diffusion is projected and also the position of a particular type of yoga within the world at large. I am going to address some of the hidden assumptions in these studies from the perspective of the anthropology of globalisation. As will be shown below, one crucial shortcoming of academic studies on the worldwide dissemination of yoga is their tendency to reduce the complex interplay of behaviour, perception and categories of experience, silencing the contingency of the body. When theorizing on global flows, I argue, we need to consider the sentient human body as a source in its own right for re-contextualisation and meaning production rather than solely its symbolic capacity.

The basic intention of sharing these reflections is to substantiate the conceptual and methodological basis of what Elizabeth De Michelis (2004) called Modern Yoga Studies as an interdisciplinary field in the social sciences and the humanities. Furthermore, I wish to contribute to anthropological debates on cultural flows and global circulation by reconnecting insights from the dissemination of yoga to more general ways of conceptualizing traveling bodily prac-

2 A phrase taken from an early popular yoga manual (Zebroff 1971).
3 In this paper, I focus solely on contemporary forms and brands of yoga. I therefore prefer anglicised spellings of Sanskrit words common among yoga providers and practitioners. I would use academic transliterations (with the usual diacritics) only in cases where the continuity with Indian concepts is to be stressed.
4 For an anthropological perspective on biomedicine see Lock & Nguyen 2010.

tices. While the scholarly focus has been on several aspects which shape processes of cultural appropriation – modification, shifting contextualisation, frictions – the body as an instrument and agent of perception, as well as the corporeality of experience and its impact on cultural flows and related dynamics of meaning production have been largely neglected. In the following, I shall combine well-known basic approaches, concepts and analytic strategies from the anthropology of globalisation with those raised in the context of an anthropology of the body, taking modern postural yoga as a prime example. With reference to a case study from Germany on chanting mantras during yoga classes, I will argue for a more nuanced way of analysing the transcultural appropriation of "body techniques" (Mauss), body movement and "somatic modes of attention" (Csordas). In conclusion I will sketch what kinds of concept and research strategies we need to recognise and explore the intrinsic dynamics of traveling body practices, not only with respect to yoga, but regarding the global flow of any cultural practice determined by the experiential possibilities of the human body.

2. Models of Dissemination

First let me look at some of the recent studies about the spread and popularity of modern yoga and distinguish two broad patterns in which the circulation of yoga discourses and practices has been conceptualised. When I speak of models here I do not suggest that the authors mentioned below were subscribing to a deductive method or were following these models as part of their research agenda. I wish neither to simplify nor to belittle their contribution. Rather I believe that certain forms of systematisation and generalisation are necessary, an important step in the hermeneutic process and, like any academic findings, also a reflection of time-specific research paradigms.

There are several publications on the twentieth-century dissemination of postural yoga in a particular national context, such as Germany, the United Kingdom, France and the United States.[5] These studies, written from the scholarly standpoint in the host nation, either implied or explicitly suggested that a hitherto foreign set of ideas and practices was part of a gradual process of cultural absorption. Christian Fuchs' (1990) study on yoga in Germany is a good example. Fuchs, who has a background in Indology and religious studies, distinguishes four major periods of cultural absorption. Against the background of selected pre-war beginnings, he points to the consolidation of widely dispersed individuals interested in yoga after 1945, followed by the gradual institutionalisation of yoga instruction between 1956 and 1966, the organisation of a yoga

5 Fuchs 1990; De Michelis 2004; Newcombe 2008; Ceccomori 2001; Syman 2010.

movement from 1967 onwards, and finally the professionalisation of yoga teaching in the nineteen-eighties.[6] His study terminates in 1989. A similar stepwise development was suggested by De Michelis (2004) in her ground-breaking study on the modern history of yoga in which she argues that modern yoga emerged from a dialogical *exchange* between a modernist Hindu elite and American esotericists in the nineteenth century. Then, with reference to the development of yoga in post-World War II Britain, she stresses a unidirectional development and identifies three distinct periods: the popularisation of yoga in the nineteen-fifties, its consolidation from the mid-nineteen-seventies onwards, and the period of acculturation of yoga since the nineteen-eighties "to date", i. e., prior to the publication of her study in 2004.

Studies along this line, focussing on the rising popularity and cultural assimilation of yoga at a particular nation state, tend to blur the range of foreign, local, and reciprocal influences to only one external source and reference point. The authors follow what I label a "model of linear diffusion", as if the dissemination of yoga in the course of the twentieth century had been primarily bilateral and a one-way transfer from India. As Mark Singleton (2010) in his illuminating study *Yoga Body* has shown, this historical process was much more complex and intertwined. At any rate, regional studies of this kind are of great significance since they highlight the social conditions that invited and accompanied the gradual acceptance of yoga in Europe and North America. Moreover, they often focus on "cultural brokers", i. e., individuals who were familiar with (at least) two cultural worlds and thus able to communicate, transfer, and rationalise yoga in new settings, such as spiritual seekers, dedicated teachers and emigrated gurus.

A focus on the cultural integration of yoga in nations beyond South Asia comes at a price. The notion of acculturation originated in the early twentieth century and proved to be a central concept in the analysis of "culture contact" and its impact on development and social change. First warnings regarding the limits of this concept were already raised in the nineteen-forties.[7] "Acculturation" related to the idea of clearly demarcated separate cultures – organic wholes in the Durkheimian sense – all of them fitting together to form a sort of worldwide mosaic. In historical perspective this way of thinking about culture(s) is linked to the invention of nation states in nineteenth-century Europe.[8] Ac-

6 Fuchs 1990. Bernd Wedemeyer-Kolwe 2004 provided further details on the ways in that yoga already influenced sub-cultures during the Weimar Republic. With regard to my argument the exact beginning of yoga reception in Germany is secondary.

7 In 1940 the Cuban anthropologist Fernando Ortiz proposed to speak of "transculturation" rather than "acculturation" since transformation resulted from the encounter *between* interconnected cultures rather than from the acquisition of or the adjustment to hitherto foreign cultural features (see Hannerz 1997).

8 Barth 1969.

cording to diffusionist and culture area theorists alike each culture had the potential to absorb foreign elements or traits and to integrate them within their own cultural repertoire, which by this process became more advanced and complex. In this line of thinking, "Indian yoga", projected as a consistent system, required "adaption" to the needs of "Western society" and "modern times", to use phrases common in yoga manuals after WWII to the nineteen-seventies.[9] Today this container-model of culture is heavily criticised for its misleading emphasis on stable and homogeneous entities and thus the essentialisation of cultural difference.[10] Although the notion of yoga traveling "from East to the West" is meaningful for yoga practitioners, if we wish to grasp the globalisation of yoga from a scholarly perspective, to conceive of yoga's dissemination process in the twentieth century in terms of a linear diffusion is problematic, and even more so with regard to the twenty-first century. It is not only obsolete since recent studies emphasised multilateral and mutual influences in the emergence of today's yoga (in particular Singleton 2010), but also since scholarly modes of thinking about cultural difference had to change in the view of rapidly expanding global interrelatedness.

Another common way to imagine yoga's worldwide spread resembles a global distribution network of a multinational company with headquarters and branch offices in various countries. For instance, Sarah Strauss (2005) explored how Sivananda Yoga is learned, conceptualised and adopted to personal biographies and living conditions in India, Germany, Switzerland and the United States. Her empirical study focuses on a *transnational community* of people, their yoga practice and discourses as an exemplary yoga culture. Furthermore, Jennifer Lea (2008) and Anne Koch (2013) have considered *temporary yoga collectives* with international participation in deterritorialised spaces, in their case fairly uniform environments of spiritual holiday resorts. In contrast, the geographer Anne-Cécile Hoyez (2005) has developed a multi-layered analysis of how the circulation of yoga influenced the social construction of global space, considering the worldwide distribution of yoga centres, the selective travel routes of yoga gurus and practitioners, the spread of yoga providers in a locality, as well as its impact on urban landscapes. Her study differentiates overlapping networks and discourses - local and transnational - and emphasises *interlinked systems of relations* rather than distinct communities.

The latter type of studies suggests a standardisation of yoga (systems) on a global scale: Sivananda Yoga in Zurich resembling Sivananda Yoga in Rishikesh, Iyengar Yoga in Paris resembling Iyengar Yoga in Melbourne, yoga holidays in Spain resembling yoga holidays in Thailand. This perspective on globalised yoga

9 See the popular yoga manuals by Yesudian & Haich 1953 and Zebroff 1971.
10 See Hannerz 1992; Abu-Lughod 1991.

projects a joint yoga world with various coexisting canonical forms of yoga (schools, styles, systems), which serve as international brand names to advertise specific products to specific types of consumers. Each canonical form comes with its own, partially overlapping view on the meanings of yoga, on yoga practitioners as a human kind, and on yoga's role in contemporary society. This joint yoga world is of course not only an idealised space or an academic construct but corresponds to merging networks of social relations and yoga-related institutions from the nineteen-nineties onwards. Roughly two decades later we have a plurality of yoga cultures, each defined by transregionally distributed and shared discourses rather than ethnic identity, place of birth, place of residence and place of yoga practice. Rootedness in territory is regarded as secondary as long as people share similar intentions and morals associated with a particular type of yoga, and hence go for a "strength and flexibility workout" in Power Yoga or, conversely, follow Swami Ramdev's patriotic yoga teachings on TV.[11] These preferences are shaped by several social factors, such as religious identity, age, attitude towards consumer culture, or active participation in Anglophone discourses.

To sum up, this "model of global distribution" acknowledges several coexisting and partly blurred transnational yoga cultures as part of a joint yoga world. In this world, India is privileged as the historical homeland and the imagined centre, whereas cartographic techniques like those employed by Hoyez reveal that yoga-related communication, contacts, routes and networks culminate in specific hegemonic environments, for instance in North America, whereas most of Africa remains a yogic *terra incognita.*[12] This perspective on globalised yoga thus allows theorizing on patterns of interaction, politics of exclusion, and asymmetries of power. With regard to postural yoga in Germany, and possibly elsewhere, the assumption of distinct canonical forms is to some degree artificial. Lay practitioners are not the only ones to try out various yoga styles. Commonly, yoga teachers have also been influenced by a variety of yoga forms, if not teacher training, and as part of their personal maturation process modify some of the yoga sequences and elements if considered appropriate. Against this background conceiving solely of clearly defined, apprehensible or pure yoga systems is misleading.

Hence, both the model of linear diffusion and the model of global distribution have distinct strengths and weaknesses. They do not represent social reality but highlight only particular aspects. As will be shown in the next section, the an-

11 See Birch 1995 for slogans advertising Power Yoga; on Baba Ramdev and postural yoga in Hindu-national contexts, see Alter 1997 and Sarbacker 2014.

12 For the world-wide distribution of Bikram Yoga and of Iyengar Yoga providers, see Hoyez 2005: 207, 210.

thropological debate on globalisation offers a variety of conceptual access points, categories and approaches, which so far have not been exhausted in theorizing the transcultural dissemination of yoga practice. Moreover, both models of conceptualizing transcultural flows have in common a disregard for the intrinsically social character of the human body.

3. Fragments of the Anthropology of Globalisation

The anthropology of globalisation emerged as a distinct field of investigation around the early nineteen-nineties. One protagonist was Ulf Hannerz (1992), who argued strongly against the notion of the world as a mosaic of independent cultures. Rather, the global system is conceived as one that is stretched out along interlinked and genuinely hybrid cultures, each conceptualised again as networks of perspectives. Due to increased communication in the late twentieth century there would be a continuous flow of cultural meanings, which by this process lose their former territorially bounded character and justifiability. According to Hannerz culture is located similarly "in human minds" and in forms of externalisation. These "overt forms" (displays) and their meanings are negotiated and interpreted on a variety of interconnected scales. Anthropologists need to look at the interfaces, affinities, interpenetrations and flows between clusters of meaning and ways of managing meaning.[13] In this manner Hannerz' concept helps to explain what ethnographies on various aspects of globalisation have shown: in the course of transcultural circulation, the perception, interpretation and contextualisation of objects, technologies and representations can vary significantly. The global distribution of particular items, skills or ideas does not cause cultural homogeneity but invites multiple re-interpretations. As a result, uneven and competing networks of meanings and practices become analytically visible with centres and peripheries in various respects and spaces.

Arjun Appadurai (1996), another key figure in this debate, suggested distinct fields of global circulation. These "scapes" of circulation should be regarded as imaginary constructs rather than as locations for empirical research, i. e., as spaces that are co-produced and negotiated between socially and spatially dispersed groups and individuals within globally defined fields of possibility. These imagined spaces reflect human experience rather than observation. Appadurai distinguishes five types: ethnoscapes, technoscapes, financescapes, mediascapes and ideoscapes.[14] The analytic distinction of these imaginary fields of circulation is intended to recognise the conditions under which global flows occur and

13 Hannerz 1992: 4.
14 Appadurai 1996: 33.

interrelate, thereby mapping heterogeneous, asymmetric and disjunctive processes and configurations, each following its own rules and dynamics (like some of the yoga networks described by Hoyez). If we use these categories in the analysis of postural yoga and its global circulation, these interlinked and disjunctive spheres of meaning production as well as the asymmetries involved become particularly clear. We could employ the category ethnoscape to focus on the imagined transnational community of yoga practitioners (as Strauss has done in her study). The term technoscape would stress essentialised ways of attending to the yogic body (e.g., posture practice) and thus highlight processes in which yoga is distinguished from other kinds of physical movement, mental activity and fields of practice. The category of the financescape might prove as a useful lens for considering flows of money associated with yoga and thus contribute to the understanding of proprietary claims on yoga teaching, yoga-related services and goods, as well as "boundary work" between competing yoga providers on the Indian subcontinent and elsewhere.[15] The perspective of a mediascape would substantiate the power of traveling media representations and their social efficacy, for instance regarding the association of yoga with particular lifestyles. Finally, the routes of circulating ideas and ideologies related to yoga could be captured as ideoscape, thinking, for example, of the trope of a specific yogic attitude towards business. However, the intention is not to objectify each of these categories. Rather, Appadurai suggested a conceptual tool to recognise disjunct sources and contexts of meaning production, as well as hierarchies of social processes in which yoga emerges as a globalised asset. At any rate, the focus on scapes reveals simplified models of yoga's cultural transmission as obsolete. Instead, it highlights the potential multicentricity of flows and counterflows.

The methodological procedure to explore cultural interrelatedness on a global scale was fostered by George E. Marcus (1995) under the heading of "multi-sited ethnography". In contrast to long-term stationary fieldwork, anthropologists are advised to follow different territorial and discursive routes along strategic hints such as "follow the people", "follow the thing", "follow the metaphor", "follow the plot, story or allegory", "follow the life or biography" and "follow the conflict". This opens up a range of methodological possibilities.

On this basis, here compressed to the approaches of Hannerz, Appadurai and Marcus, the anthropological agenda in exploring global interconnectedness provides many access points, avenues and research strategies for Modern Yoga Studies. Some of these ideas already influenced the work by Strauss, Koch and Hoyez while looking at transnational social communities or by considering overlapping imaginary and communicative networks. Their studies are indeed more complex than I could show in the previous section. At any rate, my in-

15 On proprietary claims in the field of yoga see Fish 2006.

tention is shedding light on a significant gap in theorizing global interconnectedness, and this gap is particularly relevant to the understanding of traveling bodily practices. In Hannerz' analytic concept physical movement is representative of something, and this sign quality may travel on a global scale. The meaningfulness of the human body is, whether intended or not, reduced to its semiotic capacity, to a "public meaningful form", which according to Hannerz "can most often be seen or heard, or ... [is] somewhat less frequently known through touch, smell, or taste, if not through some combination of senses"[16]. Although multisensory perception is assumed, meaning is regarded as negotiable only with respect to the body as a representation. Hannerz neither acknowledges the embodied character of culture (in this view located "in human minds") nor the sentient body as a site of perception by itself, and in this respect the body as a socially informed source for creating meaning. Again Appadurai's concept of scapes is totally confined to imaginary constructs and the discursive sphere. Although his approach can inspire several interesting research questions, it also silences the human body as both an instrument and as agent of perception.

What if the translocal circulation of bodily practices varies in its possibilities and dynamics of being appropriated, contextualised and modified from other cultural products that disseminate across national boundaries? Although there certainly are studies on systems of bodily movement and their global spread (e.g., dance), to my knowledge there has been no attempt so far in theorizing on corporeality in its impact on cultural flows and related conditions of meaning production.[17] Traveling bodily practices – forms of physical activity, clothing, body decoration, nutrition or personal hygiene – are seen primarily as modes of symbolisation rather than as experiential sites by themselves, producing distinct realities, feelings and judgements. Looking at the long-distance transmission of corporeal practices as if they were objects or mechanical procedures is problematic, last but not least if we consider insights from the anthropology of the body.

4. The Contingency of the Body

There is no natural way in which human beings relate to their body. Already Marcel Mauss (2005) in his seminal essay on "techniques of the body" drew our attention to the fact that any physical action or mode of behaviour, its transmission, classification and psychosocial assessment is culturally patterned, in-

16 Hannerz 1992: 3–4.
17 On embodiment as a paradigm for anthropology see Csordas 1990.

cluding forms of walking, sitting and sleeping.[18] In this line Mary Douglas (1973) emphasised the mutual interdependency of the "physical body" and the "social body", i.e., of body perception on the one hand and of socially communicated ways of body experience on the other. Social categories modify and restrain how the body as a physical entity is rationalised, perceived and experienced. The somatic experience again reinforces these categories.[19] Following the phenomenological approach of Thomas Csordas (1990), the human body cannot be reduced to an object or an instrument of perception but has to be regarded as an integral part of the experiencing subject and as such is the base not only of specific physical techniques but of culture in general.[20]

These insights need to have consequences for the ways in which we project the long-distance transmission of bodily practices. The ethnography of performance and the history of sport have indeed confirmed an extraordinary variability in which systems of bodily movement blur regional and above all classificatory boundaries. Whether a particular series of human postures is regarded as religious expression, as gymnastic exercise, as physical therapy, as a type of dance, as art, game or as political statement depends on the sociocultural context. There are well-known case studies to illustrate this, e.g., the transformation of a competitive game like cricket into a ritual dance on the Trobriand Islands (PNG), the public display of qigong exercises as part of Falon Gong political activism, the spirit possession by Korean shamans at international theatre festivals, or the extreme sport bungee jumping originating from a Melanesian initiation rite.[21] Seen from this angle bodily experience is highly contingent. Bodily practices from afar can be copied in mimetic and kinetic respects, yet they are likely to raise experiences configured by the time and environment of the current practitioner rather than any intrinsic meaning. Returning to yoga it is thus unclear to what extent its performance will evoke similar (if not universal) somatic reactions and interpretations. This is not passing judgement on its health benefits. No doubt, stretching and the repeated tension of particular muscles have their own training effects on the body. However, particular ways of sitting and breathing, folding hands and bowing down, educating the body as such, or the performance of acrobatic poses may have their own significance and connotations. Moreover, Indian yoga discourses relate to specific notions of a "subtle body".[22]

---

18 Mauss 2005, first published in 1934.

19 Douglas 1973: 69.

20 Csordas 1990: 36.

21 On Trobriand cricket see Taussig 1993: 243–246; on qigong performances by the Falun Gong see Bell (2004); and on the genre crossing of Korean shamans see Kendall (2009). Following Lipp (2008), bungee jumping originated in male tests of courage rather than in an initiation proper.

22 On South Asian ideas and practices involving "subtle bodies" see Samuel & Johnston (2013).

Let us look at one case study from today's yoga world. When German friends plan to take a course in (Neo) Hatha Yoga, they also consider whether the instruction will include the chanting of mantras.[23] In a city like Hamburg – with 1.7 million inhabitants the second-largest city in Germany – this practice can range from the simple humming of Om (Aum), the utterance of abstract syllables (e. g., Soham) to complex verses with hymn-like character (e. g., Ad Gure Nameh, Jugad Gure Nameh, Sat Gure Nameh, Siri Guru Dev-e Nameh).[24] People who feel reminded of liturgy commonly avoid yoga tuition with mantras; others appreciate them as an access point to Hindu spirituality.[25] A third group joins the chanting as a part of their "mind–body practice" (*ganzheitliche Körperarbeit*), and in this framework cultivate attentiveness towards various sensorial spaces within their body that resonate to these phonetic impulses. They regard the somatic sensation of chanting mantras as a pleasant effect, rationalizing the force of collective vibration as an effect of group energy (*Gruppenenergie*). In courses classified by providers and practitioners as Hatha Yoga, teachers explain the usage of mantras with reference to "tradition" and sound as a "type of energy".[26]

What surprises at first sight is the openness of the third group to chanting mantras. Following Pierre Bourdieu (1977) I assume that this willingness is related to a socially acquired sense, which helps to assess whether the uttering of syllables might fit in with an exercise system to improve health and wellbeing. This openness towards mantra chanting is grounded in the body, although it is not a subjective feeling. In Bourdieu's terms it resonates to a

23 There is extensive literature on the significance of mantras in ancient India, in Hindu, Jain and in Buddhist contexts (for an introductory essay see Padoux 2003). Literally, the Sanskrit term *mantra* refers to sounds, syllables, words and verses believed to have sacred and magical powers. They are to be repeated either vocally or in silence. While some mantras convey abstract meanings, others have a distinct theistic reference. The recitation of a series of mantras can constitute a hymn (*japa*). Both mantras and *japa-s* are preferably heard rather than read, still they are distinguished from the category of sacred sound (*nada*) as such. Since I focus on mantras in German contexts, I render the respective formulas in the spelling suggested by German-speaking yoga teachers and found in popular digests. I therefore ignore the diacritics employed in the academic transliteration of Sanskrit.

24 The largest yoga provider in Germany, Yoga Vidya (influenced by Sivananda Yoga), promotes meditating on "Soham". The quoted hymn is chanted in Kundalini Yoga classes offered by the 3HO, an international registered society with a strong affiliation to the Neo Sikh guru Yogi Bhajan (1929–2004). In 2001 the 3HO held the monopoly for teaching prenatal yoga in Hamburg.

25 On the usage of mantras among Sufis and Sikhs in the United States see Coward & Goa 2004: 68–82.

26 In 2007 I began frequenting a Hamburg yoga studio on a regular basis, looking back at earlier experiences with yoga in Germany (2001) and India (1985). Since 2009 I have repeatedly turned into an ethnographer of the German yoga scene, primarily by means of participant observation. Doing fieldwork at home, however, has its own dynamics: "headnotes" (Ottenberg) generally outnumber fieldnotes, memories of narrative interviews predominate recorded conversations.

> "[...] system of inseparably cognitive and evaluative structures which organizes the vision of the world in accordance with the objective structures of a determinate state of the social world: this principle is nothing other than the *socially informed body*, with its tastes and distastes, its compulsions and repulsions, with, in a word, all its *senses*, that is to say, not only the traditional five senses–which never escape the structuring action of social determinisms – but also the sense of necessity and the sense of duty, the sense of direction and the sense of reality, the sense of balance and the sense of beauty, common sense and the sense of the sacred, tactical sense and the sense of responsibility, business sense and the sense of propriety, the sense of humor and the sense of absurdity, moral sense and the sense of practicality, and so on."[27]

The notion of sense refers to a system of enduring dispositions (habitus), constituting the collective and unconscious principle for the generation and structuring of practices and representations. In this way yoga practitioners can "sense" a form of meaning and a benefit that resonates within their familiar cultural categories and structures.

The following section will show that the sonic-somatic sensation of chanting mantras is in principle in line with a variety of therapeutic forms that were developed in German speaking countries at the nexus of voice training, breath therapy and autosuggestive techniques, popular in the search for stage proficiency, personality development, occultist powers and holistic health.[28] The technical term for this body technique is not "to sing" but *tönen*, i. e., to modulate sounds during exhalation in order to evoke vibrations in various parts of the body. Only recently the English verb "to chant" is more common. In the nineteen-fifties the overall concept became known as *Vokalatmung*, literally: vowel or rather vocal breathing – the German term *Vokal* refers to both a vowel and the respective vocal sound.

5. Mantras and *Vokalatmung*

In the course of the twentieth century, Germans could follow several training systems based on the assumption that the uttering of sounds involved an energetic, if not healing dimension. Without doubt, vague visions of Indian yoga had been influential even in early German-speaking therapeutic circles and often contributed to the development of hybrid systems. Let me introduce a few exemplary systems of *Vokalatmung* in the chronological order in which they were developed:[29]

27 Bourdieu 1977: 124, emphasis in the original.

28 On the impact of autosuggestive techniques, Couéism and positive thinking see Wedemeyer-Kolwe 2004: 150–151, 171.

29 This list is not exhaustive. Moreover, even before the turn of the twentieth century voice

- In the 1910s Benno Max Leser-Lasario[30], a respiratory therapist and opera singer in Vienna, suggested a self-controlled form of exhalation as a prophylactic technique to improve breathing, voice and tone. While exhaling the patient had to perform lip "gestures" (*Gebärden*) miming one vowel at a time (u, o, a, e, i), consequently this method was called *Vokalgebärden-Atmung*. According to Leser-Lasario it caused subtle vibrations ("electromagnetic waves") that improved blood circulation, massaged glands as well as inner organs.[31]
- The singer Clara Schlaffhorst (1863–1945) and the musician Hedwig Andersen (1866–1957) integrated Leser-Lasario's *Vokalgebärden* into their own holistic system of breath gymnastics and education. They developed a method that consisted of circling, swinging, rhythmic movement, breathing and *tönen* with the aim to train posture-breath coordination. In 1916 they founded a training institute where they taught this method of *Tonschwingübungen* (sound-swing-exercises) for improving speech, voice, artistic performance and physical regeneration until the 1940s.[32]
- In 1928 the esotericist and theosophist Peryt Shou[33] (1873–1953) went on a lecture tour in Germany and Austria, teaching *Praktische Mantramistik* (practical mantracism), an occult practice to evoke the hidden powers of *Vokalatem* (vocal breath). It consisted of chanting combinations of particular syllables, for instance "Om", "A-him-sa", but also "Je-ho-va", "E-lo-him", "Chr-is-tos" etc.[34] According to Shou, these mantras were an essential part of yoga, here understood as a system of controlled breathing that was accompanied by visualisation techniques (no posture practice).[35] Following Shou, mantras released tension and cramps. Moreover, "mantracistic prayers" called upon "divine magic" and were appreciated as means to develop supernatural powers, mind control and telepathy.[36]
- In 1952 Shrimant Balasahib Pandit Pratinidhi's (1868–1951) book *The Ten-Point Way to Health* came out in German translation.[37] Here mantras are

exercises were known in Europe and North America, often in combination with breathing gymnastics (*Atemgymnastik*), see Wedemeyer-Kolwe 2004: 145.

30 Year of birth and death unknown.

31 Leser-Lasario 1954: 16. Following Leser-Lasario, his therapeutic system originated in Egypt.

32 Schlaffhorst & Andersen 1928; see Lang & Saatweber 2011: 155–166, 361–396.

33 Peryt Shou is a synonym of Albert Christian Georg Schultz.

34 Shou 2008a: 6, 15–16, 19–22, 26, 38; 2008b.

35 Shou 2008a: 29.

36 Shou 2008a: 50–51; Shou 2008b; see Wedemeyer-Kolwe 2004: 142, 145.

37 The first English edition was published 1928 in India, followed by an edition in the United Kingdom in 1938 and translations in several languages. To my knowledge, further German editions were published in 1955, 1957, 1964, 1967, 1972, 1974, 1977, 1985, 1988, 1994 and 1995 (marked as the eighteenth edition).

promoted for their health-related effects, if practised jointly with a series of body movements known as the sun salutation (presented as a secular type of drill exercise).[38] Pratinidhi proposes the chanting of specific kinds of mantra such as "hram", "hrim", "hrum", "hraim", "hraum" and "hrah" as preventive and curative practice.[39] For instance, the uttering of "hram" would help purifying the blood, strengthening the rib cage and the respiratory tract, support the alimentary canal and heal asthma as well as bronchitis. "Hrim" is recommended to stimulate the oral and nasal area, the upper part of the heart and to cleanse the respiratory and digestive system from phlegm secretions. "Hrum" helped strengthening the liver, spleen, stomach and intestines, "hraim" would normalise rectal function and "hrah" improve throat and chest.[40] The book was a tremendous success with regular new editions appearing until 1995. Moreover, Pratinidhi's section "Health Through Speech" was copied verbatim in the revised edition of *Hatha Yoga,* originally by Max Wilke and extended by Krishna S. Kadam in 1953.[41] Whereas Wilke still conceived of yoga as an occult system of breathing techniques to create willpower, Kadam also added a few passages on the sun salutation.

- In the same year, Felix Riemkasten (1894–1969), a German writer, theosophist and self-made yoga-teacher in the post-World War II period, published a Hatha Yoga manual of its own – in accordance with the changing view on yoga, including a chapter on posture practice (*āsana*). It also teaches *Vokal-Gebärden-Atmung* (referencing "Lesser-Lasario" [sic]) and specific clues as to the medical use of each vowel.[42] The breathing sound of "i" prevented headache, "e" stimulated the thyroid and improved a sore throat, "a" strengthened and ventilated the lungs, "o" stimulated the heart, "ö" influenced the dia-

38 The sun salutation is a rather new addition to yoga (Singleton 2010: 124). At the Mysore court, which in the 1930s promoted Sri T. Krishnamacharya and his revival of posture practice, the sun salutation was still regarded as a separate exercise system and distinguished from (Neo) Hatha Yoga. However, Pratinidhi (the "Rajah of Aundh") was an enthusiastic physical culturist. In his youth he learned Indian martial arts and wrestling, later bodybuilding as fashioned by the then world-famous German Eugen Sandow (Singleton 2010: 124).

39 Pratinidhi 1952: 60–65.

40 It is not known from where Pratinidhi learned this particular set of mantras and their claimed benefits. At any rate, in the Tantric tradition mantras are employed to perform *nyāsa*, a preliminary rite for worship to sanctify the body. Following the Mahānirvānatantra, an 18th-century *śākta* text, the utterance of *hrāṃ, hrīṃ, hrūṃ, hraiṃ, hrauṃ, hraḥ* is required for consecrating various body parts as implicitly identical to those of the supreme goddess (Wheelock 1989: 104). On Tantric notions of the imaginary body in the Indic Haṭha Yoga tradition see Padoux 2011: 103–110. In short, these mantras were not proposed to attain health; the reference point was the cosmic, not the human body.

41 Wilke 1953: 39–44. At first glance the book appears like a new edition of Wilke's publication in 1919. However, the section on healing mantras was apparently added by Krishna S. Kadam, who in his introduction acknowledged Pratinidhi's work.

42 Riemkasten 1966: 81–98.

phragm, heart, liver and stomach, "u" acted on the lower abdomen, and "ü" improved the kidneys. Furthermore Riemkasten developed phonetic exercises such as "a ha ha ha ha", "aaaa-eee-i-hiii" or "spla, sple, spli, splo, splu, splahi, sprohi, splahu".[43] These combined sounds and syllables were not regarded as mantras but derived, according to Riemkasten, from the "mental dimension of breath".[44] Riemkasten suggests doing these vocal exercises together with affirmations, visualisation and relaxation techniques (loosening-up exercises, swinging, singing). In his view, the "wavelength" of each sound evoked a specific organic effect, originating from a respiratory centre located in the back of the human skull.[45] In a brief excursus on "Mantram" at the end of his book, Riemkasten also discusses "Om" and abstract mantras such as "Om hram", "Om hrihm", "Om hruhm", "Om hrahim", "Om hramhum" and "Om hraaaahhh".[46] Chanting these, Riemkasten claims, increased blood circulation and resulted in an "inner vibration massage". Still these mantras were not associated with any specific curative function but recommended as a support of any recovery and, above all, as a way to cope with mental suffering and to achieve mental peace.[47] For the same purpose, Riemkasten suggests the recitation of the (Buddhist) mantra "Om mani padme hum".

- During the 1950s Ilse Middendorf (1910–2009) developed the concept for *Der erfahrbare Atem* (1984, lit. the perceptable breath), a training system to cultivate breath and body awareness, taught at her Berlin institute from 1965 onwards. Being a gymnastics teacher, Middendorf had studied the Schlaffhorst-Andersen method and in the 1930s also breathing techniques associated with yoga.[48] From this she developed her own respiratory therapy in which she taught breathing as a holistic embodied experience.[49] Its goal is to sense subtle inner movements that occur with breath as it is allowed to come and go. Middendorf thus underlines breathing as a sensuous experience of its own as opposed to either unconscious or deliberate respiration. According to Middendorf, the silent contemplation on a vowel provided the means to evoke

43 Exercises like "a ha ha ha ha" (1966: 85) allude to what at the end of the twentieth century became known as laughter yoga, promoted by the Indian medical practitioner Madan Kataria (2002).

44 Riemkasten 1966: 58.

45 Riemkasten 1966: 81.

46 Riemkasten 1966: 211–218, see p. 216 in particular.

47 Riemkasten 1966: 217.

48 Wedemeyer-Kolwe 2004: 92, 150. Middendorf's teacher, Emil Bäuerle (Aurelius) was clearly associated with the Mazdaznan movement, which combined elements from breath gymnastics, *Lebensreform* (life reform), notions of purity, posture practice, vocal exercises and autosuggestion before it was prohibited in 1935, and finally in 1941 (on the Mazdaznan movement see Wedemeyer-Kolwe 2004: 153–174 and pp. 159, 161 for Middendorf).

49 Middendorf 1984.

> vibrations and thus to locate the respective inner *Vokalraum* (vowel space), before it also created an outer sonic space (*Tonatemraum*). Middendorf distinguishes "u-", "e-", "i-", "o-", "a-", "ä-", "ö-" and "ü-space" from bodily sensations caused by combined vowels, consonants and syllables.[50] These acoustic sound waves helped to create awareness of inner vowel space. As opposed to Leser-Lasario, Middendorf stresses the flow of breath and its harmonizing effects rather than its impact on organs. From the 1990s onwards Middendorf 's breathwork became a modern classic for any type of voice and respiratory training.

This is not the occasion to contextualise each approach, to assess similarities and differences, highlight pathways and misunderstandings, or to discuss the health benefits of the proposed exercises. Rather, I want to show that in the course of the twentieth century several, partly overlapping therapeutic systems circulated in German-speaking areas alone, each suggesting that the uttering of sounds and syllables is in some way beneficial for physical and mental health. Keeping in mind that in German language the terms "voice" (*Stimme*), "tune" (*stimmen*) and "mood" (*Stimmung*) are linked phonetically and semantically, these repeated attempts to popularise mantras and voice training as a healing method does not come as a surprise.[51] Moreover, whereas some training systems employ the term "mantra" to specify these vocal exercises, others refer to *Vokalatmung*, possibly to differentiate it from explicitly Hindu and occult practices. This nexus of voice training, mantra chanting and yoga continues to the present with only varied terminology. On the one hand, self-help manuals on breath gymnastics emphasise various forms of sound generation, of *tönen* and of *Phonationsatmung* (phonetic breathing) and, in very unobtrusive ways, also hint at or even include Hatha Yoga postures.[52] On the other hand, recent yoga manuals intended for health protection again emphasise the chanting of mantras. Whereas "breathwork" has risen to an acknowledged alternative therapy, the notion of "mantra" expanded to include a wide range of formulas, positive assertions and guiding principles. A good example is the popular *Mantra Box* (2013), which includes a booklet, a CD and fifty cards with "healing mantras for body, mind and soul", each giving directions for application, affirmation and intonation.[53]

---

50 Middendorf 1984: 61–77.

51 It is beyond the scope of this chapter to consider similar terms and ideas in other languages (e.g., the semantic field of "to tune"). Since Germans are not the only ones to have their own soundscape and pronunciation, any crosslingual transfer of voice exercises is likely to create interferences.

52 See, exemplarily, Edel & Knauth 1993 and Höfler 1991.

53 Freund & Trökes 2013.

To come back to the aim of my paper: yoga practitioners (like all human beings) assess any of their somatic sensations in relation to previous experiences and sociocultural categories, which shape an experiential repertoire and limit its possibilities, i. e., whether a particular series of physical movements, sounds or vibrations is considered awkward, gentle, exhausting, artistic, obscene, healthy and so on. In principle, this applies not only to posture practice in a strict sense, but to any form of learned controlled movement, ranging from the alignment of eyes (gaze) or the use of voice, to eating habits and forms of personal hygiene experienced through and by the means of the body. It is the social categories that modify and restrain somatic experience. With respect to Hatha Yoga practitioners in Germany, and in particular the third group of people who have integrated chanting mantras into a healthy mind-body practice, I contend that the various forms of vocal breathing in the twentieth century have paved the ground for what Bourdieu termed "a system of enduring dispositions". They shaped collective (cultural) categories of perception, classification and experience, which allowed the integration of "energetic vibrations" as causal effect of uttering mantras and postural yoga within the larger framework of health care. Whether chanting mantras is culturally approved of at a specific yoga site is therefore not a matter of successful translation – a cognitive process explaining its meaningfulness – but of somatic assessment: it needs to feel right. In this case study, the idea of chanting mantras for mental and physical benefit has seemingly superseded previous concepts of vocal therapy. The role of mantras in modern postural yoga and the various personal approaches to chanting mantras, here shown with regard to a German metropolis, illustrate the relevance and power of somatic assessment for the transcultural circulation of Hatha Yoga and related practices. Chanting mantras in a German yoga course for pregnant women substantially differs from the experiential scope of someone who grew up in a pious Hindu (or Sikh) family. This might go without saying, yet with regard to academic debates on global flows and interconnectedness, the human body and somatic processes as device in meaning production is heavily under-theorised.

6. Conclusion

Let me return to my central argument: In this chapter, I have looked at some of the premises that come with the conceptualisation of yoga as a global practice and I have examined the explanatory force of related models of thinking. What kind of epistemic tools (metaphors, concepts, perspectives) might help to understand and explain the complexity and variability of yoga as a social phenomenon common and still disseminating further in various parts of our interconnected world? No doubt, the anthropology of globalisation has a lot to offer to Modern Yoga Studies and to research on current transformations in yoga at various cultural sites. Above all, it clearly shows that we cannot reduce transnational flows of and in yoga to unilinear diffusion or to multinational brand(s) disseminating from only one centre. Whenever we speak or write about cultural flows in the yoga world we also need to question our own (hidden) assumptions on the ways we imagine global interconnectedness. Moreover, attention should be given to the plurality of perspectives, the partiality of flows as well as the organisation of diversity, not as an exception, but as the normal state and ground of experience.

In the second part of the chapter, I turned to the specific perceptual conditions that accompany the cultural appropriation of bodily practices as a specific type of cultural form, possibly following other options, rules and dynamics of being appropriated than objects, images, ideas or technologies that circulate and constitute globalisation. Does the long-distance transmission of bodily practices differ, and if so how? On the one hand, any transcultural invention is accessed with and through the body, i. e., it involves various senses and habitual cultural patterns (e. g., using a mobile phone). Already Hannerz acknowledged this, although he emphasised the cognitive dimension and conceived of traveling items as "public meaningful forms".[54] On the other hand, the embodied character of culture is clearly missing in both Hannerz' and Appadurai's approach to grasp the dynamics that define globalisation. Situated meaning production as a non-individual and non-intended social process is shaped not only in terms of representation and discourse. The informed body (in Bourdieu's sense) is crucial to approve the validity and hierarchy of possible meanings. Therefore it can be both a significant obstacle to innovation and also the most powerful agent "to sense" new meanings altogether.

In order to analyse the transcultural dissemination of postural yoga this is crucial. The discussion of mantra chanting within the realm of yoga in twentieth-century Germany has shown repeated attempts in establishing vocal exercises as a type of holistic therapy. The pathways and motion logics were, however, shaped by discontinuities rather than a gradual "cultural absorption". A selected blend of familiar approaches to healing (e. g., breathing gymnastics) met with vague and in post-war German usage fairly undefined terminology ("mantras", "yoga"), combined and promoted by innovative teaching personalities, free of any commitment to specific yoga lineages. After the rising popularity of postural yoga seemingly superseded *Vokalatmung*, the recognition of holistic breath work again allowed the re-integration of vocal exercises and confirmed yoga as health protection. Acknowledging the body as an own source of meaning production, the case study has pointed to today's ambiguity of mantra chanting as both a

54 Hannerz 1992: 3–4.

spiritual and secular method that evokes immediate wellbeing, thereby suggesting some therapeutic efficacy in line with discourses on alternative medicine. Moreover, this openness to chanting mantras in yoga classes also reflects a widened understanding of health and self-care, last but not least coined by self-optimisation.

What would we gain by considering the corporeality of experience in the study of transcultural circulation? At first, it would complicate the recognition of cultural flows and raise methodological questions: How to explore somatic experience, and if so, how to convey these insights in academic writing? The exploration of the sentient body is in many respects still a challenge for social scientists.[55] Nevertheless, returning to Marcus' directives for a multi-sited ethnography, I propose to add programmatically the demand: "Follow the body!" Body experience should not be taken for granted but needs to be explored empirically, to begin with by means of interviews and contextualisation. Furthermore, this research strategy requires a comparative and self-reflexive analysis of the practitioner-anthropologist and her or his embodied experience, informed by "methodological atheism" (Peter Berger) rather than belief in a universally shared sensorium. Although bodily skills and modalities are commonly objectified (e.g., as sport or as religious act) and hence may function as signs, they neither consist of prediscursive "natural" components nor constitute technologies in a mechanistic sense. When systems of bodily movement travel across large distances, the process of meaning production is not only shaped by new environmental factors (such as patterns of demands, institutional structures, discourses) but also by embodied dispositions. Social conventions of attending to the human body will influence in what ways bodily practices can provoke or integrate. After all, Indian cleansing techniques associated with yoga – nasal irrigation (*jal netī*), self-induced vomiting of water (*vāman dhauti*), or strong purgative techniques (*virecan*) – (still) resist migration to larger audiences.

References

Abu-Lughod, L. (1991). Writing Against Culture. In R. G. Fox (Ed.), *Recapturing Anthropology: Working in the Present* (pp. 137–162). Santa Fe: School of American Research Press.

Alter, J. (1997). A Therapy to Live by: Public Health, the Self, and Nationalism in the Practice of a North Indian Yoga Society. *Medical Anthropology, 17,* 309–335.

55 On socio-cultural explorations of the human body see, for instance, Mascia-Lees 2011.

Appadurai, A. (1996). *Modernity at Large: Cultural Dimensions of Globalization.* Minneapolis: University of Minnesota Press.

Barth, F. (Ed.). (1969). *Ethnic Groups and Boundaries: The Social Organization of Culture Difference.* London: Allen & Unwin.

Bell, C. (2004). Körperliche Übung, Ritual und politische Abweichung: Die Falun Gong. In Ch. Wulf & J. Zirfa (Eds.), *Die Kultur des Rituals: Inszenierungen. Praktiken. Symbole* (pp. 237–246). München: Wilhelm Fink Verlag.

Birch, B. B. (1995). *Power Yoga: The Total Strength and Flexibility Workout.* Photographs by Nicholas DeSciose. New York: Simon & Schuster.

Bourdieu, P. (1977). *Outline of a Theory of Practice*, trans. R. Nice. Cambridge Studies in Social Anthropology 16. Cambridge: Cambridge University Press (French original: P. Bourdieu, *Esquisse d'une théorie de la pratique: précédé de trois études d'ethnologie kabyle.* Travaux de droit, d'économie, de sociologie et de sciences politiques 92. Genève: Droz, 1972).

Ceccomori, S. (2001). *Cent ans des yoga en France.* Collection Orient et Occident 1. Paris: Edidit.

Coward, H. G. & Goa, D. J. (2004). *Mantra: Hearing the Divine in India and in America.* New York: Columbia University Press.

Csordas, Th. J. (1990). Embodiment as a Paradigm for Anthropology. *Ethos, 18,* 5–47.

De Michelis, E. (2004). *A History of Modern Yoga: Patañjali and Western Esotericism.* London: Continuum.

Douglas, M. (1973). *Natural Symbols: Explorations in Cosmology.* London: Barrie & Jenkins.

Edel, H. & Knauth, K. (1993). *Atemtherapie.* Berlin: Ullstein.

Fish, A. (2006). The Commodification and Exchange of Knowledge in the Case of Transnational Commercial Yoga. *International Journal of Cultural Property, 13,* 189–206. DOI: 10.1017/S0940739106060127.

Freund, L. & Trökes, A. (2013). *Die Mantra-Box. 50 heilende Mantras für Körper, Geist und Seele.* München: Gräfe & Unzer.

Fuchs, Ch. (1990). *Yoga in Deutschland: Rezeption – Organisation – Typologie.* Stuttgart: Kohlhammer Verlag.

Hannerz, U. (1992). *Cultural Complexity: Studies in the Social Organization of Meaning.* New York: Columbia University Press.

Hannerz, U. (1997). Flows, Boundaries and Hybrids: Keywords in Transnational Anthropology. WPTC-2K-02. Stockholm. Department of Social Anthropology, Stockholm University.

Hauser, B. (2013). Introduction: Transcultural Yoga(s): Analyzing a Traveling Subject. In B. Hauser (Ed.), *Yoga Traveling: Bodily Practice in Transcultural Perspective* (pp. 1–34). Heidelberg: Springer.

Höfler, H. (1991). *Atemtherapie und Atemgymnastik: Durch richtiges und bewusstes Atmen zu mehr Harmonie und Energie im Leben.* Stuttgart: Trias-Thieme.

Hoyez, A.-C. (2005). *L'espace-monde du yoga: Une géographie sociale et culturelle de la mondialisation des payasages thérapeutiques.* Unpublished PhD Thesis. University of Rouen.

Kataria, M. (2002). *Lachen ohne Grund: eine Erfahrung, die Ihr Leben verändern wird*, trans. U. Kraemer. Petersberg: Via Nova (English original: *Laugh for no Reason*. Mumbai: Madhuri International, 1999).

Kendall, L. (2009). *Shamans, Nostalgias, and the IMF: South Korean Popular Religion in Motion*. Honolulu: University of Hawai'i Press.

Koch, A. (2013). Yoga as a Production Site of Social and Human Capital: Transcultural Flows from a Cultural Economic Perspective. In: B. Hauser (Ed.), *Yoga Traveling: Bodily Practice in Transcultural Perspective* (pp. 225–248). Heidelberg: Springer.

Lang, A. & Saatweber, M. (2011). *Stimme und Atmung: Kernbegriffe und Methoden des Konzeptes Schlaffhorst-Andersen und ihre anatomisch-physiologische Erklärung*. Idstein: Schulz-Kircher.

Lea, J. (2008). Retreating to Nature: Rethinking "Therapeutic Landscapes". *Area, 40*(1), 90–98. DOI: 10.1111/j.1475-4762.2008.00789.c.

Leser-Lasario, B. M. (1954). *Lehrbuch der Original-Vokalgebärden-Atmung*. 2. Auflage. Büdingen: Lebensweiser.

Lipp, Th. (2008). *Das Turmspringen der Sa in Vanuatu: Ritual, Spiel oder Spektakel?* Münster: Lit.

Lock, M. & Nguyen, V.-K. (Eds.). (2010). *An Anthropology of Biomedicine*. Chichester: Wiley-Blackwell.

Marcus, G. E. (1995). Ethnography in/of the World System: The Emergence of Multi-Sited Ethnography. *Annual Review of Anthropology, 24,* 95–117.

Mascia-Lees, F. E. (Ed.). (2011). *A Companion to the Anthropology of the Body and Embodiment*. Chichester, West Sussex: Wiley-Blackwell.

Mauss, M. (2005). Techniques of the Body. In M. Fraser & M. Greco (Eds.), *The Body: A Reader* (pp. 73–77). London: Routledge.

Middendorf, I. (1984). *Der erfahrbare Atem: Eine Atemlehre*. Paderborn: Junfermann.

Newcombe, S. (2008). *A Social History of Yoga and Ayurveda in Britain, 1950–1995*. Unpublished PhD Thesis. University of Cambridge.

Padoux, A. (2003). Mantra. In G. Flood (Ed.), *The Blackwell Companion to Hinduism* (pp. 478–492). Oxford: Blackwell.

Padoux, A. (2011). *Tantric Mantras: Studies on mantrasastra*. Routledge Studies in Tantric Traditions. London: Routledge.

Pratinidhi, Sh. B. P., Rajah von Aundh (1952). *Das Sonnengebet: Yoga-Übungen für jedermann*. Stuttgart: Günther.

Riemkasten, F. (1966). *Yoga für Sie: Lehrbuch zur praktischen Ausübung des Hatha Yoga*. Fünfte verbesserte Auflage. Gelnhausen: Schwab.

Samuel, G. & Johnston, J. (Eds.). (2013). *Religion and the Subtle Body in Asia and the West: Between Mind and Body*. London: Routledge.

Sarbacker, St. R. (2014). Swami Ramdev: Modern Yoga Revolutionary. In M. Singleton & E. Goldberg (Eds.), *Gurus of Modern Yoga*. (pp. 351–571). New York: Oxford University Press.

Schlaffhorst, C. & Andersen, H. (1928). *Atmung und Stimme*. Wolfenbüttel: Möseler Verlag.

Shou, P. (2008a). *Praktische Mantramistik: Das Mantram und die Vokal-Atmung. Wesen und Praxis der Konzentration und der Meditation*. Graz: Edition Geheimes Wissen.

Shou, P. (2008b). *Praktischer Mantram-Kursus*. Graz: Edition Geheimes Wissen.

Singleton, M. (2010). *Yoga Body: The Origins of Modern Posture Practice.* Oxford: Oxford University Press.

Strauss, S. (2005). *Positioning Yoga: Balancing Acts Across Cultures.* Oxford: Berg Publishers.

Syman, St. (2010). *The Subtle Body: The Story of Yoga in America.* New York: Farrer, Straus and Giroux.

Taussig, M. (1993). *Mimesis and Alterity: A Particular History of the Senses.* New York: Routledge.

Wedemeyer-Kolwe, B. (2004). "*Der neue Mensch*": *Körperkultur im Kaiserreich und in der Weimarer Republik.* Würzburg: Königshausen & Neumann.

Wheelock, W. T. (1989). The Mantra in Vedic and Tantric Ritual. In H. P. Alper (Ed.), *Mantra* (pp. 96–122). Albany, NY: State University of New York Press.

Wilke, M. (1953). *Hatha Yoga: Die Lebenslehre der Inder.* Neu bearbeitet von K. S. Kadam. Lindau i. B.: Rudolph.

Yesudian, S. & Haich, E. (1953). *Yoga and Health,* trans. J. P. Robertson. London: Allen & Unwin.

Zebroff, K. (1971). *The ABC of Yoga.* New York: Arco Publications.

Chapter 14

Living4giving: Politics of Affect and Emotional Regimes in Global Yoga

Anne Koch

Contents

1. Introduction 531

2. Framing Conditions: Eventisation, Charitisation, Mediatisation 533

3. The Particular Configuration of "Global Yoga" 535

4. The Emotional Complex of Yoga Aid 538
- 4.1. Theoretical Considerations 538
- 4.2. The Obligation to Give Back in a Moral Global Economy 539
  - 4.2.1. Owing – Being Indebted 541
  - 4.2.2. The Feeling of Meaningfulness: Living4giving 542
  - 4.2.3. Gratitude 542
  - 4.2.4. Competing 543
  - 4.2.5. Connectedness 544
  - 4.2.6. Self-Empowerment 544

5. Conclusion: The Cosmopolitan Mood of Living4giving 545

References 547

Anne Koch

Chapter 14: Living4giving: Politics of Affect and Emotional Regimes in Global Yoga

1. Introduction

Yoga is of great significance to the life of many practitioners I met during my fieldwork in Tokyo, Fukui, Miami, Munich, and Koh Samui. Why is this so? Where do the strong emotional ties in yoga practice originate from? It would be of great interest to better understand yoga in the context of late modern spirituality. This is especially important where it seems to differ strikingly from the mainstream, for example in hedonism, competition and profit-increase (even if only for charitable donations), or when altruism supersedes self-realisation, as in the following field study.

Searching for theories of emotion, one quickly makes a find, especially in the most recent history of emotions.[1] But when looking for literature on specific emotions in late modern spirituality, information is sparse. Certainly, there are many characterisations of alternative spirituality from sociology of religion, such as holistic, mainly private, individualised, consumerist, meeting a large variety of different needs, self-empowering, interested in alternative healing, a niche for elderly women, etc.[2] But they seldom offer insights into the interwoven play of emotions and psychology of religion, mainly stressing the coping and self-help function of spirituality as we know it from the role of religion in psychic crisis and illness. What we need is empirical work on the specific emotional constellations of spiritual performances.

To reach our goal we will refer to those fields of research which do not lack analytical categories and employ an analytic distinction: that of the aesthetic and affective pattern of yoga experience within specific traditions, the so-called emotional regime,[3] and that of politics of affect, in order to reveal the embedd-

1 Hitzer 2011.
2 E.g., Heelas & Woodhead 2005.
3 This concept was introduced by William Reddy to denote the dominant norms of feeling accompanied with a code of behaviour and controlled by the reigning class (2001). It was later

edness of emotional regimes within emotional cultures in a wider societal field. Questions to address the emotional regime would be: What are typical yogic emotions during practice and which emotions and which handling of emotions are trained through regular practice? Is it the popular view of a Buddhist detachment from feelings that is acquired? Or is it, in keeping with secularist wishes, the relaxation, the meditative intensification of the moment, the experiencing of the self and of one's own body? The latter touches on further emotional cultures and forms of subjectivity in a pluralistic setting of values and spiritual providers. This context will determine the options and constellation of the politics of affect that are successful and in which emotional regimes may collide and conflict with other sets of emotional regimes. The difference between the concepts of emotional regime and politics of affect is a subtle one. It is not inwardness as opposed to outwardness. Both of them denote the habitual result from an interplay of socio-economic structures, body styles, strategic goals and milieu-specificities. But whereas emotional regimes are employed here to follow more closely the subgroup of specific institutionalised behavioural and attitudinal aspects, the notion of politics of affect gives rigor to the battle over interests in which strong emotional relations to symbols (charismatic individual, brands, values, "traditions") often stand. So the conceptual difference is more of scale and perspective. Politics of affect is a societal-wide emotional regulation with players from economy to art and politics. It may even dissolve the public vs. private life distinction in evading both by strong emotionalisation. Politics of affect is a perennial battlefield where adaptation and conflict of the plurality of emotional regimes take place. The two concepts converge regarding the constructive character of emotional complexes. According to the praxeological social theories of Pierre Bourdieu and others, emotions are "a practical engagement with the world".[4] They are likewise the expression of individual "feeling"[5] and of social norms.

As yoga is such a highly heterogeneous phenomenon we will not attempt to answer all these questions in general but in light of a very specific yoga practice. It is certainly special insofar as it is a collective practice of a huge scale with a global dimension. This chapter will analyse an event in global yoga that took place from 2005 to 2012. Launched in Sydney, Australia, it had spread to more than thirty countries all over the world by 2012, and combined yoga practice, the raising of money for charities and an imagination of the global. Our study is concerned with the twenty-four-hour event Yoga Aid World Challenge (YAWC). I will

criticised for setting overly fixed entities, whereas emotions may vary widely. Riis and Woodhead rely on it in their *A Sociology of Religious Emotion* (2010).

4 Scheer 2012: 193.

5 Reddy 2001.

elaborate on the emotional structure of this event that introduces slight changes to local Western positional yoga regimes and builds up the emotional regime of a global yoga. As we will see, this is not a radical new story, as it reflects partly an enhancement of familiar emotional regimes and partly the inauguration of new symbolic and embodied ascriptions of meaning through this particular form of communication.

2. Framing Conditions: Eventisation, Charitisation, Mediatisation

For the distinctive emotional complex of Yoga Aid it is indispensable to take into account the overall processes of eventisation, charitisation, and mediatisation. An event is a new possibility of transcultural engagement through performance. Eventisation addresses the social structure as well as its aesthetics. The sociology of event sees in events a congenial form of postmodern community building that is fluid, only temporary and low in commitment.[6] Enjoyment and fun, sometimes role-plays with costumes and a slogan or theme serve to connect together the participants for a set period of time, e. g., "Help us raise $1 million for charities around the world" – "Join the fun" in the case of Yoga Aid. Professionals of our contemporary experiential and fun markets, like marketing and tourism agencies, mostly organise and orchestrate these events with their aesthetic instruments. This makes events players in the "market of intense experiences".[7] Examples are global church youth meetings, music and dance festivals, neo-pagan or brand-cult gatherings. Events create an in-group that is familiar and identify with the mission of the event without having to profess a deep belief in its mission. What is sought is an intense and holistic experience beyond those offered by an ever more fragmented world and fragmented subjectivity.

Charitisation can be illustrated by recent initiatives in the field of yoga that explicitly raise donations as the main goal of a meeting. Charity initiatives that act in the global fundraising market are important global players. They follow religious, secularist, national or nonreligious ideologies. With the money raised and material donations the donor can transfer his/her institutions of education, medical knowledge, and humanitarian beliefs. The impact on the recipient's situation is not to be undervalued. The redistribution of financial support and governance works through emotions, which is why one could call the event's strategic action a politics of affect. Besides this political aspect, it is other-regarding behaviour that is deeply involved in this kind of performance and that,

6 Hepp & Vogelgesang 2003.
7 Schulze 2005: 417–457.

besides the politics of affect, also changes the narrative and emotional regimes of the participants on the occasion of this global yoga event.[8] A trigger for charitable action is the claim that there is an obligation to give something back in exchange for the gift of yoga by Indian yogis. In the imagination of the organisers and the participants, India and yoga are permeated by nostalgia for mystic and highly spiritual pasts.

A third and important context in which the particular format of the "new" global yoga performs is that of mediatisation. Media societies communicate in mediatised formats, be it print, analogue or digital media.[9] In media societies one is forced to mediatise one's mission in order to be perceived as and be a part of public life. Governance heavily relies on this mode of communication, which is highly accessible and available. There are many subdivisions of media formats providing specialised forms of communication in which specific milieus in society express and constitute themselves. The event discussed in this case study is marked by the communicational conventions of social media.

This chapter cannot go into all the details and relevant circumstances of contemporary yoga.[10] Rather, it focuses on the politics of affect on the widely mediatised representative level and the assumption that the emotional regime was slightly altered in this specific event. These two aspects constitute a wide ground to cover and we will partly depart from empirical research in order to develop hypotheses that require future testing. The distinction and concomitant relatedness of global and local yoga scenes, milieus and even narratives deserve attention. Against this backdrop I introduce YAWC as a self-reflexive "specific configuration" within world society (part 2). I will elaborate on this argument by analysing the emotional complex within the basic narrative of the event ("giving back") and the structuring of further emotions (part 3). What arises from this is what I will call "living4giving", a well-tuned cosmopolitan mood driving the event (conclusion).

8 "Other-regarding" is a term in opposition to "self-regarding behaviour" that was regularly attributed to yoga practitioners in the West from the polemic perspective during the last decades. Other-regarding behaviour is meant here as a general term with regard to findings in behavioural economics that distinguish altruist, reciprocal, fair or unfair and maximizing behaviour. Therefore altruist behaviour is more specific than other-regarding (see Koch 2015: 74–75).

9 Hepp & Krönert 2009.

10 See also Koch 2015.

3. The Particular Configuration of "Global Yoga"

There is no doubt that yoga has spread all over the globe in various ways. It is even practised in Muslim societies – mostly in gyms. In 2012 the participating countries of YAWC mostly chose the "Africa Yoga Project. Educate. Empower. Elevate", a New York based non-profit organisation that aims at bringing all the benefits of yoga to East African countries and offering yoga teachers from all over the world opportunities to do volunteer work there. The Africa Yoga Project explicitly expresses its aim as "expansion of the market" for yoga practitioners and teachers.[11] This initiative works simultaneously on both the demand and supply sides. It increases the supply by offering teacher training and sending volunteers, and augments the demand by attracting pupils and promoting yoga as a universal practice for a multitude of purposes. The benefits of yoga are seen in "physical, mental and emotional health, facilitating authentic personal expression, building supportive communities, and inspiring positive action."[12] At the same time, yoga has spread over many social classes and milieus. Even if yoga is practised most frequently by urban middle-class younger women, many initiatives also bring the practice to veterans, ex-criminals, drug addicts, the poor and disadvantaged, as well as to employees and self-employed persons.

Besides mere geographic and societal expansion, yoga has a transcultural transfer history: between India and British colonisers in India, especially British military gymnastics; between India and US-American religious, therapeutic and sporting culture at the end of the nineteenth century, and with many other countries in the course of the following decades. Furthermore, we find well-established translocal scenes, retreats and resorts with dedicated travelling practitioners and a multitude of international schools, certificates and styles. World society is the very context of these global networks, which influences agents and institutions beyond the local ones.[13] Rudolf Stichweh has introduced the concept of "particular configurations" (*Eigenstruktur*) within world society to address structures that have emerged on a global scale over the last 500 to 600 years (2008). Particular configurations overlap with older communicative structures and minimise their relevance over time. Functional systems, the delocalisation of networks, the global production of knowledge and world events, world urban space, and a world public realm are all connected to this world system. We can observe the development of such a global configuration in pos-

11 Africa Yoga Project, About, Our Model. See http://www.africayogaproject.org/pages/our-model (accessed 1 December 2012).

12 Africa Yoga Project, About, What we do. See http://www.africayogaproject.org/pages/what-were-up-to (accessed 20 February 2013).

13 Meyer 2010.

tural yoga, which is parallel to countless local yoga scenes and at the same time distinct from them in regards to some relevant features.

One such particular configuration is Yoga Aid Challenge, founded in Australia in 2007 by the Sydney-based yoga teacher Clive Mayhew and his Japanese wife Eriko Kinoshita. Yoga Aid Challenge is held twice annually. Yoga Aid Challenge matured to Yoga Aid *World* Challenge in about thirty-five countries around the world in the spring and autumn of 2012, when the last event was held.[14] My research data on the YAWC, that took place in September 2012, are based on participant observation, guided interviews with participants and organisers in Tokyo and (in 2013) in Miami, the homepage of YAWC and their Facebook page. The advertising by the Japanese section of Yoga Aid provides a good expression of the event's spirit:

> Join us for Yoga Aid World Challenge Japan! Join hundreds of yogis and some of Japan's most influential teachers on Sunday September 9th in the Yoga Aid World Challenge: a 24-hour global yoga-relay. Beginning in Sydney, the World Challenge will follow the sun west, tour through 20+ countries at 200+ events, and end at sunset in Los Angeles. In a network of simultaneous community events across the country, we will celebrate the collective power of yogis by practicing together in this global event and fundraising for charity.[15]

A global particular configuration may be associated with the following elements:
- The self-understanding of some yoga events or discourses as global: global imaginations and global narratives. The image of the continents in the form of a globe on the Yoga Aid Homepage can serve as an example of such an imagination of yoga[16] – the front page, for example, shows a globe with the continents. The background pattern, showing how yoga has radiated throughout the world, has its centre in Australia where the founders of Yoga Aid live and started the charity. Human figures with hands raised, as in performing sun salutations, are coloured according to the flags of the countries where they are placed. Following the course of the sun, the practice mainly consists of sun salutations, as well as yoga classes with a sequence of *āsana*-s. The event centres around a remarkable imagination of cosmopolitan space: from Sydney to Los Angeles, yoga is performed from sunrise to sunset; from an Anglo-Saxon remote corner of the Euro-Anglo world to some Anglo-American place on the fringe of the wide Pacific Ocean.

14 Mayhew and Kinoshita will now focus on other projects of their private Sydney Yoga Foundation (talk with Kinoshita January 2014).

15 Yoga Aid, Homepage, Japan. See http://www.yogaaid.com/japan (accessed 29 July 2012).

16 The homepage was discontinued at the beginning of 2014 but snapshots can be accessed with ArchiveOrg. See http://archive.org/web/. Insert there: http://www.yogaaid.com; then choose a date.

- The role of specific events and a social milieu of globally minded people have been described (for LOHAS, new middle class, holistic spirituality or cultural creative, see Hero 2008).
- The specific configuration links to global media productions (e.g., international films like "Yogawoman"[17] and "Der atmende Gott / Breath of the Gods"[18]; several yoga journals, virtual communication on Facebook sites, social media, yoga blogs, etc.).
- Specific configurations also fall into place through global movements (social, cultural, eco-friendly, spiritual): raw food, vegan and healthy food, holistic medicine, body-therapies, breathing therapy and other self-therapies to name just a few.
- Furthermore, these configurations evolve towards a similar structural background of economic culture, like Yoga Aid in the context of neoliberalism and the recent financial market crisis, global charity-markets and charity culture.
- The change resulting from mediatised communication can hardly be underestimated: the structural level is massively influenced by the typical virtual communication habits and patterns of user content production and social media use, with considerable competition for mass participation.
- And last but not least, the language of this global yoga, as of other spiritual movements like meditation trends, is "guru English"[19] with a special yoga vocabulary: global yogis will know specific words such as tailbone, diaphragm, and pubic bone. Formulae such as "Let it go" or "I wish you a good practice" are common. Particular intonations have also developed, like the prolonged "a" in "relaaaax". This global-yoga English has also developed a particular tone through digital communication. An analysis of Facebook posts on the Yoga Aid site would be revealing in this regard.

According to the logic of a particular configuration, YAWC differs from some local practices in modern Western positional yoga. YAWC shifts remarkably from private cosy yoga studios to public space and seeks high visibility.[20] Yoga

17 Movie available in eight languages on women and yoga worldwide with the subtitle "Never underestimate the power of the inner peace". See http://www.yogawoman.tv/the-crew (accessed 1 May 2017). The film is promoted by yogawoman.tv; see also the subpage on yoga women giving back to the yoga community: http://www.yogawoman.tv/giving-back-to-the-community.

18 German language movie (with English subtitles) about the life and teachings of T. Krishnamacharya directed by J. Schmitt-Garre. See http://www.breathofthegods.com (accessed 1 May 2017).

19 Aravamudan 2006.

20 Many of these phenomena are not altogether new. They have existed in neo-Hindu movements or Indian yoga during the last two centuries. Public and collective yoga camps took place in twentieth-century India ("shivir"; see Alter 2008).

Aid takes place on meadows; for example in Sydney at the bay with a view of Harbour Bridge, in Jerusalem at the Western temple wall or in Tokyo in March 2012 behind Midtown, a high-end mall and office building. As a consequence, Yoga aid was regularly performed as a collective practice with hundreds of yogis. Then, the focus on other-regarding behaviour and charity, instead of a primal interest in self-development, is salient and has to be interpreted. The biggest influence is that Yoga Aid heavily adapts to known forms of collecting donations worldwide. Examples of global social activism are disaster relief and Aids charity events like the Band Aid and Life Aid traditions from the 1980s onwards, which combine music and charity. The configuration of multi-sited global charity events was already established prior to Yoga Aid. Above all, professional fund-raiser communication through social media preponderates, introducing icons and a corporate identity aesthetics. Events and charity activism also have historical forerunners in neo-Hindu charities (e.g., Sivananda's Indian and Sri Lankan tour for peace and unity of men in 1950, or Vishnu Devananda's world peace mission in 1971). Admittedly, there is a great deal of competition in yoga history (just think of yoga Olympics). Cultural critique, as implicit in YAWC, also appeared towards the end of the nineteenth century, when Western elites behaved critically towards society and politics in general by promoting many of the elements of past and present yoga, like vegetarianism, an educated self-ideal, and cultivated body work in the "life reform" movement. This has led Karl Baier to see in YAWC a "globalized update" of early Western yoga.[21]

4. The Emotional Complex of Yoga Aid

4.1. Theoretical Considerations

To understand the culture of giving it is necessary to bring into focus the symbolic and social payoffs that Ole Riis and Linda Woodhead approach via the concept of emotional regimes in any given religion. By emotional regimes of practitioners we understand their habitual set of related emotions and modes of experiencing. They structure the emotional programme of given groups.[22] Based on their observations, Riis and Woodhead have developed a middle way between the two main sociological and culture theories of emotions in modernity: one that sees a rationalisation of low if-at-all-emotional bureaucratic procedures and another stressing the high emotionality of modern expressive subjects. But seemingly strong emotional displays may also be post-emotional, insofar as they are eval-

21 Email to the author, 9 August 2012.
22 Riis & Woodhead 2010: 180.

uated as aestheticised mass styles and part of consumerism.[23] In individualist late modern spirituality, some emotional regimes are strongly connected to authenticity, the experiencing of oneself, and consequently to persons who stand for "contact with oneself" or the individual ability to stand up against alienating pressures. Inasmuch as symbols are self-reflexive and come along with the awareness of constructed signs, the symbol system and associated emotional regimes are bereft of a traditional religious beyond. A single emotion that is less valued than traditionally religious or moral emotions, such as happiness, personal fulfilment or a balanced self, becomes the ultimate goal.[24] On the other hand, these emotional goals are often attained through therapeutic methods that have become accessible by self-help literature and the spread of psychotherapies. The context of economisation may stress material values and the aesthetisation of life styles and emotional regimes.

In his monograph on religious affects Donovan Schaefer takes up Sara Ahmed's concept of affective economies by which he understands "economies driven by a complex matrix of compulsions that do not necessarily follow predictable watercourses of functional clarity" (2015: 173). Affects are driven by uneven and queer desires of embodied agents that cannot be reconstructed in an arithmetic rationality but are motivated by unintentional enjoyment of embodied states. This poststructuralist approach warns against a rationalised reconstruction of affect economies according to assumed evolutionary necessities and instead promotes the consideration of chaotic triggering surroundings as well as affects that break rules and habits.

What we learn from these theoretical approaches as well as from the empirical plurality of present emotions is that there are several emotional registers and modes that can overlap, contradict or enhance each other in multiple ways. One option for structuring the diversity is discussed below, based on a narrative with its politics of affect and the fine-grained interrelation of emotions.

4.2. The Obligation to Give Back in a Moral Global Economy

The politics of affect requires a global imagination of yoga. This is why we so carefully introduced the specific configuration of global yoga. The global scale is anchored in the founding narrative of YAWC. It says that the founding couple, while travelling through India, stayed with a "wonderful swami", the Pujya Swami

23 Meštrović 1997.
24 Riis & Woodhead 2010: 181.

Chidanand Saraswatiji, who taught them yoga.[25] The swami said it was "time to give back" and he "planted a seed" into their hearts. The Facebook timeline indicates this meeting as the birth of Yoga Aid in March 2006 at the International Yoga Conference in Rishikesh. Gift and gift-return occurs here on an intercultural scale: between India and the rest of the global yoga world. A charity is seen as a cultural return mode for a gift. The setting of the swami and the Westerners, as in ancient myths of two people inhabiting the known world, is telling. India is still the imagined land of yoga origin and is often represented visually in yoga institutions[26] even though much of their practice derives from modern Western yoga. Yoga and Qigong have both been advertised "in literature that accompanies such training courses as Indian or Chinese 'gifts to the world'".[27] Van der Veer takes this as a sign that these practices have gone global while at the same time staying connected to national identities – at least in the imaginary.[28] The metaphor of the growing seed is a very ancient image of surplus, a harvest that grows on its own by natural energy supply. However, it can also easily connect with the neoliberal and capitalistic idea of generating a surplus. The seed is multiplied in the globalisation of Yoga Aid.

The motivating feeling heavily relies on an imagination of globality and community and not on an instantaneous, actual outbreak of collective harmonious feeling in the sense of Emil Durkheim's effervescence, which he takes to be the religious master feeling. The politics of affect has therefore been conceptualised as a moral economy from the interlinkage of state and intergenerational values (for instance by Edward P. Thompson). Even if these feelings might be evoked on the event day, face-to-face gatherings take place beforehand. Even so, one could argue that regular yoga classes evoke an everyday emotionality of connection with other yogis. This is probable, but the dynamic here works on a different level insofar as this connectedness is habitual and carried out by symbols and embodied practice from case to case by the explicit teachings of yoga teachers.

The central emotion in the event narrative of Yoga Aid is the desire to give back. What might be the elements of this emotion? Is it a feeling of guilt, the feeling of owing something to somebody? To whom does the couple want to give something back? To the Indian people, the wise men who develop *āsana*-s, the poor and exploited postcolonial countries? Is there a transcultural obligation? Or

25 Robertson 2012. See also Facebook YogaAid, Timeline, Birth; www.facebook.com/YogaAid (accessed 3 August 2012).

26 Hoyez 2007: 115, despite the fact that three-fourths of the French teachers have never been to India.

27 Van der Veer 2009: 263.

28 Ibid.

is it not important to single out one recipient because the main purpose is to recognise the phrasing of giving back as a narrative sequence?

4.2.1. Owing – Being Indebted

The emotion or formula of owing is tacit. It is inherent in the mission to give back. With a hermeneutics of suspicion one could claim that owing is a hidden or even repressed emotion or narratological sequence to make a motivational structure plausible. If owing indeed underlies the "giving back" narrative, then it is important to talk about guilt more generally. Guilt for the YAWC is a collective feeling, not an individual matter. It has to be compensated and amended in a joint effort. Some scholars characterise shame as a feeling of the self that endangers its integrity with dissolution, whereas guilt is seen as a feeling of a person strong enough to harm others.[29] There are further options: concerning YAWC, there is good reason to see the addressee of the guilt in a self-relational circle of an exchange economy: it is the gift of yoga to which one is duty bound. "Yoga" in this formula takes on the meaning of a substitute. It represents the entirety of a long-standing tradition, millions of practitioners and endless narratives of existential self-finding. One is "I owe yoga so much"; it is a feeling of finding peace, values, oneself, or even a life through yoga. Self-development is still an aim but now it includes the reconciliatory work of giving back.

Sun salutations are the main practice at events in public spaces (some studios just give regular yoga classes). According to the introduction given by yoga teachers and the practitioner's imagination, sun salutations can be performed with an attitude of devotion. This prostration-like form of bending down invokes an outward other that is addressed: that is, the sun, enabling life on earth with its warmth and light and representing a higher force in the mind-set of practitioners. This externalisation of attention can create an emotion of dedication towards this outside, beyondness or however it might be called.[30] Through this symbolic as well as embodied level of performance, a strong sense of being indebted is triggered insofar as it is directed.

In the history of religions, the sense of being indebted regularly includes deities. Believers owe care, fostering and service to their gods, spirits and ancestors. The connection between deeds and consequences is a very common multi-variant pattern in history and seen to be valid in inter-human relations as well as in relationships with superhuman beings or inter-generational dependents. A vast anthropological literature has described merit-making in relation to class or status, hegemony, and morality in many localities. But the karma

29 E.g., by Helen Lynd according to Scheff 2000.
30 Nevrin 2008.

framework seems to be more prevalent in autobiographical interpretations than as a motivational structure for giving in the observed milieu.

4.2.2. The Feeling of Meaningfulness: Living4giving

How can someone feel that by giving she/he can receive *meaning* in return? Giving appears to be a main purpose of life. This connection is worthy of explanation. How closely the meaning of life – or even in a sense, "our life" – connects with giving is manifested in the Yoga Aid advertisement on Facebook: "What we get makes our living, but what we give makes our life." Life is interpreted holistically as giving. Giving is what makes sense, and in this way it is equated with meaningful life. The quest for a sense of fulfillment and for quality of life, which are so fundamental in the subjective culture of alternative and secularist spiritualties, is expressed through the act of giving, sharing and dividing up of what one has in abundance. Another advertising image from the Yoga Aid Facebook site has triggered some controversial debate in the commentaries. The event slogan in the corporate identity design of Yoga Aid reads: "The smallest good deed is better than the greatest intention."[31] The problem for some of the commentators is that intention, their central concept, is now devaluated against action. The conflict arises when the emotional economy is outdated in comparison with the political moral economy. We can observe that supporters of a more individualistic understanding of yoga feel harassed by this: the emotional economy of high and proper intentions that remains self-sufficient is questioned by Yoga Aid activism. Therefore, the point of the advertisement is not to dishonour intention (which is a central term in yoga philosophy), but to ask for engaged monetary and other-regarding behaviour.

4.2.3. Gratitude

Gratitude is at the heart of everything. In this logic of gratitude, those in need serve with a sense of fulfillment for those who give. Fulfillment is the immaterial good received in return for giving away surpluses. Perhaps this desire to give back arises from the privileged situation of a generation that has prospered through the lifework of their parents and has accumulated huge wealth in the long period of peace after World War II in many industrialised societies? This feeling of gratitude towards ancestors or society in general is then directed towards those who are in need. One might see this intentionalist concept of gratitude as an

31 Facebook YogaAid. See https://www.facebook.com/photo.php?fbid=445258682181483&set=a.108787219161966.4617.107643195943035&type=1&theatre (accessed 9 January 2014).

exuberance of emotions regularly promoted in many yogic meditations. Yoga Aid posts: "The Attitude of Gratitude is the Highest Yoga. Yogi Bhajan."[32]

Where and when did this idea of "giving back" originate? Leza Lowitz, now a yoga studio owner in Tokyo and one of the leaders of Yoga Aid Japan, originally comes from California. In her view, the "wish to share" arises from many sources: the indigenous traditions of the US and Canada, as well as the California spirit of "free boxes" in the streets for exchanging second-hand articles: "This is the spirit of my childhood in Berkeley, the ancient spirit of the indigenous peoples of the U.S. and Canada, the people of Australia and Africa and Asia and America – people all over the world who wish to share what they have with others in the spirit of giving. As Clive and Eriko put it, these are 'The People of Love'."[33] Noticeably, Europeans do not appear in this enumeration. This naturalisation of a feeling and the autobiographic narratives of the YAWC founders nicely show to what degree a certain autobiographical interpretation may be a resource for social action. This form of engaged spirituality is a combination of biography, social milieu and a sense of identity. They are the background for a specific experiencing of spirituality and how to embed it in everyday life so that it will develop – as Gregory C. Stanczak learned in interviews with practitioners across religions and beliefs in the USA – on their motivation for social action (2006). In distinguishing between institutional religion and more experience-based, emotional spirituality, the latter is seen to follow rules of its own and to be a critical power for transforming everyday life. Thus, spirituality may be a hidden cultural power for social transformation with effects on a larger scale.

4.2.4. Competing

The self-centred practice of self-perfection is combined with competition for donations (2015). For some years now, instead of being a gentle practice, forms of power yoga and military-like instructions have appeared in the international yoga scene. "Help us raise 1 million for charities around the world": the imperative slogan astonishingly sets a clear financial aim. To reach this goal, hundreds of teams in countries all over the world competed to raise as much money as possible in advance of and on the day of the event. Competition between teams and fundraisers is an integral part of this process and of the strategy of the Yoga Aid organisers. Competition works as an incentive to instill a sporting spirit for a good cause. The sporting spirit may be inferred from the following wording: "team", "challenger", "top fundraiser" and "top team" charts. One might imagine

32 Facebook YogaAid. See https://www.facebook.com/YogaAid (accessed 6 March 2013).
33 Lowitz, L., The global spirit. See http://blog.yogaaid.com/?p=185, posted 28 June 2012 (accessed 2 March 2013).

that this kind of competition, which in the end relies on the social network of the challengers and makes them clearly visible on the Yoga Aid homepage, easily fuels latent competition between yoga teacher teams and studios. They appear with their photo or logo and a short pledge to donate on the Yoga Aid homepage, and every donor appears with his or her name on the subsite of the challenger. Even if the donations are for a good cause, this channelling of donations on the Yoga Aid homepage cannot be totally uncoupled from the fundraisers' personality and charisma.

4.2.5. Connectedness

The desire to give back might also be motivated by another feeling: being connected and the connectedness that results from helping and giving. The donors play an active role; they are behaving properly; they are good people. In this way, they include themselves in an imagined and self-empowering community of people of good will. The dream of interconnectedness in a metaphysical dimension of the New Age cosmology, where everything is interwoven, might also play a role in some practitioners' emotional regime. At the very least, this giving adds to the feeling of companionship. The yogi donor is not alone in a global world of anonymous contractual relations and corporations. It is not the imagination of an idyllic Indian ashram, so common in yoga studios worldwide. It is the image on the front page of Yoga Aid homepage of a human chain of people in different colours and raising their arms up as in sun salutation posture. "Together we make a difference" is another event-slogan. They constitute a moral community of those of good will. They are experiencing pleasure, as in Luke 2.14 in the Bible. Regardless of whether this pattern of people of good will stems from Christian mainstream societies like the USA and Australia, what counts is that a moral community is constituted.

4.2.6. Self-Empowerment

Giving for reasons of interconnectedness establishes a gift economy, in which the position of those who are giving-back is one of power and force: they are able to give back. The Yoga Aid marketing discourse is guided by the positive and empowering idea of each donor and their wealth, their "having too much". This surplus means vitality, health and opportunities that are easy to share or easy to implement for a good cause and the advantage that there is no need of drastic renunciation. Just practice, just pay for the yoga class on that day as usual and your teacher will transfer the revenues from the class to a good cause! This reversion of direction is typical for the charity strategy of global yoga: the charities stay in the background as subsites of the homepages. It is above all the activism, the fun of performing, and the promise of a good mood arising out of gathering with other like-minded people. First, one feels privileged to enjoy this glorious practice – and then there are some only vaguely know people in need to whom one can give. Therein lies the ambivalence of the event: an oscillation between the need for self-realisation and other-regarding behaviour. The multiple event spaces bind people together on a particular day, and the global imagination of a chain of people standing together can offer an "invigorating social space" providing empowerment.[34]

Yoga Aid succeeds in erecting an emotional signifier within the global yoga arena: redemption through joyful yoga practice and spreading this gift to others amidst the global economic debt crisis. The overall mission is the self-ascription of giftedness: one is gifted with the wonderful tool of yoga. That way one's life is meaningful. From this perspective, the event appears as the confirmation of being powerful. In this sense, one finds other-regarding motivations in a more sophisticated self-interested way but also in a pro-social manner.

5. Conclusion: The Cosmopolitan Mood of Living4giving

Yoga Aid's inaugurated social bonds of its politics of affect may be interpreted along Ulrich Beck, Natan Sznaider and Edgar Grande's concept of cosmopolitanism that exceeds dualisms, such as foreign-domestic and national-international, and differs from the global or world system.[35] Cosmopolitanism only loosely integrates very different styles and local places. Yoga Aid as an uncontrollable non-state actor favours many local and independent charity organisations. In a system-inherent manner it strengthens yoga by regularly choosing the yoga-specific charities instead of more general humanitarian organisations from a list of options. The communicative templates of YAWC are embossed by the highly mediatised virtual communication we are familiar with from social media and commercial user-generated contents. Their experts with a "predisposition to 'cosmopolitanism'"[36] stem from the new middle class of freelancers in marketing, graphic design, consulting and personal growth markets that are familiar with negotiating symbolic goods. According to these communicative templates, competition seems to be an apt means of motivating action. By having found a way to institutionalise certain feelings, Yoga Aid can express a cosmopolitan mood, even if only episodically, and initiate an iconic-affective "marker of certainty" (Shmuel Eisenstadt).

34 Nevrin 2008: 130.
35 Beck & Sznaider 2006; Beck & Grande 2007.
36 Altglas 2014: 18.

Most central to the politics of affect of our yoga narrative is guilt. We find a similar element of guilt in the politics of affect in some of today's eco-spirituality, which rediscovers the "indigene" treasures of wise men and women parallel to postcolonial movements. An awareness of closeness to nature, seasons and subsistence economy, as well as a feeling of dependence on nature, go hand in hand with the feeling of owing nature what industrialisation took away. Renaturation and the removal of technological and artificial devices provide redemption for our sins against nature. In our field study, guilt is seen to result from a feeling of living in a privileged situation that is turned into gratitude.

For our interpretation of guilt, we have relied on the prominence of the positive thinking approach in alternative spirituality: I am gifted and I can share. We find this in current bestsellers such as Jonathan Haidt's *Righteous Mind* (2012) or in Martin Seligman's Europe tour 2014 on positive psychology. Riis and Woodhead see this "crude distinction of positive and negative emotions" as typical for contemporary emotional regimes[37] and Altglas introduces psychologisation as the process by which exotic resources like Hindu yoga become a helpful resource for self-realisation in the standardizing context of therapy societies.[38] The reduction of the emotional repertoire or the prominence of a "cool" emotional style do not apply to Yoga Aid. But Yoga Aid meets the high expectations for existential fulfillment and answers the longing for a moral community.

In our yoga case study the practice is contextualised in an event that turns the focus from self-perfection towards other-regarding behaviour. It resonates with global challenges and neoliberalism-opposing movements of generosity. By opposing greedy capitalism and the two factions of winners and losers of globalisation, "pockets" of generosity have emerged over the past decades. This opens up moral communities, as in James Farrer's concept of cosmopolitanism as a virtue that includes hospitality (2012). Thomas J. Scheff sees a symptom of alienation in shame being narrowed and love broadened in public discourse, whereas the contrary direction of change would indicate solidarity (2000). The rationale behind Scheff's thesis is that shame arises from endangered social bonds and that this kind of shame is a taboo in individualised societies that permanently endanger the collective. Interesting as this is, in the outlined politics of affect the envisioned other-regarding aims are resolved on an activist level and the emotion of love is not as central as fun is. But, with the strong feeling of interconnectedness, the relational world of practitioners worldwide takes up much space in the imaginary of YAWC against individualisation. Therefore, a lack of solidarity, even with a model of suppression and emotional reversion,

37 Riis & Woodhead 2010: 186.
38 Altglas 2014: 201–238.

cannot be found. Nevertheless, shame could be seen in close connection to alienation from modern invisible and incomprehensible finance market capitalism. Bruno Latour sees a "feeling of crisis" as being responsible for the loss of social belonging, resulting in new forms of "reassembling" in networks.[39] He criticises sociological explanations that "begin with society or other social aggregates, whereas one should end with them. They believed the social to be made essentially of social ties, whereas associations are made of ties, which are themselves non-social"[40] – such as collective moods and emotional practices. The chapter has shown how several non-social ties come together in the reassembling of YAWC: an emotional regime in the sense of a recognizable subcultural pattern, virtual and marketing communication, a corporate identity aesthetics, the globally imagined "artefact-space-structuration"[41] and body practices.

My aim was to demonstrate some major aspects of transformation within this specific yoga configuration: the transformation of social belonging, the offer of a specific purpose in life, and a politics of affect with other-regarding behaviour in its ambivalence as something distinct from late modern spirituality and at the same time a self-empowerment concordant with it.

References

Alter, J. (2008). Yoga Shivir: Performativity and the Study of Modern Yoga. In M. Singleton & J. Byrne (Eds.), *Yoga in the Modern World: Contemporary Perspectives* (pp. 36–48). Oxford: Routledge.

Altglas, V. (2014). *From Yoga to Kabbalah: Religious Exoticism and the Logics of Bricolage.* Oxford: Oxford University Press.

Aravamudan, S. (2006). *Guru English: South Asian Religion in a Cosmopolitan Language.* Princeton: Princeton University Press.

Beck, U. & Grande, E. (2007). Cosmopolitanism: Europe's Way Out of Crisis. *European Journal of Social Theory, 10,* 67–85.

Beck, U. & Sznaider, N. (2006). Unpacking Cosmopolitanism for the Social Sciences: A Research Agenda. *The British Journal of Sociology, 56*(1), 1–23.

Farrer, J. (2012). Cosmopolitanism as Virtue: Toward an Ethics of Global City Life. *Policy Innovations. A Publication of Carnegie Council.* http://www.policyinnovations.org/ideas/commentary/data/000166. Accessed 1 February 2014.

Heelas, P. & Woodhead, L. (2005). *The Spiritual Revolution: Why Religion is Giving Way to Spirituality.* Oxford: Oxford University Press.

Hepp, A. & Krönert, V. (2009). *Medien – Event – Religion: Die Mediatisierung des Religiösen.* Wiesbaden: Springer VS.

39 Latour 2005: 7.
40 Ibid.
41 Reckwitz 2012: 251ff.

Hepp, A. & Vogelgesang, W. (Eds.). (2003). *Populäre Events: Medienevents, Spielevents, Spaßevents.* Opladen: Leske und Budrich.
Hero, M. (2008). Religious Pluralization and Institutional Change: The Case of the Esoteric Milieu. *Journal of Religion in Europe, 2,* 200–226.
Hitzer, B. (2011). Forschungsbericht: Emotionsgeschichte – ein Anfang mit Folgen. 11/23/2011, *HsozuKult.* http://hsozkult.geschichte.hu-berlin.de/forum/2011-11-001#note5. Accessed 17 July 2014.
Hoyez, A.-C. (2007). The "World of Yoga": The Production and Reproduction of Therapeutic Landscapes. *Social Science & Medicine, 65,* 112–124.
Koch, A. (2015). Competitive Charity: A Neoliberal Culture of "Giving Back" in Global Yoga. *Journal of Contemporary Religion, 30,* 73–85.
Latour, B. (2005). *Reassembling the Social: An Introduction to Actor-Network-Theory.* Clarendon Lectures in Management Studies. Oxford: Oxford University Press.
Meštrović, St. G. (1997). *Postemotional Society.* London: Sage.
Meyer, J. W. (2010). World Society, Institutional Theories, and the Actor. *Annual Review of Sociology, 36,* 1–20.
Nevrin, K. (2008). Empowerment and Using the Body in Modern Postural Yoga. In M. Singleton & J. Byrne (Eds.), *Yoga in the Modern World: Contemporary Perspectives* (pp. 119–139). Oxford: Routledge.
Reckwitz, A. (2012). Affective Spaces: A Praxeological Outlook. *Rethinking History: The Journal of Theory and Practice, 16*(2), 241–258.
Reddy, W. M. (2001). *The Navigation of Feeling: A Framework for the History of Emotions.* Cambridge: Cambridge University Press.
Riis, O. & Woodhead, L. (2010). *A Sociology of Religious Emotion.* Oxford: Oxford University Press.
Robertson, D. (2012). Interview with Clive Mayhew (and his wife Eriko Kinoshita). *Helloyoga* 15 June 2012. http://www.helloyoga.com/2012/06/15/clive-mayhew-co-founder-director-yoga-aid/. Accessed 22 February 2013.
Schaefer, D. O. (2015). *Religious Affects: Animality, Evolution, and Power.* Durham: Duke University Press.
Scheer, M. (2012). Are Emotions a Kind of Practice (and Is That What Makes Them Have a History)? A Bourdieuian Approach to Understanding Emotion. *History and Theory, 51* (2), 193–220.
Scheff, Th. (2000). Shame and the Social Bond. *Sociological Theory, 18*(1), 84–98.
Schulze, G. (2005). *Die Erlebnisgesellschaft: Kultursoziologie der Gegenwart.* 2nd ed. Frankfurt: Campe.
Stanczak, G. C. (2006). *Engaged Spirituality: Social Change and American Religion.* New Brunswick: Rutgers University Press.
Stichweh, R. (2006). Strukturbildung in der Weltgesellschaft: Die Eigenstrukturen der Weltgesellschaft und die Regionalkulturen der Welt. In Th. Schwinn (Ed.), *Die Vielfalt und Einheit der Moderne: Kultur- und strukturvergleichende Analysen* (pp. 239–258). Wiesbaden: Springer VS.
Veer, P. van der (2009). Global Breathing: Religious Utopias in India and China. In Th. J. Csordas (Ed.), *Transnational Transcendence: Essays on Religion and Globalization* (pp. 263–279). Berkeley: University of California Press.

Chapter 15

Spaces of Yoga: Towards a Non-Essentialist Understanding of Yoga

Suzanne Newcombe

Contents

1. Introduction 551

2. The Stage and Yoga Performance 554

3. Yoga in Schools: Encinitas School District Yoga 557

4. Mappings of Space: Maps and the Spatial Theory 560

5. Private Space and the Imagined Yoga Tradition 563

6. The Studio Space 567

7. Conclusions 569

References 570

Suzanne Newcombe

Chapter 15: Spaces of Yoga: Towards a Non-Essentialist Understanding of Yoga[*]

What yoga is can only become clear within a specific context.
(Maya Burger)[1]

1. Introduction

This chapter will examine some of the spaces that yoga occupies in the contemporary world, both physical and social. By looking at yoga through the focus of particular, contested spaces and locations, it will be argued that overarching essentialist definitions of yoga are impossible, although individuals and social groups can and do create essentialist definitions that are more or less useful for particular purposes. By exploring these narratives and boundaries in the context of specific locations, we can better understand what people are doing with the collection of beliefs and practices known as yoga.[2]

Since the 1990s, in much of the developed and cosmopolitan areas of the world, there has been an obvious proliferation of purpose-built yoga centres, with

* Some of the research for this chapter was carried out as part of the AYURYOG Project (http://www.ayuryog.org/). This project has received funding from the European Research Council (ERC) under the European Union's Horizon 2020 research and innovation programme (grant agreement No 639363-AYURYOG). I would like to extend my gratitude to Karl Baier, Philipp A. Maas and Karin C. Preisendanz, as well as to Alexandra Böckle who organised the conference "Yoga in Transformation: Historical and Contemporary Perspectives on a Global Phenomenon" (Vienna, 19–21 September 2013) and for providing the inputs and support without which this paper would not have been written. I also thank the comments of all the conference attendees who helped me think about these ideas further, especially, but by no means exclusively, the constructive criticism and encouragement on the themes of this paper from Joseph Alter, Karl Baier, Maya Burger, Anne Koch, Elizabeth De Michelis, David Gordon White, Dagmar Wujastyk and Dominik Wujastyk. I would particularly like to thank Cathryn Keller and Kim Knott for sharing their interests and enthusiasm.

1 This was an astute comment Maya Burger made in contextualizing her presentation "Sāṃkhya Interpretation in a Transnational Perspective: Śrī Anirvāṇa and Lizelle Reymond" on 20 September 2013 at the conference "Yoga in Transformation" mentioned in n. *. Cf. also her contribution to its proceedings in the present volume.

2 Andrea Jain (2012) and Andrew Nicholson (2013) have also explored similar themes based on historical analysis of yoga traditions.

a preference for white walls, wooden floors and high ceilings. But people also describe "doing yoga" in ashrams, gyms, at Hindutva camps, Indian temples (mandirs), inside ritually prepared fires, in schools, in homes, on surfboards, in prison cells and hospital beds. In fact, someone has probably done something he or she might describe as yoga, just about everywhere.

And, there is also likely to be someone willing to say that whatever is described as yoga is *not* yoga – or at least not "true yoga". The removal, or glossing over, of the historical Indian religious and philosophical context to yoga is seen as perverting the essence of yoga by many Hindu activist groups.[3] The perceived commercialisation, commoditisation and sexualisation of yoga are considered objectionable by many – secular practitioners and Hindu activist groups alike.[4] Some Christian groups and Muslim clerics have argued that yoga practices are potentially undermining to their faith (a view shared by some Hindus).[5] Followers of one particular guru might reject the insights of followers of another guru, although the contradictory insights are sometimes achieved by using very similar practices.

The general absence of specific religious imagery reflects the multicultural, cosmopolitan areas where yoga studios proliferate, with vaguely Buddhist or "Om" symbols being more likely than any references to specific Hindu deities. Except in the case of yoga spaces in more sectarian *sampradāya*-s (teaching lineages), any such symbols are likely to be underplayed and presented as "optional" in the contemporary context. The minimalistic aesthetics popular in many practice and teaching spaces, may suggest an openness to creativity, to personal transformation, to interpretation and re-interpretation.

But as already implied, the modern, non-religious nature of the contemporary yoga space is not without controversy. This overtly "empty" room in which yoga is taught and practised is seen as disingenuously neutral by many religious groups, particularly more conservative forms of Christianity and Islam. The lack of imagery is believed to be a trick, where Hindu or at least "un-Christian"

3 For examples see Occupy Yoga (2014) which is re-printed on the National Council of Hindu Temples (UK) website (2014) and the Hindu American Foundation's (HAF) Take Back Yoga campaign which began in 2010 (HAF 2014a, 2014b and Vitello 2010).

4 For a case study of these types of re-occurring controversy, the concept of commercial copyright and yoga was discussed in depth by Allison Fish (2006) in the context of Bikram Yoga, which has since been associated with cases of sexual impropriety (Vanity Fair 2013 and Forshee 2016). An overview of many areas of controversy and yoga is also provided by Gwilym Beckerlegge (2013). Also see Jain's analysis (2012).

5 For examples see Tedjasukmana 2009 on yoga in Indonesia and Fleetwood 2012 for the distinctions the Catholic Church has made between different kinds of "Eastern Meditation" including yoga, and Catholic orthodoxy; Mohler 2010 for a Southern Baptist position and Shukla 2010 for a Hindu "yoga purist" position. However, a more nuanced Hindu American Foundation position on yoga in schools is that "*āsana*-s" are okay but "yoga as a whole" is not (2014c). Jain (2014a) has also analysed the oppositional dialectics of two of these positions.

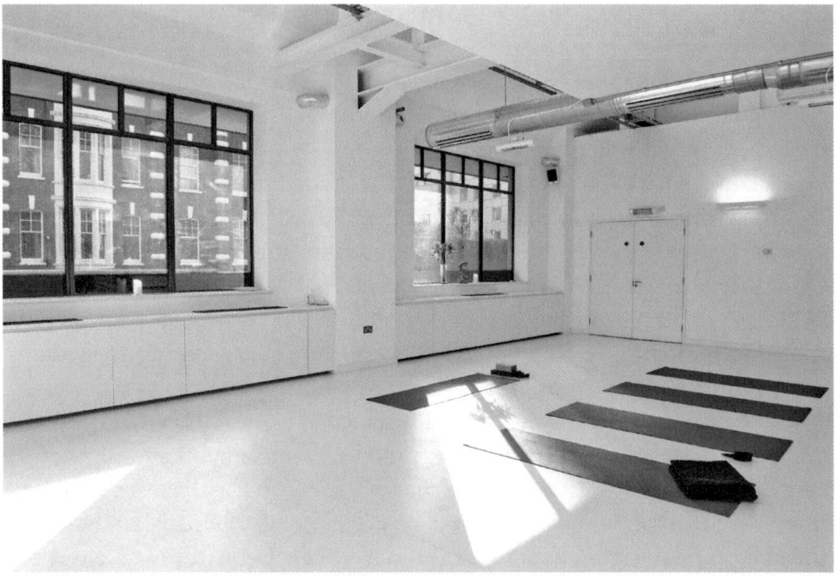

Figure 1: A typical contemporary "yoga studio" space in 2014 (photograph of triyoga Chelsea in London, used with the permission of triyoga).

indoctrination lies subtly beneath the surface of activities conducted therein. Simultaneously, some Hindutva groups see the absence of religious signifiers as a dilution and corruption of their sacred traditions.[6] In this way, physical space becomes an exceptionally useful focus for understanding controversy, contested meanings and the complex and multivalent place of yoga in contemporary society.

Before returning to the aesthetics found in contemporary yoga centres, it would be helpful to examine a few other locations where yoga has been controversial. Looking at the origins of the controversy in a particular case can help us discover the boundaries and contested concepts embroiled in the term yoga. If one starts to look at specific places of yoga practice, one quickly becomes enmeshed in narratives of what yoga is and is not in the eyes of both practitioners and other interested commentators.

6 See Jain 2012.

2. The Stage and Yoga Performance

Most understandings of yoga assume that the practice must be taught or transmitted in some way from an adept, guru or teacher, to the neophyte or student (*śiṣya*). This is often imagined as a private exchange between two individuals and not a public experience. But in the modern period yoga has become associated with more performative, public demonstrations. Yoga as performance has a long history; during the colonial period feats of physical daring and contortion were reported in street performances.[7] This association gave yoga practices a particularly unsavoury connotation – being associated with low-life cheats, street performers and beggars. This performative aspect of yoga also is associated with the scientific demonstrations of Swami Kuvalayananda, the Mysore palace demonstrations by Krishnamacharya and his students and the promotion of yoga as an "Olympic" event by Bikram Choudhury.[8] In some of these contexts, there is also a stage, a space where experts or virtuosos are raised above, or at least separated from, an audience of spectators. This can be a particularly controversial as some find the stage offensive; its use is seen as exhibitionist and antithetical to a more introverted essence of yoga, often assumed to be historically, or more authentically, a personal transmission from a single teacher (*guru*) to an individual student (*śiṣya*).

When B. K. S. Iyengar (1918–2014) came to Britain to promote yoga in the 1960s, he attempted to make use of every platform he could in order to inspire interest in the subject. His stages included the living rooms of the elite in Highgate, the Everyman's Theatre in Hampstead, the stage offered by BBC television broadcasting, the large stage of London's Quaker Meeting Hall in Euston, and a sell-out demonstration at the Barbican in London (a major classical music venue) in 1984. Some during this period took offense at Iyengar's performance of physical virtuosity, which they considered to be violent, exhibitionist, and exemplifying contortionism rather than yoga.[9] However, Iyengar's performances did inspire considerable interest in the subject of yoga and his promotion contributed to making physical-posture oriented yoga a more normal activity in the West.

Even after the initial goal of popularizing yoga had been achieved, Iyengar continued to make pedagogical and practical uses of the stage as a teaching tool. Stages were sometimes built into the multi-purpose schoolrooms, theatres, and meeting rooms that were used to teach yoga. The majority of spaces in which the

7 White 2009 and Singleton 2010: 35–54.

8 For early twenty century examples of performative yoga see Alter 2004 and 2008, Singleton 2010 and Sarbacker 2014; for Bikram Yoga see Hauser 2013, Fish 2006 and Vanity Fair 2013.

9 Newcombe 2008: 99 and Thompson 2004.

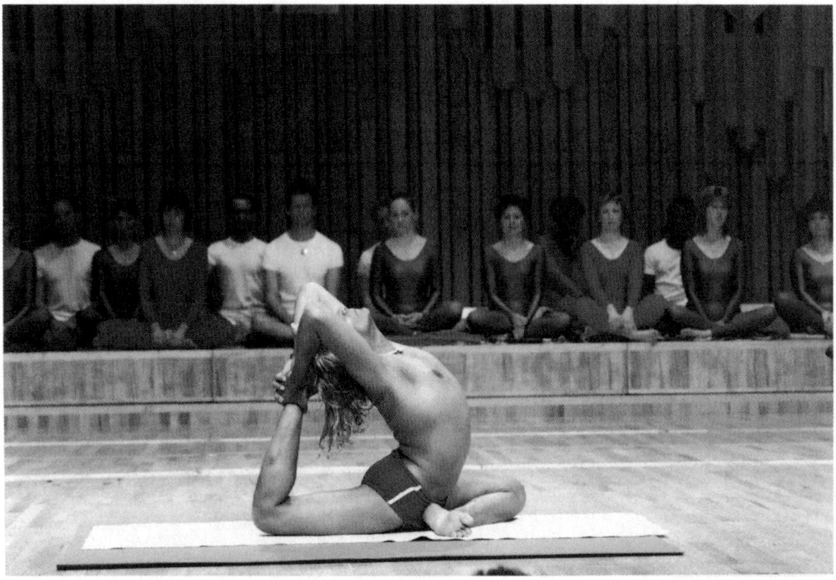

Figure 2: B. K. S. Iyengar on stage at the Barbican Theatre in Central London in 1984 (photograph courtesy of the Iyengar Yoga Institute Maida Vale in London).

Iyengar method of yoga is taught do not contain a stage-like structure. However, a stage area does feature at the Iyengar "home institute" in Pune (Ramamani Iyengar Memorial Yoga Institute or RIMYI). The yoga studio here is a purpose-built room which also features eight columns to symbolise Patañjali's *aṣṭāṅga* (eight limbed) description of yoga. In addition to serving as a traditional stage for events and celebrations, during the course of a normal class, RIMYI teachers and their students may stand on the stage to demonstrate "correct" actions, extensions and alignment to be visible to the entire class. In the pedagogical model of the Iyengar method of yoga, the correct actions, extensions and alignments must be felt proprioceptively, but also teachers must be able to see if their students are embodying subtle physical actions. The performance of particular *āsana*-s by students forms part of the pedagogic framework to enable a multi-faceted understanding of *āsana*. The stage is also used in Iyengar classes as a piece of equipment to assist and enhance the actions of particular postures: to drop back to, or lean over with in backbends, to hang over in an inversion, or perhaps as a ledge for leg raises. From the early 1970s Iyengar was well known for emphasizing how household objects and walls, as well as gymnasium equipment could be used as an aid towards improving yoga *āsana*-s.[10]

10 There are a series of articles about Iyengar teaching with "found" props such as walls, in *Yoga & Health* (1971–1975).

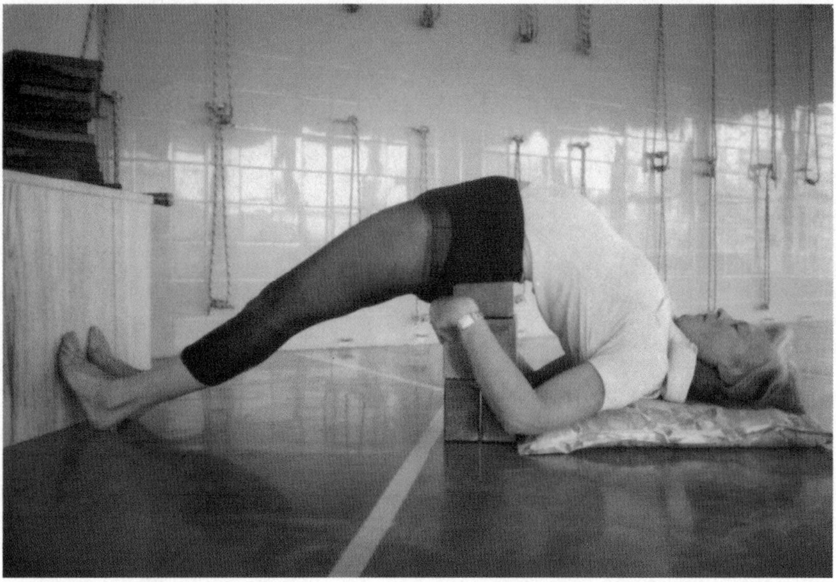

Figure 3: Diana Clifton using the stage at RIMYI in Pune as a "prop" for self-practice in 1977 (photograph courtesy of the Iyengar Yoga Association [UK] Archives Committee).

Lefebvre's analysis of the production of space emphasises the social construction and re-construction of spaces (1991). This can be seen to be recapitulated in the above uses of the stage – the architects, builders and engineers designed the structure to function for certain expected uses (for people to stand and perform upon), but the structure is re-used for different purposes (e.g., as a yoga prop), and the same space is imagined to hold different meanings by different people (an area for clarity in demonstration, the popularisation of a sacred art or an exhibition of contortionism). What the stage *is* can only be understood in context of what it is doing. While a "functional" stage necessitates a separation between performers and audience, this difference can serve a variety of purposes (e.g., art performance, teaching, exhibitionism, attracting attention for a political campaign etc.) and of course it is experienced and evaluated in many different ways by the individuals involved. Meanwhile, the physical object of the stage in Iyengar classes is also reinvented as a ledge for sitting, a "prop" for backdrops or backbends, or its edge can form a wall for the foot to push against. Here the physical object itself is conceptualised as a tool for teaching and assisting in the development of inner proprioceptive awareness.

The diversity of uses for the stage in Iyengar's presentation of yoga is illustrative of a contentious area – is yoga primarily internal or external? Is it for public presentation or a matter of sacred, inner contemplation and experience?

3. Yoga in Schools: Encinitas School District Yoga

Another place where yoga is periodically controversial is when it appears in children's educational establishments.[11] Schools are a particularly emotionally charged physical and social space, where a community sends its children to learn the skills and values considered most essential to successful participation in that particular society. As in other locations, central to the debate on what yoga is are concerns where to draw the lines between public and private; sacred and profane; religious and secular. A particularly salient example of how exploring yoga in a particular physical space can illuminate the multiplicity of social and conceptual placements of yoga is encapsulated in the lawsuit brought against the teaching of yoga in California's Encinitas School District during 2013.

In 2011, the Encinitas School District accepted a grant from an organisation called the Jois Foundation to teach a version of its yoga programme to school children.[12] The Jois Foundation was established in 2011 largely on the initiative of Sonia Tutor Jones, a practitioner of the yoga taught by Pattabhi Jois (1915–2009), described as Ashtanga Vinyasa Yoga or often just "Ashtanga" yoga. Sonia Tutor Jones is also the wife of billionaire hedge-fund investor Paul Tutor Jones II of Tudor Investment Corp. The beliefs and practices of Jois' very physical, flowing yoga practice-lineage have received a fair amount of academic attention since becoming an influential "style" of yoga outside India since the 1970s, becoming particularly popular from the 1990s onwards.[13] This was an interesting place from which to launch a large yoga-in-schools initiative as the Jois lineage is not the most secular of contemporary Modern Postural Yoga schools[14] with many senior practitioners emphasising that strict adherence to the series of postures, done correctly over many years, will solve both physical ailments and lead to liberation. However, the Jois Foundation took a more flexible approach to its initiative to promote yoga in schools with aims to promote a "holistic" and "mind-body" approach to students' health and wellbeing. The Taylor Jones' have also given large donations to the Contemplative Sciences Centre at the University of Virginia who are seeking to empirically examine the effectiveness of various "contemplative" activities that are widely believed to promote health and well-

---

11 In general the role of yoga and educational institutions has been under-researched from social scientific and social historical perspectives. But for the development of Iyengar yoga in the British Adult Education framework see Newcombe 2007, 2008, and 2014, and for comments on yoga in German schools Augenstein 2013.

12 The first classes were piloted in Capri Elementary School in Encinitas, California in 2011 and expanded into more elementary schools in 2012. The original grant was for US$ 533,720 over three years to cover teaching for up to 5,600 students in the Encinitas Union School District (Spagat 2013).

13 Burger 2006; Byrne 2014; Nichter 2013; Nevrin 2008; Smith 2004, 2007, 2008.

14 De Michelis 2004: 187–189.

ness. In fact, the Taylor Jones' philanthropic agenda is broader than simply an alliance to the lineage of Pattabhi Jois' teaching, which was reflected in a change of name from the Jois Foundation to the Sonima Foundation in 2013.

The yoga programme offered in the Encinitas School District was introduced as a "life skills curriculum" that included discussions of ethics, nutrition, general wellness and character development. The school district and supportive parents emphasised the promotion of health and well-being as the goal of the programme and denied it having a religious nature. The Foundation argued that through two thirty-minute yoga sessions a week and some "character training" sessions based on the ethical principles of the *yama* and *niyama,* there might be widespread benefits for students. Everything from reductions in diabetic symptoms, behaviour problems in class, a decline in obesity, and higher standardised test scores were suggested as potential benefits. In addition to offering the money for the classes, the Jois Foundation intended to test specific health and wellness claims with University of San Diego-led research on the efficacy of the programme in meeting these goals (CEPAL 2014).

However, even before the pilot class was launched in the Capri Elementary School, parents of some students were objecting to the very idea that yoga could be taught to their children. The "Sedlock parents" represented a group of objecting parents supported pro-bono by The National Centre for Law and Policy (NCLP), an non-profit legal group supporting "the protection and promotion of religious freedom, the sanctity of life, traditional marriage, parental rights, and other civil liberties" which is closely associated with ideological positions of contemporary neo-conservative politics and conservative Christian faith (NCLP 2014). They argued that the Jois Foundation was deeply committed to "Ashtanga Yoga" which, the plaintiffs asserted, has its roots in Hinduism and therefore was inseparable from Hinduism.[15] The religious studies scholar Candy Gunther Brown argued for the plaintiffs; in her expert witness statement she testified that in Hinduism, bodily movement and ritual carry an essence of religiosity independent of beliefs. She held that any *āsana* – for example, the sun salutation – is infused with the essence of "Hindu" religiosity (Brown 2013a).[16] Here, Brown is offering an example of an essentialist understanding of yoga, based on her own ideological and political positioning.

In response to Brown's essentialist proposal, it is important to also consider the significance of the internal meaning to the actor. For example, walking into a church and sitting still is not necessarily a religious act – one can enter from any

15 DiBono 2013; Broyles 2013.

16 Her testimony can also be seen as publicity for her book (Brown 2013b) that discusses how the healing involved with a variety of alternative and complementary medicine practices entails beliefs and worldviews that might have complex and contested relationships with other belief systems – particularly Christianity.

number of internal positions – as a sceptic, as a sociologist, as a sympathetic friend, or for private prayer and contemplation. An internal position may shift unexpectedly – but it is equally inappropriate to assume a religious or a secular meaning to any physical movement made by an individual as far as the internal experience of the individual is concerned. It may also be relevant to consider the internal position of the "teacher" as significant for those who wish to participate or critique the practice – something that may or may not be obvious in the way the material is presented.[17] The significance of this point will be discussed further in the next section of the chapter.

The presiding judge made his judgment on the case of Sedlock vs. Baird on 1 July 2013; this was not a jury trial. Judge Meyer agreed with the plaintiff's expert witness, Candy Gunther Brown, that yoga (in principle) was religious. However Judge Meyer applied a legal precedent, called the Lemon Test (*Lemon v. Kurtzman* 1971), to argue that the programme (1) was not undertaken with the intention of propagating religion, (2) that there wasn't strong evidence that a view of "pro-Eastern religion" or "anti-Western religion" was taught and that (3) the school district has complete control over the curriculum and teachers. It was considered particularly significant that the intention was neither to propagate nor denigrate any religious beliefs and that the school district, not the funding body, had ultimate control over the curriculum taught.[18] Therefore Judge Meyer found that the classes did not represent a challenge to the US legal requirement that there be a separation between church and state.[19] This provides an (arguably) clear legal position relative to the concepts of religious and secular of what Judge Meyer termed "EUSD yoga – that is – Encinitas United School District yoga".[20]

Judge Meyer's conclusion highlighted that the objecting parents had defined yoga through their Christian beliefs and what they had read about yoga on the Internet – the Judge specifically called the plaintiffs' complaints "Trial by Wikipedia" and believed that the legal fiction of an "objective child" would not "perceive religion in EUSD yoga".[21] Judge Meyer implied that the plaintiffs' po-

17 This point was also made by a journalist in relation to the Encinitas Yoga trial (Thompson 2013).

18 The issue of control of curriculum was seen as an essential difference from *Malick vs. Yogi* (1978) which ruled that teaching yoga in form of the Maharishi Mahesh Yogi's Science of Creative Intelligence in the New Jersey public school system was a violation of the First Amendment; here the curriculum in question was neither open to public scrutiny nor modification by the school district.

19 Meyer 2013: 13–16.

20 Although the expert witness Brown disagrees; she wrote an article in the *Huffington Post* in response to the verdict (Brown 2013c). The 2015 appeal decision more unambiguously stated that, "After reviewing the evidence, the court of appeal agreed that a reasonable observer would view the content of the district's yoga program as being entirely secular" (Aaron 2015).

21 Meyer 2013: 19.

sition was ideologically and not experientially based; their objections to yoga were based in their own ideas of what yoga is or is not. In Encinitas you can clearly see the same curriculum – which all sides agree to call "yoga" – being defined in an essentialist way as "religious" by the plaintiffs and non-religious by the defendants. In contrast, the judge took what I am going to call a situationalist definition, considering a unique case by specific criteria.

The result of this trial is revealing of the complex and contested positioning that yoga holds in contemporary society. The same curriculum, called "yoga" by both the plaintiffs and defendants in this case, was held to be radically different in nature by each group. For the plaintiffs, yoga is essentially religious and for the defendants yoga (at least in this case) is a secular way to promote health and well-being. So how can we understand what yoga is conceptually?

In order to understand the situational, and contested definitions exemplified by *Sedlock v. Baird*, I will borrow from Kim Knott's spatial theories, in particular Knott's diagram of "The Religious/Secular Field and its Force Relationships" which helps envision a more metaphorical spatial relationship between the religious, the secular, and the post-secular.[22]

4. Mappings of Space: Maps and the Spatial Theory

As one looks at particular local articulations of religious or spiritual meaning, the more these concrete (physical locations) and abstract realms (ideological positions) become interconnected. In his far-reaching Marxist spatial analysis Lefebvre declares that "its [space's] effects may be observed on all planes and in all the interconnections between them [...]" and that the effect and importance of space cannot be restricted to any single methodology or academic discipline.[23] Drawing on Lefebvre, Kim Knott has been interested in understanding religion through what she calls a "spatial analysis". Her analysis began at looking where religion is located both in geographical locations and built-environment places, but quickly realised the importance of considering "cultural spaces" and "ideological positions". As many commentators on architecture and space have pointed out, while in some respects human activity is constrained by the immediate physical environment, humans constantly recreate, and subvert apparent restrictions. For example, a building's usages change and adapt from the original building plans; spaces are re-designed to suit new social uses.

Kim Knott has used her model of spatial analysis to illustrate the contested areas of religious, secular and "post-secular" understandings in contemporary

22 Lefebvre 1991 and Knott 2005: 125.
23 Lefebvre 1991: 412.

societies. To better conceptualise and "map" the dialectical relationships between sacred and secular, Knott has created a triangular diagram reconstructed below:

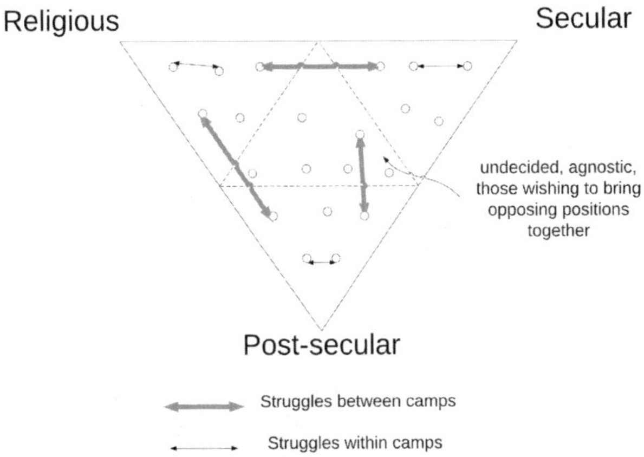

Figure 4: From Kim Knott's "The Religious/Secular Field, and its Force Relationships" (2005: 125). Reprinted with permission from Kim Knott.

The small dots represent individuals or institutional actors. Everyone in every place could potentially be mapped onto this grid, holding some kind of position in relation to the religious. Knott holds that within this field "four areas or camps can be seen: religious, secular, post-secular and the middle-ground – which includes the undecided, the deliberately agnostic, and those who desire to build bridges."[24] The downward point of Knott's triangle is labelled "post-secular". This is a way of addressing the activities, popular in the "late-modern West", that are neither the traditionally religious, nor clearly secular and might include things classified as new age, spiritual, holistic or other ways of "returning" to the sacred influenced by post-modern understandings of the world. While this idea of "post-Secular" might be a useful way of characterizing one "polarity" of the religious vs. secular dialectic in contemporary Western society more generally, James Beckford had skilfully demonstrated how it is also a problematic concept.[25]

While Lefebvre was primarily concerned with how the space of neo-liberal, capitalistic society was produced, Knott has applied the idea of spatial analysis to the subject of specifically religious and spiritual locations and practices. Knott suggests this diagram describes a field where power and knowledge is expressed and contested, in which "deeply held views and values […] mark out the territorial areas and lines of engagement within it". These controversies "occur in

24 Knott 2005: 125.
25 Knott 2005: 71–77 and Beckford 2012.

space and, as such, the places they occupy are amenable to spatial analysis".[26] Knott holds that there is no position outside these relationships; all actors and commentators are somehow positioned in this "field" that is dialectical and not merely oppositional. That is to say, although some positions, or actors, in yoga may present themselves as antagonistic to other actors, closer analysis can show that both positions are created through relationship with the other, and many positions also depend on relationships which are much less antagonistic. All the various actors and understandings are positioned in dialogue with other possible positions and the complexity of the relationship between positions must be considered for a more comprehensive synthesis of meaning to emerge.

Thinking more closely about the physical and metaphorical spaces that yoga occupies in the contemporary world, I have adjusted Knott's diagram:

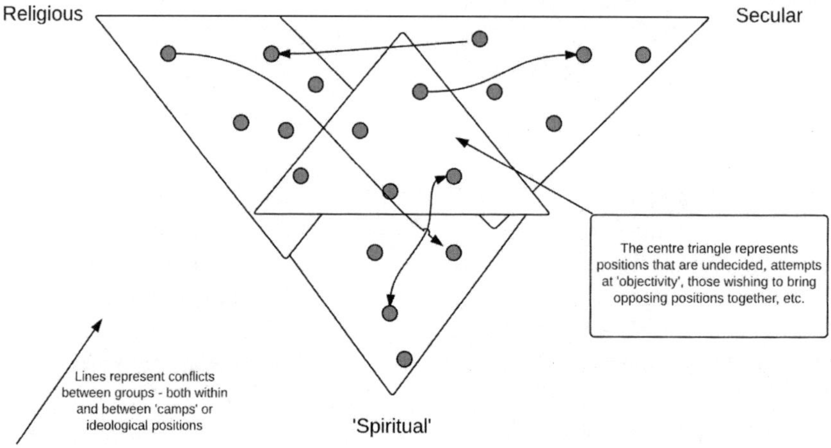

Figure 5: Yoga Religious/Secular Field and its Force Relationships.

This spatial analysis of yoga creates a less tidy "map" than Knott's template. The Yoga Sacred vs. Secular Field contains the dialectics of Knott's triangle. The "post-secular" pole at the bottom has been replaced with "spiritual" as many yoga teachers report their practice to be "spiritual but not religious" or variations on that idea.[27] The significant central triangle area in this map incorporates some academic positions, but at times, academic positions are coloured by underlying assumptions and ideological positions on one of the "poles" or points of the triangle. Additionally yoga practitioners, whose personal practice has a definite placement on the triangle, might also adopt more "objective", "neutral" and

26 Knott 2005: 125.

27 This was a theme in my oral history interviews of yoga practitioners in Britain (Newcombe 2008: 197–226).

bridge-building perspectives as they interact with others or attempt to understand more objectively the history and diversity of what is called "yoga". This overlap necessitates the incorporation of Venn-diagram style overlaps of the internal triangles. Although this is certainly not the only way to conceptualise yoga, every local expression, personal practice, or ideological placement of what yoga "is" could be understood as having a place somewhere in the largest triangular field. Any one position is determined, in part, through a dialogue and interaction with other positions on the diagram.

Thinking about the Encinitas yoga trail, this diagram helps one understand how each opposing side placed the same EUSD yoga curriculum definitively in different places in this diagram. Each side had a deeply held belief about what yoga is, but in practice, the yoga curriculum was modified due to parental objections and the lived experience changed because of the public debate and lawsuit. Looking at this case as a whole, yoga cannot be seen as a fixed thing – depending on where you stand, like in a hall of mirrors, what people are *doing* as yoga can be viewed as resting in quite a few different places in the map. This spatial mapping of yoga is messy, imprecise, and subject to debate. However, by introducing this Religious vs. Secular mapping to yoga (and the idea of special analysis more generally), a conceptual framework begins to emerge where the complex positioning of individuals and traditions in the contemporary world can be visualised, discussed and acknowledged.[28]

We will now turn our attention to another contested location for yoga in contemporary society.

5. Private Space and the Imagined Yoga Tradition

Many individuals who have been involved with teaching or practising yoga for decades have a particular understanding and definition of "authentic yoga" based on their own involvement with the subject. Sometimes this sentiment finds expression in contrast with what is considered "not yogic" or at least "not *real* yoga". Most of these practitioners have had profound and transforming personal experiences that they have experienced by practising something called yoga.[29]

28 As much as I would like to have a "bird's eye view", as Knott (2005) emphasises, in arguing this position I am attempting to position myself in the central triangle of this spatial diagram – that of someone who wishes to build bridges and bring antagonistic positions towards a more common understanding. From this central position, I attempt to accurately observe and understand all other positions within the descriptions of "yoga" as accurately as possible.

29 Since 2002, I have formally interviewed over thirty people who were involved in forming the practice of yoga in Britain from the 1960s to the 1990s and dozens more who are involved in a contemporary yoga practice.

There are two aspects of this – the first is that often when people speak of what yoga is or is not, they have some idea of what yoga should be. This idea in their head is an ideal from which they judge their practice – and how they judge the practice of others. Wilfred Clark, founder of the British Wheel of Yoga, talked a lot in the early journals about "True Yoga" with a capital "T" – that could not be divorced from the study of philosophy. True Yoga for Wilfred Clark and many others equates to "union with God".[30] This mental positioning of a "True vs. False" yoga, can also be understood as a continuation of the narrative of yogis coming out of colonial India – which populated popular imagination of "yogis" with deceitful fakirs, dangerous magicians as well as ideas of respectable teachers and highly realised ascetics with super-natural abilities.[31]

In my research I found a tendency for people in the yoga world to say, agreeably, "it's all yoga" except when they find something they disagree with – which is then categorised as not being "TRUE yoga". This conceptual framework of "True vs. False" yoga contains many similarities across traditions – "true" yoga is usually something "more than physical" and makes reference to Patañjali's *Yogasūtra, samādhi,* and/or an idea of "union with the divine". Usually objections have to do with accusations of commodification, sexualisation, westernisation, or secularisation of the practices.[32] But there are also passionate differences on both goals and techniques, what are appropriate *kriya* (cleansing) practices, how much emphasis there should be on the "more than physical" aspects of the practice, if postures (*āsana*-s) and/or breathing techniques (*prāṇāyāma*-s) should be practised before a firm grounding in the ethical framework (*yama* and *niyama*) is established. Each and every one of these practices has been described by someone as "True Yoga" or "real yoga" – in contrast to an imagined "fraudulent yoga".

Every individual's "True Yoga" differs in shade and colour to the next person's; some are populated by deities, others by emptiness, yet others by the primacy of health and wellness as goals. Some of these places are reached by intense physical practice, others by mystical visions within quiet contemplation or relaxation. Although it could be also argued there is great conformity in assumptions about yoga's aims and means, practitioners can become passionate about seemingly minor differences in doctrine or practice. While in some contexts, this differentiation could be read as a marketing technique,[33] practitioners are also often making deeply felt theological and practical distinctions. This

30 Newcombe 2008: 72 and 198–206.

31 White 2009 and Singleton 2010: 35–54.

32 Matthew Remski (2014) is in the process of doing interesting work on the experience and rationalisation of injury by contemporary yoga practitioners.

33 Jain 2014b.

imagined positioning of "True Yoga" is important to take note of – and to take seriously.

Yet, if we want to present ourselves as aiming for an objective understanding – positioning ourselves in the centre of this spatial triangle metaphor – it is important that we remember the "No-True-Scotsman Move" or logical fallacy. This error of argument was well described by the British philosopher Anthony Flew, who explained "the essence of the move consists in sliding between two radically different interpretations of the same or very similar forms of words."[34] A short way of explaining this fallacy is as follows:

Person One: Every Scotsman loves whiskey.

Person Two: But my friend is Scottish and he hates whiskey.

Person One: Oh, but every TRUE Scotsman loves whiskey.

In contemporary yoga milieus there is both a superficial tolerance for a diversity of traditions and practices as well as a logical move to set apart and define a specific practice as more "yogic" than the alternatives.

In some respects, the experiential referent of the word "yoga" is unique for every individual. Used in this way the word yoga could be seen as an example of Wittgenstein "private language".[35] Yoga is a symbol that refers to real experiences – but experiences that are essentially untranslatable. There are clear patterns and resemblances to do with the way the word "yoga" is used; we know the sort of thing people are talking about. Again following Wittgenstein, the word yoga can be understood as a kaleidoscopic pattern of family resemblances[36].[37] Practitioners derive their understanding of "True Yoga" from a particular tradition and personal experiences. Teachers and students of a particular yoga will understand and present that tradition somewhat differently from the guru and other practitioners of that school. It is a mistake therefore to use private experience and personal understanding as a basis of an essentialist definition of what Yoga "truly is".

However, "True Yoga" is a sacred place – in the Durkheimian sense of the word – a place set apart and forbidden.[38] In what way forbidden? In my experience, it is

34 Flew 1975: 48.

35 Wittgenstein 2001, §§ 243–271.

36 Wittgenstein 2001, §§ 65–71.

37 Although central to Wittgenstein's philosophy, the basic idea of family resemblances also predates Wittgenstein and has been found in the work of John Stuart Mills, Friedrich Nietzsche, Lev Vygotsky and Władysław Tatarkiewicz, amongst others. Another way of understanding might be offered by Hilary Lawson's concept of "linguistic closure", which, Lawson (2001) argues, is what we do to make sense of a world that is open. When we present one definitional understanding of yoga, it either incorporates or excludes other possibilities – it is a decision to make a task, or understanding more manageable.

38 Durkheim (1995: 44): "A religion is a unified system of beliefs and practices relative to sacred things, that is to say, things set apart and forbidden."

an imagined understanding often approached with metaphors and stories, but consisting of insights that are hard to verbalise and share with others. Perhaps here is the heart of many religious experiences. As such, the place of "True Yoga" needs to be treated with both respect and curiosity. This is a description of a place of deep meaning and transformation for those who articulate it. The idea of "True Yoga" for the practitioner is an attempt to identify and protect an experience of holiness and meaning, that may have deep significance for their lives and worldview.

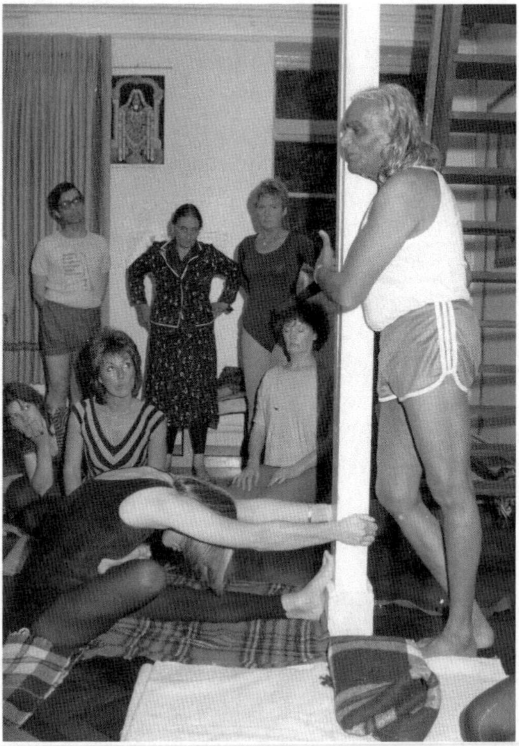

Figure 6: B. K. S. Iyengar teaching in the first Iyengar Yoga Institute in Maida Vale in 1983, a former artists' studio. Note the use of the existing pillar for pedagogical purposes (photograph: Silvia Prescott, courtesy of the Iyengar Yoga Institute Maida Vale, London).

The ubiquitous "yoga mat" which appeared sometime in the 1980s has become associated with a portable sacred space. A number of these mats are seen clearly in Figure 1, they are slightly sticky to avoid sliding while holding various postures. They separate out the "personal space" of each individual in the room and give a sense of privacy to the internal experience of the person on the mat. Elizabeth De Michelis has described the ritual elements of contemporary globalised yoga as a "healing ritual of secular religion".[39] The yoga mat has become a ritual space where physical and psychological re-orientations (often experienced as "healing") are enacted. Although often performed in public, the limits of a personal mat are often experienced as a deeply personal location. There is a sacredness of this experience, that many practitioners feel must be guarded from prying eyes and disrespectful thoughts in order for the practitioner's journey to continue. All the tension and acrimonious allusions between yoga practitioners of "this is not yogic", "yoga teachers should not sell their skills for profit – that's not True Yoga", "True Yoga is never [...]" could be seen as individuals protecting their sacred space.

6. The Studio Space

As touched upon in the introduction, there are a wide variety of ways of physically accommodating a space for yoga within the home – from a dedicated practice room with religious iconography, to an empty corner with space for a yoga mat, to no obvious space at all for the practice, which is somehow fitted around oversized furniture and television screens. Lefebvre argued that every society produces its own unique arrangement of space and that it would be surprising to find a real society that did not produce a distinctive space. Although yoga can be found potentially in any space, the culture of contemporary yoga practice *is* producing a particular kind of physical space: the yoga *studio.*

"Studio" is a particularly apt description of many of the physical spaces used for a dedicated yoga practice in the developed world. The word "studio" became popular in English in the nineteenth century to describe the work place of artists. But it is also a word with other meanings: is also used to describe the work places of filmmakers, musicians, and one-room living quarters. Many commercial yoga spaces and also martial arts centres are referred to as studios. In contemporary English-speaking countries the yoga "studio" may refer just to the entire centre or simply the room where yoga is practised. In a commercial yoga venue, there may be several such studio rooms, while the building as a whole is known by a brand name. In large commercial yoga venues there is usually an entrance space (where monetary transactions occur), toilets, and an area or room(s) for changing clothes. Larger centres also may have small shops for yoga-related books and equipment, cafes, meditation rooms, and possibly therapy rooms for other complementary treatments, e.g., massage, osteopathy, chiropractic, and/or Ayurvedic treatments. Rather than studios, these areas for therapy are typically called "treatment rooms", perhaps underlying the active involvement of the

39 De Michelis 2004: 252–257.

practitioner in the yoga experience, in contrast to an individual being a passive recipient of the work of a therapist in the other rooms. Some studio spaces can be mapped explicitly on the religious side of the conceptual triangle, including images of deities and/or guru figures. Other studio spaces are absent of overt ideological symbols, aiming for a more secular impression. Often there is a fudging of relatively neutral symbols, like the sound Om in Sanskrit or a figure that is meditating, which leave a "post-secular" or "spiritual" impression without pointing towards any specific affiliation. The ubiquitous spacious and "blank" aesthetics found in contemporary yoga studios, described at the beginning of this chapter lend themselves to a multitude of creative interpretations.

Like the contemporary yoga studio, there is a curious bridging of dichotomies in the space conceptualised as an artist's studio. A studio is the private space of creation and a space sometimes opened to the public for the sale of art, in order to support more creation. Here the controversy about the sale of yoga finds a close parallel. Do artists "sell out" when they produce popular, but inferior works to feed themselves? Artists often seek out light and space for their studio spaces – like the rooms of modern yoga practitioners. There is also a curious continuum between cluttered and empty workspaces where the art is produced. Yoga spaces often aim a feeling of spaciousness, while also sometimes moving towards clutter with images of deities and props to assist the transformative process. It is not without accident that some of the first dedicated yoga-teaching spaces in Europe, e.g. the space used by Selvarajan Yesudian in Geneva during the 1940s and the first dedicated Iyengar Yoga Institute in London were previously used by artists as studios.[40]

The artists' studio, like the yoga studio is a space of creation and transformation, of highly disciplined practices and of unpredictable insight and creativity. In these spaces, yoga practitioners seek to transform themselves – often in ways that they can only intuit and not necessarily articulate. Contemporary yoga practitioners work on themselves as they might on a work of art, where the process itself is often viewed as significant as anything that is actually produced. What the actual work is, what it aims to create and represent, and how others see it is as varied for the yoga practitioner as it is for the artist.

40 I would like to thank Cathryn Keller for sharing this historical information on Yesudian and her enthusiasm about studio spaces more generally.

7. Conclusions

The spaces that yoga occupies in contemporary society are many and various. This presentation only touched upon some of the many activities called yoga by different groups of people. I hope that by looking at some of the places where yoga is practised and at the meanings given to the use of those spaces, some of the narratives about what "is" and "is not" yoga will be enriched by a broader understanding. Yoga is presented in particular ways depending on the requirements of particular social or physical locations.

Although there is an ideal that yoga can be practised anywhere, at any time, some spaces cost money, others need to maintain an income in order to focus on their practice – the space of the market place puts pressure on the shape and places occupied by yoga. Likewise, the intentions and internal experiences behind any practice are hard to access. The imagined meanings and significance of the practice add another layer of complexity to understanding the placement of yoga in contemporary society.

Yoga cannot be reduced to a religious practice. It cannot be reduced to a spiritual practice, or a secular practice. It is often intensely private, but it can also be a social and political act. It has genealogies of historical continuity and spontaneous re-inventions that are glossed with narratives of tradition. Conceptualizing yoga as a lived space occupying all positions from sacred to secular – public and private – opens up a view of yoga that is non-linear and non-essentialist. If one looks at yoga from all the spatial positions it can occupy it is obvious that yoga is immensely flexible and amorphous.

In academic articles and media reports alike, there is pressure to define yoga. A standard narrative might touch on Indus valley seals, ascetic practices in the first century BCE, the codification of Patañjali's *sūtra*-s, various Tantric and Haṭha developments, into more modern accommodations with scientific worldviews. Writing this linear introduction to what yoga is often feels unavoidable and perhaps it is necessary. But this standard piece places the researcher in an ideological position that may obfuscate other aspects of critical observation. The essentialist, linear narrative legitimates *and* delegitimises a variety of political positions of actors involved with yoga globally.

With this analysis I hope to draw attention to the positioning of academic researchers, as well as yoga practitioners into this highly contested field of definitions, narratives and politics. Historical narratives and normative discourses defining what yoga "is" and "is not" can both reveal and obfuscate ideological positioning and underlying assumptions of the speakers. Often unspoken assumptions and essentialist understandings of yoga lead to different traditions speaking at cross-purposes, unable to engage in dialogue, or actively antagonistic towards other understandings of the practice.

Complicating definitions of yoga – understanding yoga in non-essentialist, but in instrumental, situational terms – is important. These diverse practices called "yoga" can be a space for radical transformations of consciousness, the expression of religious sentiment, means for commercial profit, a way of crafting the physical body or establishing a social persona and every space in between. If we enquire more into where yoga is practised and what people are doing with their practices, rather than what yoga *is*, we might find more space for dialogue. It is only by considering yoga in precise locations that statements about yoga's significance and effects can have any meaning.

References

Aaron, J. (2015). *Sedlock vs Baird.* The Court of Appeal of the State of California Fourth Appellate District, Division One. (14 C.D.O.S. 3394) 6 April 2015. http://www.therecorder.com/id=1202722729490/Sedlock-v-Baird?slreturn=20160431051312. Accessed 31 May 2016.

Alter, J. (2004). *Yoga in Modern India: The Body Between Science and Philosophy.* Oxford: Princeton University Press.

Alter, J. (2008). Yoga Shivir: Performativity and the Study of Modern Yoga. In M. Singleton & J. Byrne (Eds.), *Yoga in the Modern World: Contemporary Perspectives* (pp. 36–48). London: Routledge.

Augenstein, S. (2013). The Introduction of Yoga in German Schools: A Case Study. In B. Hauser (Ed.), *Yoga Traveling: Bodily Practice in Transcultural Perspective* (pp. 155–172). Heidelberg: Springer.

Beckerlegge, G. (2013). Chapter 3: Unifying Consciousness, Unifying the Nation: Competing Visions of the Future of India and Yoga Tradition. In H. Beattie (Ed.), *Controversial Futures* (pp. 94–140). Milton Keynes: Open University Press.

Beckford, J. (2012). SSSR Presidential Address Public Religions and the Postsecular: Critical Reflections. *Journal for the Scientific Study of Religion, 51*(1), 1–19.

Brown, C. G. (2013a). Declaration of Candy Gunther Brown. *Sedlock v. Baird.* Case No. 37-2013-00035910-CU-MC-CTL. ICJ: C-61. Superior Court of the State of California for the County of San Diego – Central Division. 8 February 2013. http://www.nclplaw.org/wp-content/uploads/2011/12/DECLARATION-OF-CANDY-BROWN-FINAL.pdf. Accessed 3 July 2014.

Brown, C. G. (2013b). *Healing Gods: Complementary and Alternative Medicine in Christian America.* New York: Oxford University Press.

Brown, C. G. (2013c). Yoga Can Stay in School: Looking More Closely at the Encinitas Yoga Trial Decision. *The Huffington Post,* 2 July 2013. http://www.huffingtonpost.com/candy-gunther-brown-phd/what-made-the-encinitas-p_b_3522836.html. Accessed 3 July 2014.

Broyles, D. R. (2013). Verified Petition for Writ of Mandamus; Complaint for Injunctive and Declaratory Relief. *Sedlock v. Baird.* http://www.casewatch.org/civil/yoga/complaint.pdf. Accessed 1 July 2014.

Burger, M. (2006). What Price Salvation? The Exchange of Salvation Goods Between India and the West. *Social Compass, 53*(1), 81–95.

Burger, M. (2013). Sāṃkhya Interpretation in a Transnational Perspective: Śrī Anirvāṇa and Lizelle Reymond. Paper given at "Yoga in Transformation: Historical and Contemporary Perspectives on a Global Phenomenon", University of Vienna, 20 September.

Byrne, J. (2014). "Authorized by Sri K. Pattabhi Jois": the Role of *Paramparā* and Lineage in Ashtanga Vinyasa Yoga. In M. Singleton & E. Goldberg (Eds.), *Gurus of Modern Yoga* (pp. 107–121). New York: Oxford University Press.

CEPL – Centre for Education Policy and Law at the University of San Diego (2014). Yoga in Public Schools: Evidence from the Encinitas Union School District's Yoga Program 2012–2013. https://lib.sandiego.edu/soles/documents/EUSD%20Yoga%20Student%20Effects%202012-13%20Formattedforwebsite.pdf. Accessed 2 July 2014.

De Michelis, E. (2004). *A History of Modern Yoga: Patañjali and Western Esotericism.* London: Continuum.

DiBono, M. (2013). District Adds Yoga to All Schools Despite Opposition. KSWB San Diego News (Fox5 SanDiego.com), 3 January 2013. http://www.coastlawgroup.com/portfolio/district-adds-yoga-to-all-schools-despite-opposition/. Accessed 2 July 2014.

Durkheim, E. (1995). *The Elementary Forms of Religious Life*, trans. K. E. Fields. New York: The Free Press.

Fish, A. (2006). The Commodification and Exchange of Knowledge in the Case of Transnational Commercial Yoga. *International Journal of Cultural Property, 13*(2), 194–201.

Fleetwood, P. (2012). Podcast: Mgr Peter Fleetwood on Eastern Meditation. *The Catholic Church in England and Wales.* http://www.catholicnews.org.uk/Home/Podcasts/Catholic-News/Catholic-News-Podcasts-2012/Eastern-Meditation. Accessed 1 July 2014.

Flew, A. (1975). *Thinking About Thinking or, Do I Sincerely Want to Be Right?* London: Fontana Press.

Forshee, S. (2016). GC of Bikram Yoga Wins $7.3 Million in Sexual Harassment Case. *Law.Com* http://www.law.com/sites/articles/2016/01/26/gc-of-bikram-yoga-wins-7-3-million-in-sexual-harassment-case/#ixzz4ADspG2gY. Accessed 31 May 2016.

Hauser, B. (2013). Touching the Limits, Assessing Pain: On Language, Performativity, Health and Well-Being in Yoga Classes. In B. Hauser (Ed.), *Yoga Traveling: Bodily Practice in Transcultural Perspective* (pp. 109–134). Heidelberg: Springer.

Hindu American Foundation (HAF) (2014a). Yoga Beyond Asana: Hindu Thought In Practice. http://hafsite.org/media/pr/yoga-hindu-origins. Accessed 20 May 2014.

Hindu American Foundation (HAF) (2014b). Take Back Yoga. http://hafsite.org/media/pr/takeyogaback. Accessed 20 May 2014.

Hindu American Foundation (HAF) (2014c). Yoga in Public Schools: An Addendum. http://hafsite.org/media/pr/yoga-public-school. Accessed 20 May 2014.

Jain, A. (2012). The Malleability of Yoga: A Response to Christian and Hindu Opponents of the Popularization of Yoga. *Journal of Hindu-Christian Studies, 25,* 3–10.

Jain, A. (2014a). Who Is to Say Modern Yoga Practitioners Have It All Wrong? On Hindu Origins and Yogaphobia. *Journal of the American Academy of Religion, 82*(2), 427–471.

Jain, A. (2014b). *Selling Yoga: From Counterculture to Pop Culture.* New York: Oxford University Press.

Knott, K. (2005). *The Location of Religion: A Spatial Analysis.* Durham: Acumen.

Lawson, H. (2001). *Closure: A Story of Everything.* London: Routledge.
Lefebvre, H. (1991). *The Production of Space,* trans. D. Nicholson-Smith. Oxford: Blackwell Publishing.
Lemon v. Kurtzman ("*Lemon*") (1971). 403 U.S. 602.
Meyer, Judge J. S. (2013). Statement of Decision. *Sedlock v. Baird.* Case No. 37-2013-00035910-CU-MC-CTL. ICJ: C-61. Superior Court of the State of California for the County of San Diego – Central Division. 23 September 2013. http://kpbs.media.clients.ellingtoncms.com/news/documents/2013/10/31/https___roa.sdcourt.ca.gov_roa_faces_userdocs_0202A0DAD9F6549993F3B9E36003F72F_37-2013-00035910-CU-MC-CTL_ROA-113_09-23-13_Statement_of_Decision_1383242027390.pdf. Accessed 4 July 2014.
Mohler, A. (2010). The Subtle Body: Should Christians Practice Yoga? http://www.albertmohler.com/2010/09/20/the-subtle-body-should-christians-practice-yoga/. Accessed 2 July 2014.
National Centre for Law and Policy (NCLP) (2014). Homepage. http://www.nclplaw.org/. Accessed 2 July 2014.
National Council of Hindu Temples (UK) (2014). Yoga – Not a Part of Hinduism? http://www.nchtuk.org/index.php/extensions/s5-image-and-content-fader/yoga-not-a-part-of-hinduism. Accessed 20 May 2014.
Nevrin, K. (2008). Empowerment and Using the Body in Modern Postural Yoga. In M. Singleton & J. Byrne (Eds.), *Yoga in the Modern World: Contemporary Perspectives* (pp. 119–139). London: Routledge.
Newcombe, S. (2007). Stretching for Health and Well-Being: Yoga and Women in Britain, 1960–1980 *Asian Medicine: Tradition and Modernity, 3*(1), 37–63.
Newcombe, S. (2008). A Social History of Yoga and Ayurveda in Britain, 1950–1995. Unpublished PhD dissertation. University of Cambridge.
Newcombe, S. (2014). The Institutionalization of the Yoga Tradition: 'Gurus' B. K. S. Iyengar and Yogini Sunita in Britain. In M. Singleton & E. Goldberg (Eds.), *Gurus of Modern Yoga* (pp. 147–170). New York: Oxford University Press.
Nicholson, A. (2013). Is Yoga Hindu? On the Fuzziness of Religious Boundaries. *Common Knowledge, 19*(3), 490–505.
Nichter, M. (2013). The Social Life of Yoga: Exploring Transcultural Flows in India. In B. Hauser (Ed.), *Yoga Traveling: Bodily Practice in Transcultural Perspective* (pp. 201–224). Heidelberg: Springer.
Occupy Yoga (2014). Homepage. http://www.occupyyoga.org/. Accessed 20 May 2014.
Remski, M. (2014). WAWADIA: A Prospectus. 1 November. http://matthewremski.com/wordpress/wp-content/uploads/2014/10/WAWADIA-Prospectus.pdf. Accessed 31 May 2016.
Sarbacker, S. R. (2014). Swami Ramdev: Modern Yoga Revolutionary. In M. Singleton & E. Goldberg (Eds.), *Gurus of Modern Yoga* (pp. 351–372). New York: Oxford University Press.
Shukla, A. (2010). Dr. Chopra: Honor Thy Heritage. *Washington Post,* 28 April 2010. https://web.archive.org/web/20130121010842/http://newsweek.washingtonpost.com/onfaith/panelists/aseem_shukla/2010/04/dr_chopra_honor_thy_heritage.html. Accessed 1 July 2014.
Singleton, M. (2010). *Yoga Body: The Origins of Modern Posture Practice.* New York: Oxford University Press.

Smith, B. R. (2004). Adjusting the Quotidian: Ashtanga Yoga as Everyday Practice. *The Online Proceedings from Everyday Transformations: The 2004 Annual Conference of the Cultural Studies Association of Australasia* [Online]. http://www.mcc.murdoch.edu.au/cfel/docs/Smith_FV.pdf. Accessed 12 April 2009.

Smith, B. R. (2007). Body, Mind and Spirit? Towards an Analysis of the Practice of Yoga. *Body & Society*, *13*(2), 25–46.

Smith, B. R. (2008). "With Heat Even Iron Will Bend": Discipline and Authority in Ashtanga Yoga. In M. Singleton & J. Byrne (Eds.), *Yoga in the Modern World: Contemporary Perspectives* (pp. 140–160). London: Routledge.

Spagat, E. (2013). California Judge Allows Yoga in Public Schools. *The Associated Press: Big Story*. http://bigstory.ap.org/article/calif-judge-says-public-school-yoga-not-religious. Accessed 1 July 2014.

Tedjasukmana, J. (2009). Indonesia's Fatwa Against Yoga. *Time Magazine*, 29 January 2009. http://content.time.com/time/world/article/0,8599,1874651,00.html. Accessed 1 July 2014.

Thompson, B. (2013). Is Yoga Religion? It Depends on the Person. *UT San Diego*, 18 April 2013. http://www.utsandiego.com/news/2013/apr/18/is-yoga-religion-it-depends-on-the-person/. Accessed 3 July 2014.

Thompson, K. & Thompson, A. (2004). Trustees of the British Wheel of Yoga. Personal Interview. 28 November 2004.

Vanity Fair (2013). Bikram Yoga's Embattled Founder: The Alleged Rapes and Sexual Harassment Claims Against Guru Bikram Choudhury. *Vanity Fair*, 5 December 2013. http://www.vanityfair.com/online/daily/2013/12/bikram-yoga-sexual-harassment-claims. Accessed 20 May 2014.

Vitello, P. (2010). Hindu Group Stirs a Debate Over Yoga's Soul. *New York Times*, N.Y./Region, 27 November 2010. http://www.nytimes.com/2010/11/28/nyregion/28yoga.html?src=me&ref=homepage&_r=0. Accessed 20 May 2014.

White, D. G. (2009). *Sinister Yogis*. Chicago, IL: Chicago University Press.

Wittgenstein, L. (2001). *Philosophical Investigations*, trans. G. E. M. Anscombe. 3rd ed. Oxford: Blackwell Publishing.

Yoga & Health (1971–1975). Published by Astrian Public Relations, 344 South Lambeth Road SW8, London.

Chapter 16

Nāga, Siddha and Sage: Visions of Patañjali as an Authority on Yoga

Gudrun Bühnemann

Contents

1. Introduction 577

2. Two-armed Representations of Patañjali in the Tradition of the Naṭarāja Temple at Cidambaram 578

3. Patañjali as a Four-armed Figure in the Tradition of T. Krishnamacharya 583

4. Patañjali as a Meditating Sage in the South Indian *Siddha* Tradition 590

5. Patañjali Associated with the Syllable *Oṃ* 591

6. A Brief Look at Recent Innovative Representations of Patañjali 591

References 592

Figures 596

Gudrun Bühnemann

Chapter 16: *Nāga, Siddha* and Sage: Visions of Patañjali as an Authority on Yoga*

> India is believed to be the mother of civilization. Patañjali is known as the father of yoga. In our own invocatory prayers, we call him a patriarch, spiritual father of many generations, and a revered sage.
> (Iyengar 2002: 289)

1. Introduction

Patañjali has emerged as an important figure in modern yoga[1] whose visual representations are often installed in yoga studios. Believed to be the author of the *Yogasūtra,* which has attained canonical status in many yoga traditions, Patañjali is eulogised with invocations in Sanskrit. The invocation of the king of divine serpents Ananta (often identified with Patañjali) at the beginning of yoga practice is already attested in Brahmānanda's nineteenth-century commentary[2] on the *Haṭhayogapradīpikā.* It was prescribed again in the twentieth century by the influential yoga master Tirumalai Krishnamacharya (1888–1989) in his book on yoga titled *Yogamakaranda.*[3] While in the teachings of Krishnamacharya's

---

* I would like to thank Gerd Mevissen for material concerning the Patañjali statues at the Naṭarāja Temple in Cidambaram. I am indebted to Rosemary J. Antze and Martine Burat for generously providing information and material from the tradition of T. Krishnamacharya and T. K. V. Desikachar. For photographs, I would like to thank G. Mevissen, R. Sathyanarayanan Sarma, Dominik Ketz, Corinna Wessels-Mevissen, Gudrun Melzer, R. J. Antze, M. Burat, Emily Malavenda and Melissa Athens. A separate monograph on the iconography of Patañjali is in preparation.

1 M. Singleton (2008) has analysed in detail how Patañjali, considered the author of the *Yogasūtra,* became the figurehead of modern yoga. S. R. Sarbacker (2015) further examines the role of Patañjali and his visual representations in modern yoga. For the reception history of the *Yogasūtra* in India and the West, see White 2014, especially ch. 1–9, 11 and 12.

2 Brahmānanda's commentary *Jyotsnā* on *Haṭhayogapradīpikā* 2.48 quotes a stanza prescribing that the practitioner bow to the lord of divine serpents, Ananta, at the beginning of yoga practice to ensure success in (the practice of) postures (*pīṭha,* i.e., *āsana*): *deśakālau ca saṃkīrtya saṃkalpya vidhipūrvakam | anantaṃ praṇamed devaṃ nāgeśaṃ pīṭhasiddhaye ||* .

3 The following statement is found in an excerpt from the *Yogamakaranda* in Mohan 2010: 146: "For success in the practice of asanas … [p]ray to Adisesha before starting the practice."

son T. K. V. Desikachar (b. 1938) the stanzas to Patañjali are recited before studying the *Yogasūtra*,[4] Krishnamacharya's long-time student Srivatsa Ramaswami[5] (b. 1939), the traditions of Krishnamacharya's former students K. Pattabhi Jois (1915–2009) and B. K. S. Iyengar (1918–2014), for example, practise the recitation of the stanzas in praise of Patañjali before commencing *āsana* practice. The status of the *Yogasūtra* and the recitation of stanzas describing Patañjali's visual form generated an interest in visual representations of Patañjali. Statues and images of the sage are installed in yoga centres, where they function as objects of reverence. At the same time they serve as links between the practice of *āsana*-s commonly taught there and the teachings of the *Yogasūtra* (see Figures 1–4). The late B. K. S. Iyengar contributed considerably to the popularisation of the figure of Patañjali during his long teaching career. The prefatory matter of his book *Light on the Yoga Sūtras of Patañjali* encapsulates Iyengar's devotion to Patañjali in the following dedication: "This work is my offering to my Invisible, First and Foremost Guru Lord Patañjali." Iyengar inaugurated a special day for celebrating the sage, the Patañjali-jayantī, and even built a temple for Patañjali in his native village of Bellur in Karnataka, South India (see Figure 5).

In this paper I will trace the development of Patañjali's iconography, starting with the earliest representations as a two-armed half-human half-serpentine devotee of Śiva in the tradition of the Naṭarāja Temple at Cidambaram in Tamilnadu, South India. I will then examine the more recent iconography of Patañjali as a four-armed manifestation of Ādiśeṣa/Ananta/Viṣṇu in the tradition of Krishnamacharya; as an accomplished being (*siddha*), absorbed in meditation; and as an authority on yoga associated with the syllable *oṃ*. Finally, I will take a brief look at two representations of Patañjali experimenting with new forms.

2. Two-armed Representations of Patañjali in the Tradition of the Naṭarāja Temple at Cidambaram

The earliest iconography of Patañjali is derived from a myth narrated in the *Cidambaramāhātmya*,[6] a religious text extolling the importance of the temple complex in the town of Cidambaram in South India. According to the myth, Patañjali is a manifestation of the king of divine serpents (*nāga*), Ananta or Śeṣa,

4 I would like to thank R. J. Antze (email message dated 7 January 2016) and M. Burat (email message dated 14 January 2016) for this clarification.

5 See Ramaswami 2000: 95, 96 and 208 for the practice of paying obeisance to Ananta (also referred to as Ādiśeṣa or Nāgarāja and identified with Patañjali) at the beginning of yoga practice.

6 See Kulke 1970: 8–103 for a detailed analysis of the myth.

on whom the god Viṣṇu rests.[7] The cosmic serpent, we are told, desired to witness Śiva's dance at Cidambaram. Assuming a half-human half-serpentine form, he manifested himself as Patañjali by falling into the cupped hands (*añjali*) (forming the womb) of Anasūyā, the sage Atri's wife, who thereby became Patañjali's mother.[8] Yoga teachers in the tradition of Krishnamacharya such as Ramaswami[9] and Iyengar[10] transmit another version of the story of Patañjali as a manifestation of Ādiśeṣa who fell into the cupped hands of Goṇikā, as told in the *Patañjalicarita*[11] (or *Patañjalivijaya*), a *mahākāvya* based on diverse legends, which was composed by the South Indian poet Rāmabhadra Dīkṣita in the seventeenth or early eighteenth century.[12] Patañjali, whose name is popularly derived from the forms *patat* or *patita* of the verbal root *pat* ("to fall") and the word *añjali* ("cupped hands") and is explained as "fallen into/from the cupped hands (*añjali*)",[13] became an ardent devotee of the Dancing Śiva.

The tradition of the Naṭarāja Temple at Cidambaram views Patañjali as a great yogi in the service of Śiva. At the same time, it identifies him with the grammarian of the same name and with an authority on the Indian medical system of Āyurveda. The three authors cannot be identical. The *Vyākaraṇa-Mahābhāṣya,* a commentary on Pāṇini's *Aṣṭādhyāyī* written by Patañjali, considered by the later tradition as one of the three sages (*munitraya*) of the Pāṇinian tradition of Sanskrit grammar, dates from c 150 BCE. The compiler of the *yogasūtra*-s, however, is likely to have flourished around the fourth century CE. Not much reliable information is found about the Patañjali considered to be the author of a medical text.[14]

7 For interpretations of the word *ananta* as referring to the cosmic serpent Ananta in the context of the *Yogasūtra*-s, see the chapters by Wujastyk (p. 33f.), Maas (p. 83f.) and Birch (footnote 50) in this volume; for the visualization of Ananta as "the divine yoga couch" of Nārāyaṇa and Śrī, see Rastelli's chapter (p. 250).

8 *Naṭeśavijaya* 3.66 also narrates the story of Anasūyā and Atri as Patañjali's (foster) parents.

9 See Ramaswami 2000: 22–29.

10 See, for example, Iyengar 2002: 2 and Iyengar 2000–2010: I/201, V/186 and VII/ 58.

11 For a detailed discussion of the *Patañjalicarita,* see Thiruvengadathan 2002: 27–55. The text and translation of the relevant passage on the birth of Patañjali from the *Patañjalicarita* (canto 2, stanzas 7–10) can be found in Roodbergen 1984: 371–372, n. 16. For a summary of the contents of the passages on Patañjali's life from the *Patañjalicarita,* see Ramaswami 2000: 22–29. A retelling of the contents of the passages on Patañjali included in the *Patañjalicarita* combined with information from the *Naṭeśavijaya* written by Rāmabhadra Dīkṣita's contemporary Veṅkaṭakṛṣṇa Dīkṣita can be found in Balasubramanian 1992: 2–4 (with line drawings).

12 For this date, see Thiruvengadathan 2002: 9.

13 A summary of different derivations of the name Patañjali by Indian grammarians can be found in Bhattacharya 1985: 85–89.

14 For a summary of the different accounts relating to Patañjali as the author of medical texts, see Filliozat 1964: 22–25, Bhattacharya 1985: 98–99 and especially the very detailed references provided in Meulenbeld 1999–2002: I A/141–144 (with the notes in I B/231–234). According to

There is evidence that already in the tenth century the three Patañjali figures[15] had become amalgamated in the Indian tradition. The identity of the three authors, which is also expressed in the design of a commemorative postal stamp issued by India Post in 2009 (see Figure 26), is firmly assumed by most modern yoga masters. It is suggested by the text of the first of two stanzas in Sanskrit recited in praise of Patañjali by some teachers in the tradition of Krishnamacharya, for example, by Desikachar and Iyengar.[16] The stanza (1.1) is also inscribed on the pedestals of Patañjali statues (see Figures 2–3) and on the outside wall, to the left of the entrance, of the Patañjali Temple at Bellur (see Figure 5):

> I bow with clasped hands to Patañjali, the most excellent of sages, who removed the impurity of the mind by yoga, (that) of speech by grammar and (that) of the body by the science of medicine.[17]

---

some authorities, Patañjali's treatise focused on metallurgy (*lohaśāstra*) and its medical application; others consider Patañjali as the redactor of the *Carakasaṃhitā* or even identify him with Caraka (Meulenbeld 1999–2002: I A/142–143).

15 For the amalgamation of the three Patañjali figures from the tenth century onward, see Bhattacharya 1985: 101–102. J. Filliozat (1964: 22) argues that the invocation of Patañjali as author of a work on yoga, grammar and medicine found in Cakrapāṇidatta's eleventh-century commentary *Āyurvedadīpikā* on the *Carakasaṃhitā* (p. 1, ll. 14–16, introductory stanza 4) "does not signify that the three works are of one and the same author; the three authors could also have been considered as the three successive incarnations of Śeṣa." It seems, however, that most modern yoga authorities assume the identity of the three authors. One of the later sources relevant here is canto 5 of Rāmabhadra Dīkṣita's seventeenth- or early eighteenth-century *Patañjalicarita,* a work in which the three Patañjalis are also considered identical (see stanzas 3–24 for Patañjali the grammarian and stanza 25 for the author of the *Yogasūtra* and explanations [*vārttika*] on a medical treatise). For a detailed analysis of the contents of canto 5, see Thiruvengadathan 2002: 34–37. For textual material referring to Patañjali as an incarnation of Śeṣanāga, see Deshpande 1997: 449–450. Different points of view on the hypothesis that the grammarian Patañjali hailed from Gonarda and the eastern part of India are discussed, for example, in Cardona 1980: 269–270 and Aklujkar 2008b. A. Aklujkar (2008a: 69 and 2008c) argues for Kashmir as the geographical area where the grammarian may have flourished; M. Deshpande (1994: 113–114) suggests a link to South India. On other authors named Patañjali, see Bhattacharya 1985: 99–100 and 103–106 and Larson & Bhattacharya 2008: 52 ff.

16 The stanza is not recited in the Ashtanga Yoga tradition of K. Pattabhi Jois.

17 *Yogena cittasya padena vācāṃ malaṃ śarīrasya ca vaidyakena | yo 'pākarot taṃ pravaraṃ munīnāṃ patañjaliṃ prāñjalir ānato 'smi ||* . This stanza, composed in the Upajāti metre, appears as the fourth benedictory stanza (with the *varia lectio tu* instead of *ca* in the second *pāda*) at the end of the commentary *Pātañjalayogaśāstravivaraṇa* (p. 370, ll. 11–12) attributed to Śaṅkara, where it may be an interpolation. It is also found in some manuscripts of the text of the prefatory part to the *Mahābhāṣya* (Woods 1914: xiv), where it may have been likewise interpolated. The stanza is cited in Śivarāma's eighteenth-century commentary *Darpaṇa* on Subandhu's *Vāsavadattā* (p. 239, ll. 5–8) with the *varia lectio tu* instead of *ca*. It is furthermore part of the hymn to the deities in the Naṭarāja temple at Cidambaram (see *Cidambarakṣetrasarvasva* I/ 207).

In addition to being considered to be the author of the *Mahābhāṣya*, the *Yogasūtra* and a medical treatise, the tradition of the Naṭarāja Temple at Cidambaram attributes to Patañjali five manuals[18] in Sanskrit outlining the worship rituals conducted at the temple, the *Cidambaranaṭeśvarapañcapūjāsūtrāṇi* of the *Cidambarakṣetrasarvasva*, which he is said to have composed for the officiating priests, known as the Dīkṣitar-s ("initiated ones"). In addition to the other initiations (*dīkṣā*) passed on to Śaiva teachers, these priests are said to receive a special initiation, the *patañjalidīkṣā*.[19]

At one time, at least six stone sculptures of Patañjali were found at or in the Naṭarāja Temple at Cidambaram. Originally, one sculpture of Patañjali was installed on the outside wall of each of the four temple towers (*gopura*),[20] all of them dating to the end of the twelfth or beginning of the thirteenth century.[21] The sculptures were symmetrically paired with sculptures of Vyāghrapāda (Tiger-Foot), installed on the opposite side. Vyāghrapāda, a sage named for his tiger feet, is another devotee of Śiva with a half-animal body. Additionally, a stone sculpture of Patañjali dating to the early twelfth century[22] is found in the Nṛttasabhā, the Hall of Dance, of the Naṭarāja Temple. It is installed in a niche (see Figure 7) to the right side of the figure of Kaṅkālamūrti, a fierce form of Śiva with a corpse skewered on his trident (see Figure 8). The sculpture is again paired with Vyāghrapāda on the opposite side.

In Cidambaram, Patañjali is adorned with five serpent hoods and his body from the waist down is represented as that of a coiled serpent. He is shown in the standing position, with his hands clasped in the *añjali* gesture. The representation on the eastern temple tower of the Naṭarāja Temple shows him with fangs and holding a beaded chaplet between the palms (see Figure 6). The *añjali*

18 The five manuals are (1) the *Cidambareśvara-* (or *Naṭeśa-)Nityapūjāsūtra*, (2) the *Naṭeśanaimittikapūjāsūtra*, (3) the *Citsabheśa-* (or *Naṭeśa-)Utsavapūjāpātañjalasūtra*, (4) the *Prāyaścittapūjāsūtra* and (5) the *Naṭeśapratiṣṭhāpātañjalasūtra* (or *Pātañjalapratiṣṭhāsūtrasaṃgraha*) (see *Cidambarakṣetrasarvasva* II, editor's introduction, p. 2 [unnumbered].) They are also referred to as *Patañjalisūtra*-s (*Cidambarakṣetrasarvasva* I/113). The following stanza, composed in the Vasantatilakā metre and printed on an unnumbered page prefixed to vols. I and II of the *Cidambarasarvasva*, ascribes the *Cidambaranaṭeśvarapañcapūjāsūtra*-s to Patañjali who authored treatises on medicine, yoga and grammar: *śrīmaccidambaranaṭeśvarapañcapūjāsūtrāṇy akāri muninā phaṇināyakena* | *taṃ vaidyayogapadaśāstrakaraṃ vareṇyaṃ śrīmatpatañjalimunīśvaram ādyam īḍe* || .

19 See Younger 1995: 42, n. 26, and 160, and Younger 2004: 62.

20 Only the sculptures of Patañjali on the northern and eastern temple towers can be seen nowadays. The sculptures on the southern and western temple towers have disappeared. So far only the Patañjali figure on the eastern tower has been published, since the one on the northern tower is hard to access and photograph. I would like to thank G. Mevissen for this information (email message dated 29 April 2012).

21 See Mevissen 2004: 89–90 with fig. 5 [map].

22 See Mevissen 1996: 365, 377–379 and 2002: 63.

gesture, which indicates a subordinate status, characterises him as Śiva's devotee. Patañjali is always represented as a member of the group of sages (*ṛṣi*). In a much later, circa eighteenth-century stone relief[23] (see Figure 9) in the inner courtyard of the Citsabhā, the holiest shrine in the Cidambaram temple, Patañjali is grouped with the other great devotees who witnessed Śiva's dance at Cidambaram, the sages Jaimini, founder of the Mīmāṃsā school of Indian philosophy (left) and Vyāghrapāda (in the centre, carrying an implement used for picking flowers and fruit as offerings).

Patañjali's iconography in Cidambaram is that of a divine serpent (*nāga*) in the service of Śiva. There are no specific features characterizing him as an authority and teacher of yoga. In the absence of his companion sages or an identifying inscription, one cannot easily distinguish these South Indian representations of Patañjali from those of other divine serpents making the *añjali* gesture, such as the *nāga* and *nāginī* in the famous seventh-century Mamallapuram bas-relief (showing either Arjuna's or Bhagīratha's penance) (see Figure 10).

Only a few examples from the earlier time period are known where Patañjali's iconography deviates from the above. One twelfth-century bronze sculpture[24] from the Naṭarāja Temple at Cidambaram (see Figure 11) shows Patañjali, with the lower body and hoods of a serpent, displaying the gestures of teaching (*cinmudrā*) and wish-granting, while the *añjali* gesture is absent. Here, it seems, Patañjali has emerged from the role of a devotee of Śiva and assumed the role of a teacher in his own right.

In later representations Patañjali sometimes appears as a bearded figure. The beard characterises him as an ancient sage and sets him apart from other *nāga* figures. This iconography of Patañjali is seen in South Indian sculptures and paintings, such as the seventeenth-century sculpture from the temple town Avudaiyarkoil (Āvuṭaiyārkōvil) in Tamilnadu (see Figure 12). As in a seventeenth-century[25] bronze, now in the Ashmolean Museum in Oxford (acc. no. EA2005.11) (see Figure 13), the bearded sage lacks the serpent hoods.

A seventeenth-century wall painting (see Figure 14) and sculpture (see Figure 15) from the Narumbunathar Temple at Tiruppudaimarudur (Tirupputaimarutūr) in Tamilnadu also show the bearded Patañjali. His lower body is fully

23 See Mevissen 1996: 378, n. 75 and 379, n. 79.

24 R. Nagaswamy (1995: 123) dates the sculpture to 1130 CE, B. Natarajan (1994: plates 135–136) to 1150 CE.

25 This date was assigned by staff members of the Ashmolean Museum. J. F. Staal (1972: 28, with plate II on p. 29) dated the bronze, which was part of a private collection before it was acquired by the Ashmolean Museum in 2005, to the fourteenth or fifteenth century.

human but a *nāga* is wound around his waist and shelters the sage with its five hoods.[26]

In an early nineteenth-century painting from a portfolio of sixty-three paintings of deities, the bearded Patañjali and the bearded sage Tiger-Foot worship the Dancing Śiva (see Figure 16), who has placed his right foot on Apasmārapuruṣa. To Śiva's left is his consort Śivakāmasundarī. In a representation of the Kedāra musical mode (*rāga*) from an eighteenth- or nineteenth-century illustrated manuscript of the *Svaracūḍāmaṇi* (p. 119) (see Figure 17), Patañjali, Vyāghrapāda, Śuka and other sages worship a form of Śiva called Yoga-Dakṣiṇāmūrti. Patañjali and the other sages except for Śuka are bearded. The deity is seated atop a mountain on which ascetics practise yoga postures or worship *śivaliṅga*-s.

As we have seen, in all but one representation (see Figure 11) discussed in this section Patañjali clasps his hands in the gesture of obeisance (*añjali*), which is characteristic of many *nāga*-s and marks him as a subordinate figure. According to the *Cidambaramāhātmya,* he turned into a devotee of the Dancing Śiva, although originally he was a manifestation of Ananta on whom god Viṣṇu rests and thus a Vaiṣṇava figure. This appropriation of Patañjali by Śaiva authorities may well be interpreted as an attempt to establish the superiority of Śaivism, as I will discuss in more detail in my forthcoming monograph on Patañjali. In contrast, the much later iconography discussed in the next section is characterised by mostly Vaiṣṇava attributes.

3. Patañjali as a Four-armed Figure in the Tradition of T. Krishnamacharya

Some later representations furnish Patañjali with an extra pair of hands which holds Vaiṣṇava attributes. Here we encounter two major iconographic types. The first type displays the *añjali* gesture, which is often seen with *nāga*-s and is the characteristic attribute of the images from Cidambaram. The two extra hands hold the Vaiṣṇava attributes conch and wheel. The second type does not exhibit the *añjali* gesture and the four attributes are mostly identifiable as Vaiṣṇava.

The four-armed iconography is popular with teachers in the tradition of Krishnamacharya. Visual representations of this iconography appear to emerge from the 1980s onward among students of Desikachar. These representations seem to have been commissioned to conform to the textual descriptions recited in the tradition. Exceptions are replicas of the two-armed Patañjali sculpture on

26 For this iconography, see also the seventeenth-century sculpture from the Ranganathaswamy Temple Museum, Śrīraṅgam, reproduced in Sivaramamurti 1981: fig. 72.

the eastern tower (*gopura*) of the Naṭarāja Temple in Cidambaram (see Figure 6), which are also installed by teachers in this tradition. One such replica (but without the snake fangs),[27] made by a stone sculptor from Mahabalipuram, is installed in the Krishnamacharya Yoga Mandiram, Chennai, which was established by Desikachar in 1976 to honour his father Krishnamacharya.

Krishnamacharya regularly gave instructions in Patañjali's *Yogasūtra.* He dictated his own Sanskrit commentary on the text titled *Yogavallī* to his students when he was already advanced in age.[28] As a Vaiṣṇava in the Viśiṣṭādvaita tradition, he explained the text in accordance with this philosophical system. It has been said that Krishnamacharya wrote two compositions eulogizing Patañjali.[29] A closer look, however, shows that both compositions mainly focus on the *nāga* king Ananta/Ādiśeṣa on whom Viṣṇu rests.

The earlier composition is the following set of two stanzas (2.1–2) composed in 1980 "when the Krishnamacharya Yoga Mandiram published the 'Yoga Sutra Work Book'."[30] Here the occasion warranted a focus on Patañjali. However, only the second stanza refers to Patañjali and does not describe his visual form:

> I salute Ananta, the King of the cobras who is revered by all, who, with a thousand hoods, each distinct and grand, has in his hands a disc as bright as the sun and a conch as pleasant as a full moon.
> I offer my respects to the sage Patañjali whose very name, when remembered, dissolves all impurities of body, speech and mind.[31]

The first stanza pays homage to the *nāga* king Ananta who holds the wheel and conch, two typical Vaiṣṇava attributes. Here Krishnamacharya does not describe Ananta as a four-armed figure as he does in the text prefixed to his *Ādiśeṣāṣṭaka* (see stanzas 3.1–2 quoted below, p. 588). The second stanza eulogises Patañjali as the great sage who removes the impurities of body, speech and mind. It is thus similar in content to the stanza quoted above (1.1, see p. 580). The stanza does not shed light on the iconography of Patañjali. Krishnamacharya's composition does not link or identify Ananta and Patañjali in any way, although it is generally assumed that the latter is a manifestation of the former, even if he does not necessarily exhibit the same physical characteristics.

27 For a photograph of the replica, see Desikachar 1998, plate after p. 48, and Sarbacker 2015: 21, fig. 1.2.

28 For the *Yogavallī*, see Mohan 2010: 134–136.

29 See Krishnamacharya 1992: 11.

30 Krishnamacharya 1992: 11.

31 *Karayugavidhṛtābhyāṃ cakraśaṅkhābhidhābhyāṃ karayugavidhṛtābhyāṃ cakraśaṅkhābhidhābhyāṃ mihiraśaśinibhābhyām āyudhābhyāṃ pradīptam | daśaśatavitatābhiḥ prasphuṭābhiḥ phaṇābhiḥ suyutam akhilavandyaṃ bhogirājaṃ bhaje 'ham || yasya smaraṇamātreṇa dehavāṅmanasāṃ malāḥ | līyante tam ahaṃ naumi patañjalimahāmunim ||* . Text and translation are quoted from Krishnamacharya 1992: 11.

Krishnamacharya's other composition said to concern itself with Patañjali[32] is the *Ādiśeṣāṣṭaka,* written in October 1984 at the request of Desikachar. As will be discussed further below, it specifies four hand-held attributes (conch, wheel, mace, sword) for Ādiśeṣa but does not mention Patañjali's name.

Of great significance for the development of the four-armed iconography of Patañjali is a description of unknown origin[33] recited by practitioners in the tradition of Krishnamacharya. It merely lists three of four expected attributes (conch, wheel, sword).

One statue of Patañjali at the Ramamani Iyengar Memorial Yoga Institute, Pune (see Figure 2) corresponds to the iconography of type 1. It shows the four-armed sage displaying the familiar *añjali* gesture with his two lower hands and holding the Vaiṣṇava attributes conch and wheel with the upper hands. On the statue's pedestal, two stanzas in Sanskrit are inscribed in Devanāgarī script.[34] The text and translation of the first one were provided earlier (see stanza 1.1 above, p. 580 with n. 17). The second stanza (1.2) gives a description of Patañjali, which does not correspond with the iconography of the statue (i. e., the conch and wheel and the *añjali* gesture). This second stanza, which Krishnamacharya apparently taught but did not compose himself,[35] is recited by practitioners in his tradition.[36] It is also inscribed on the outside wall of the Patañjali Temple at Bellur (see Figure 5) even though the iconography of the sculpture in the temple does not correspond with the stanza's description. It is sometimes ascribed to the introduction to Bhoja's commentary[37] on the *Yogasūtra,* but I was unable to locate it in that text. It is, however, possible, that this simple stanza in Anuṣṭubh metre was later prefixed to or inserted into a popular edition of the commentary: "I bow to

32 See Krishnamacharya 1992: 13.

33 See the stanza quoted below, p. 588.

34 The pedestal of the Patañjali statue (see Figure 3) installed in the Iyengar-Yoga-Institut Rhein-Ahr e.V. in Cologne, which is similar to the one installed in the Ramamani Iyengar Memorial Yoga Institute in Pune (see Figure 2), has the two stanzas in Sanskrit inscribed in transliteration.

35 The anonymous editor of Krishnamacharya 1992 lists the stanza as a "traditional prayer" and adds that its author is unknown (see Krishnamacharya 1992: 16).

36 As noted before, in the teachings of Desikachar the stanza is recited before studying the *Yogasūtra.* However, some other teachers such as Ramaswami, Jois and Iyengar recite the stanza before commencing *āsana* practice. Iyengar specifically requested his students to recite both stanzas (1.1 and 1.2) in praise of Patañjali at the beginning of yoga classes and defended the practice against criticism; for details, see Iyengar 2000–2010: I/234–235 and V/184–187. The stanza describing the iconography of Patañjali is included in the prefatory matter to Iyengar's *Light on the Yoga Sūtras of Patañjali* and to each of the eight volumes of his *Aṣṭadaḷa Yogamālā.*

37 The stanza is ascribed to Bhoja's commentary on the *Yogasūtra,* for example, in Bryant 2009: 288 (and quoted in White 2014: 35). The translation of the stanza provided in Bryant 2009: 288 (see also White 2014: 35) omits the sword attribute, which is clearly mentioned in the Sanskrit text cited in Bryant 2009: 542.

Patañjali, of human form down to the arms, who holds a conch, wheel and sword, who has a thousand hoods (and) is white."[38]

The stanza describes Patañjali as holding the two Vaiṣṇava attributes conch (*śaṅkha*) and wheel (*cakra*), along with a sword (*asi*). In this description no attribute is specified for Patañjali's fourth hand. It should also be noted that Patañjali's (like Ananta's/Śeṣa's) complexion is specified as white, whereas many Patañjali statues are made of black stone.

The problem of assigning the three attributes listed in the stanza to Patañjali's hands was resolved in different ways. One free translation of the stanza transmitted by Desikachar specifies three hand-held attributes (conch, wheel, sword) but assigns the sword to Patañjali's two (front or lower) hands.[39] In contrast, Iyengar[40] explains that Patañjali holds the disc and conch in his (upper) right and left hands, makes the *añjali* gesture and that the sword is tied to his waist "and kept in a scabbard" (Iyengar 2000–2010: VII/58). He adds that he found "the picture in a book called *Religion on Earth.* There is also a temple of the Śeṣāvatāra in Koregaon, Maharashtra, in which the idol is similar to Lord Patañjali." Iconographically, the representation of a sword inserted into a scabbard with its tip facing downwards is highly unusual.

One modern sculpture of Patañjali (see Figure 18) at the Ramamani Iyengar Memorial Institute, Pune, corresponds with the stanza's iconography but does not agree with these two interpretations. The statue holds the conch and wheel in the upper hands and the sword (with its tip facing downwards) in the left lower hand. The unknown artist has supplied the gesture of protection as the fourth attribute.

I have found several other modern representations of Patañjali which repeat this iconography and are based on the description in this widely-recited stanza. They, too, show the gesture of protection as a fourth attribute but the sword is raised and not inserted into a scabbard with its tip pointing downwards. The iconography of some of these representations (see Figures 19–21) deviates in yet another way: Patañjali's lower body is fully human. The sage is seated, and that also in the full lotus posture, which characterises him as a yogi.

---

38 *Ābāhupuruṣākāraṃ śaṅkhacakrāsidhāriṇam | sahasraśirasaṃ śvetaṃ praṇamāmi patañjalim ||*. The text is transmitted without any variants in numerous publications (see Krishnamacharya 1992: 16) and on Internet sites. The translation is mine.

39 According to the text of a handout transmitted by Desikachar and ascribed to an "oral tradition" (sent to me by R. J. Antze; email message dated 7 December 2015), Patañjali holds "a conch in his left hand, a disc in the right, and a sword in the other two."

40 See, for example, Iyengar 2000–2010: V/185 and VII/58. An image of the corresponding Patañjali statue is reproduced in VII/60 (plate 2), next to one of a statue showing the more common iconographic attributes, conch and wheel and the *añjali* gesture.

A stone sculpture (see Figure 20), commissioned by Professor W. Skelton (1923–2009) in Mahabalipuram, South India, in 1996[41] on the basis of a batik (see Figure 21) he had made[42] to conform to the description in stanza 1.2, shows the sword-wielding Patañjali exhibiting the gesture of protection and holding conch and wheel but oddly lacking a human face. The stone sculpture's ten (instead of five or seven) serpent hoods are another non-traditional feature. The batik shows a large number of hoods instead. A *kalamkārī* textile with a Patañjali figure similar to the one on Skelton's batik, which was made by the daughter of one of Desikachar's American students,[43] hung on a wall of Desikachar's home and was occasionally used for instructional purposes[44]. Instead of the gesture of protection the sword-wielding Patañjali displays the *cinmudrā*.

Line drawings of the sword-wielding iconographic type (with minor variations) have appeared in various places, including the cover of Krishnamacharya's *Dhyānamālikā*. The booklet was published by the Krishnamacharya Yoga Mandiram, Chennai, in November 1998 and the well-known illustrator and painter Maniam Selvan is credited with the artwork.

The prototype for Skelton's batik and stone sculpture may have been a line drawing (see Figure 19) made by the artist K. M. Gopal of Cholamandal, an artists' village near Chennai. It was first published in 1982.[45] The drawing was later reproduced in other places, including Krishnamacharya 1992: 15. Even a corresponding bas-relief[46] was commissioned in South India. The drawing shows the four-armed Patañjali with a human face, exhibiting the gesture of protection and holding a wheel, conch and sword. The four male figures paying homage to Patañjali with their hands clasped in the *añjali* gesture are an interesting feature of this representation. They are Patañjali's four disciples: (from the left) "Mastakāñjali, Kṛtāñjali, Baddhāñjali, Pūrṇāñjali as conceived by Krishnamacharya".[47] Mastakāñjali's hands are clasped in the *añjali* gesture and placed on top of

41 I would like to thank R. J. Antze for this information (email message dated 7 December 2015). For a photograph of the sculpture, see also Desikachar 1998, plate after p. 192. The sculpture is now in the possession of Kerry Koen, Hamilton, New York.

42 I thank M. Burat for this information (email message dated 8 December 2015). It is not known when the batik was made.

43 According to information from R. J. Antze (email message dated 7 December 2015). See the textile described below, p. 588.

44 According to information from R. J. Antze (email message dated 13 December 2015).

45 See Desikachar 1982, plate after p. 38.

46 For a photograph, see Moors 2007: 18.

47 Quoted from the text accompanying the line drawing (Desikachar 1982: 39). The drawing is also reproduced on the cover of the now discontinued quarterly journal *Darsanam* (vol. 1[3] August 1991) published by the Krishnamacharya Yoga Mandiram and in Krishnamacharya 1992, where we read (on p. 15): "… Krishnamacharya has stated on several occasions that Sri Patanjali had four disciples namely Krtanjali, Baddhanjali, Purnanjali and Mastakanjali. It is not clear as to what the source of this information is, since this is not found in any traditional

his head (*mastaka*) to account for his name. The representation of the four students corresponds to Krishnamacharya's teaching that Patañjali wrote each of the four parts of the *Yogasūtra* for one of his disciples, taking the student's mental development into account. The first part (*samādhipāda*) was composed for Kṛtāñjali, the second one (*sādhanapāda*) written for Baddhāñjali, the third part (*vibhūtipāda*) for Mastakāñjali and the fourth (*kaivalyapāda*) for Pūrṇāñjali.[48]

Another interpretation of Patañjali's iconography referred to by Desikachar[49] specifies the *cinmudrā* (not the gesture of protection) as Patañjali's fourth attribute. In this *mudrā*, which is also displayed by the statue in Figure 11, the tip of the index finger touches the tip of the thumb.[50] This gesture is seen in the aforementioned *kalamkārī* textile, which was done by the daughter of an American student of Desikachar. The *cinmudrā* is apparently a creative interpretation on the part of the student who made the fabric.

Elsewhere Desikachar (1998: 54) lists the mace, another Vaiṣṇava attribute, as the fourth attributes of "one form" of Patañjali, along with the wheel, conch and sword. This iconography can be traced back to the description in two stanzas (3.1–2) that detail the iconography of Ādiśeṣa on whom Viṣṇu rests. These two stanzas (erroneously labelled as one single *dhyānaśloka*) are prefixed to and form an integral part of the *Ādiśeṣāṣṭaka*, a devotional hymn composed by Krishnamacharya in October 1984.[51]

> Known as Ādiśeṣa, having a head consisting of a thousand hoods and holding with [his] four hands [successively] a conch, a wheel, a mace and a sword, he is the permanent bed for Śrīpati. He is eternally absorbed in service to Śrīkānta. May the resplendent king of the *nāgas* always shine in my heart.[52]

---

text known to us. The adjoining illustration of Sri Patanjali and his four disciples as conceived by Sri T. Krishnamacharya [was] drawn by the artist K. M. Gopal of Cholamandal. It appeared for the first time in the book 'Yoga of T. Krishnamacharya' published by Krishnamacharya Yoga Mandiram."

48 See Krishnamacharya 1992: 15 and Marechal 2013–2014: 53 for this information.

49 According to information provided by Desikachar to R. J. Antze and a group of students in India in 2006 (email message from R. J. Antze dated 7 December 2015).

50 For a description of the *cinmudrā* and a line drawing, see Desikachar 1980: 175 with fig. 77.

51 On p. 3 of the preface to the publication *Pātañjalayogadarśanam* dated March 1985, Desikachar notes that the *Ādiśeṣāṣṭaka* was "conceived and dictated by him (i. e., Krishnamacharya) last October". According to Krishnamacharya 1992: 13, the year of composition is estimated as 1986.

52 *Nityaśayyā śrīpater yaḥ ādiśeṣa iti śrutaḥ | phaṇāsahasramūrdhā ca śaṅkhacakragadāsidhṛt || hastaiś caturbhiḥ śrīkāntanityakaiṃkaryadīkṣitaḥ | bhātu me hṛdaye nityaṃ nāgarājo mahādyutiḥ ||* . The text of the stanzas and a modified translation are quoted from the publication *Pātañjalayogadarśanam,* issued by the Krishnamacharya Yoga Mandiram in 1985. The text is found on p. 10, the original translation on p. 11. The book has been reprinted several times. The text and a slightly different translation of the hymn are also found in Krishnamacharya 1992: 12–14.

Stanza 2 contains a reference to the well-known Ranganathaswamy Temple with seven *prākāra* walls, which is located at Śrīraṅgam and houses the image of Raṅganātha, the form of Viṣṇu reclining on Ādiśeṣa. In stanzas 3 and 6 of this hymn (not quoted here) Ādiśeṣa is praised as the author of the *Mahābhāṣya* and Aṣṭāṅga Yoga and thus confounded with the figure of Patañjali but there is no mention of Patañjali in the hymn.

That the four attributes (conch, wheel, mace and sword) of Ādiśeṣa are those of Viṣṇu/Nārāyaṇa becomes clear, for example, from the following description in *Harivaṃśa* 92.33ab: "Viṣṇu, Nārāyaṇa, the god holding a conch, wheel, mace and sword."[53]

Elsewhere the conch of Kṛṣṇa/Viṣṇu is specified as Pāñcajanya, Viṣṇu's wheel as Sudarśana, his mace as Kaumodakī and his sword as Nandaka.

Of the four attributes of Ādiśeṣa in Krishnamacharya's hymn (stanzas 3.1–2), namely the conch, wheel, mace and sword (*śaṅkhacakragadāsi-)*, three are also found in the description of Patañjali in stanza 1.2 quoted above (p. 585 f.), namely the conch, wheel and sword (*śaṅkhacakrāsi-).* Thus Patañjali as described in the widely-recited stanza 1.2 represents a form of Ādiśeṣa holding Viṣṇu's attributes. As noted before, the invocation/worship of Ananta/Ādiśeṣa at the beginning of yoga practice is recommended in Brahmānanda's nineteenth-century commentary *Jyotsnā* on *Haṭhayogapradīpikā* 2.48 (see n. 2) and is prescribed again in Krishnamacharya's *Yogamakaranda* written in 1934. It is therefore not surprising that the tradition of Krishnamacharya emphasises the iconography of Ādiśeṣa/Ananta which is Vaiṣṇava. Krishnamacharya is also quoted as having stated that Patañjali (in fact, rather Ādiśeṣa!) personifies the two qualities of yogic posture (*āsana*) which are specified in *Yogasūtra* 2.46 as stable (*sthira*) and comfortable (*sukha*),[54] since he carries the universe on his hoods, which requires stability, and since he serves as Viṣṇu's couch, which calls for comfort.[55]

The problem that a text lists only three attributes for a four-armed form of Viṣṇu is not new. Goudriaan (1978: 142–144) discusses at length the common sequence of three attributes, conch, wheel and mace (*śaṅkhacakragadā-*), to which a fourth attribute or gesture was added later, which was variously a sword (*asi*), the gesture of protection or the wish-granting gesture. In descriptions or visual representations of Patañjali, the Vaiṣṇava attribute mace does not seem to be attested. Visual representations often show the gesture of protection and, in one case, the *cinmudrā* as fourth attribute. The wish-granting gesture is part of the iconography of the stone sculpture of Patañjali in the Patañjali Temple in-

53 *Viṣṇur nārāyaṇo devaḥ śaṅkhacakragadāsibhṛt* | .

54 On *Yogasūtra* 2.46, see the chapter by Philipp Maas in the present volume.

55 See Krishnamacharya 1992: 18 ("The Significance of the Form of Sri Patanjali"), Desikachar 1998: 54 and Marechal 2013–2014: 53.

augurated by Iyengar in the South Indian village of Bellur in 2004 (see Figure 22), which represents yet another iconographic type. The sage displays the common gestures of wish-granting and protection with his lower hands, and holds the Vaiṣṇava attributes conch and wheel in the upper hands.

4. Patañjali as a Meditating Sage in the South Indian *Siddha* Tradition

Another tradition portrays Patañjali as a meditating sage; serpentine features are often minimised. These representations seem to emerge when Patañjali, considered the author of the *Yogasūtra,* is included in groups of *siddha*-*s* or accomplished persons, according to Tamil traditions.[56] Patañjali appears as one of the 18 *siddha*-s in a possibly nineteenth-century Tamil tradition but his name is occasionally also included in other lists of *siddha*-s. A contemporary poster (see Figure 23) shows Patañjali adorned by serpent hoods as one of the 18 *siddha*-s.

At least two places in South India claim to be sites where the *siddha* Patañjali left his body while absorbed in deep meditation (*samādhi*). One of them is located in Rameshwaram,[57] the other in a temple in Tirupattur near Trichy in Tamilnadu.

A devotional picture (see Figure 24) associated with the second site (the Patañjali Jeeva Samadhi at the Brahmapureeswarar Temple in Tirupattur) shows Patañjali as an older, emaciated, almost naked sage with long hair, a beard and totally human features. He is meditating, with his hands resting on his knees. Light appears above his head, suggesting an enlightened state of consciousness.

A sculpture with somewhat similar features (see Figure 25) is installed on the premises of the Patañjali Yogapīṭha in Haridwar in North India, an institution that teaches yoga and promotes the medical system of Āyurveda. The long-haired, bearded sage is seated in meditation, with his hands forming the *cinmudrā* and resting on his knees. He wears a long garland of beads around his neck and a shorter one around his upper left arm and right wrist. This iconography includes characteristics one would expect from an authority of yoga: mastery of meditation, knowledge, wisdom and self-control.

The sculpture is included in the design on a commemorative postal stamp issued by India Post in 2009 (see Figure 26) on the occasion of the birthday of an

---

56 More research is needed on the important topic of South Indian *siddha* traditions. Some useful information on Tamil *siddha* traditions can be found in Venkatraman 1990. For lists of *siddha*-s that include Patañjali, see Zvelebil 1973: 132, n. 11, and Venkatraman 1990: 6 (n. 39), 199, 202 and 205.

57 For Patañjali's association with Rameshwaram, see Venkatraman 1990: 210.

associate of yoga-guru Rāmdev at the Patañjali Yogapīṭha. The stamp illustrates well how the Indian tradition has amalgamated different authorities named Patañjali, a fact I referred to earlier in this paper (p. 579ff.). The text (in grey letters) in the background is taken from the *Yogasūtra* ascribed to Patañjali. The small figure on the left is Patañjali, the *siddha*. He is seated in the full lotus posture and *cakra*-s are visible on his body. The paper scroll and feather pen, although anachronistic, likely allude to the *Mahābhāṣya*, the work authored by the grammarian Patañjali. The mortar filled with medical herbs, which is surrounded by fruits and plants, symbolises Patañjali's authority within the medical tradition of Āyurveda.

5. Patañjali Associated with the Syllable *Oṃ*

A modern stone sculpture (see Figure 27) shows Patañjali with fully human features seated on a *nāga* throne. The sage, sheltered by five serpent hoods, is seated in the full lotus posture and clasps his hands in the *añjali* gesture. The sculpture's pedestal is inscribed with the sacred syllable *oṃ*. This syllable, often recited at the beginning of yoga classes, is frequently associated with Patañjali. However, it plays only a minor role in the *Yogasūtra*, where it is recommended as one among other objects of meditation in *sūtra* 1.27. The syllable *oṃ* also features prominently on the pedestal of the Patañjali statue in the Iyengar-Yoga-Institut Rhein-Ahr e.V., Cologne (see Figure 3), where it precedes (with three repetitions) and follows the two inscribed stanzas (see stanzas 1.1–2 treated above).

In a modern poster (see Figure 28), a serpent, assuming the shape of the syllable *oṃ*, appears behind the figure of Patañjali. The sage has a serpentine lower body and is sheltered by serpent hoods. The serpent is also suggestive of the awakened *kuṇḍalinī* energy that has ascended from the bottom of the spine to the crown of the head, although the *kuṇḍalinī* is not known to the *Yogasūtra*. Patañjali is seated atop a globe, possibly alluding to the worldwide network of the International Yoga Federation, which uses the painting for advertising purposes.

In both of these cases, the basic representation of Patañjali with his two hands clasped in the *añjali* gesture follows the tradition of the Cidambaram temple.

6. A Brief Look at Recent Innovative Representations of Patañjali

A contemporary piece of jewellery, a pendant, shows Patañjali's head directly attached to the body of a coiled serpent (see Figure 29). His head is enveloped by a circle of light and his gaze is directed upwards as if in deep concentration. The long white beard reinforces the stereotype of an ancient sage.

I would like to conclude with a discussion of a painting of Patañjali the yogi and *siddha* by the Indian artist Kalathi Adiyen Aadi Nandhi (see Figure 30), completed in 2003. The painting uses traditional elements in an innovative way. The long-haired, bearded, emaciated and naked Patañjali is seated in a squatting position, his arms raised above his head and his hands held below a canopy of serpents that shelters him. Light radiates from the area of his third eye on the forehead, spreading above his head and all around him. To the front, a swirling river is visible. It is the fierce river of cyclic existence (*saṃsāra*) that needs to be crossed, which is frequently described in Indian literature. As the text accompanying the painting explains:

> Crossing the river of karma through grace and surrender,
> digesting all sacred as light sitting in the doorway of the eyebrows,
> ascend above to be Siva.

In this painting we recognise the serpent canopy, which is part of Patañjali's *nāga* iconography. At the same time, the serpent evokes the symbolism of the awakened *kuṇḍalinī* serpent energy that has ascended upwards. The energy centre (*cakra*) on the forehead radiates a mass of light. Apparently another energy centre is indicated in the area of the sage's navel. The squatting posture is in deviation from the earlier iconographies, which show Patañjali either standing or sitting in a cross-legged meditation posture.

In this way, different traditions and individual artists continue to engage with the image of the king of divine serpents (*nāga*), accomplished being (*siddha*) and sage (*muni, ṛṣi*) Patañjali to create new meaning for changing contexts. Since the cult of Patañjali as an authority on Yoga appears to be spreading, we are likely to see more experimentation with his visual form in the near future.

References

Primary Sources

Ādiśeṣāṣṭaka by T. Krishnamacharya
see *Pātañjalayogadarśanam* 1985.
see also Krishnamacharya 1992: 12–14.

Carakasaṃhitā
The Charakasaṃhitā by Agniveśa: Revised by Charaka and Dṛidhabala, with the Āyurveda-Dīpikā Commentary of Chakrapāṇidatta, ed. by J. Trikamji Āchārya. 3rd ed. Bombay: Satyabhāmābāi Pāndurang for the Nirṇaya Sāgar Press, 1941.

Cidambarakṣetrasarvasva
Śrīcidambarakṣetrasarvasva, ed. by Somasetu Dīkṣita. 2 vols. Cidambaram: M. S. Trust, 1977, 1982.

Harivaṃśa
The Harivamsha: Being the khila or Supplement of the Mahābhārata, ed. P. L. Vaidya et al. 2 vols. Poona: Bhandarkar Oriental Institute, 1969–1971.

Haṭhayogapradīpikā
The Haṭhayogapradīpikā of Svātmārāma with the Commentary Jyotsnā of Brahmānanda and English Translation. Madras: Adyar Library and Research Centre, 1972 (repr. 1975).

Naṭeśavijaya
Natesa Vijayam by Venkatakrishna Dikshita. Srirangam: Sri Vani Vilas Press, 1912.

Pātañjalayogadarśanam
Pātañjalayogadarśanam: Text with Chant-notation in Sanskrit and Roman Script and Ādiśeṣāṣṭakam of Sri T. Krishnamacharya. Madras: Krishnamacharya Yoga Mandiram, 1985.

Pātañjalayogaśāstravivaraṇa
Pātañjala-Yogasūtra-Bhāṣya-Vivaraṇam of Śaṅkara-Bhagavatpāda, ed. Polakam Rama Sastri & S. R. Krishnamurthi Sastri. Madras: Madras Law Journal Press, 1952.

Patañjalicarita
The Patañjali Charita of Ramabhadra Dikhit, ed. Mahāmahopādhyāya Paṇḍit Śivadatta et al. 2nd ed. Bombay: Pāndurang Jāwajī, 1934.

Svaracūḍāmaṇi
Svaracūḍāmaṇi Śrī-Tattva-nidhi of Krishṇaraya Woḍeyar III of Mysore. Vol. 1: *Svarachūḍāmaṇi (Rāgamālā Paintings)*, ed. S. K. R. Rao. Hampi: Kannada University, 1993.

Vāsavadattā
The Vásavadattá, a Romance by Subandhu; accompanied by Śivaráma Tripáṭhin's Perpetual Gloss, Entitled Darpaṇa, ed. F. Hall. Calcutta: Baptist Mission Press, 1855–1859 (repr. Osnabrück: Biblio Verlag, 1980).

Yogamakaranda by T. Krishnamacharya (excerpt)
see Mohan 2010: 139–146.

Yogasūtra attributed to Patañjali
see Bryant 2009.
see Moors 2007.
see *Pātañjalayogadarśanam*.

Secondary Sources

Aklujkar, A. (2008a). Patañjali's Mahābhāṣya as a Key to Happy Kashmir. In M. Kaul & A. Aklujkar (Eds.), *Linguistic Traditions of Kashmir: Essays in Memory of Paṇḍit Dinanath Yaksha* (pp. 41–87). New Delhi: D. K. Printworld.

Aklujkar, A. (2008b). Gonardīya, Goṇikā-putra, Patañjali and Gonandīya. In M. Kaul & A. Aklujkar (Eds.), *Linguistic Traditions of Kashmir: Essays in Memory of Paṇḍit Dinanath Yaksha* (pp. 88–172). New Delhi: D. K. Printworld.

Aklujkar, A. (2008c). Patañjali: A Kashmirian. In M. Kaul & A. Aklujkar (Eds.), *Linguistic Traditions of Kashmir: Essays in Memory of Paṇḍit Dinanath Yaksha* (pp. 173–205). New Delhi: D. K. Printworld.

Balasubramanian, A. V. (1992). Sri Patanjali. *Darsanam: A Quarterly Journal from the Krishnamacharya Yoga Mandiram, 2*(1), February 1992: 2–10.

Bhattacharya, R. S. (1985). *An Introduction to the Yogasūtra.* Delhi: Bharatiya Vidya Prakasana.

Bryant, E. F. (2009). *The Yoga Sūtras of Patañjali: A New Edition, Translation, and Commentary with Insights from the Traditional Commentators.* New York: North Point Press.

Cardona, G. (1980). *Pāṇini: A Survey of Research.* Delhi: Motilal Banarsidass (first Indian ed.).

Deshpande, M. (1994). The Changing Notion of Śiṣṭa from Patañjali to Bhartṛhari. In S. Bhate & J. Bronkhorst (Eds.), *Bhartṛhari: Philosopher and Grammarian. Proceedings of the First International Conference on Bhartṛhari (University of Poona, January 6–8, 1992)* (pp. 95–115). Delhi: Motilal Banarsidass.

Deshpande, M. (1997). Who Inspired Pāṇini? Reconstructing the Hindu and Buddhist Counter-Claims. *Journal of the American Oriental Society, 117,* 444–465.

Desikachar, T. K. V. (1980). *Religiousness in Yoga: Lectures on Theory and Practice,* ed. M. L. Skelton & J. R. Carter. Washington, D. C.: University Press of America.

Desikachar, T. K. V. (1982). *The Yoga of T. Krishnamacharya.* Madras: Krishnamacharya Yoga Mandiram.

Desikachar, T. K. V. (with R. H. Cravens). (1998). *Health, Healing and Beyond: Yoga and the Living Tradition of Krishnamacharya.* New York: Aperture Foundation.

Filliozat, J. (1964). *The Classical Doctrine of Indian Medicine: Its Origins and its Greek Parallels,* trans. D. R. Chanana. Delhi: Munshiram Manoharlal (French original: *Doctrine classique de la médecine indienne: ses origines et ses parallèles grecs.* Paris: Imprenterie Nationale, 1949).

Goudriaan, T. (1978). *Māyā Divine and Human: A Study of Magic and its Religious Foundations in Sanskrit Texts, with Particular Attention to a Fragment on Viṣṇu's Māyā Preserved in Bali.* Delhi: Motilal Banarsidass.

Iyengar, B. K. S. (2000–2010). *Aṣṭadaḷa Yogamālā (Collected Works).* 8 vols. Mumbai: Allied Publishers.

Iyengar, B. K. S. (2002). *Light on the Yoga Sūtras of Patañjali.* London: Thorsons.

Krishnamacharya (1992). N. N. (Ed.), Selected Works of T. Krishnamacharya: 2. Sri T. Krishnamacharya on Sri Patanjali. *Darsanam: A Quarterly Journal from the Krishnamacharya Yoga Mandiram, 2*(1), February 1992, 11–18.

Kulke, H. (1970). *Cidambaramāhātmya: Eine Untersuchung der religionsgeschichtlichen und historischen Hintergründe für die Entstehung der Tradition einer südindischen Tempelstadt.* Freiburger Beiträge zur Indologie 3. Wiesbaden: Otto Harrassowitz.

Larson, G. J. & Bhattacharya, R. S. (Eds.). (2008). *Yoga: India's Philosophy of Meditation.* Encyclopedia of Indian Philosophies 12. Delhi: Motilal Banarsidass.

Marechal, C. (2013–2014). Teachings of Professor Krishnamacharya. *Nāmarūpa: Categories of Indian Thought, 18,* 52–59.

Meulenbeld, G. J. (1999–2002). *A History of Indian Medical Literature.* 3 vols. (in five parts). Groningen Oriental Studies 15. Groningen: Egbert Forsten.

Mevissen, G. J. R. (1996). Chidambaram – Nṛttasabhā: Architektur, Ikonographie und Symbolik. *Berliner Indologische Studien, 9/10,* 345–420.

Mevissen, G. J. R. (2002). The Nṛtta-sabhā at Chidambaram. Some Remarks. In R. Nagaswamy (Ed.), *Foundations of Indian Art: Proceedings of the Chidambaram Seminar on Art and Religion, Feb. 2001* (pp. 61–71). Chennai: Tamil Arts Academy.

Mevissen, G. J. R. (2004). Chola Architecture and Sculpture at Chidambaram. In V. Nanda with G. Michell (Eds.), *Chidambaram: Home of Nataraja* (pp. 82–95). Mumbai: Marg Publications.

Mohan, A. G. (2010). *Krishnamacharya: His Life and Teachings.* Boston: Shambala.

Moors, F. (2007). *Yoga-Sūtra de Patañjali: Traduction et Commentaire.* Les cahiers de Présence d'esprit 9. Lyon: Étude et Pratique du Yoga & Présence d'esprit.

Nagaswamy, R. (1995). On Dating South Indian Bronzes. In J. Guy (Ed.), *Indian Art & Connoisseurship. Essays in Honour of Douglas Barrett* (pp. 100–129). Middletown etc.: Indira Gandhi National Centre for the Arts in association with Mapin Publishing.

Natarajan, B., assisted by Venkataraman, B. and Ramachandran, B. (1994). *Tillai and Nataraja.* Madras: Mudgala Trust.

Ramaswami, S. (2000). *Yoga for the Three Stages of Life: Developing your Practice as an Art Form, a Physical Therapy, and a Guiding Philosophy.* Rochester, Vermont: Inner Traditions International.

Roodbergen, J. A. F. (1984). *Mallinātha's Ghaṇṭāpatha on the Kirātārjunīya, I–VI.* Part 1: *Introduction, Translation and Notes.* Leiden: Brill.

Sarbacker, S. R. (2015). The Icon of Yoga: Patañjali as Nāgarāja in Modern Yoga Traditions. In T. Pintchman & C. G. Dempsey (Eds.), *Sacred Matters: Material Religion in South Asian Traditions* (pp. 15–37). Albany, New York: State University of New York Press.

Singleton, M. (2008). The Classical Reveries of Modern Yoga: Patañjali and Constructive Orientalism. In M. Singleton & J. Byrne (Eds.), *Yoga in the Modern World: Contemporary Perspectives* (pp. 77–99). London: Routledge.

Sivaramamurti, C. (1981). *Ṛishis in Indian Art and Literature.* New Delhi: Kanak Publications.

Staal, J. F. (1972). *A Reader on the Sanskrit Grammarians.* Studies in Linguistics 1. Cambridge, Massachusetts: The Massachusetts Institute of Technology Press.

Thiruvengadathan, A. (2002). *Ramabhadra Diksita and his Works: A Study.* Chennai: The Kuppuswami Sastri Research Institute.

Venkatraman, R. (1990). *A History of the Tamil Siddha Cult.* Madurai: Ennes Publications.

White, D. G. (2014). *The Yoga Sutra of Patanjali: A Biography.* Princeton, New Jersey: Princeton University Press.

Woods, J. H. (1914). *The Yoga-System of Patañjali Or the Ancient Hindu Doctrine of Concentration of Mind: Embracing the Mnemonic Rules, Called Yoga-sūtras, of Patañjali and the Comment, Called Yoga-bhāshya, Attributed to Veda-vyāsa and the Explanation, Called Tattva-vāiçāradī, of Vāchaspati-miçra, transl. from the orig. Sanskrit by J. H. Woods.* Harvard Oriental Series 17. Cambridge, Massachusetts: Harvard University Press.

Younger, P. (1995). *The Home of Dancing Śivan̲: The Traditions of the Hindu Temple in Citamparam.* Oxford: Oxford University Press.

Younger, P. (2004). Ritual Life of the Nataraja Temple. In V. Nanda with G. Michell (Eds.), *Chidambaram: Home of Nataraja* (pp. 60–69). Mumbai: Marg Publications.

Zvelebil, K. V. (1973). *The Poets of the Powers.* London: Rider.

Figures

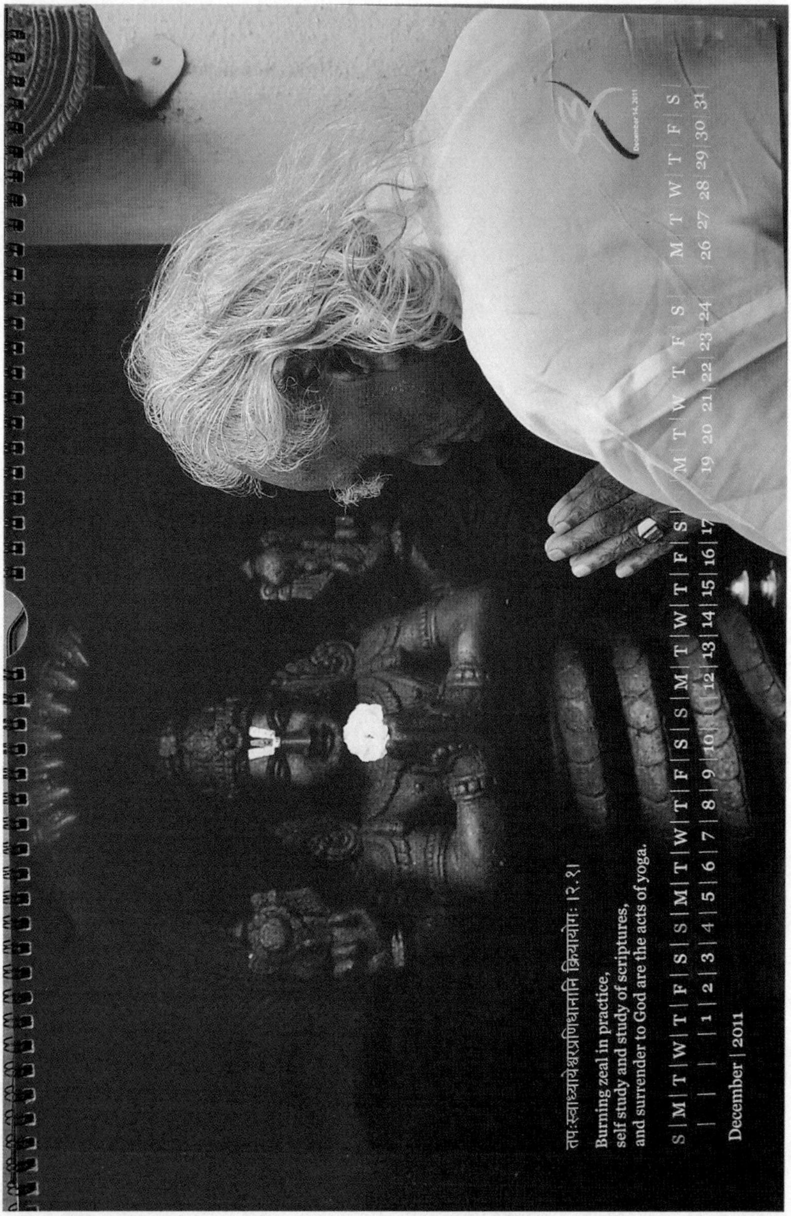

Figure 1: Calendar image: B. K. S. Iyengar worships Patañjali (photograph: Gudrun Bühnemann).

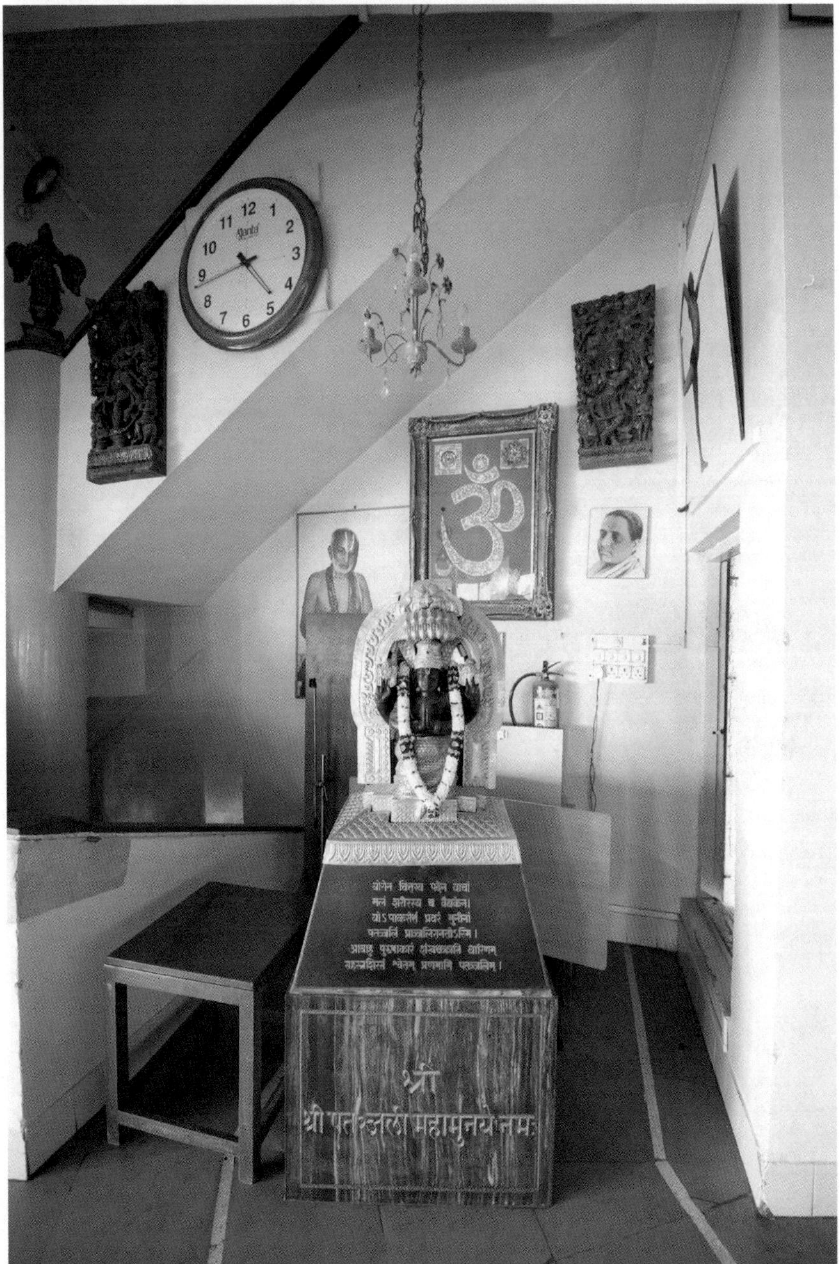

Figure 2: Patañjali sculpture in the Ramamani Iyengar Memorial Yoga Institute, Pune (photograph courtesy of Dominik Ketz).

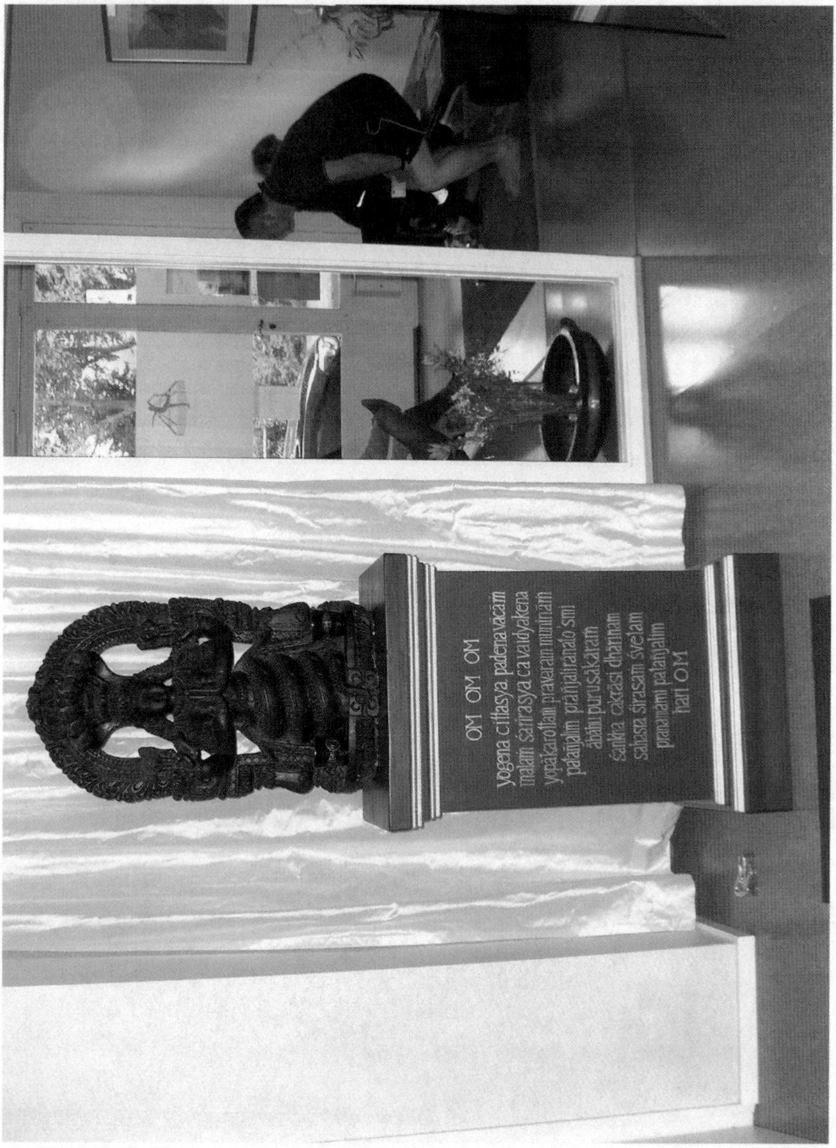

Figure 3: Patañjali sculpture in the Iyengar-Yoga-Institut Rhein-Ahr e.V., Cologne (photograph: Gudrun Bühnemann).

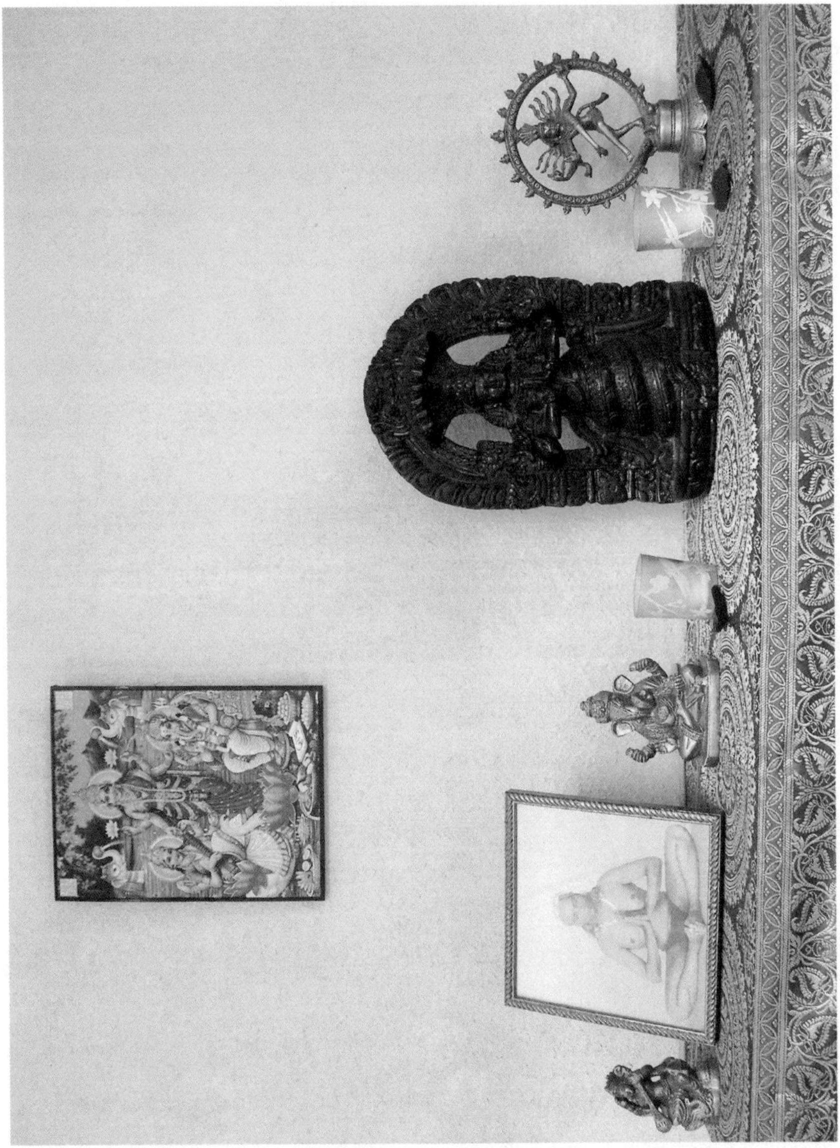

Figure 4: Altar with a statue of Patañjali and a photograph of B. K. S. Iyengar; Iyengar-Yoga-Zentrum, Cologne Centre (photograph: Gudrun Bühnemann).

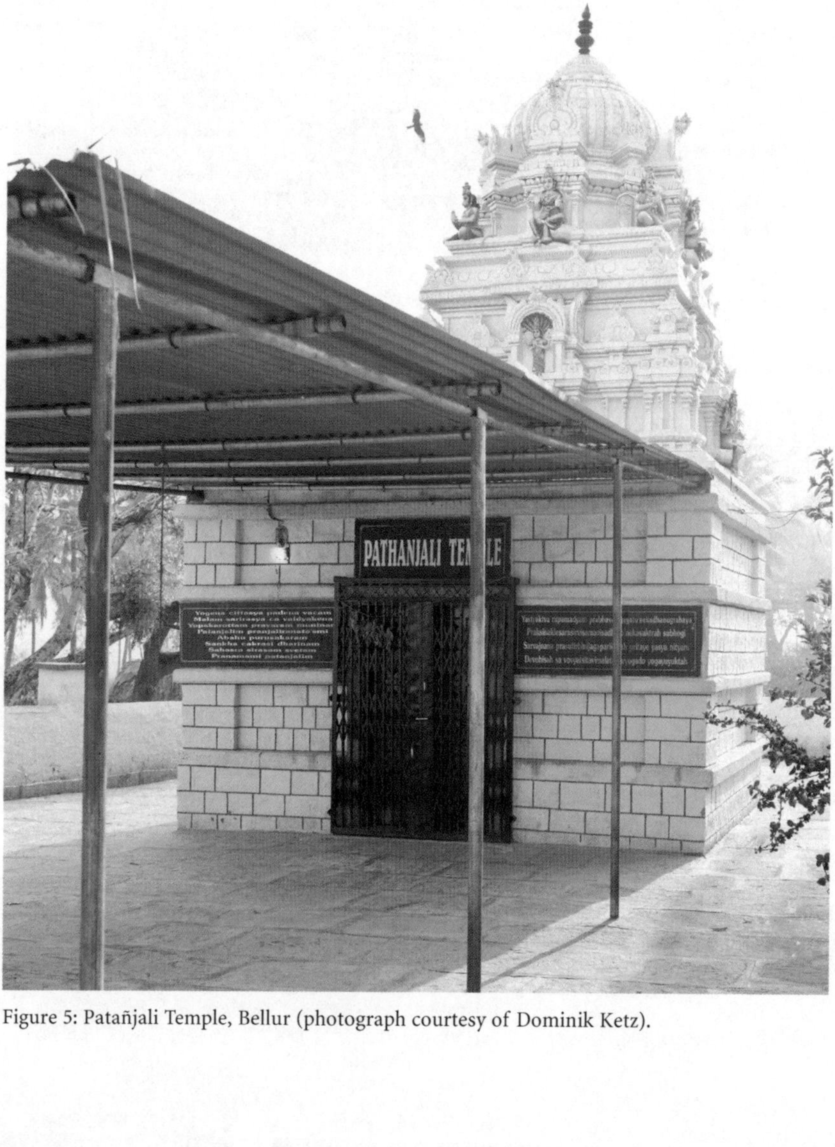

Figure 5: Patañjali Temple, Bellur (photograph courtesy of Dominik Ketz).

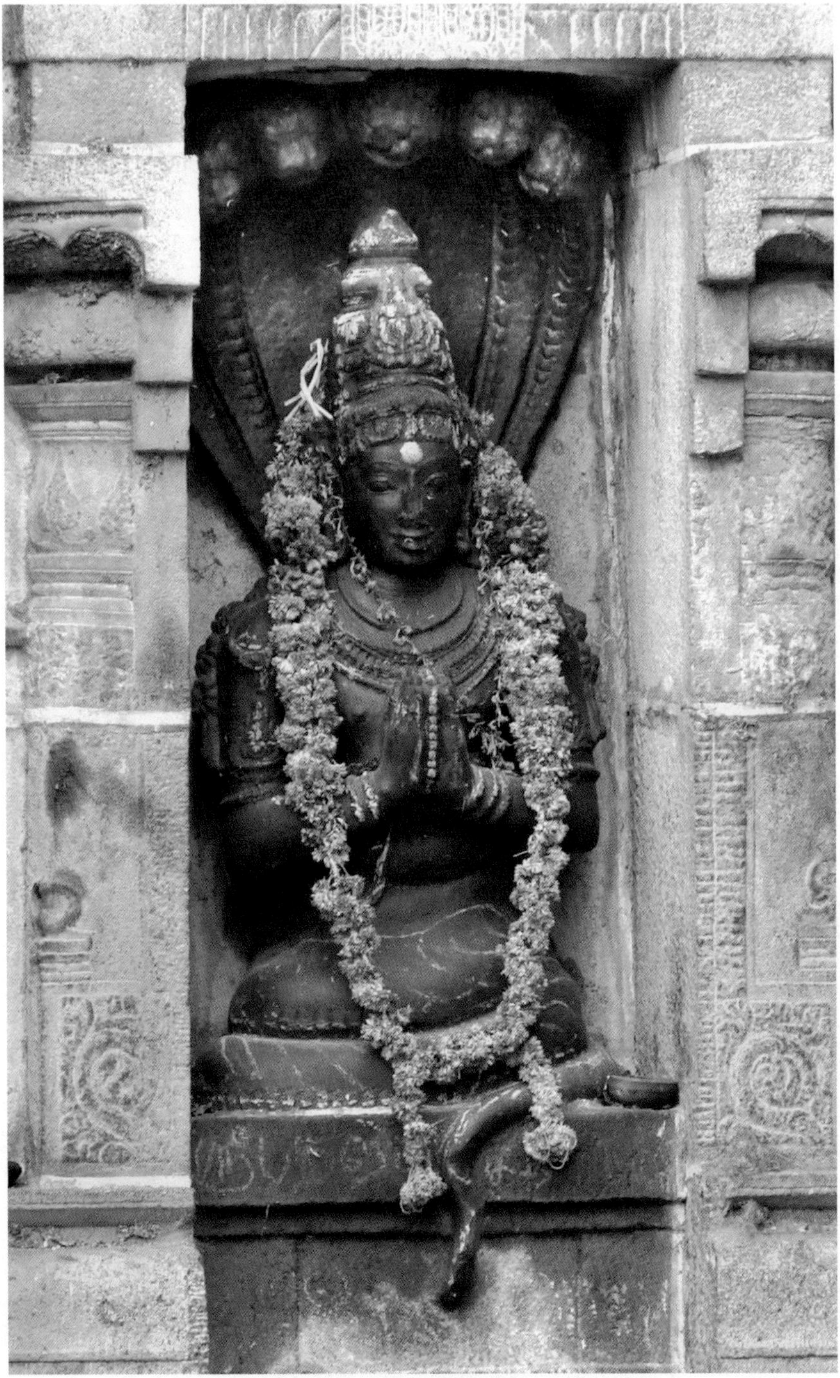

Figure 6: Patañjali sculpture on the eastern temple tower of the Naṭarāja Temple, Cidambaram (photograph courtesy of Gudrun Melzer).

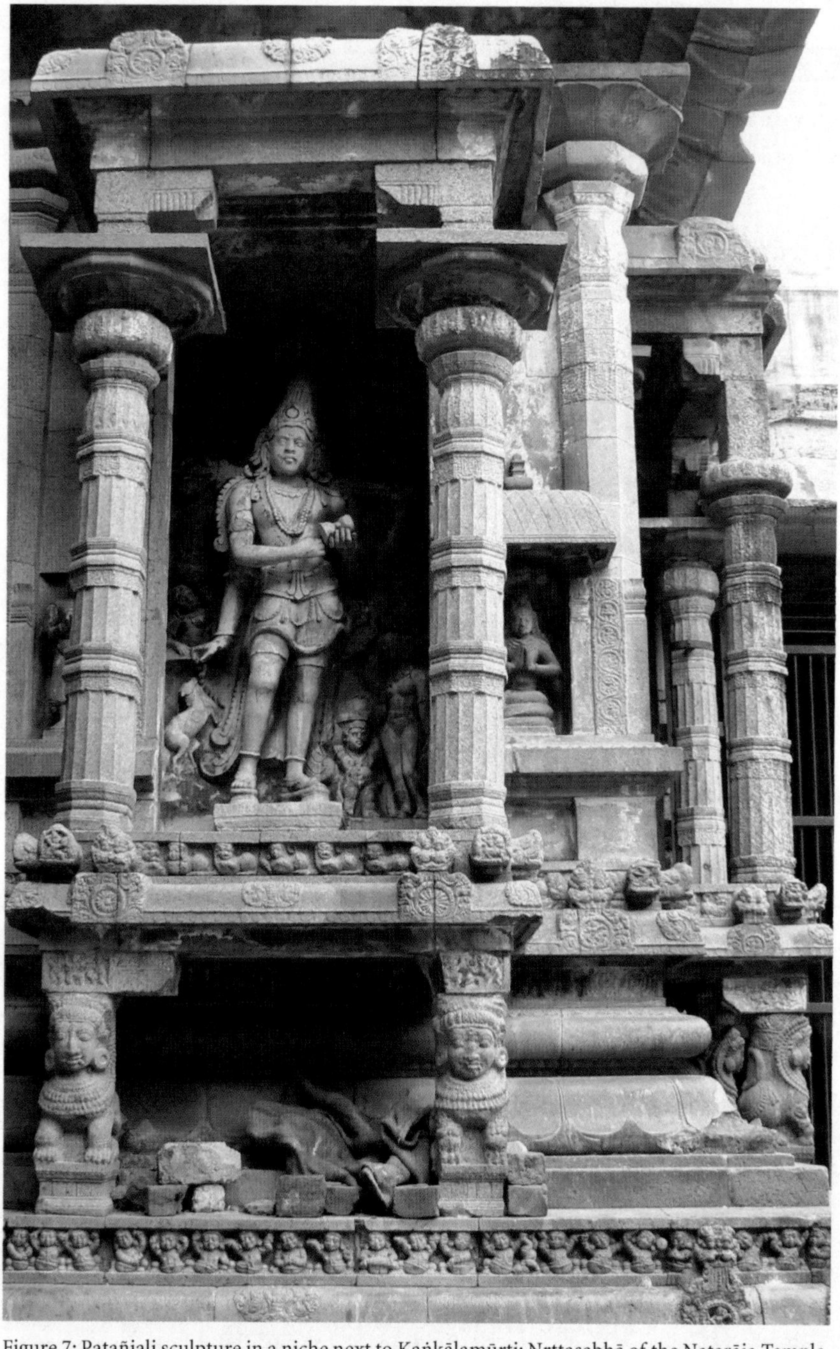

Figure 7: Patañjali sculpture in a niche next to Kaṅkālamūrti; Nṛttasabhā of the Naṭarāja Temple, Cidambaram (photograph courtesy of Corinna Wessels-Mevissen).

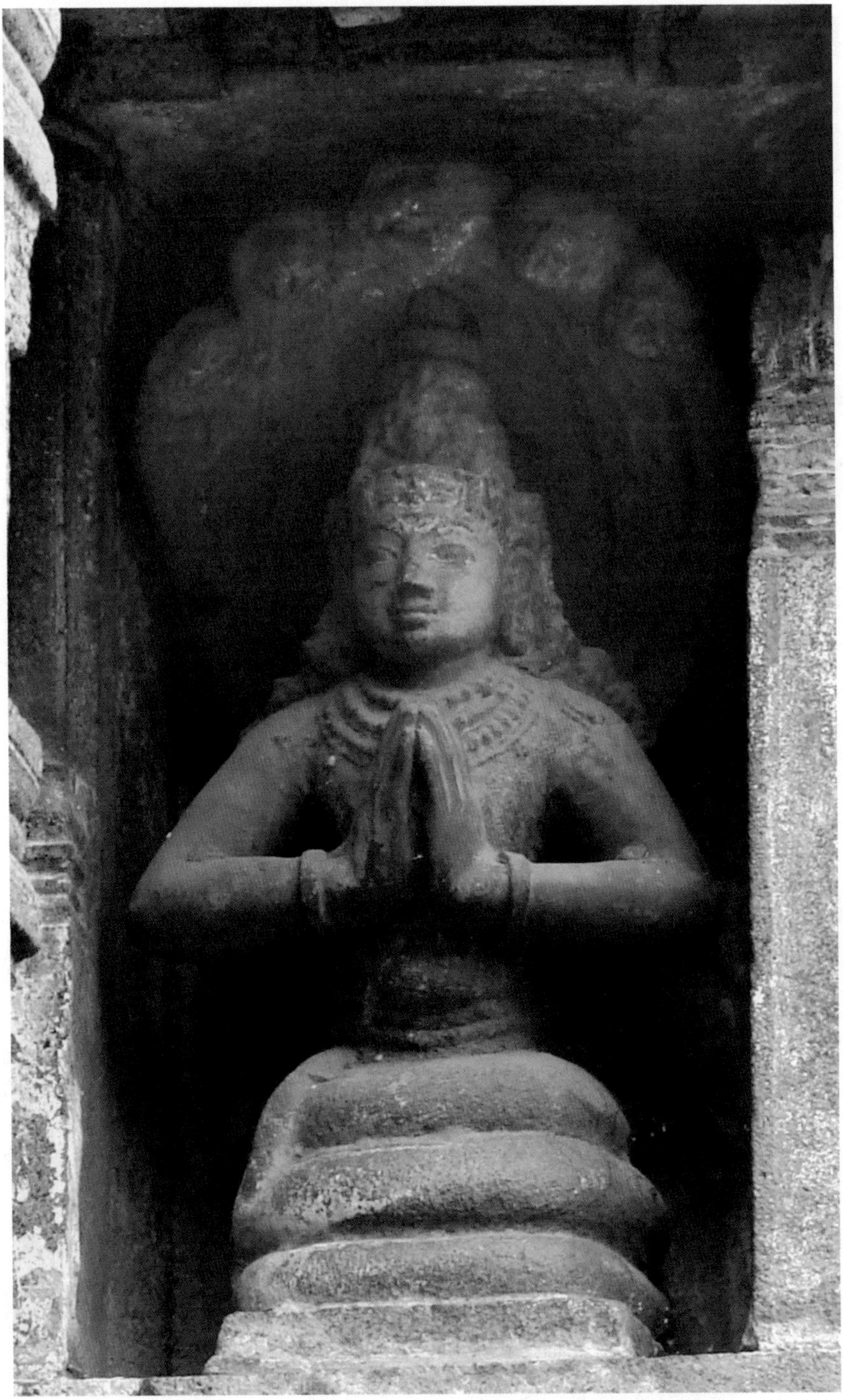

Figure 8: Detail of Figure 7 (photograph courtesy of Corinna Wessels-Mevissen).

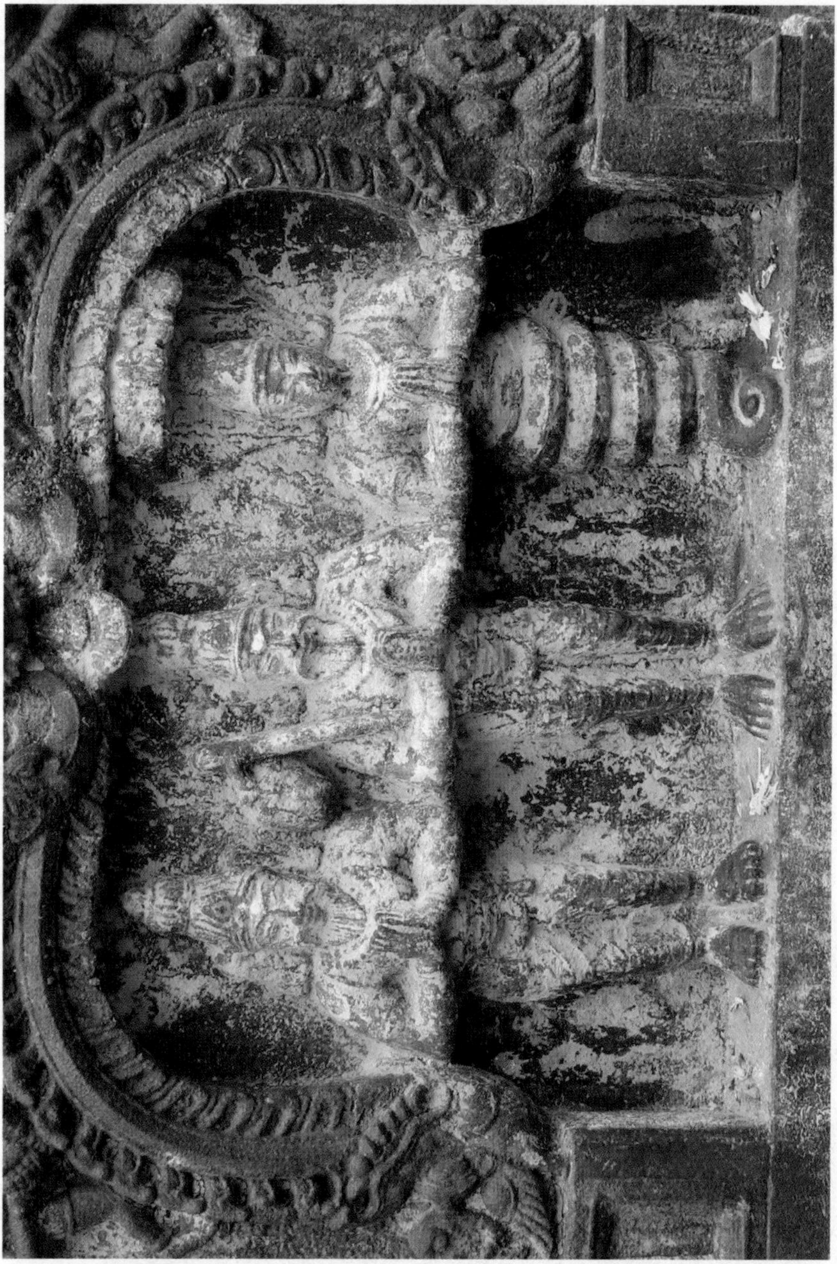

Figure 9: Patañjali grouped with the sages Vyāghrapāda ("Tiger-Foot") and Jaimini; Citsabhā of the Naṭarāja Temple, Cidambaram (photograph courtesy of Corinna Wessels-Mevissen).

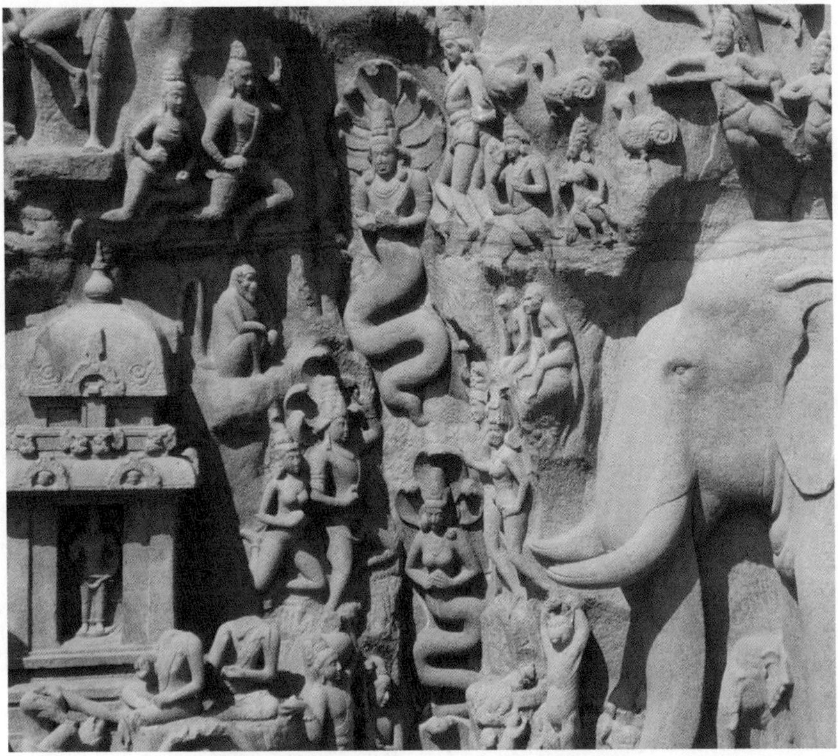

Figure 10: *nāga* and *nāginī*; Mamallapuram bas-relief (photograph courtesy of Gerd Mevissen).

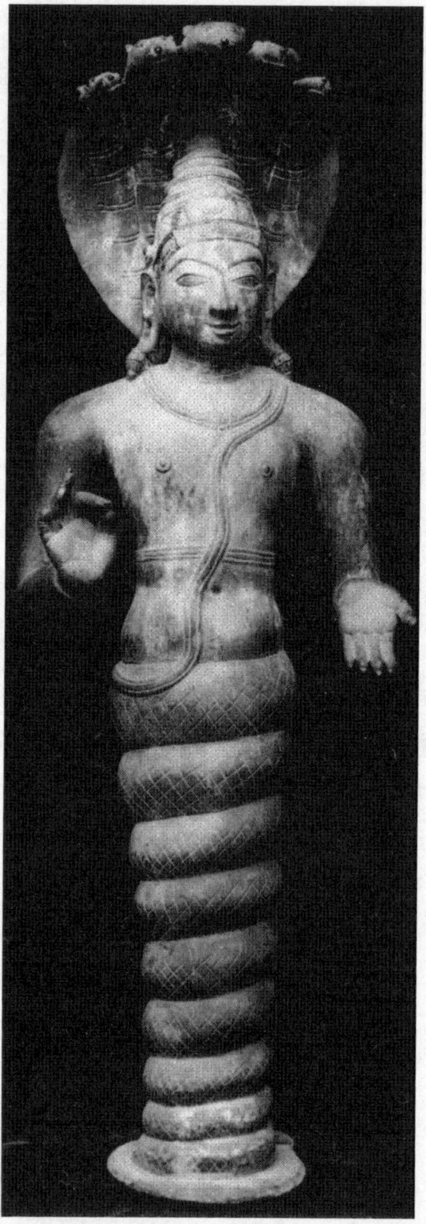

Figure 11: Patañjali; after Nagaswamy 1995: fig. 21.

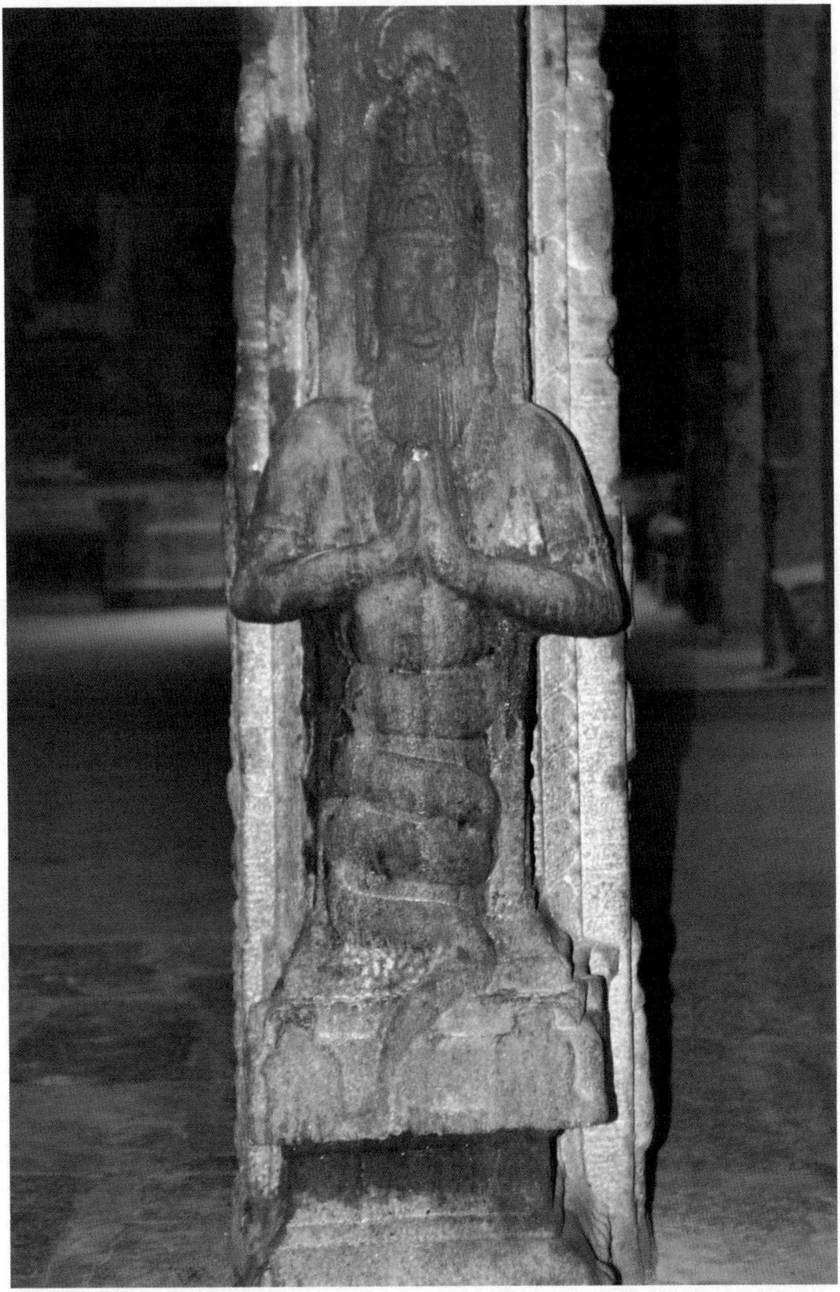

Figure 12: Patañjali sculpture from the temple town Avudaiyarkoil (Āvuṭaiyārkōvil) (photograph courtesy of the École Française d'Extrême-Orient, Pondicherry).

Figure 13: Bronze sculpture showing Patañjali; Ashmolean Museum, Oxford, acc. no. EA2005.11 (photograph courtesy of the Ashmolean Museum).

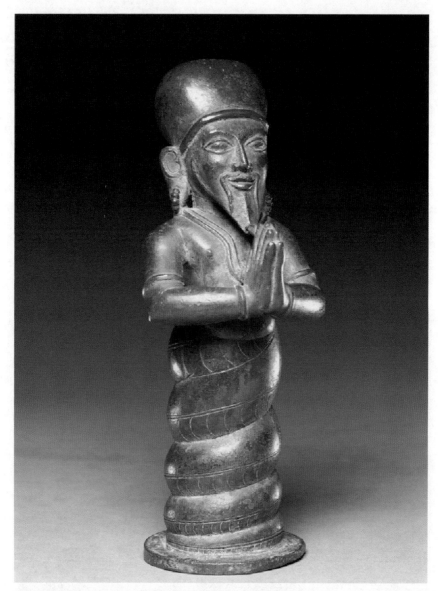

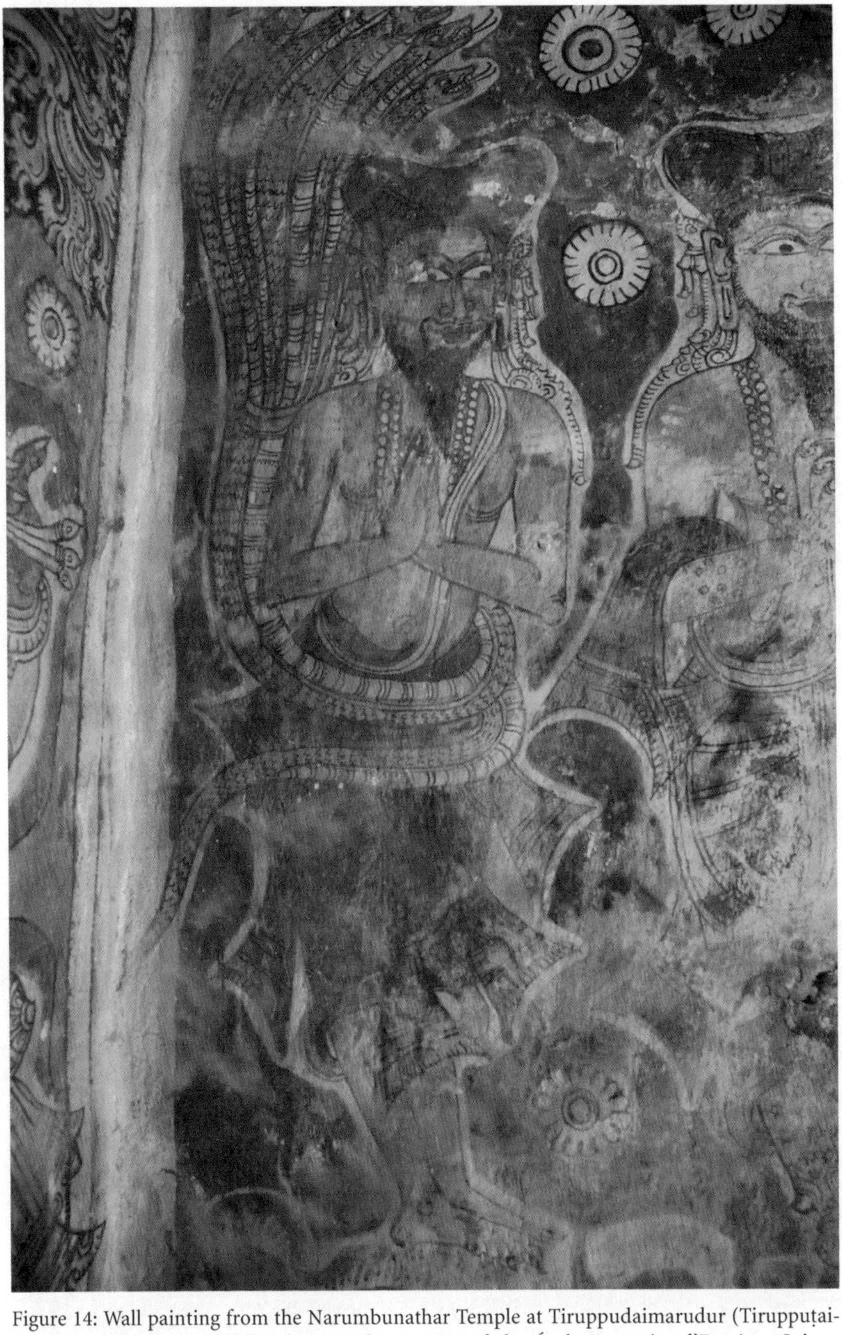

Figure 14: Wall painting from the Narumbunathar Temple at Tiruppudaimarudur (Tirupputai-marutūr) showing Patañjali (photograph courtesy of the École Française d'Extrême-Orient, Pondicherry).

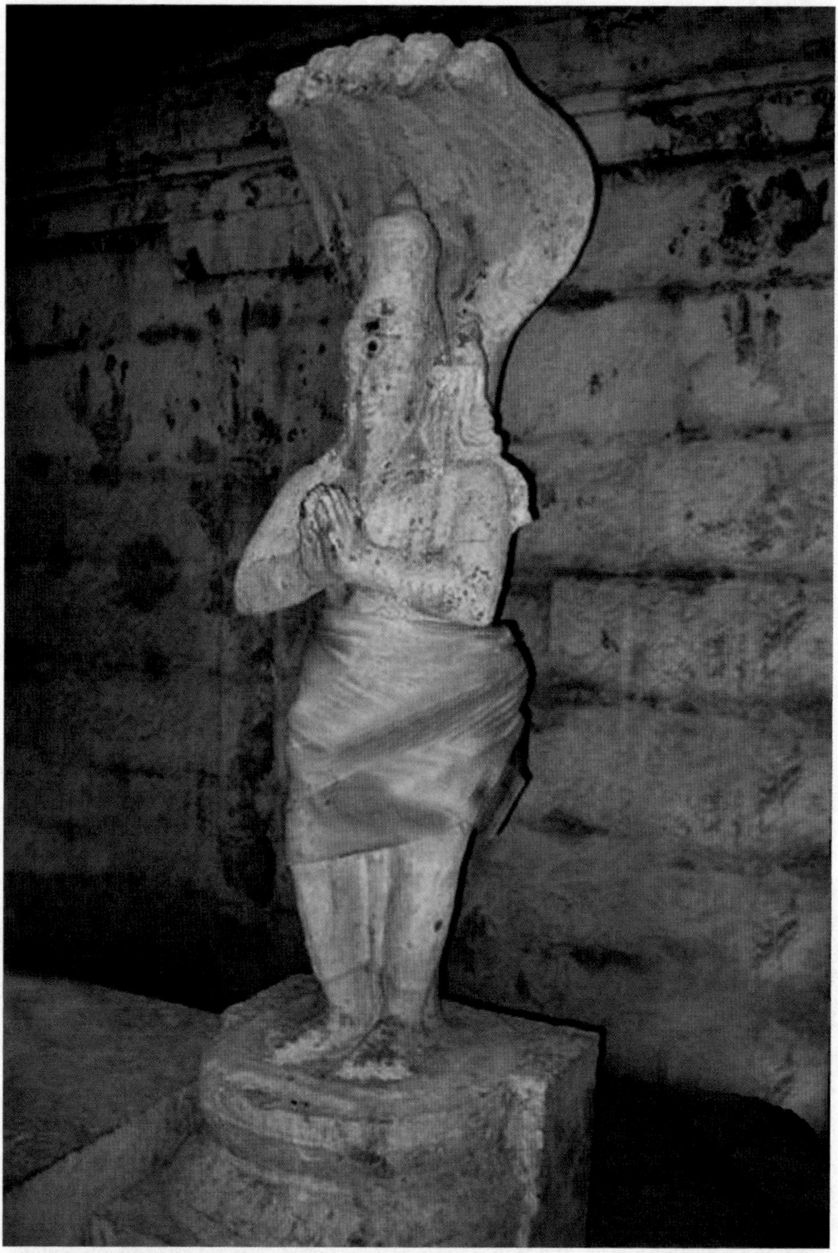

Figure 15: Patañjali sculpture from the Narumbunathar Temple at Tiruppudaimarudur (Tiruppuṭaimarutūr) (photograph courtesy of the École Française d'Extrême-Orient, Pondicherry).

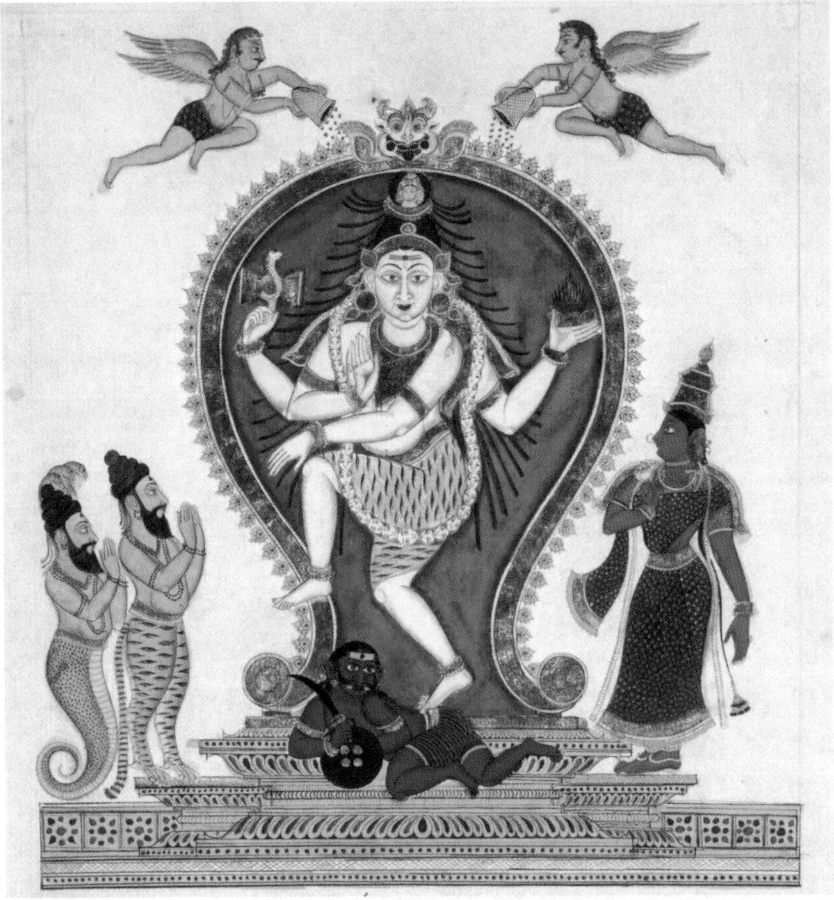

Figure 16: Patañjali and Vyāghrapāda worshipping the Dancing Śiva; gouache painting on paper, c 1820; collection of the British Museum, acc. no. AN356267001 (photograph courtesy of the British Museum).

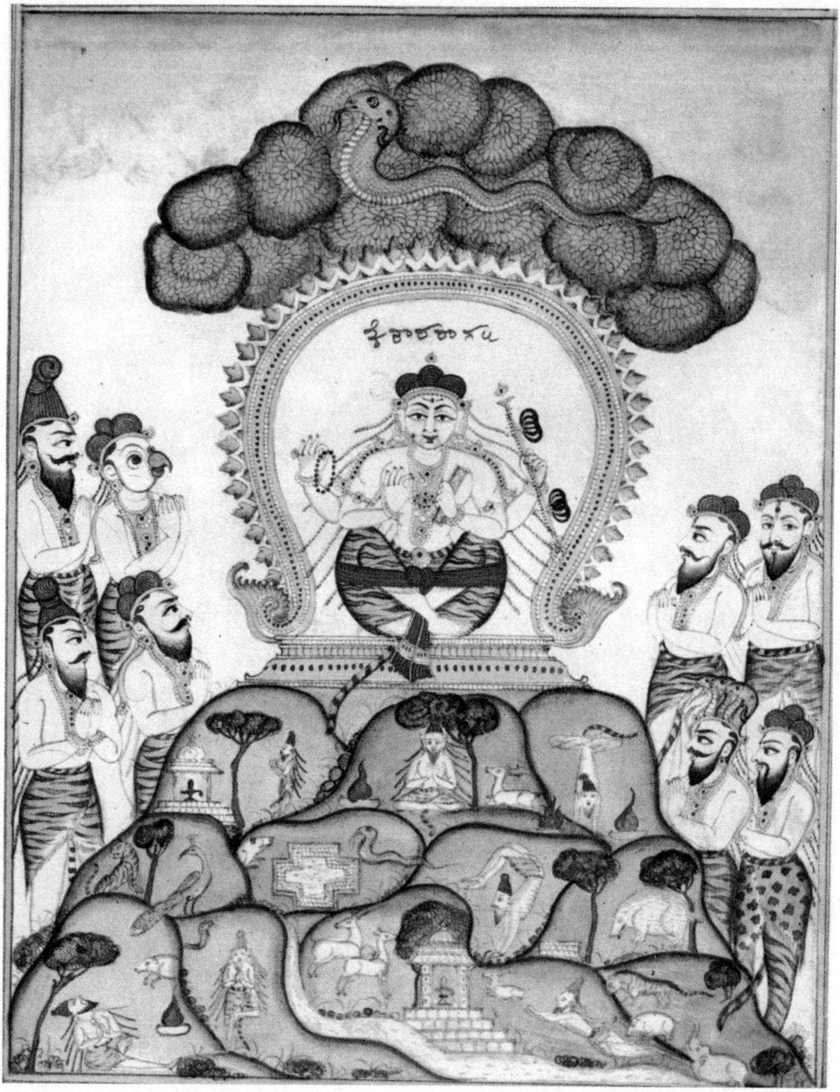

Figure 17: Yoga-Dakṣiṇāmūrti worshipped by Patañjali and other sages (photograph after Svaracūḍāmaṇi p. 119).

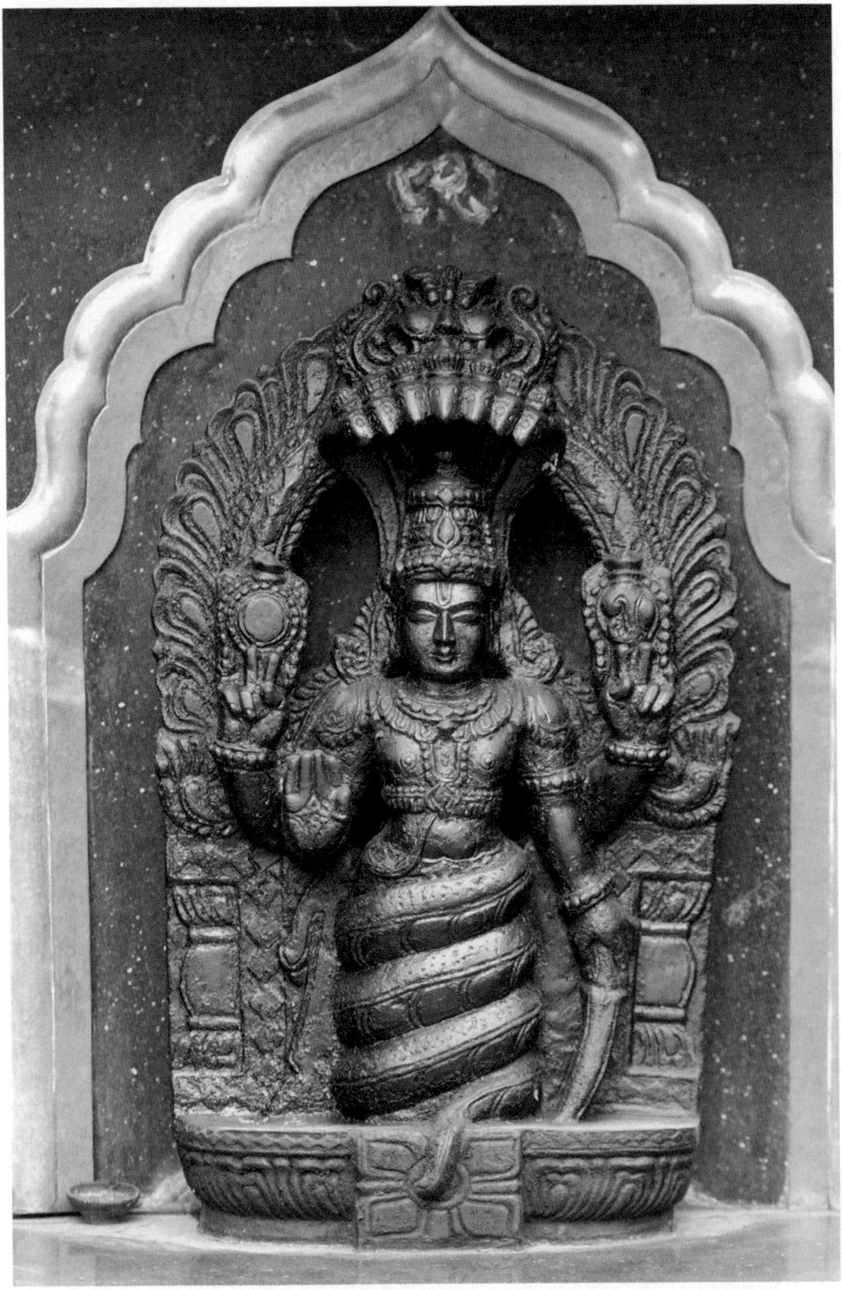

Figure 18: Four-armed Patañjali holding a sword; Ramamani Iyengar Memorial Yoga Institute, Pune (photograph courtesy of Dominik Ketz).

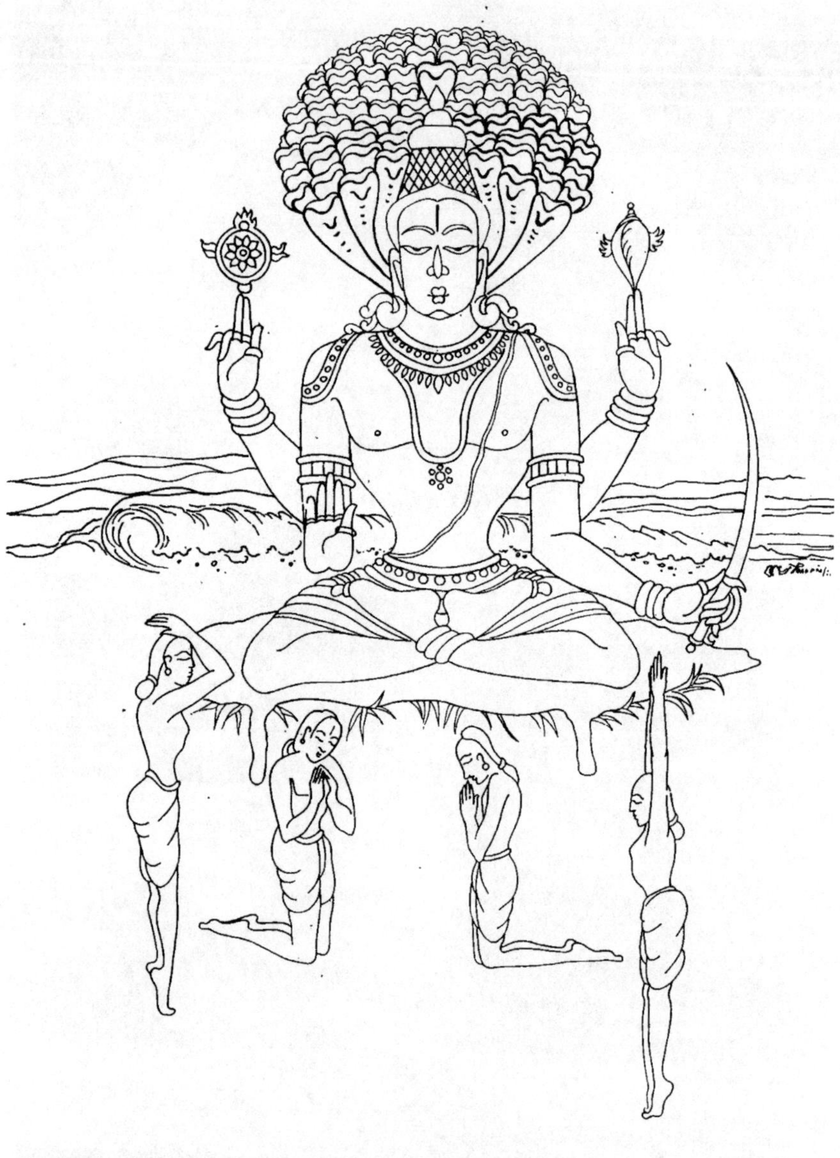

Figure 19: Four-armed Patañjali holding a sword, worshipped by Mastakāñjali, Kṛtāñjali, Baddhāñjali and Pūrṇāñjali (Desikachar 1982, plate after p. 38).

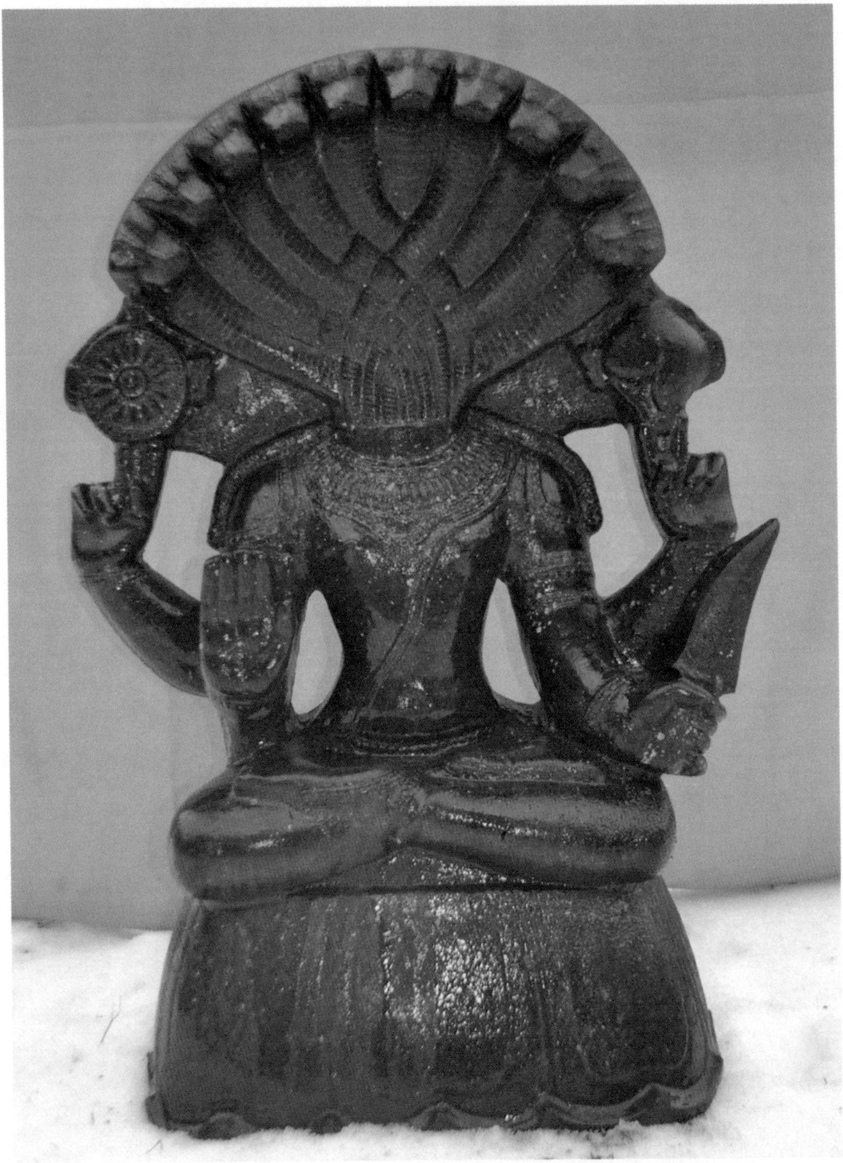

Figure 20: Four-armed Patañjali holding a sword; stone sculpture, commissioned in c 1996 (photo courtesy of Martine Burat).

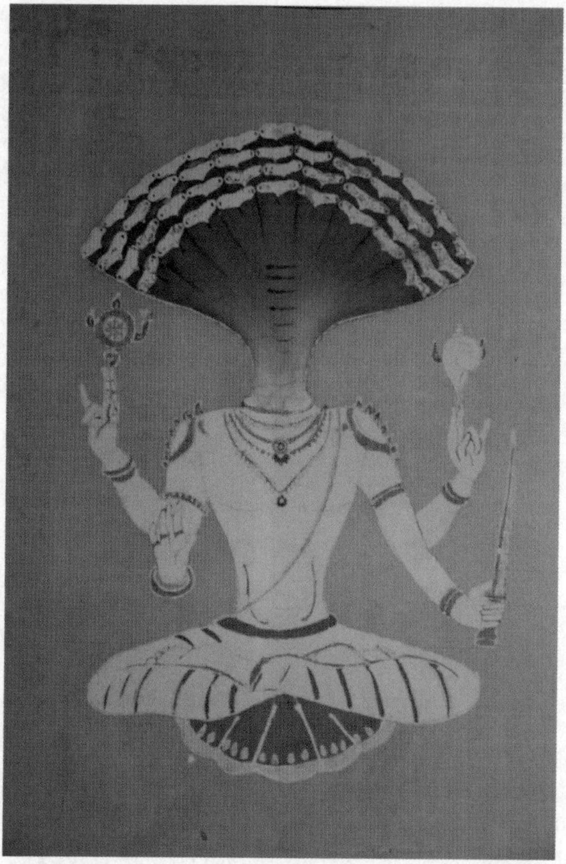

Figure 21: Four-armed Patañjali holding a sword; batik made by W. Skelton and kept in the Upstate Yoga Institute, Fayetteville, New York (photo courtesy of Emily Malavenda).

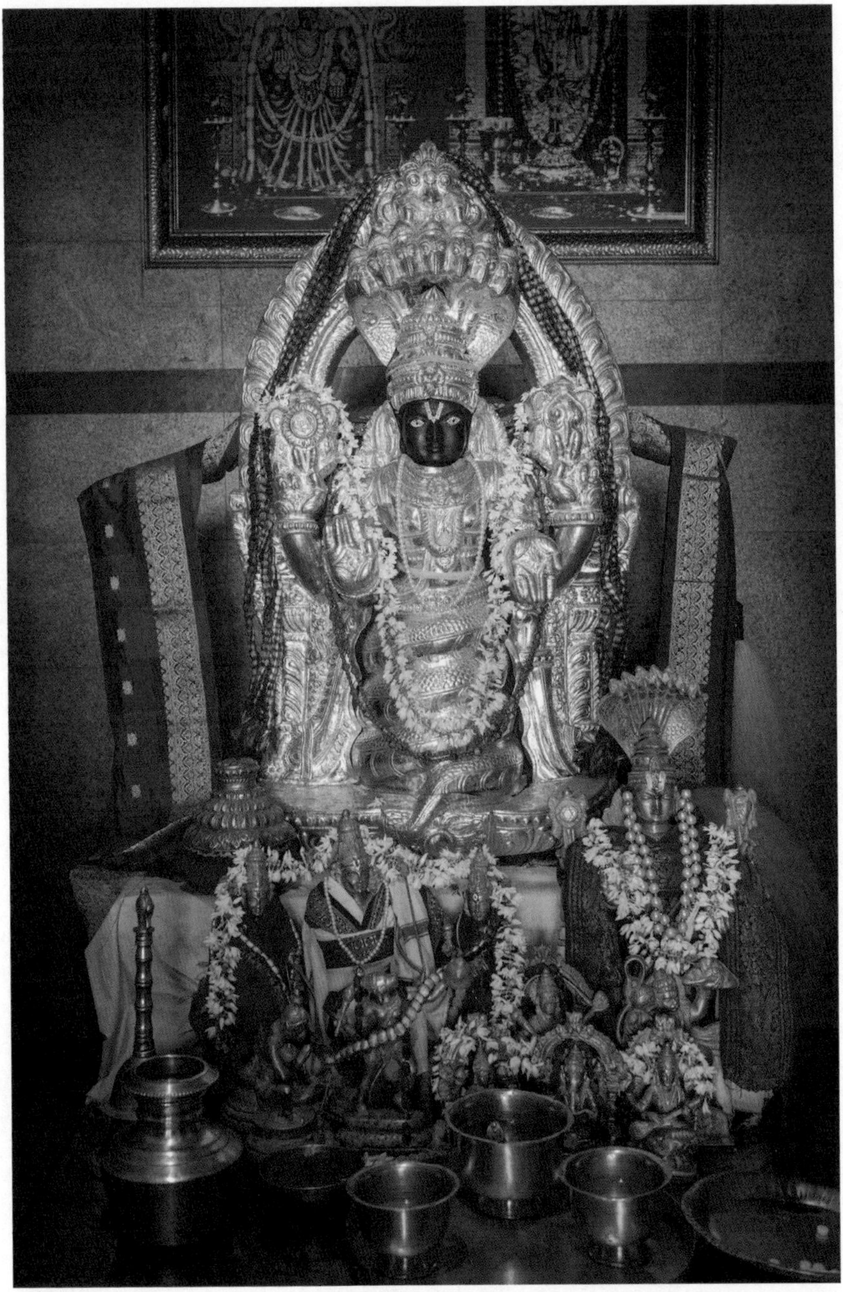

Figure 22: Patañjali sculpture in the Patañjali Temple at Bellur (photograph courtesy of Dominik Ketz).

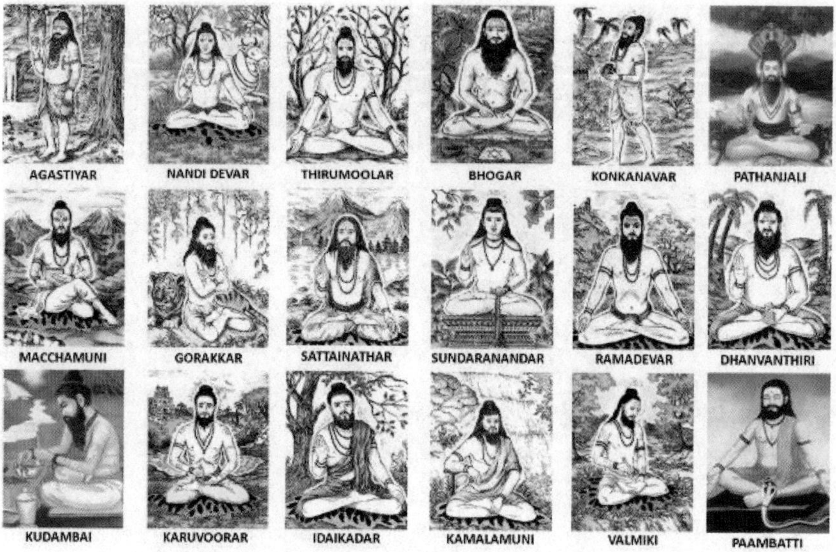

Figure 23: Patañjali as one of the 18 *siddha*-s; modern devotional print.

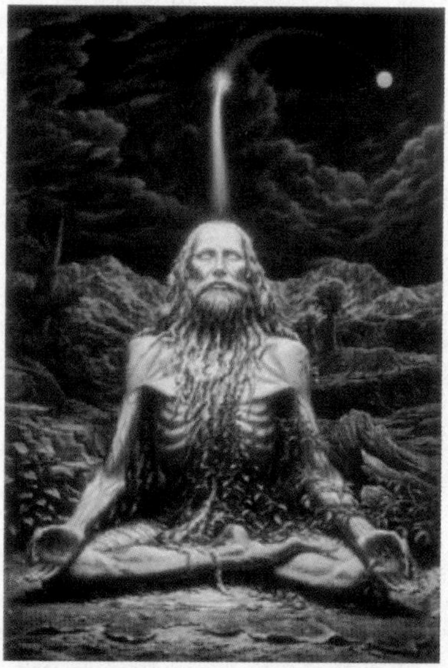

Figure 24: Patañjali; modern devotional print associated with the Patañjali Jeeva Samadhi at the Brahmapureeswarar Temple, Tirupattur.

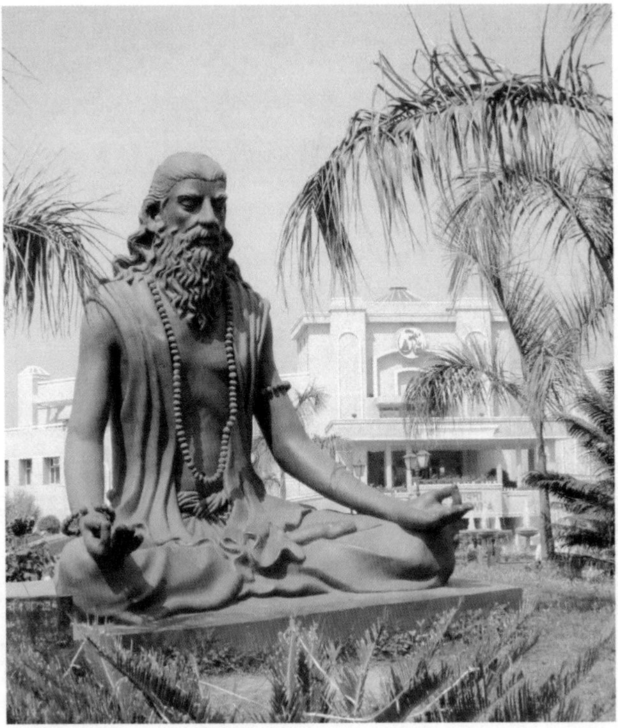

Figure 25: A statue of Patañjali installed on the premises of the Patañjali Yogapīṭha in Haridwar, North India (photograph: Gudrun Bühnemann).

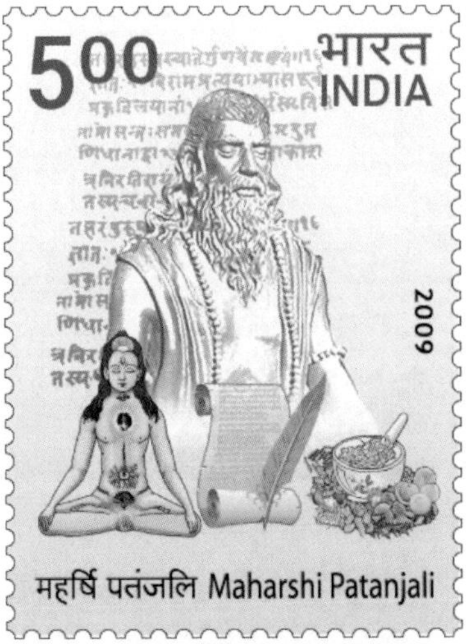

Figure 26: Patañjali; commemorative postal stamp issued by India Post.

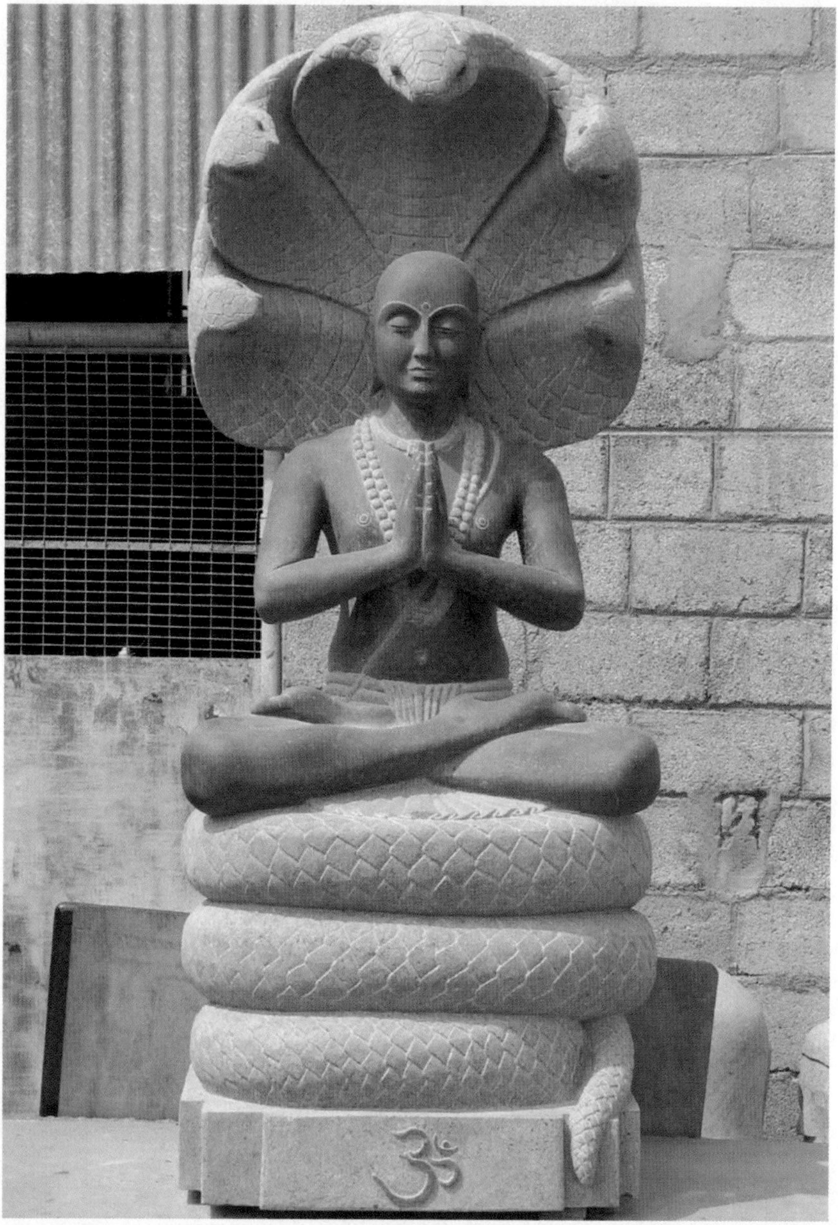

Figure 27: Modern stone sculpture of Patañjali (photo courtesy of Kyle Tortora, www.lotus sculpture.com).

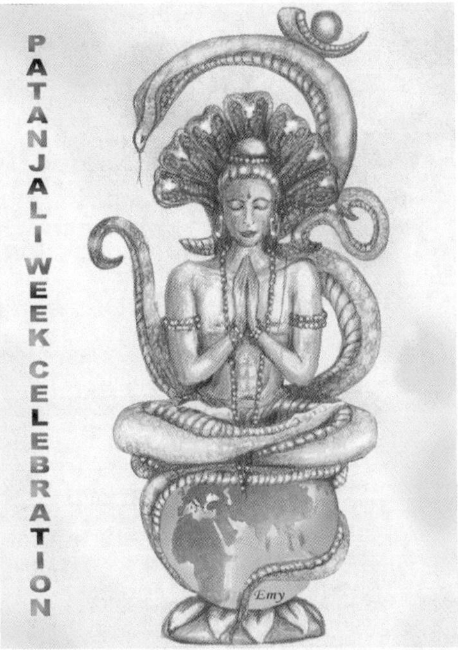

Figure 28: Patañjali with a serpent that assumes the shape of the syllable *oṃ* (poster designed by Erny Blesio; photo courtesy of Suryanagara, Milano).

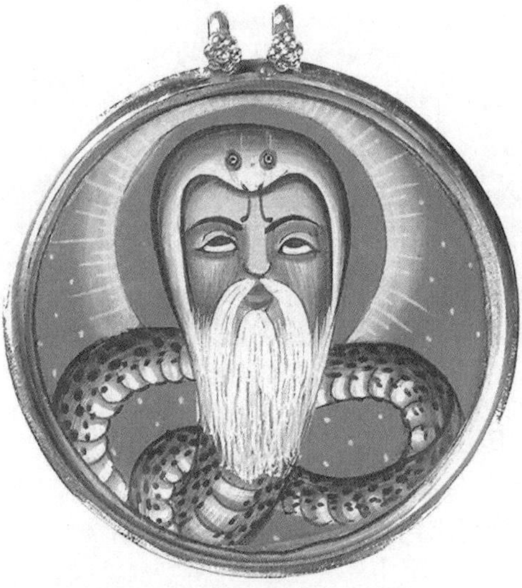

Figure 29: Pendant featuring Patañjali (photograph courtesy of Exotic India (http://www.exotic india.com).

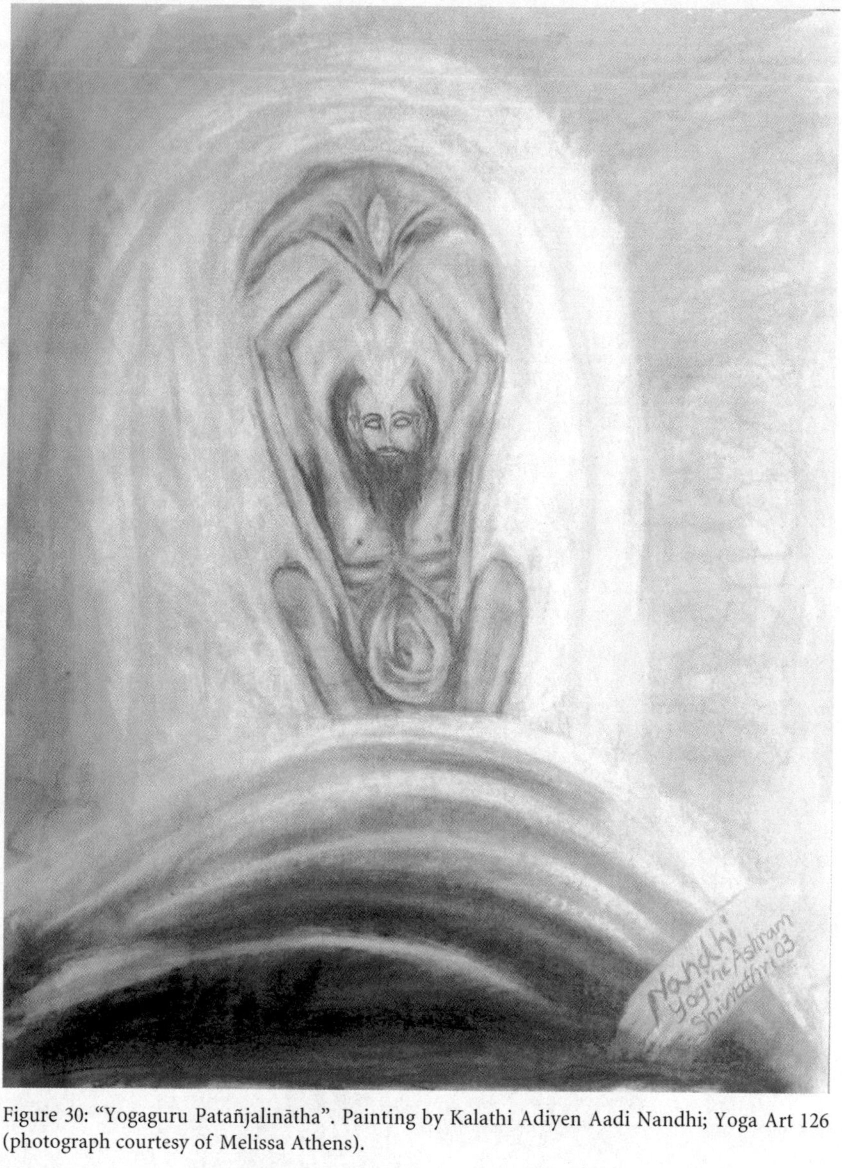

Figure 30: "Yogaguru Patañjalinātha". Painting by Kalathi Adiyen Aadi Nandhi; Yoga Art 126 (photograph courtesy of Melissa Athens).

Contributors

Joseph S. Alter

Joseph S. Alter is Professor of Anthropology at the University of Pittsburgh. His research is on the medicalisation of yoga and the cultural history of yoga's development within the institutionalised structure of Nature Cure in contemporary India. Having published on yoga in relation to sexuality, athleticism and Ayurvedic medicine, Joseph is currently studying the way in which yoga and Nature Cure establish an "ecology of the body" within the rubric of Public Health.

His publications include *Yoga in Modern India* (2004), *Moral Materialism* (2011) and "Medicine, Alternative Medicine and Political Ecologies of the Body" (in M. Singer [Ed.], *A Companion to the Anthropology of Environmental Health*, 2016, pp. 121–142).

Anand Amaladass

Anand Amaladass is Professor emeritus of the Satya Nilayam Jesuit Faculty of Philosophy, now part of the Loyola College, Chennai. He learnt the rudiments of yoga through *The Christian Yoga* by Jean-Marie Dechanet and as a student was initiated into yoga practice as part of the general training he received from his Jesuit formators. Later he taught a course on the Tamil Cittar tradition at the University of Vienna, which led him to the study of different yoga texts like the *Tirumantiram, Pātañjalayogaśāstra* and *Haṭhayogapradīpikā.*

His research interests are diverse. Anand translated selected hymns of the Tamil Cittars in *Śiva tanzt in Südindien* (2009) and studied the feminine aspect of the Divine, based on Sanskrit and Tamil texts on the Goddess phenomenon where yogic symbols play a great role. In this connection, he also translated a Tamil text in his *Abhirāmi Antāti: Die weibliche Dimension der Gottheit. Eine indische Perspektive* (2004). His focus was on the role of the body, which includes, among others, aesthetic and religious dimensions. This led to the publication of selected Tamil and Sanskrit texts on Śiva in translation in *Der tanzende Gott Śiva* (2004).

Karl Baier

Karl Baier is a Professor of Religious Studies and Head of the Department of Religious Studies at the University of Vienna. He has published on the history of the reception of yoga in the West, modern yoga research and the European history of meditation (including influences from South and East Asian traditions). Besides his university employment he works as a certified Iyengar Yoga teacher.

His publications on yoga include the books *Yoga auf dem Weg nach Westen: Beiträge zur Rezeptionsgeschichte* (1998) and the two-volume *Meditation und Moderne: Zur Genese eines Kernbereichs moderner Spiritualität in der Wechselwirkung zwischen Westeuropa, Nordamerika und Asien* (2009), and the paper "Theosophical Orientalism and the Structures of Intercultural Transfer: Annotations on the Appropriation of the Cakras in Early Theosophy" (in J. Chajes & B. Huss [Eds.], *Theosophical Appropriations: Esotericism, Kabbalah, and the Transformation of Traditions,* 2016, pp. 309–354).

Ian A. Baker

Ian Baker is an anthropologist, art curator, and cultural historian and the author of seven books on Tibetan art history, traditional medicine, sacred geography, and Buddhist practice, including *The Heart of the World: A Journey to the Last Secret Place* (2004) and *Tibetan Yoga: Secrets from the Source* (forthc. 2019). His published academic articles include "Embodying Enlightenment: Physical Culture in Dzogchen as revealed in Tibet's Lukhang Murals" (*Asian Medicine, 7,* 2012, pp. 225–264). His current research interests concern bodymind disciplines in Tantric Buddhism and their adaptations across cultures and traditions. He was lead curator of the Wellcome Trust's 2015–2016 exhibition "Tibet's Secret Temple: Body, Mind and Meditation in Tantric Buddhism", London, and is currently affiliated with the Centre for the Social History of Health and Health Care (CSHHH) at the University of Strathclyde, Glasgow, Scotland.

Jason Birch

Jason Birch is a Postdoctoral Research Fellow at the School of Oriental and African Studies, University of London, where he works on the history of physical yoga on the eve of colonialism. In 2013, he completed a DPhil in Oriental Studies (Sanskrit) at the University of Oxford with a doctorate on the *Amanaska,* the earliest known Rāja Yoga work. Jason has published on the early history of Haṭha Yoga, liberation-in-life in Yoga traditions, the shared terminology, theory and praxis of Ayurveda and Yoga, and the revival of yoga in recent years in the Jain Terāpanthī sect. Jason is also a professional yoga teacher for more than ten years. He collaborates with Jacqueline Hargreaves to share his research with yoga practitioners on a blog called "The Luminescent".

His publications include the papers "The Meaning of *haṭha* in Early Haṭhayoga" (*Journal of the American Oriental Society, 131*(4), 2011, pp. 527–554), "Rājayoga: The Reincarnations of the King of All Yogas" (*International Journal of Hindu Studies, 17*(3), 2013, pp. 401–444) and "The Yogatārāvalī and the Hidden History of Yoga" (*Nāmarūpa, 20,* 2015, pp. 4–13).

Gudrun Bühnemann

Gudrun Bühnemann is a Professor of Sanskrit and Indic Religions in the Department of Asian Languages and Cultures at the University of Wisconsin–Madison, USA. She has published extensively on Tantric iconography and ritual.

Her work on yoga includes the book *Eighty-four Āsanas in Yoga: A Survey of Traditions* (2007; 2nd edition, 2011) and the papers "The Identification of an Illustrated Haṭhayoga Manuscript and its Significance for Traditions of 84 Āsanas in Yoga" (*Asian Medicine: Tradition and Modernity* 3 [Special Yoga Issue], 2007, pp. 156–176) and "The Śāradātilakatantra on Yoga: A New Edition and Translation of Chapter 25" (*Bulletin of the School of Oriental and African Studies, 74*(2), 2011, pp. 205–235). Her current research projects include a monograph on the iconography of Patañjali.

Maya Burger

Maya Burger is Professor at the Department of South Asian Studies of the University of Lausanne, where she teaches early modern South Asian literatures (in Braj and Hindi) and history of Indian religions, with a focus on yoga and the exchange between India and Switzerland.

Her publications include the papers "La Sarvāṅgayogapradīpikā de Sundardās: une classification des chemins du yoga au 17e siècle" (*Asiatische Studien / Études Asiatiques, 68*(3), 2014, pp. 683–708), "Jayatarāma's Jogapradīpakā: Between Hāṭha-yoga and Bhakti in Eighteenth Century North India" (in I. Bhanga [Ed.], *Bhakti in Current Research,* 2013, pp. 177–190), "Illustrating Yoga: From the Master to the Book" (in B. Beinhauer-Köhler et al. [Eds.], *Religiöse Blicke – Blicke auf das Religiöse: Visualität und Religion,* 2010, pp. 165–184), and "Une posture inversée: le yoga global" (in M. Burger & C. Calame [Eds.], *Comparer les comparatismes: perspectives en histoire et sciences des religions,* 2006, pp. 161–188).

Beatrix Hauser

Beatrix Hauser is a senior lecturer at the Institute for the Study of Religion and Religious Education, University of Bremen. She holds a PhD in Social Anthropology from the University of Hamburg (1997) and in 2009 obtained the habilitation degree at the University of Halle. Her main research interests lie in the anthropology of the body, ritual studies, Hinduism and gender. Her current research focuses on the mutual influence of health seeking behaviour and spiritual aspirations in the present postsecular age, taking postural yoga as a prime example and considering case studies from Germany and India.

She has published several articles and books. In particular, she is the editor of *Yoga Traveling: Bodily Practice in Transcultural Perspective* (2013).

Catharina Kiehnle

Catharina Kiehnle is a retired faculty member of the Department of Indology and Central Asian Studies, University of Leipzig, where she taught Sanskrit, Marathi and Hindi language and literature. She did her PhD in Vedic Studies, and her DLitt on "Songs on Yoga" and anonymous songs from the tradition of the Maharashtrian national saint and Nāth yogi Jñāndev. Her work includes numerous publications on Bhakti and Yoga literature, most importantly the two monographs *Songs on Yoga: Texts and Teachings of the Mahārāṣṭrian Nāths* and *The Conservative Vaiṣṇava: Anonymous Songs of the Jñāndev Gāthā,* both published in 1997, and the paper "The Secret of the Nāths: The Ascent of Kuṇḍalinī according to Jñāneśvarī 6.151–328" (*Bulletin d'Études Indiennes, 22–23,* 2004–2005, pp. 447–494). Her special interests are yoga practice and Sanskrit recitation.

Anne Koch

Anne Koch is Professor of Religious Studies at Salzburg University, with a focus on contemporary religion in Europe and entangled global discourses of religion. Her main areas of research are method and theory, economics of religion, and aesthetics of religion / embodied cognition with current research on *prāṇāyāma.* She has conducted a number of fieldwork projects on cosmopolitan spirituality, with case studies of global urban yoga in Tokyo, Thailand and Germany over a period of two years.

Her publications include the papers "Competitive Charity: A Neoliberal Culture of 'Giving Back' in Global Yoga" (*Journal of Contemporary Religion, 30,* 2015, pp. 73–85) and "Yoga as a Production Site of Social and Human Capital: Transcultural Flows from a Cultural Economic Perspective" (in B. Hauser [Ed.], *Yoga Traveling: Bodily Practice in Transcultural Perspective,* 2013, pp. 225–248).

Philipp A. Maas

Philipp A. Maas is Research Associate at the Institute for Indology and Central Asian Studies, University of Leipzig, following previous appointments at the Universities of Vienna and Bonn. The traditions of Sanskrit manuscripts on Yoga, Indian philosophy and Ayurveda figure prominently among his areas of research interest. His establishment of the first critical edition ever of the first chapter of the *Pātañjalayogaśāstra* deserves special mention. In addition, Philipp published widely on the reception history of Patañjali's Yoga in pre-modern South Asia and in modern academic research, on yogic mediation, on Yoga philosophy and on the early history of South Asian religions.

His publications include the book *Samādhipāda: Das erste Kapitel des Pātañjalayogaśāstra zum ersten Mal kritisch ediert. The First Chapter of the Pātañjalayogaśāstra for the First Time Critically Edited* (2006) and the papers "A Concise Historiography of Classical Yoga Philosophy" (in E. Franco [Ed.], *Periodization and Historiography of Indian Philosophy*, 2013, pp. 53–90) and "From Theory to Poetry: The Reuse of Patañjali's Yogaśāstra in Māgha's Śiśupālavadha" (in E. Freschi & Ph. A. Maas [Eds.], *Adaptive Reuse: Aspects of Creativity in South Asian Cultural History*, 2017, pp. 27–60).

James Mallinson

James Mallinson is Senior Lecturer in Sanskrit and Classical Indian Studies at the School of Oriental and African Studies, University of London. He has a BA in Sanskrit and Old Iranian from the University of Oxford, an MA in Area Studies (South Asia) from SOAS and a DPhil in Sanskrit from the University of Oxford. His doctoral supervisor was Professor Alexis Sanderson. James is currently leading a five-year research project on the history of Haṭha Yoga funded by the European Research Council. James' research work has focused on the history of yoga and its practitioners.

His publications include *The Khecarīvidyā: A Critical Edition and Annotated Translation of an Early Text of Haṭhayoga* (2007, a revision of his doctoral thesis), translations of the *Gheraṇḍasaṃhitā* (2004) and *Śivasaṃhitā* (2007), and *Roots of Yoga* (Penguin Classics, 2017, co-authored with Mark Singleton) as well as several articles. In addition to text-critical study, James' research draws on fieldwork in India with traditional yogis, in whose communities he has spent several years, and art-history.

Suzanne Newcombe

Suzanne Newcombe is a Lecturer in Religious Studies at the Open University in the United Kingdom and a Research Fellow at Inform, based at the London School of Economics and Political Science. She researches yoga and Ayurveda from a sociological and social-historical perspective. Suzanne is currently a postdoctoral researcher on the European Research Council project "AYURYOG: Entangled Histories of Yoga, Ayurveda and Alchemy in South Asia" at the Department of South Asian, Tibetan and Buddhist Studies of the University of Vienna. From her work at Inform, she also has extensive experience in sociology of religion specializing in new and minority religious movements in contemporary Britain.

She has a forthcoming book on the history of yoga in Britain in press with Equinox and has published chapters on yoga in edited books and journals including *The Journal of Contemporary Religion*, *Religion Compass* and *Asian Medicine*.

Marion Rastelli

Marion Rastelli is deputy director and senior research fellow at the Institute for the Cultural and Intellectual History of Asia of the Austrian Academy of Sciences, Vienna, and lecturer at the Department of South Asian, Tibetan and Buddhist Studies of the University of Vienna. Her research focuses on the teachings, ritual, and yoga of the Vaiṣṇava tradition of Pāñcarātra.

Her most important publications related to yoga are chapters in her books *Philosophisch-theologische Grundanschauungen der Jayākhyasaṃhitā* (1999) and *Die Tradition des Pāñcarātra im Spiegel der Pārameśvarasaṃhitā* (2006), and the paper "Perceiving God and Becoming Like Him: Yogic Perception and Its Implications in the Viṣṇuitic Tradition of Pāñcarātra" (in E. Franco [Ed.] in collaboration with D. Eigner, *Yogic Perception, Meditation and Altered States of Consciousness,* 2009, pp. 299–317).

Noémie Verdon

Noémie Verdon's research interests comprise the transmission of ideas and knowledge in ancient and early medieval South Asia. In her doctoral research, she examined the historical context in which classical Sāṃkhya and Yoga were transmitted by al-Bīrūnī, as well as the manner in which the scholar interpreted the two philosophies into Arabic. She currently teaches Sanskrit and a course on Indian religions and philosophies at Nalanda University in Rajgir (Bihar).

Noémie's main current projects are the publication of her PhD dissertation, entitled *Al-Bīrūnī's Kitāb Sānk and Kitāb Pātanğal: A Historical and Textual Study* and several articles, one of them on al-Bīrūnī's use of Greek terminology to interpret classical Sāṃkhya and Yoga. In 2013, in collaboration with Vladimir Loncar, Noémie produced a documentary film on al-Bīrūnī entitled "Biruni, the Quill of the Invaders". She also received a one-year training as a yoga teacher at a school affiliated to the Yoga Vidya Gurukul in Nashik (Maharashtra).

Dominik Wujastyk

Dominik Wujastyk works at the University of Alberta, Canada, where he holds a professorship and the Singhmar Chair in Classical Indian Society and Polity. He was educated at the universities of London, Oxford and Pune, and has held appointments at the University of Vienna, at University College London, at the Wellcome Institute for the History of Medicine in London, and elsewhere.

His research and publications have explored the Indian tradition of formal grammar, Indian manuscript studies, the history of science and medicine in India, and the history of yoga. He has also worked in Digital Humanities and their application to Indian studies. His books include *Metarules of Pāṇinian Grammar* (1993), *The Roots of Ayurveda* (1998), and several edited volumes. He has published over sixty research articles and book chapters.